AF688378

Current Techniques in Canine and Feline Neurosurgery

To my many mentors who shaped the direction of my career and planted many seeds that every day yield the fruits of their tutelage: Drs. Frank Hoerlein, Charlie Knecht, Steve Swaim, John Oliver, Ralph Henderson, Jimmy Milton, Bill Carney, Dick Redding, Don Sorjonen, Steve Simpson, and Paul Cechner – your teachings shaped me and continue to inspire me every day.

To all the surgery and neurosurgery residents I have had the pleasure of teaching and mentoring – passing the flames of this exciting profession and knowing your talents will be the new and exciting blossoms of the future of veterinary neurosurgery.

To *all* my family – my parents that afforded me every opportunity to pursue my profession; to my children, for all the smiles you've given me, for keeping me young, and for keeping me on my toes; to my grandchildren that show me there is hope for the future; and to my wife Jessy, gracias por todo, mi amor.

Andy Shores

To my husband Sean, for his incredible patience and unwavering support, which allow me to do what I love and to reach my dreams. You are my rock.

To my wonderfully inspiring and beautiful daughter Julia who brings so much joy, laughter and balance to my life. You never cease to amaze me. You are my world.

To the residents, interns and veterinary students I have had the privilege to teach and learn from. You motivate me to push further every day and remind me that there is always something new and exciting to learn.

To Dr. David Holmberg who was an incredibly talented surgeon and a wonderful mentor and colleague. Thank you for teaching me so much about neurosurgery and inspiring me to seek the answers to what I don't yet know. You are greatly missed.

Brigitte A. Brisson

Current Techniques in Canine and Feline Neurosurgery

Edited by

Andy Shores
Neurosurgery and Neurology
Mississippi State University College of Veterinary Medicine and
The Veterinary Specialty Center
Mississippi State / Starkville
Mississippi, USA

and

Brigitte A. Brisson
Professor of Small Animal Surgery
Department of Clinical Studies
Ontario Veterinary College
University of Guelph, Guelph
Ontario, Canada

WILEY Blackwell

ACVS FOUNDATION

ACVIM
American College of Veterinary Internal Medicine

This edition first published 2017
© 2017 John Wiley and Sons, Inc.

All rights reserved. No part of this publication may be reproduced, stored in a retrieval system, or transmitted, in any form or by any means, electronic, mechanical, photocopying, recording or otherwise, except as permitted by law. Advice on how to obtain permission to reuse material from this title is available at http://www.wiley.com/go/permissions.

The right of Andy Shores and Brigitte A. Brisson to be identified as the authors of the editorial material in this work has been asserted in accordance with law.

Registered Office
John Wiley & Sons, Inc., 111 River Street, Hoboken, NJ 07030, USA

Editorial Office
John Wiley & Sons, Inc., 111 River Street, Hoboken, NJ 07030, USA

For details of our global editorial offices, customer services, and more information about Wiley products visit us at www.wiley.com.

Wiley also publishes its books in a variety of electronic formats and by print-on-demand. Some content that appears in standard print versions of this book may not be available in other formats.

Limit of Liability/Disclaimer of Warranty
The contents of this work are intended to further general scientific research, understanding, and discussion only and are not intended and should not be relied upon as recommending or promoting scientific method, diagnosis, or treatment by physicians for any particular patient. In view of ongoing research, equipment modifications, changes in governmental regulations, and the constant flow of information relating to the use of medicines, equipment, and devices, the reader is urged to review and evaluate the information provided in the package insert or instructions for each medicine, equipment, or device for, among other things, any changes in the instructions or indication of usage and for added warnings and precautions. While the publisher and authors have used their best efforts in preparing this work, they make no representations or warranties with respect to the accuracy or completeness of the contents of this work and specifically disclaim all warranties, including without limitation any implied warranties of merchantability or fitness for a particular purpose. No warranty may be created or extended by sales representatives, written sales materials or promotional statements for this work. The fact that an organization, website, or product is referred to in this work as a citation and/or potential source of further information does not mean that the publisher and authors endorse the information or services the organization, website, or product may provide or recommendations it may make. This work is sold with the understanding that the publisher is not engaged in rendering professional services. The advice and strategies contained herein may not be suitable for your situation. You should consult with a specialist where appropriate. Further, readers should be aware that websites listed in this work may have changed or disappeared between when this work was written and when it is read. Neither the publisher nor authors shall be liable for any loss of profit or any other commercial damages, including but not limited to special, incidental, consequential, or other damages.

Library of Congress Cataloging-in-Publication Data

Names: Shores, Andy, 1952– editor. | Brisson, Brigitte A., 1973– editor.
Title: Current techniques in canine and feline neurosurgery / edited by Andy Shores and Brigitte A. Brisson.
Description: Hoboken, NJ : John Wiley & Sons, Inc., 2017. | Includes bibliographical references and index. |
Identifiers: LCCN 2017025970 (print) | LCCN 2017027047 (ebook) | ISBN 9781118711460 (pdf) |
ISBN 9781118711521 (epub) | ISBN 9781118433287 (cloth)
Subjects: | MESH: Neurosurgical Procedures–veterinary | Dogs–surgery | Cats–surgery
Classification: LCC SF913 (ebook) | LCC SF913 (print) | NLM SF 981 | DDC 636.089/7–dc23
LC record available at https://lccn.loc.gov/2017025970

Cover images: courtesy of Andy Shores. For more details, please see the figure captions in chapter 11 for (left) Figure 11.9, (middle) Figure 11.3A–D, and (right) Figure 11.1.
Cover design by Wiley

Set in 9/11pt Minion by SPi Global, Pondicherry, India

10 9 8 7 6 5 4 3 2 1

Contents

Contributors, vii

ACVS Foreword, ix

ACVIM Foreword, xi

About the Companion Website, xiii

Section I: Diagnostics and Planning

1 Neurosurgical Instrumentation, 3
Michelle Oblak and Brigitte A. Brisson

2 Orthopedic Implants in Neurosurgery, 11
Noel M.M. Moens

3 Minimum Database for Intracranial Surgery, 21
Theresa E. Pancotto

4 Advanced Imaging: Intracranial Surgery, 29
Simon Platt and J. Fraser McConnell

5 Cisternal Cerebrospinal Fluid Taps, 55
Nora Ortinau

6 Minimum Database: Spinal Surgery, 59
Luis Gaitero and Brigitte A. Brisson

7 Advanced Imaging: Spinal Surgery, 71
Stephanie Nykamp

8 Lumbar Cerebrospinal Fluid Taps, 85
Luis Gaitero

9 Muscle and Nerve Biopsy, 93
Michaela Beasley

Section II: Intracranial Procedures

10 Transfrontal Craniotomy, 99
Ane Uriarte and Rodolfo Cappello

11 Lateral (Rostrotentorial) Craniotomy/Craniectomy, 109
Andy Shores

12 Suboccipital Craniectomy/Foramen Magnum Decompression, 115
Erin Y. Akin and Andy Shores

13 Surgical Treatment of Skull Tumors, 121
Michelle Oblak and Andy Shores

14 Shunt Placement and Marsupialization in Treatment of Hydrocephalus and Quadrigeminal Diverticula, 129
William Thomas and Jill Narak

Section III: Spinal Procedures

15 Atlantoaxial Subluxation, 141
Fred Wininger

16 Dorsal Cervical Decompression (Laminectomy/Hemilaminectomy and Laminotomy), 149
James M. Fingeroth

17 Ventral Cervical Decompression, 157
Ronaldo C. da Costa

18 Lateral Cervical Approach, 163
Amy Fauber and Robert Bergman

19 Cervical Distraction and Stabilization, 169
Bianca Hettlich

20 Thoracolumbar Hemilaminectomy, 179
Andy Shores

21 Pediculectomy/Mini-Hemilaminectomy, 183
Brigitte A. Brisson

22 Intervertebral Disc Fenestration, 191
Brigitte A. Brisson

23 Thoracolumbar Lateral Corpectomy, 199
Pierre Moissonnier

24 Dorsal Laminectomy in the Thoracolumbar Region, 205
Cory Fisher and Andy Shores

25 Vertebral Fracture and Luxation Repair, 209
Bianca Hettlich

26 Lumbosacral Decompression and Foraminotomy, 223
Trevor Bebchuk

27 Surgical Management of Spinal Neoplasia, 235
Mark S. Levy

Section IV: Postoperative Care and Rehabilitation

28 Guidelines for Postoperative Medical Care of the Neurosurgical Patient, 245
Debbie Reynolds and Brigitte A. Brisson

29 Physical Rehabilitation of the Neurological Patient, 257
María Pérez Hernández and Ruby Lynn Carter

Index, 269

Contributors

Editors

Andy Shores
Mississippi State University College of Veterinary Medicine and the Veterinary Specialty Center, Mississippi State / Starkville, Mississippi, USA

Brigitte A. Brisson
University of Guelph, Ontario Veterinary College, Guelph, Ontario, Canada

Chapter Authors

Erin Y. Akin
Bush Veterinary Neurology Service, Woodstock, Georgia, USA

Michaela Beasley
Mississippi State University, College of Veterinary Medicine, Mississippi State, Mississippi, USA

Trevor Bebchuk
Great Plains Veterinary Surgery, Winnipeg, Manitoba, Canada

Robert Bergman
Carolina Veterinary Specialists, Charlotte, North Carolina, USA

Rodolfo Cappello
North Downs Specialist Referrals, Brewerstreet Dairy Business Park, Bletchingley, Surrey, UK

Ruby Lynn Carter
Mississippi State University, College of Veterinary Medicine, Mississippi State, Mississippi, USA

Ronaldo C. da Costa
Ohio State University, Veterinary Medical Center, Columbus, Ohio, USA

Amy Fauber
Purdue University, School of Veterinary Medicine, Department of Clinical Science, West Lafayette, Indiana, USA

James M. Fingeroth
Orchard Park Veterinary Medical Center, Orchard Park, New York, USA

Cory Fisher
Bluff City Veterinary Specialists Memphis, Tennessee, USA

Luis Gaitero
University of Guelph, Ontario Veterinary College, Guelph, Ontario, Canada

Bianca Hettlich
Ohio State University, College of Veterinary Medicine, Department of Clinical Science, Columbus, Ohio, USA

Mark S. Levy
NYC Veterinary Specialists, New York, New York, USA

J. Fraser McConnell
University of Liverpool, Small Animal Teaching Hospital, Leahurst, Neston, Wirral, UK

Noel M.M. Moens
University of Guelph, Ontario Veterinary College, Guelph, Ontario, Canada

Pierre Moissonnier
Service de Chirurgie de L'enval Fort, Pole Chirugical du Chuva Chirurgie, France

Jill Narak
Veterinary Referral Surgical Practice, Roswell, Georgia, USA

Stephanie Nykamp
University of Guelph, Ontario Veterinary College, Guelph, Ontario, Canada

Michelle Oblak
University of Guelph, Ontario Veterinary College, Guelph, Ontario, Canada

Nora Ortinau
VCA Aurora Animal Hospital, Aurora, Illinois, USA

Theresa E. Pancotto
Virginia Tech, VA-MD Regional College of Veterinary Medicine, Blacksburg, Virginia, USA

María Pérez Hernández
Mississippi State University, College of Veterinary Medicine, Mississippi State, Mississippi, USA

Simon Platt
Watkinsville, Georgia, USA

Debbie Reynolds
Toronto Veterinary Emergency Hospital, Scarborough, Ontario, Canada

William Thomas
University of Tennessee, Small Animal Clinical Sciences, College of Veterinary Medicine, Knoxville, Tennessee, USA

Ane Uriarte
Cummings School of Veterinary Medicine, Tufts University, North Grafton, Tennessee, USA

Fred Wininger
Columbia, Missouri, USA

ACVS Foreword

The American College of Veterinary Surgeons Foundation is excited to present *Current Techniques in Canine and Feline Neurosurgery*. The ACVS Foundation is an independently charted philanthropic organization devoted to advancing the charitable, educational, and scientific goals of the American College of Veterinary Surgeons. Founded in 1965, the ACVS sets the standards for the specialty of veterinary surgery. The ACVS, which is approved by the American Veterinary Medical Association, administers the board certification process for Diplomates in veterinary surgery and advances veterinary surgery and education. One of the principal goals of the ACVS Foundation is to foster the advancement of the art and science of veterinary surgery. The Foundation achieves these goals by supporting investigations in the diagnosis and treatment of surgical diseases; increasing educational opportunities for surgeons, surgical residents and veterinary practitioners; improving surgical training of residents and veterinary students; and bettering animal patients' care, treatment and welfare.

Current Techniques in Canine and Feline Neurosurgery is edited by Drs. Andy Shores and Brigitte Brisson. Both are well recognized as experts in this field. They have chosen strong contributing authors to detail the areas of diagnostics and planning, intracranial and spinal surgery, and postoperative care and rehabilitation. We are sure you will find this reference extremely valuable.

The ACVS Foundation is proud to partner with Wiley Blackwell and the American College of Veterinary Medicine, and is honored to present this book.

R. Randy Basinger
Chair, Board of Trustees
ACVS Foundation

ACVIM Foreword

The American College of Veterinary Internal Medicine (ACVIM) advances knowledge of animal health and diseases, and fosters the continued development of specialty veterinary care in large animal internal medicine, small animal internal medicine, cardiology, neurology, and medical oncology. To achieve these purposes, the ACVIM certifies new Diplomates by guiding training programs, and ensuring fair and appropriate credentialing and examination procedures; promotes and advocates veterinary specialization; promotes continuing education and the dissemination of knowledge in veterinary cardiology, large animal internal medicine, small animal internal medicine, neurology, and oncology; and promotes the generation of new knowledge relevant to ACVIM specialties for the benefit of improved animal and human health.

Drs. Andy Shores (an ACVIM (Neurology) Diplomate) and Brigitte Brisson (an ACVS Diplomate) have collaborated on this issue to create a text which provides expertise from members of both veterinary specialty colleges. The ACVIM is proud to partner with the ACVS Foundation and with Wiley Blackwell to present this book.

Charles Vite
President, Neurology Specialty
American College of Veterinary Internal Medicine

About the Companion Website

This book is accompanied by a companion website:

www.wiley.com/go/shores/neurosurgery

The website features the following video clips:

Video 5.1 A cerebrospinal fluid (CSF) tap performed on a dog in lateral recumbency, using a 22G, 1-1/2 inch spinal needle.
Video 10.1 The transfrontal craniotomy approach is demonstrated in this video, using a sagittal to remove a diamond shaped section of the frontal bone over the frontal sinus (video courtesy of Dr. Ane Uriarte).
Video 12.1 A suboccipital craniectomy is performed in a patient with Chiari malformation.
Video 13.1 A cotton tip applicator is used to free the bone segment from the dura for removal of the tumor and surrounding normal bone en-bloc.
Video 13.2 Rotational view of a preoperative 3D CT reconstruction of a dog with cranial tumour. The image can be manipulated in multiple planes to assist in preoperative visualization and planning.
Video 15.1 A modified right parasagittal ventral surgical approach and placement of transarticular screws for the surgical management of atlantoaxial subluxation in the canine are demonstrated (video courtesy of Dr. Fred Wininger).
Video 20.1 **Part I** The dorsolateral approach to the thoracolumbar spine is demonstrated in this video. In Part I, rongeurs are used to create a left-sided hemilaminectomy at L1-L2 on a small canine patient. In **Part II**, a nitrogen powered burr drill is used to create the hemilaminectomy at L1-L2 in a larger canine patient.
Video 21.1 Pediculectomy performed at T13-L1 through a dorsolateral approach on the left side (entire procedure).
Video 21.2 Modified dorsolateral surgical approach for pediculectomy.
Video 21.3 Following the initial approach through a dorsolateral incision, the spinal musculature is elevated using a periosteal elevator to identify the appropriate site for pediculectomy at T13-L1 on the left.
Video 21.4 An air drill is used to create a pediculectomy for removal of herniated disc material from the spinal canal.
Video 21.5 After drilling through cortical, medullary and inner cortical bone, the spinal canal is entered by removing the remaining, thin inner periosteum using an iris spatula or 90 degree bent needle and #11 blade.
Video 21.6 Opening of the remaining thin inner periosteal bone and removal of herniated disc material and hemorrhage from the spinal canal using an iris spatula.
Video 21.7 Using a bent iris spatula to retrieve herniated disc material from the spinal canal. The spatula is manipulated from craniodorsal and dorsocaudal toward the mid section of the pediculectomy ventrally to avoid pushing disc away from the pediculectomy window.
Video 21.8 Surgical closure of the modified dorsolateral approach used for pediculectomy.
Video 22.1 Blade fenestration performed at T13-L1 on the left following a pediculectomy procedure.
Video 24.1 Surgery is performed on a young, paralyzed canine patient with a gun projectile lodged in the dorsal aspect of the spinal canal at the T12-T13 junction. A modified dorsal laminectomy is performed at that site to both remove the projectile and decompress the spinal cord.
Video 29.1 Therapeutic exercises used in the rehabilitation of canine patients with neurologic diseases are demonstrated with commentary on the benefits of each exercise and the recommended number of repetitions for each procedure.

SECTION I

Diagnostics and Planning

1 Neurosurgical Instrumentation

Michelle Oblak and Brigitte A. Brisson

Introduction

The surgical suite should be large enough to accommodate the patient, anesthesia machine, and one to two instrument tables. Depending on the procedure performed, the surgeon may wish to have access to fluoroscopy to confirm the surgical site, anatomical landmarks, or implant position during the procedure. Specialized equipment may vary depending on the surgical approach and procedure to be performed. Preoperative imaging should be readily available for review. Spinal models are helpful, especially for the novice surgeon, to assist with anatomy and orientation as many surgical approaches have limited exposure. Surgical loupes or an operating microscope are useful for fine dissection around the spinal cord or brain; a nonsterile assistant helps set up these devices once the surgical approach is completed (Figure 1.1). Endoscopy may be utilized under certain circumstances and the use of an exoscope has become more commonplace in recent years (Figure 1.2).

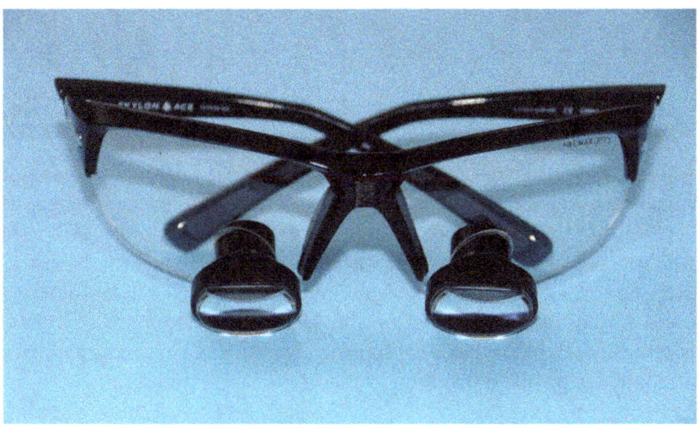

Figure 1.1 Surgical loupes can be helpful in providing magnification of the surgical site.

Basic Surgical Instrumentation

A basic neurosurgical pack includes the following instruments:

- fine rat-tooth forceps (such as Adson tissue forceps);
- Debakey forceps;
- Metzenbaum scissors;
- Mayo scissors;
- scalpel handle(s) and blade(s);
- needle holders;
- sharp-blunt scissors to cut suture;
- small-tipped mosquito forceps (curved preferred);
- Frazier–Ferguson suction tip;
- a variety of fine neurosurgical curettes, spatulas, or dental tartar scrapers;
- rongeurs (Lempert, Kerrison or others);
- electrocoagulation (bipolar preferred).

Draping and Approach

Patients are positioned according to the procedure being performed. Draping involves the placement of four paper or cloth corner drapes secured to the patient's skin with towel clamps (Figure 1.3). A self-adherent impervious drape such as Opsite® or Ioban® can be placed over the exposed skin followed by a top sheet. Monopolar and bipolar electrosurgical instruments can be used to address hemorrhage that occurs during dissection (Figure 1.4). Only bipolar cautery should be used near the spinal cord or brain. Retraction of the skin and muscle is accomplished with a variety of different self-retaining retractors. Blunt retractors including Gossett and pediatric Balfours are helpful for a ventral cervical approach (Figure 1.5). Retractors equipped with multiple blunt or sharp teeth include Weitlaner, Adson-baby, and West retractors (Figure 1.6). These retractors can occasionally lead to damage to the surrounding neurovascular and soft tissue structures, so care must be taken when placing

Current Techniques in Canine and Feline Neurosurgery, First Edition. Edited by Andy Shores and Brigitte A. Brisson.
© 2017 John Wiley & Sons, Inc. Published 2017 by John Wiley & Sons, Inc.
Companion website: www.wiley.com/go/shores/neurosurgery

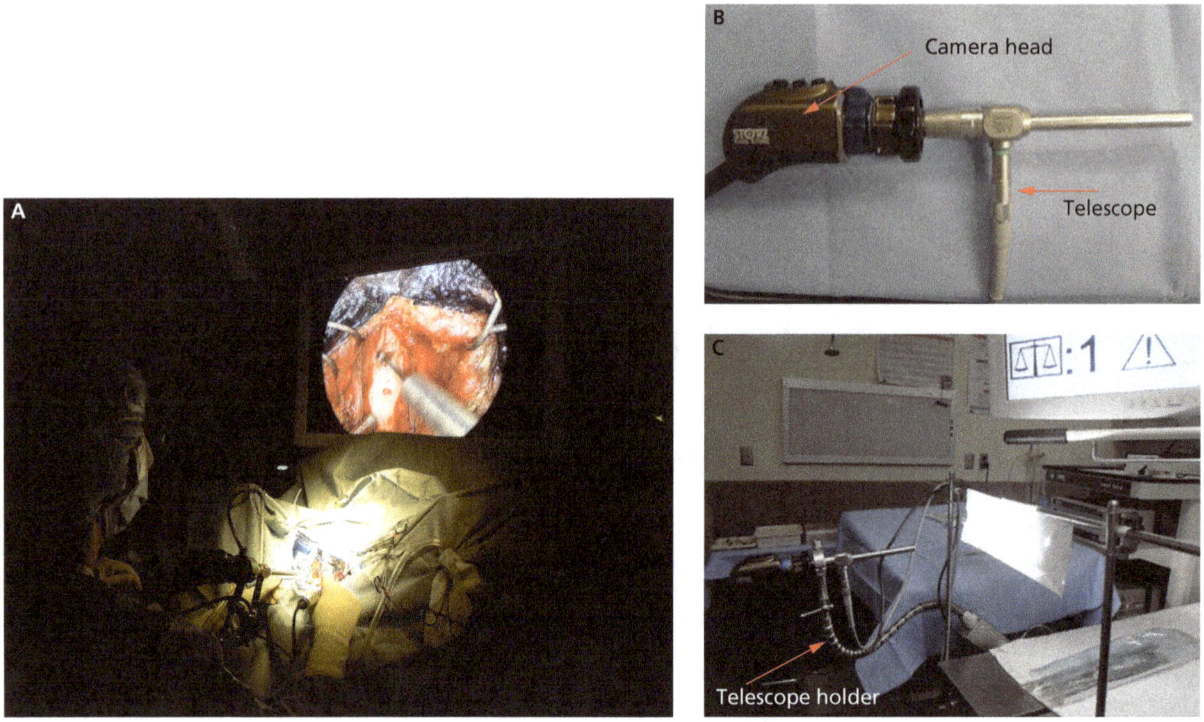

Figure 1.2 More recently, some surgeons prefer using an endoscope/exoscope for magnification during neurosurgical procedures: (A) intraoperative view of HD screen during surgery using an exoscope; endoscope and camera (B) and frame (C) used to stabilize the instrument during surgery. *Source*: Courtesy of Dr. Tina Owen, VCAWLA.

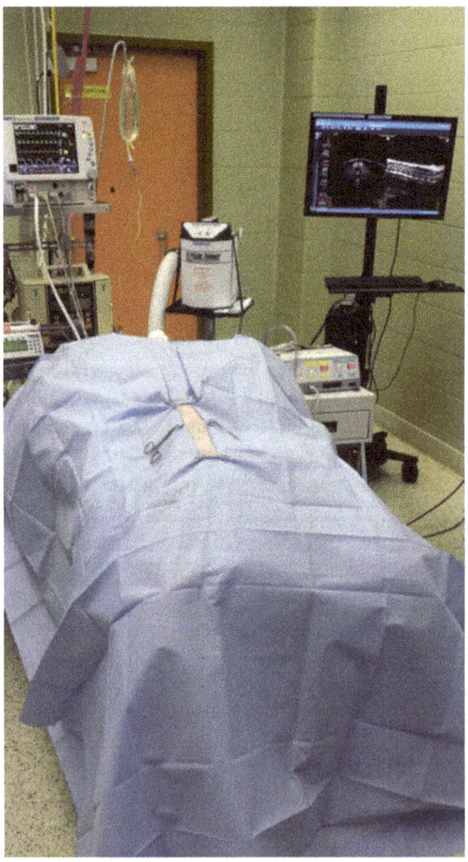

Figure 1.3 The patient is positioned and widely clipped for the surgical procedure. Following final preparation, an adhesive spray may be applied. Four half sheets are applied at the four quadrants of the surgical field and secured to the patient's skin with towel clamps. If used, an adhesive drape (such as Opsite® or Ioban®) is now applied followed by a top sheet (not yet applied in this picture).

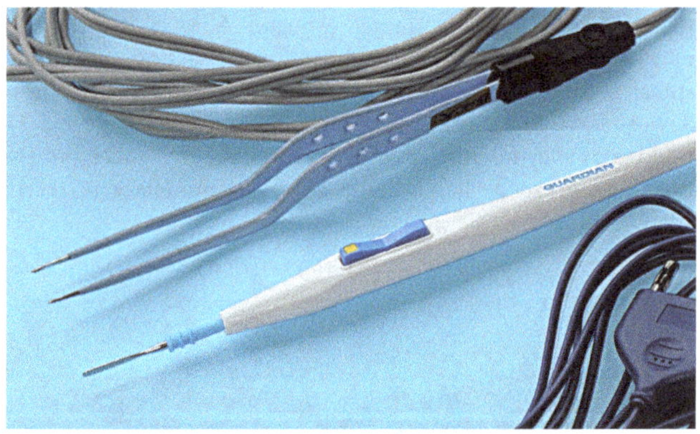

Figure 1.4 Electrosurgical instruments should be used sparingly around the spinal cord or brain. With bipolar cautery (*top*) the electric current passes between the tips of the forceps limiting lateral thermal injury compared with monopolar cautery (*bottom*) where the current passes from the instrument tip to the tissues and to the ground plate. Although bipolar cautery is the mainstay of electrocoagulation in neurosurgery, monopolar cautery is sometimes used for the initial approach when a more extensive approach is required (e.g., spinal fracture).

and removing these instruments. Like others, Gelpi retractors are available in a variety of angles and sizes. The 1-inch, 90°, medium-sized Gelpis are the authors' retractors of choice for dorsolateral approaches to the thoracolumbar spine of smaller dogs (Figure 1.7). These retractors have a sharp tip so caution must be exercised during placement and removal. Hand-held retractors, including Hohmann, Miller–Senn, Langenbeck, Army–Navy, and malleable, can also be used for exposure or to protect vital underlying structures but require an assistant (Figure 1.8). Elevation of soft tissues is performed with Freer or other periosteal elevators (Figure 1.9).

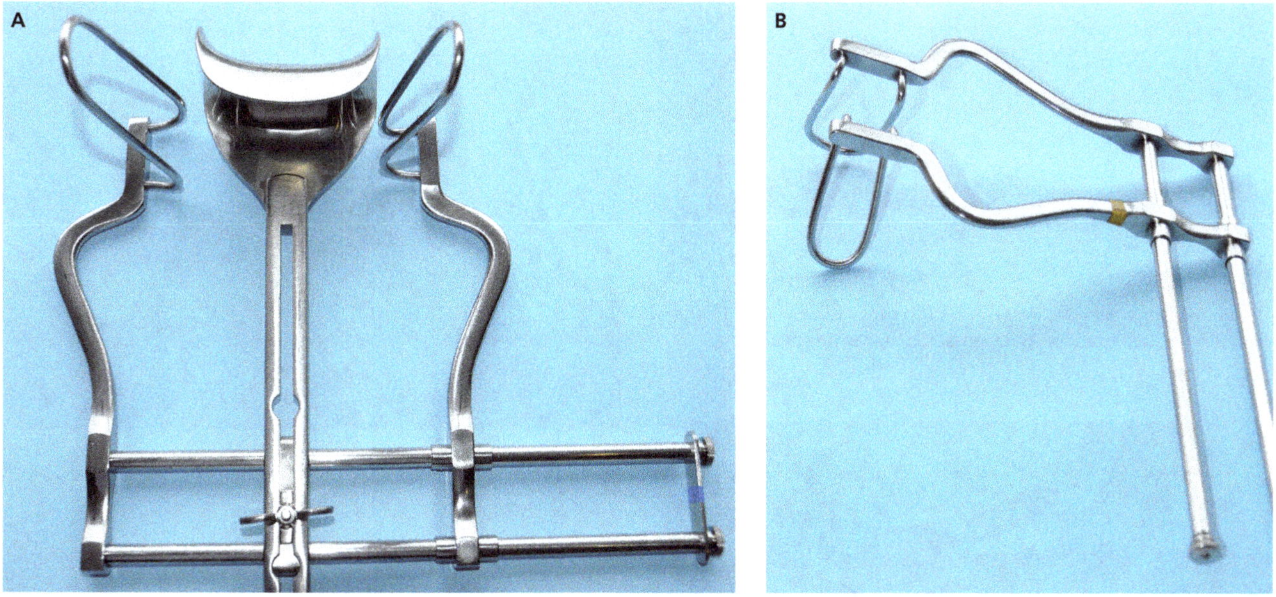

Figure 1.5 Blunt self-retaining retractors: (A) Gossett and (B) pediatric Balfour. Gossett or Balfour abdominal self-retaining retractors can be helpful for soft tissue retraction in a ventral approach to the cervical spine.

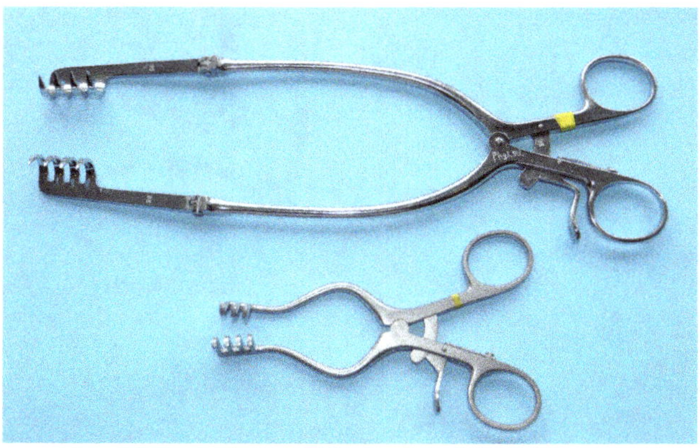

Figure 1.6 Toothed self-retaining retractors: Weitlaner (*top*) and Adson-baby (*bottom*). Weitlaner retractors are available in varying sizes. Weitlaner retractors have curved arms with varying numbers of curved (sharp or blunt) prongs on either end. A ratchet mechanism allows this instrument to remain in the spread position (with various degree of spread) after engaging the ratchet. Adson-baby retractors have a similar mechanism with varying tooth conformation.

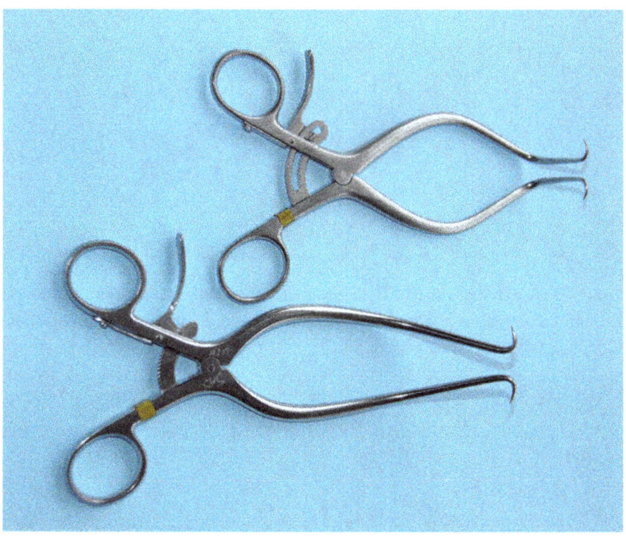

Figure 1.7 The curved arms and sharp-angled tips of Gelpi retractors provide good leverage on tissues being retracted. A ratchet mechanism allows this instrument to remain in the spread position after retraction. They are frequently used for deep muscle retraction. The 90°, 1-inch medium Gelpis (*top*) are the authors' preferred retractors for spinal procedures in small to medium-sized patients.

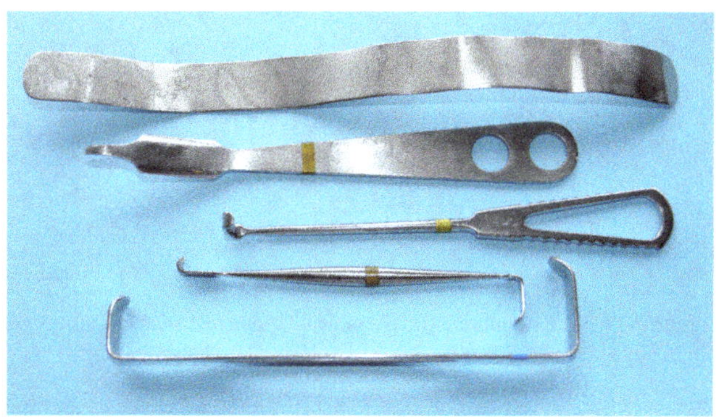

Figure 1.8 Hand-held retractors: (*in sequence from top*) malleable, Hohmann, Langenbeck, Miller–Senn, and Army–Navy retractors. Hand-held retractors require an assistant for retraction but can be helpful in areas where more precise or varied retraction is necessary. The retractor chosen is based on the depth and fragility of tissues.

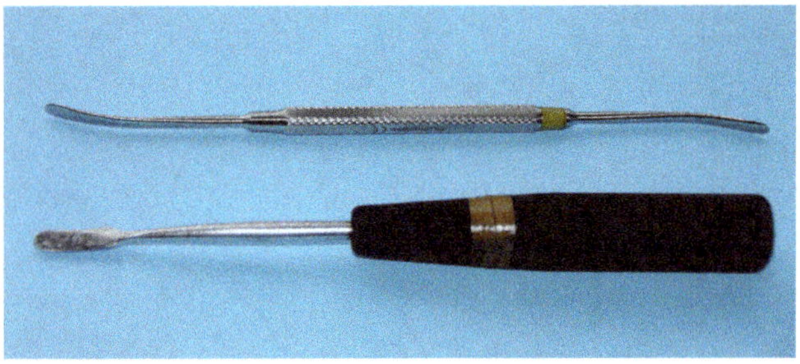

Figure 1.9 Freer elevator (*top*) and AO periosteal elevator (*bottom*). Elevators are used to elevate soft tissues from underlying bone.

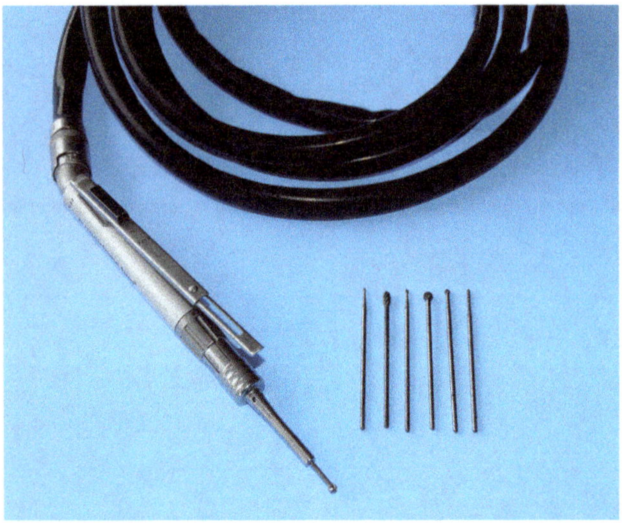

Figure 1.10 An electric (not shown) or pneumatic (illustrated) drill is used to gain access to the spinal canal. Burrs of varying sizes are available and can be varied during the various stages of the drilling process.

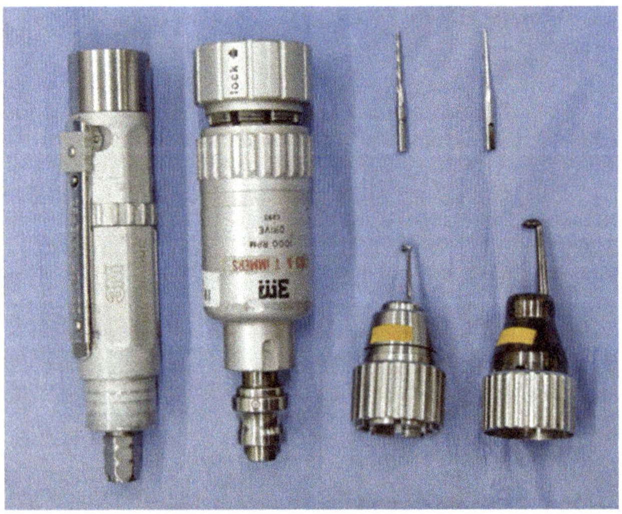

Figure 1.11 3M Craniotome (unassembled handpiece). *Source*: Courtesy of Dr. Andy Shores.

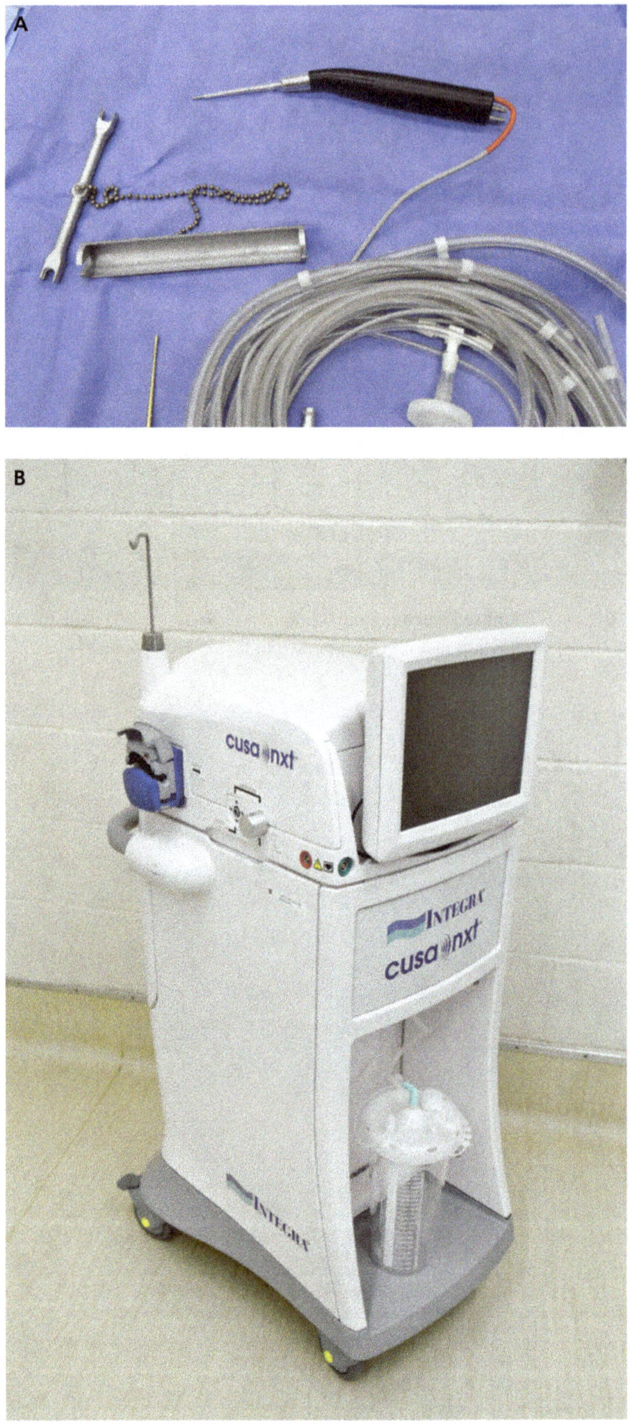

Figure 1.12 CUSA ultrasonic tissue ablation system: assembled handpiece (A) and console (B). *Source*: Permission granted by Integra LifeSciences Corporation, Plainsboro, NJ, USA.

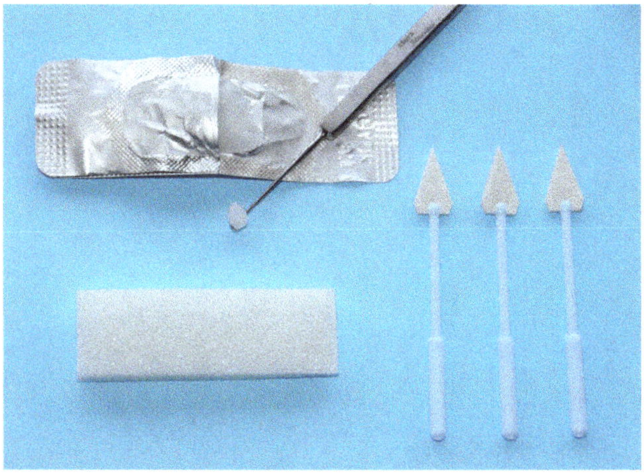

Figure 1.13 Hemostatics commonly used in neurosurgery: (*top*) bone wax; (*bottom left*) gelatin sponge; (*bottom right*) cellulose surgical spears.

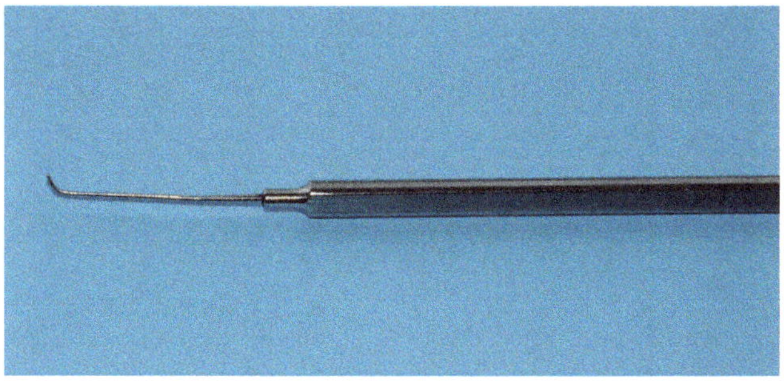

Figure 1.14 The iris spatula has a very fine tip that can be used for palpation and dissection and to retrieve disc material. Its tip is pliable, allowing the surgeon to bend it to a desired angle and length.

Access to the spinal canal is typically achieved using a pneumatic or electric drill. Burrs are available in a variety of configurations and sizes (Figure 1.10). Other specialized equipment used to penetrate the cranial bone or ablate tissues include the 3M craniotome (Figure 1.11) and CUSA (Figure 1.12). Intermittent or continuous saline irrigation should be available to remove bone dust created during burring and to decrease the heat transmitted to the bone and spinal cord. Bone wax is a sterile mixture of beeswax, paraffin, and isopropyl palmitate, a softening agent that can be used to control trabecular bone hemorrhage by acting as a mechanical (tamponade) sealant [1] (Figure 1.13). It is minimally resorbable and should be used sparingly as it can prevent bone healing, promote infection, and lead to granuloma formation [2]. As such, it should never be left in place in fusion sites and within the spinal canal and must never be used in contaminated fields [3].

Burring of the bone is continued to the level of the inner periosteum. Adequate cortical bone removal is typically confirmed by palpation with an iris spatula or other fine blunt-tipped probe (Figure 1.14). An effort is made to make an adequately sized window prior to removing the remaining thin periosteum and exposing the spinal cord. Once paper thin, the inner cortical bone/periosteum can be incised with a bent (90°) 22–25G hypodermic needle with or without the use of a #11 scalpel blade to enter the spinal canal (Figure 1.15). Once a full-thickness defect in the bone exists, it can be enlarged as needed using a burr, a Kerrison or Lempert rongeur, or a house curette (Figure 1.16). Kerrison rongeurs

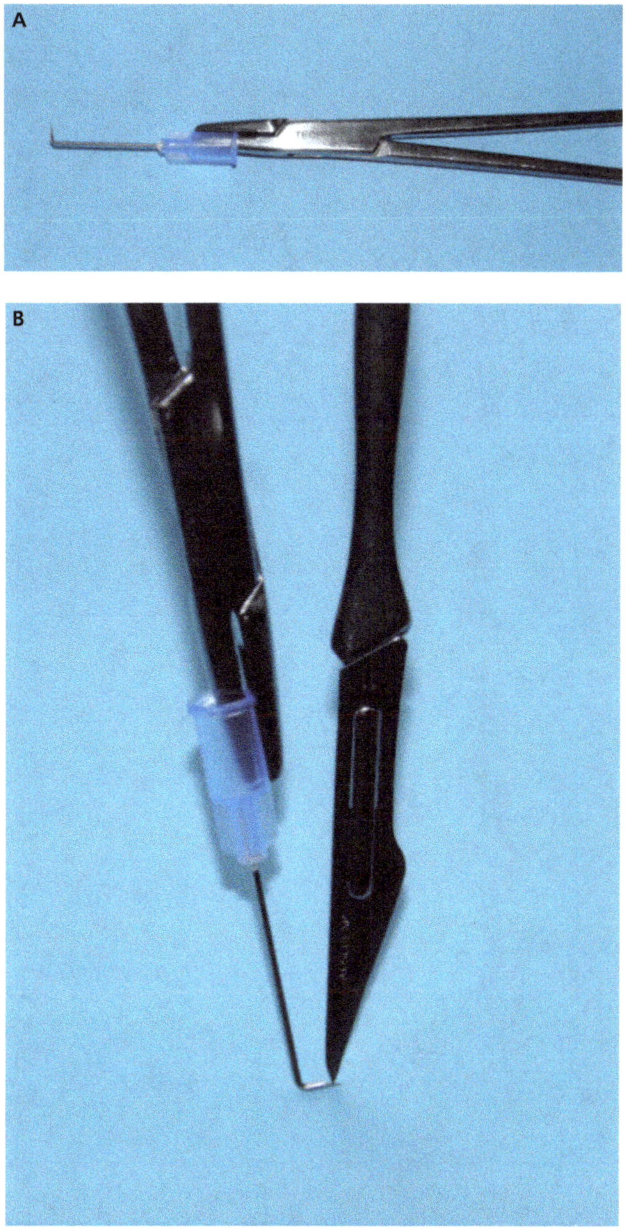

Figure 1.15 A 22G or 25G needle is bent at 90° (A) just caudal to the bevel (facing upward) and is used to penetrate and cut off the inner cortical bone/periosteum with the needle alone or with a #11 scalpel blade (B).

come in a variety of sizes and footplate thickness. Those with a low profile footplate are helpful for engaging the bony edge without damaging the spinal cord.

Retrieving disc material from the spinal canal is achieved with a variety of curettes, an iris spatula bent to the preferred angle and length, or with a dental tartar scraper (Figure 1.17). Appropriately sized brain spoons are used to mobilize brain tumors. Suction, using a Frazier–Ferguson suction tip, can facilitate the atraumatic removal of loose extruded disc fragments from the spinal canal or the removal of tumor tissue as well as hemorrhage from the surgical site (Figure 1.17). Cellulose surgical spears can be used to absorb mild hemorrhage and absorbable gelatin sponge can help control venous sinus hemorrhage

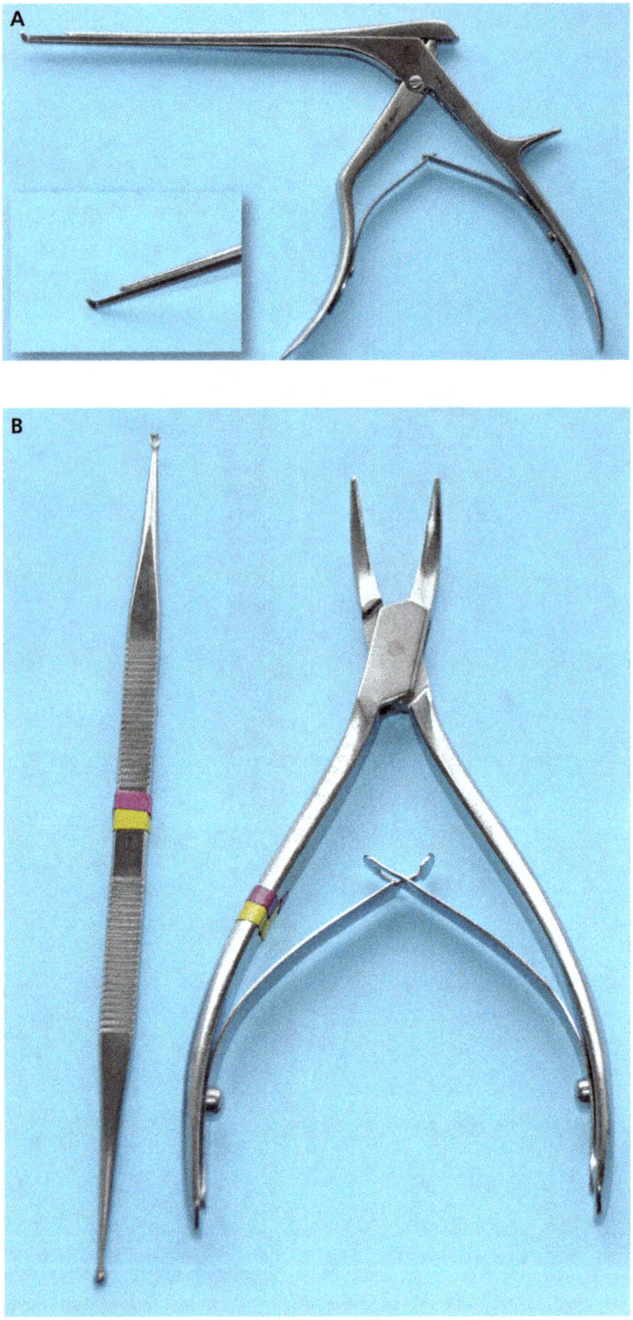

Figure 1.16 Kerrison rongeurs (A) have one long blade that ends as a footplate at the tip of the instrument while the other blade has a cutting end that meets the footplate when the instrument is closed. The footplate can be placed safely between the spinal cord and the bony lamina to allow atraumatic removal of small bony fragments at the edge of the laminectomy site. This instrument is especially useful in the cervical and lumbosacral areas because of the relatively greater space between the spinal cord/nerve roots and the bone. A house curette (B, *left*) is helpful for removing remaining endosteum when little space exists between the bone and spinal cord. Lempert rongeurs (B, *right*) with tapered jaws are used to grasp and remove smaller bone pieces along a laminectomy or craniotomy site.

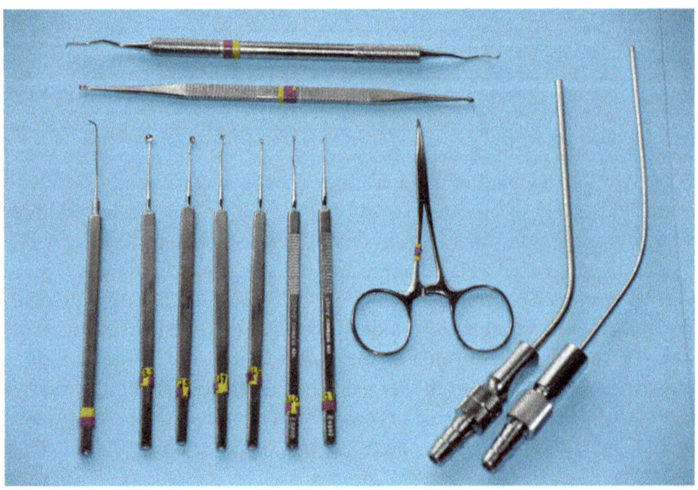

Figure 1.17 Retrieving disc material from the spinal canal is achieved with a variety of curettes, an iris spatula bent to the preferred angle and length, a dental tartar scraper, a small curved mosquito forceps, or with the use of suction through a Frazier–Ferguson suction tip.

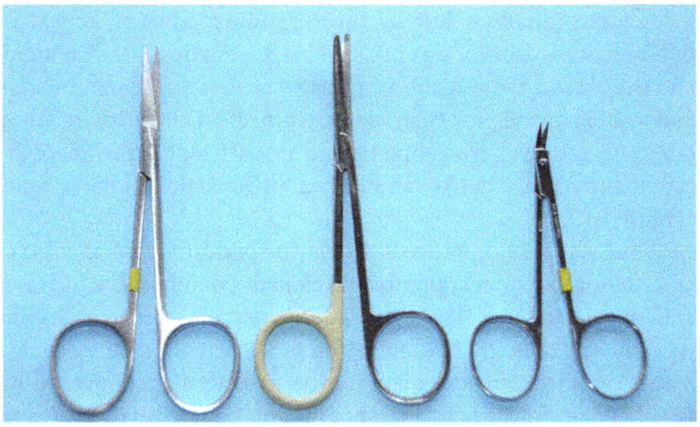

Figure 1.18 A variety of fine-tipped scissors are used in neurosurgery to cut fine, delicate tissues. Iris scissors (*left*) have sharp tips and are available in varying sizes. Tenotomy scissors (*center*) are available as straight or curved instruments and also come in a variety of sizes. Potts scissors (*right*) have a sharp tip and are angled, typically at 45°. They are designed for vascular incisions where the bottom jaw is inserted within the lumen but can be useful for durotomy.

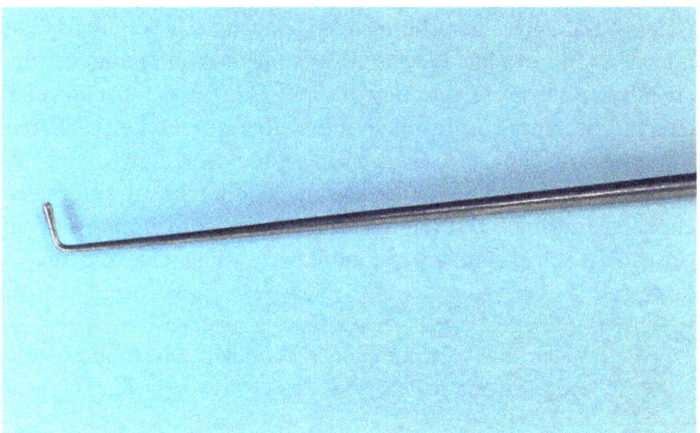

Figure 1.19 Nerve hook.

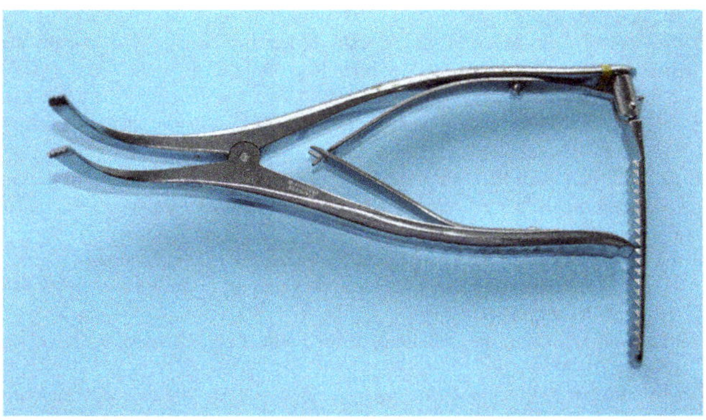

Figure 1.20 Lamina spreaders are equipped with small teeth at their tips and a ratchet mechanism that allows hands-free distraction of adjacent vertebrae. They are used for spinal distraction/stabilization procedures.

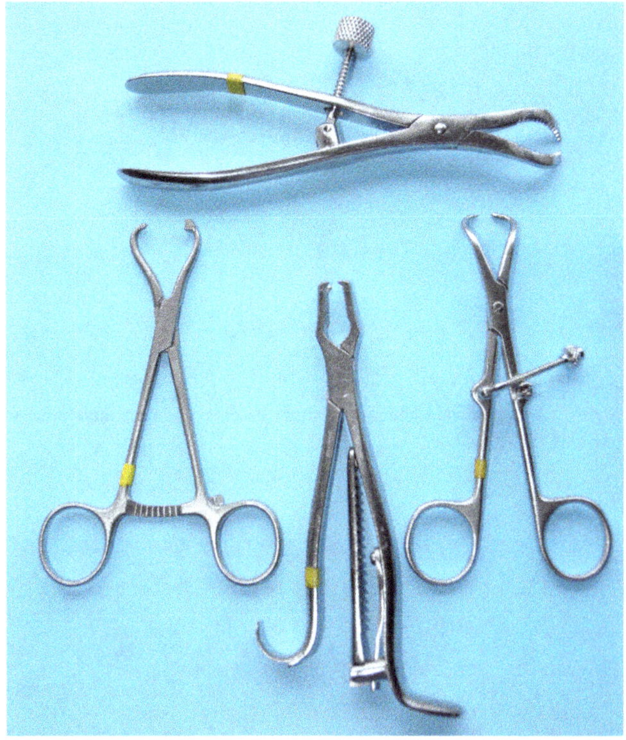

Figure 1.21 A variety of bone-holding forceps: clamshell (*top*), sharp-blunt (*bottom left*), Kern (*bottom center*), and sharp-sharp (*bottom right*). Bone-holding forceps can grasp the dorsal transverse processes or other portions of the bone during spinal distraction procedures or fracture repair.

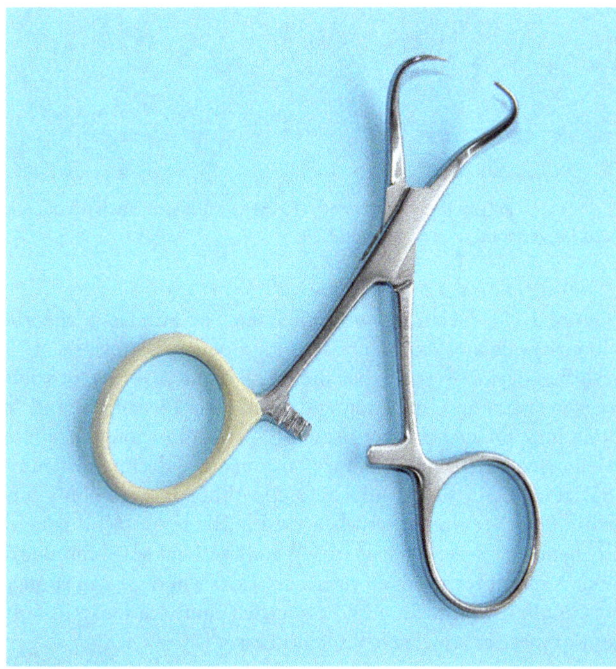

Figure 1.22 Towel clamps are occasionally used to provide distraction during spinal distraction or fracture repair.

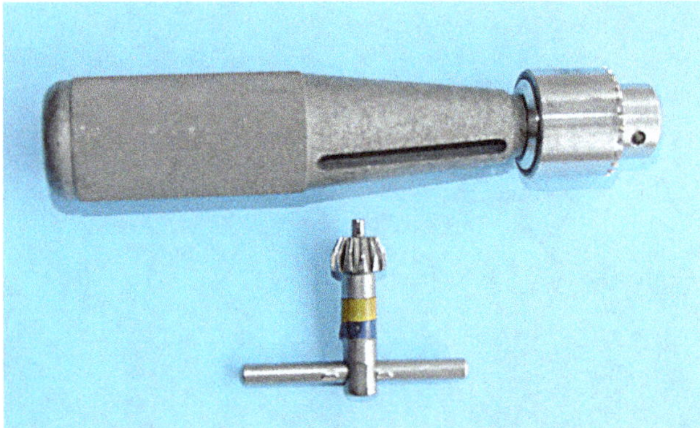

Figure 1.23 Hand-held chuck sometimes used to place implants such as pins into the spine.

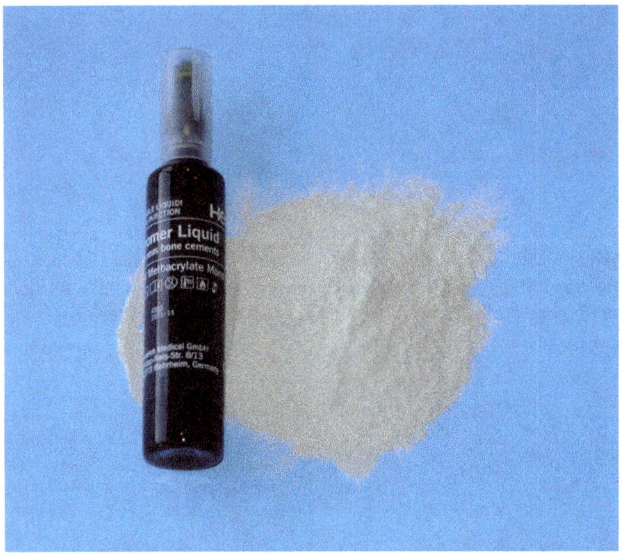

Figure 1.24 Polymethylmethacrylate (PMMA) bone cement is frequently used for vertebral fracture stabilization.

(Figure 1.13). Gelatin sponge (Gelfoam® or Surgicel®) absorbs blood, swells and exerts pressure to produce hemostasis. It is resorbed over 4–6 weeks, but should be removed where possible as it may promote infection and granuloma formation, and in bone may slow or prevent healing [3]. Gelatin sponge has also been associated with temporary postoperative decline in neurological status in some patients [3–5]. Although granuloma formation has been reported when used in the brain [6], it is used frequently by veterinary neurosurgeons without such complication. A recent review of 60 veterinary cases where gelatin sponge was used at surgery found no associated complications but only four of these cases were neurological cases [7].

To access intradural lesions, the dura is incised using Potts, iris, or tenotomy scissors or a #11 scalpel blade. (Figure 1.18). Tenotomy and iris scissors are available in a variety of sizes and tenotomy scissors come as straight or curved instruments. Unlike iris scissors, tenotomy scissors have a blunt tip and are used for cutting fine, delicate tissues. Nerve hooks can be used for retraction of nerve roots (Figure 1.19).

Spinal stabilization procedures may be performed for atlantoaxial luxations, cervical spondylomyelopathy, lumbosacral disease, and spinal fractures. These procedures require the use of several types of implants in addition to the previously mentioned equipment. Laminectomy spreaders can be used to distract overriding vertebrae or fracture fragments (Figure 1.20). Sharp-blunt and Kern bone-holding forceps can also be employed to manually distract and reduce vertebral segments (Figure 1.21). Although not intended for this purpose, towel clamps are also sometimes used for this purpose (Figure 1.22). Implants are placed with pneumatic drills or manually with a hand-held chuck (Figure 1.23). A review of orthopedic implants and techniques for implantation can be found in Chapter 2.

Polymethylmethacrylate (PMMA) is a relatively inert, strong, lightweight bone cement that is often applied to stabilize implants around the vertebral column (Figure 1.24). Antibiotic impregnation is possible and may be recommended when the site is at high risk of infection. This product is available as a polymer and monomer that are mixed prior to use, resulting in a moldable cement that polymerizes and becomes hard through an exothermic reaction. Different consistencies of PMMA are available (liquid or dough) with the same end result; either can be used depending on surgeon preference and availability. Preventing excessive heat formation, especially close to the spinal cord, is paramount when using bone cement.

> Video clips to accompany this book can be found on the companion website at:
> www.wiley.com/go/shores/neurosurgery

References

1 Bone Wax Product Insert. http://cpmedical.com/wp-content/uploads/2012/07/BONE-WAX-INSERT.pdf

2 Ozdemir N, Gelal MF, Minoglu M, Celik L. Reactive changes of disc space and foreign body granuloma due to bone wax in lumbar spine. *Neurol India* 2009;57:493–496.

3 Schonauer C. The use of local agents: bone wax, gelatin, collagen, oxidized cellulose. *Eur Spine J* 2004;13(Suppl 1):S89–S96.

4 da Costa RC, Pippi NL, Graça DL et al. The effects of free fat graft or cellulose membrane implants on laminectomy membrane formation in dogs. *Vet J* 2006; 171:491–499.

5 Brodbelt AR, Miles JB, Foy PM, Broome JC. Intraspinal oxidised cellulose (Surgicel) causing delayed paraplegia after thoracotomy: a report of three cases. *Ann R Coll Surg Engl* 2002;84:97–99.

6 Knowlson GT. Gel-foam granuloma in the brain. *J Neurol Neurosurg Psychiatry* 1974;37:971–973.

7 Charlesworth TM, Agthe P, Moores A, Anderson DM. The use of haemostatic gelatin sponges in veterinary surgery. *J. Small Anim Pract* 2012;53:51–56.

2 Orthopedic Implants in Neurosurgery

Noel M.M. Moens

Introduction

Surgical implants are routinely used in neurosurgery for the stabilization of unstable vertebral segments caused by fracture, luxation, or chronic degenerative processes and congenital malformations. Regardless of the implant being used, and for what purpose, the goals should be to achieve stable fixation and return the animal to full function in a consistent and reliable manner. This requires a basic understanding of biomechanics as well as a thorough understanding of how implants are loaded and how they should be used to ensure reliable results. This is particularly important since few implants used in neurosurgery were specifically designed for this purpose and rather were designed for fixation of long bone fractures.

This chapter is not designed to be exhaustive but to provide a quick overview of some of the different implants used in neurosurgery and to provide information on the rationale for their use and their limitations.

Pins and Wires

Surgical pins and wires are made of hardened surgical grade 316L stainless steel and come in a variety of sizes and designs. Small pins from 0.7 to 1.6 mm are often referred to as Kirschner wires or K-wires, while large-diameter pins, generally from 2 to 6 mm, are referred to as Steinmann pins. The pin or wire tips can have different configurations, with the most frequent being the trocar tip and the chisel tip (Figure 2.1). Other tip types exist but are not as common in veterinary medicine.

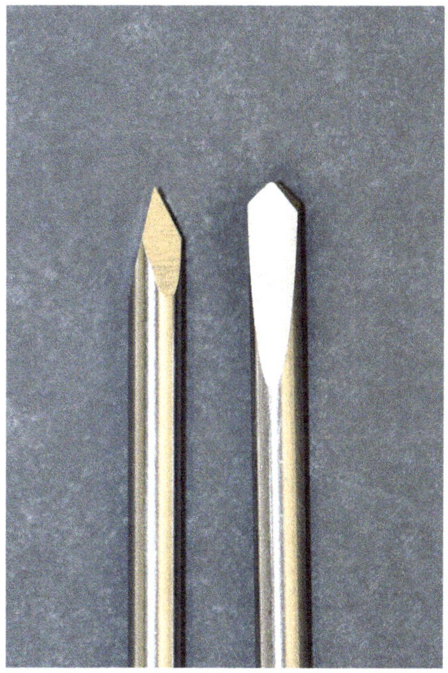

Figure 2.1 Steinmann pin tips with trocar (*left*) and chisel (*right*) tips.

The pins can either be smooth or threaded, with the threaded portion located at the end of the pin or in the middle section of the pin. Threaded pins can be either *negative profile* or *positive profile*. Negative-profile pins have the thread cut into the shaft of the pin, thereby decreasing the core diameter along the threaded portion of the pin. Although these pins provide better pull-out strength than smooth pins, their strength and bending stiffness are significantly decreased compared with smooth or positive-profile pins. Negative-profile pins are prone to breaking at the junction between the solid shaft and the threaded portion of the pin due to stress concentration at that level when loaded [1,2].

Positive-profile pins have their thread built over the pin core and have a uniform core shaft diameter along their entire length (Figure 2.2). They offer greater pull-out strength and better bending strength and stiffness than negative-profile pins. Positive-profile pins are manufactured with two different types of thread, one optimized for cortical bone, with smaller diameter and smaller pitch, the other optimized for cancellous bone with a larger thread diameter and longer pitch.

Current Techniques in Canine and Feline Neurosurgery, First Edition. Edited by Andy Shores and Brigitte A. Brisson.
© 2017 John Wiley & Sons, Inc. Published 2017 by John Wiley & Sons, Inc.
Companion website: www.wiley.com/go/shores/neurosurgery

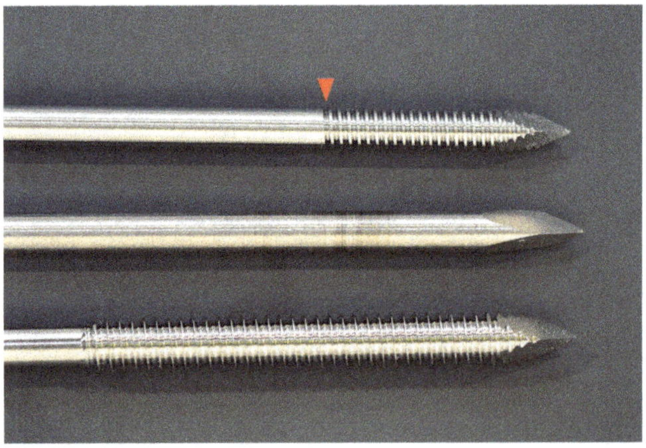

Figure 2.2 Negative-profile pin (*top*), smooth nonthreaded pin (*middle*), and positive-profile threaded pin (*bottom*). Note the decrease in core diameter of the negative-profile pin at the junction between the smooth shaft and the threaded portion (arrowhead).

Importance of the Pin–Bone Interface

In neurosurgery, pins are often used as internal fixators, where all the implants are contained under the skin: the pins are inserted into the vertebrae to provide purchase into the bone and are connected together, generally using acrylic cement (Figure 2.3).

In most cases, the pin–bone interface is the weakest link of the construct and the one aspect of the fixation that can be most easily compromised by poor surgical technique. No matter how strong the fixator, its efficacy ultimately relies on the integrity of the pin–bone interface and small, seemingly benign technical errors can easily and rapidly lead to the loss of the entire fixation. There are several ways to improve the pin–bone interface and influence long-term pin–bone stability [3].

Pin Insertion Technique

Bone is exceedingly sensitive to temperature increases, and thermal necrosis can be blamed for a significant number of fixator failures. A temperature slightly above 53 °C irreversibly damages bone and leads to necrosis, resorption, and loss of the pin–bone interface [4]. It is remarkably easy to exceed this temperature during drilling and pin insertion.

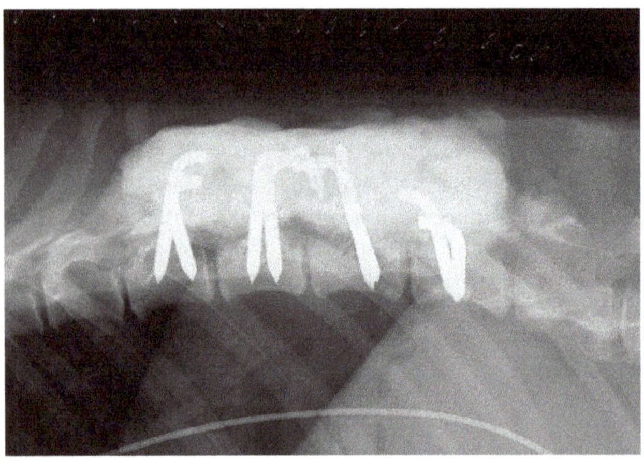

Figure 2.3 Spinal luxation in a dog stabilized using cortical positive-profile pins and PMMA cement. *Source*: Courtesy of Dr. Fiona James.

Low-speed power drill insertion (150 rpm) is the most recommended method of insertion and, if done appropriately, has been shown to keep bone temperatures within acceptable limits and is, for most applications, the preferred insertion technique [5]. Many surgical drills are designed for high-speed drilling and are therefore not ideal for pin insertion. Great care must be taken to avoid excessive speed during insertion as high-speed insertion almost invariably generates excessive heat and produces large areas of thermal necrosis of the pin track [4,5].

Manual insertion has been recommended to minimize the risk of thermal injury. However, manual insertion can also create wobble during insertion which can decrease holding strength. In a study on external fixation, smooth pins inserted manually with a hand chuck in canine tibiae demonstrated less holding power than a similar pin inserted at low speed (150 rpm) with a power drill [6]. The loss of pin purchase was blamed on the unavoidable wobble that occurs during hand insertion and the enlarged hole that ensues. The design of the pin tip also plays a role in the amount of heat that is produced during pin placement. The two most common pin types in veterinary medicine are the trocar and chisel tips. Although trocar tips are easy to manufacture and are the most common, they can generate a significant amount of heat by friction. Chisel tips are slightly more efficient and generate less heat than trocar tips but the difference has not been shown to be statistically different [7].

Predrilling

The benefit of predrilling a pilot hole into the bone prior to inserting the pin has been the topic of intense debate and remains controversial. Predrilling a hole close to, but slightly smaller than, the core diameter of the pin to be used into cortical bone has been shown to decrease the amount of microfractures produced during pin insertion and has resulted in an improved initial pull-out strength in canine tibiae [8]. However, differences in pull-out strength following predrilling were not observed in other studies [9,10]. In fact, a decrease in pull-out strength following predrilling has even been reported when predrilling was performed prior to screw insertion in bovine cancellous bone and in human vertebrae. As such, the recommendation was to drill only a short pilot hole into the vertebrae to allow the thread to engage. It is likely that the different and sometimes contradictory findings are the result of different testing methodologies, insertion sites, bone characteristics, and techniques. It appears safe to recommend predrilling with a drill bit slightly smaller than the core diameter of the pin when dense cortical bone is likely to be encountered but that predrilling vertebral bodies or cancellous bone beyond the creation of a short pilot hole may not be necessary.

Irrigation

Another method of effectively controlling temperature during insertion is to dissipate the heat produced using copious irrigation with cool sterile saline. This method has been shown to be effective at avoiding thermal necrosis in the bone [11]. It must be noted however that irrigation is much less effective on the pin tip once it has penetrated the first cortex (cis-cortex) and engages the second cortex (trans-cortex). An increase in temperature of up to 9 °C has been measured as the pin engages the far cortex [12]. As such, irrigation alone cannot replace good pin insertion technique.

Length of Bone Engagement

Holding power for screws in cancellous bone is dependent upon the diameter of the thread, characteristics of the thread design, the quality of the bone, and the length of engagement [13].

Because the resistance to pull-out is directly linked to the length of the pin engaging the cancellous bone, it is important to maximize this length. Ideally, the pin should penetrate the trans-cortex to ensure maximal bone engagement [14]; however, bicortical engagement is not always possible or advisable in neurosurgery due to the high risk of penetrating the spinal canal. The depth of penetration must be carefully controlled during insertion. Over-penetration must be avoided because it can cause irreversible damage to essential structures. Because of the thin cortices of vertebral bodies, it may be difficult to identify at which point the pin penetrates the cortical wall. Measuring the bone and the pin prior to insertion is therefore essential and will help reduce the risk of over-penetration. If a pilot hole has been drilled, the length of the hole can be measured using a depth gauge and the distance of penetration compared to the length of the threaded portion of the pin as a guide. Premeasurements from radiographs or CT images can also be very useful for determining acceptable penetration length. Backing out a pin that has been inserted too far should be avoided unless necessary, as the back and forth movement has been shown to decrease the pin–bone interface and holding strength [9].

Pin Thread Design

In long bone external fixation, the design of the pin thread appears to have a significant effect on the short- and long-term stability of fixators. Threaded pins have significantly greater initial pull-out strength than smooth pins. They are also less likely to loosen during the postoperative period. Threaded pins have been shown to have a 14-fold better pull-out strength than smooth pins 8 weeks following tibial implantation in the dog [1]. It is reasonable to assume that the same trend would be observed in vertebrae. The choice between cancellous and cortical threaded pins remains controversial and likely depends on bone characteristics, thickness, and quality. In theory, cancellous threaded pins have a larger thread diameter than cortical pins and will therefore better resist pull-out forces. They are, however, generally manufactured with a smaller core diameter than cortical pins in order to maximize thread depth, thus making them weaker in bending and shear. Because internal fixators are often loaded in bending and shear, the quest for larger thread should not come at the expense of the core diameter of the implant or failure is likely to be observed [15,16]. The pitch of a screw is the distance between two consecutive threads. Cancellous threads have a larger pitch than cortical threads in order to capture more bone between each thread. This theoretically increases pull-out strength if enough bone can be engaged, but it can result in poor holding strength if bone penetration is shallow or if the bone is thin since fewer threads actually engage the bone.

Importance of the Pin–Cement Interface

For many neurosurgical applications, pins or screws are secured using acrylic cement (polymethylmethacrylate, PMMA). Acrylic cement does not truly adhere to metal and the initial adhesion that may exist between the cement and the pins is generally short-lived. Long-term stability is provided by the creation of a more durable interlock between the cement and the implants [14,17,18]. This is particularly critical as contamination of the pin surface with blood or fat is almost unavoidable and further decreases cement adhesion. Notching the pins using a pin cutter creates grooves on the pin surface, allowing the cement to interlock with the pins and has been recommended to prevent pin loosening and migration [14]. Cutting the pin to length and bending the end of the pin may also be a good way to increase the interlock between the pin and the cement. Although it is very difficult and potentially dangerous to bend or even cut large pins in situ after implantation, it is possible to precut and to bend the pin prior to insertion. In this instance, the bent pin can be carefully inserted through a predrilled hole using a hand chuck. Care must be taken to avoid wobble that could cause deterioration of the pin–bone interface. Some small pins are specifically designed for composite fixators and their shaft surface is covered by a fine thread to improve cement interlock (Figure 2.4).

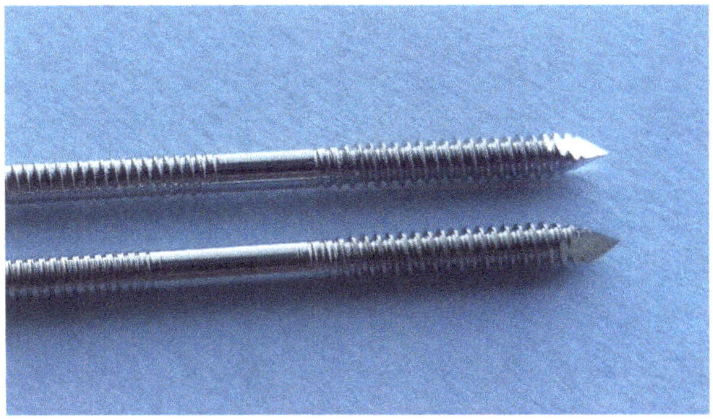

Figure 2.4 Imex Miniature Interface® pins (IMEX Veterinary Inc., Longview, TX, USA). These pins have a threaded tip and a roughened core to ensure a better grip of the acrylic cement. These are available in diameters from 0.9 to 2.4 mm.

Bone Screws

The development of new implants and new surgical techniques has been associated with a parallel evolution in bone screw design. The thin and fragile nature of the bone in maxillofacial surgery and neurosurgery has also contributed to new screw designs with better purchase in thin and poor-quality bone. The recent development of locking plate systems has also significantly changed the function of screws and their design.

In orthopedics, screws are generally used to secure bone plates to bones or provide interfragmentary compression, whereas in neurosurgery compression is rarely applied to the construct. Instead, screws are often used in combination with PMMA cement as an alternative to pins for the construction of internal fixators. Screws used in this fashion become part of an *angle-stable* construct and are subjected to different forces from traditional plate screws. This difference must be taken into account when selecting the size and type of screw for this particular use.

The main characteristics of a screw are its length, thread diameter, core diameter, and pitch. The thread diameter, also referred to as the major diameter, generally identifies the size of the screw and is the major determinant of the screw pull-out strength. The core diameter, also known as the minor diameter, is the diameter of the shaft and in most cases dictates the diameter of the hole that must be drilled into the bone before insertion. The core diameter is the main determinant of the shear strength and bending strength of the screw and has a lesser effect on the pull-out strength of the screw. The pitch is a characteristic of the thread and can be defined as the distance between two consecutive threads (Figure 2.5).

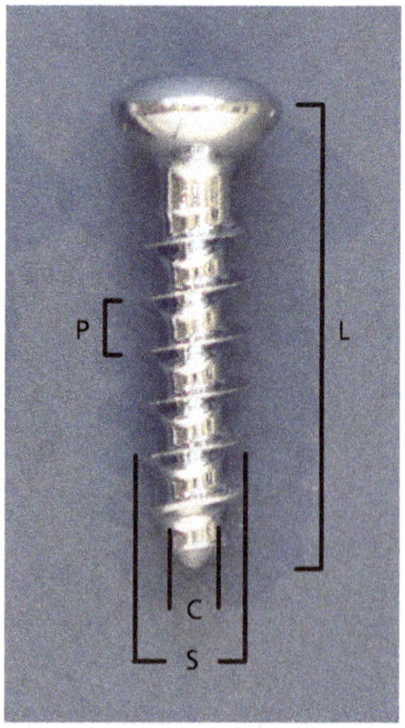

Figure 2.5 Characteristics of a bone screw. L, length of the screw. S, screw diameter, also known as major diameter or thread diameter; it is a major determinant of the pull-out strength of the screw. C, core diameter or minor diameter; the minor diameter is an important determinant of the bending and shear strength of the screw. P, pitch, the distance between two consecutive threads; in most screws with a single start-thread, it is also the distance that the screw will advance if turned 360°.

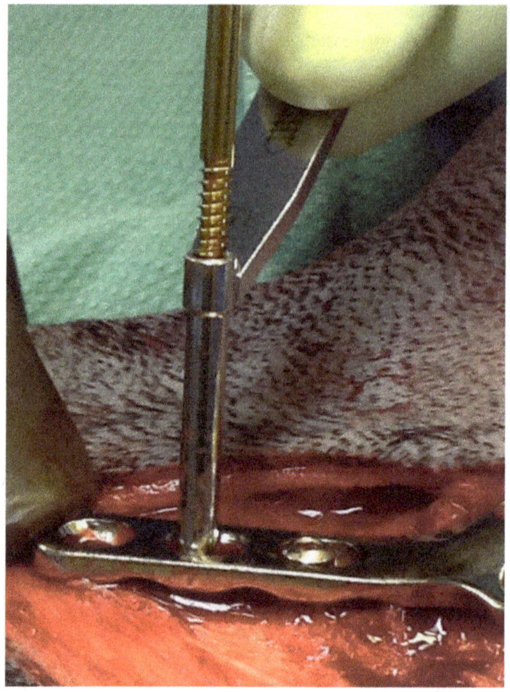

Figure 2.6 Tapping the hole with the appropriate tap is always done using a tap sleeve to minimize entrapment of the soft tissue but also to steady the tap and decrease wobble.

Screw Insertion Technique

Similarly to pins, the preservation of the bone–screw interface is essential for the long-term stability of the construct [19]. Many of the aspects of preservation of the pin–bone interface apply to bone screws and have been described earlier in this chapter. The basic sequence for bone screw insertion is drill, measure, tap, and insert.

Predrilling

Unlike pins, which have a sharp point, insertion of screws generally requires predrilling of the bone. The diameter of the hole is dictated by the core diameter of the screw. Because of the many sizes of screw available, a wide range of drill bit diameters and lengths are also available. It is essential to carefully match the drill bit to the core diameter of the screw as creating too small a hole will not allow screw insertion and creating too large a hole will automatically decrease the holding strength of the screw [19].

Drilling must be done with great care to avoid thermal necrosis of the bone and creating an unnecessarily large hole. Sharp drill bits and irrigation must be used to ensure the hole is drilled efficiently and with as little heat generation as possible. The use of a drill sleeve or drill guide during drilling is also essential to protect the soft tissues from catching, but also to minimize wobble and enlargement of the hole.

Measuring

Measurement of the length of the hole is generally performed after drilling but before tapping so as to not damage the delicate thread cut into the bone using a bone tap. This is often performed with a specialized depth gauge but can sometimes be achieved by using specifically designed graduated drill bits. Depth gauges are often graduated in 2-mm increments. For all bicortical screws, the measured length from the depth gauge is generally rounded up to the next measurement to ensure that the tip of the screw fully exits past the trans-cortex of the bone. If a monocortical screw is to be inserted, a screw slightly shorter than the measured distance is chosen to avoid contact with, or penetration of the trans-cortex. Because errors can easily occur when using the depth gauge, it is always recommended to double check the measurement against radiographic or CT measurements and to use common sense.

Tapping

Tapping is the creation of the thread in the bone using a specific instrument that exactly matches the characteristics of the chosen screw thread and cuts the thread into the bone as it is advanced. Tapping is a delicate operation that carries a high risk of damaging the hole and immediately reducing the screw's holding strength. As each type of screw has a specific thread pattern, one must choose the appropriate bone tap for the screw to be inserted. The orientation of the tap must exactly match the orientation of the drilled hole or stripping of the thread will occur. Wobble while tapping must be minimized as it enlarges the size of the hole or damages the thread. For this reason a tap guide of appropriate size is always used, even if surrounding soft tissues do not require protection (Figure 2.6).

Screw Insertion

Screw insertion must be carried out carefully in order to prevent damage to the previously created thread. The orientation of the screw must carefully match the orientation of the tapped hole or damage to the thread will occur. Over-tightening of the screw will result in stripping of the thread. Stripping of the thread during screw insertion may be the result of poor bone quality and bone mineral density, inappropriate hole preparation, or inappropriately high torque during insertion. Stripping of the thread immediately decreases the holding strength of that screw by more than 80% and presents a significant challenge to the surgeon [19]. Replacing a stripped screw by a slightly larger screw (also known as a rescue screw) has been common practice in veterinary surgery but has been shown to be of limited value, both in osteoporotic long bones and in vertebrae [20,21]. If the screw cannot be reoriented to engage undamaged bone, filling the stripped hole with PMMA prior to reinserting the screw has been used successfully for the revision of human pedicle screws and for salvage of stripped holes in feline radii [22,23].

Types of Screw

Cancellous Screws

Cancellous screws are designed to offer maximum pull-out resistance in soft and cancellous bones and therefore have a large outer diameter, a larger pitch, and a smaller core. However, because of their smaller core, they provide reduced resistance in bending and shear and may not be appropriate for use in angle-stable constructs (such as a locking plate or screws and PMMA internal fixator) [15,16]. With the exception of self-drilling screws, a pilot hole equivalent to, or slightly smaller than, the core diameter of the screw must be drilled into the bone before inserting the screw. Tapping the bone to create the bone thread has been shown to decrease pull-out strength of cancellous screws and therefore this step is often avoided in cancellous bone [24]. However, it may be useful to get the thread started in the cis-cortex by turning the tap for a couple of turns before inserting the screw. If tapping is not performed, it must be noted that if the tip of the screw contacts a strong and thick cortex on the opposite side of the bone during insertion, the screw is likely to strip the thread. If such a scenario is likely, it is recommended to fully tap the hole before insertion. Independent of bone quality, the major determinants of pull-out strength for cancellous screws are thread diameter and length of engagement of the screw [13,25]. Therefore, the larger screw diameter and the longest screw (engaging bone) that can safely be used should be used.

Cortical Screws

Compared with cancellous screws, cortical screws have a finer thread, a smaller pitch, and a relatively larger core. They are designed to provide increased pull-out strength in denser, more compact bone. Because of their larger core diameter, they are often preferred over cancellous screws for vertebral fixation with PMMA. The thread and the screw head provide good interlock with the PMMA, without the need to cut, bend or notch the pins. However, failure of the fixation by fracture or bending of the screws has been observed and large screws should be used whenever possible [14–16].

Self-tapping Screws

Many screws are now designed with a self-tapping tip (Figure 2.7). These screws cut the thread into the bone as they are inserted and do not require tapping as a separate step. This feature not only saves surgical time but may be of great importance in bone with cortices less than 1 or 2 mm thick, in which tapping with a separate instrument greatly increases the risk of enlarging the hole and decreasing pull-out strength [26]. Self-tapping screws are widely used in veterinary surgery and have been shown to provide good bone-holding characteristics [27,28]. The self-tapping tip does not contribute to the holding power of the screw and it is therefore recommended to insert those screws bicortically with the tip of the screw exiting past the far cortex by 1 to 2 mm to maximize holding strength [28,29].

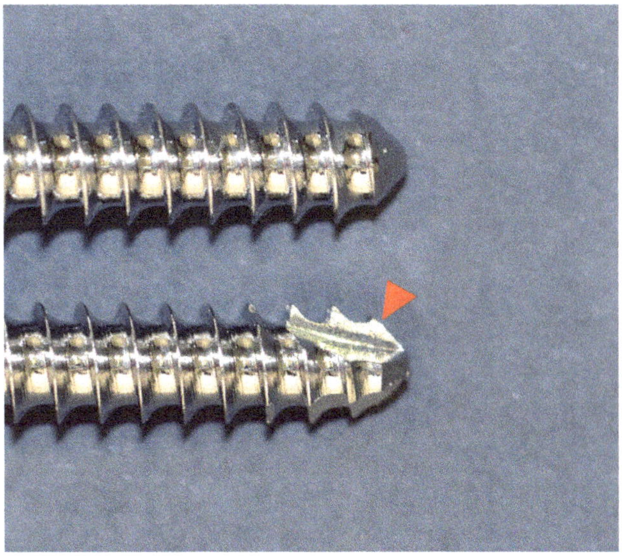

Figure 2.7 Detail of the tips of 3.5-mm regular (*top*) and self-tapping (*bottom*) cortical screws showing the cutting flute at the extremity of the self-tapping screw (arrowhead).

Self-drilling Screws

Most recently, self-drilling screws have been introduced. These screws have an elongated tip shaped like a corkscrew and are able to penetrate relatively thin bone without the need for a pilot hole. They have been designed for skull fixation in neurosurgery or for maxillofacial surgery and are generally of small size and small diameter (up to 2 mm) (Figure 2.8). Much larger self-drilling screws have been designed for stabilization of cervical vertebrae in humans [13]. Because insertion is a one-step process, it is believed to improve the bone–screw interface by minimizing the risk of enlarging the hole or by reducing heat generation [30]. However, this was not supported by Sowden and Schmitz [31] who found that the self-drilling screws produced more tearing and microfracturing of the endosteal bone than self-tapping screws. Careful measurement of the bone thickness must be performed prior to self-drilling screw insertion since there is no good way to measure the thickness of the bone during surgery. The use of self-drilling screws has been anecdotally reported in spinal fixation in miniature breeds, although their efficacy, safety, and holding power in canine vertebrae has not yet been reported. These screws are generally used with mesh to cover skull defects following craniotomy (Figure 2.9).

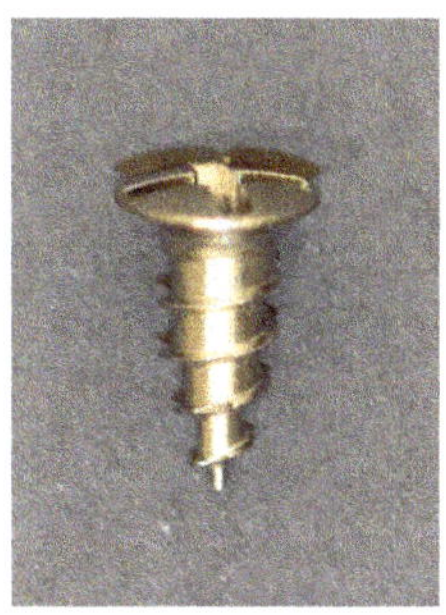

Figure 2.8 Self-drilling, self-tapping screw.

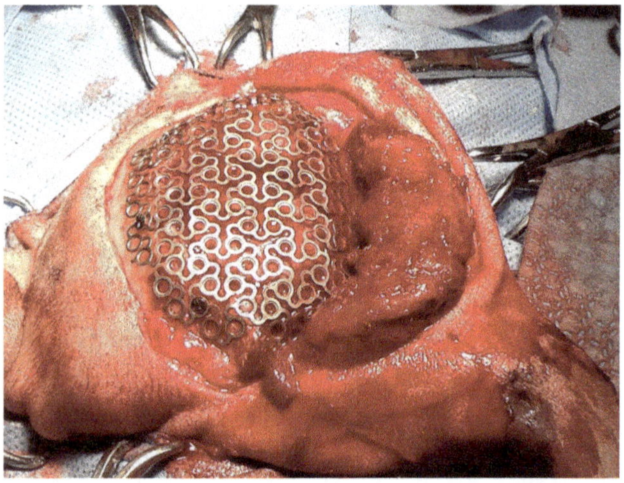

Figure 2.9 Coverage of an extensive craniectomy defect using mesh and self-drilling screws. *Source*: Courtesy of Dr. Michelle Oblak.

Locking Screws

The invention of the locking plate system has led to the parallel development of locking screws. When a locking screw is tightened, its head engages the plate and effectively locks the screw into the plate. Although some locking plates allow the surgeon to determine the screw insertion angle, once locked, the angle of the screw relative to the plate cannot be modified and acts as an angle-stable construct similar to an external fixator. Unlike traditional screws that have been designed to resist pull-out forces, locking screws are mostly subjected to bending and shear forces and have been designed to resist such forces [32]. Their core diameter has been increased to better resist bending and shear forces, while their thread has become finer and symmetrical to equally resist pull-out or push-in forces (Figure 2.10). The head of the screw has also been redesigned with a conical shape or a thread to provide a locking mechanism in conjunction with the plate hole. Locking screws are generally self-tapping. Some locking screws have a self-drilling tip and are designed to be used as monocortical screws in long bones with thick cortices [33].

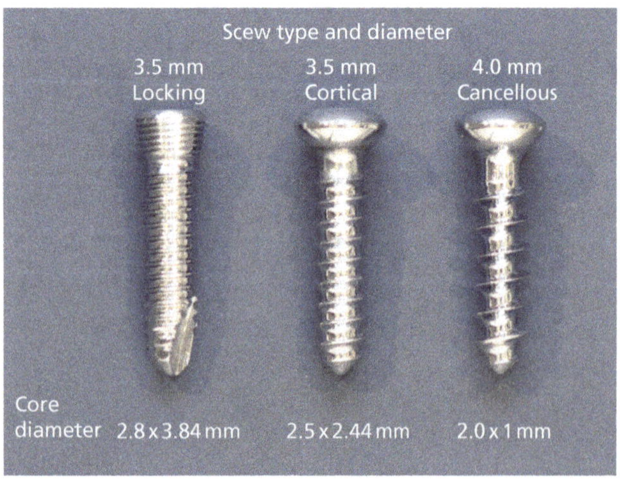

Figure 2.10 (*Left to right*) A 3.5-mm locking screw, 3.5-mm cortical screw, and 4.0-mm cancellous screw. Note the difference in core diameter of the screws and the relative increase in bending stiffness compared with the cancellous screw. Despite its overall larger diameter, the 4.0-mm cancellous screw is nearly four times weaker in bending than the 3.5-mm locking screw.

Bone Plates

In the recent years, there has been a significant paradigm shift in the way fractures are approached and treated. In orthopedic surgery, the need for perfect reconstruction and absolute stability have been progressively supplanted by indirect reduction and relative stability, and a much stronger emphasis is now placed on the preservation of the fracture biology [34,35]. Associated with this shift, recent years have seen an explosion of new technologies, plates and implant designs in both human and veterinary surgery. Bone plates now come in a variety of materials and shapes and as such we are no longer limited to the traditional straight rectangular plates used in the past for the fixation of long bones.

Nonlocking Plates

Traditional, nonlocking plates use the screws to generate compression of the plate against the bone. The friction generated between the plate and the bone provides stability. If at any time during activity the forces acting on the fracture exceed the frictional forces generated by the screws, toggling and pull-out of the screws will occur resulting in loss of reduction [32,35]. To minimize this risk of failure, the traditional bone screws are designed with a large thread and a relatively small core diameter to provide maximum pull-out strength and generate maximal compression (Figure 2.11).

To generate adequate friction, traditional bone plates require intimate contact with the bone cortex. This requires a time-consuming and sometimes difficult process of contouring the plate to match the bone surface. The large area of contact between the plate and the bone causes devascularization and osteonecrosis of the bone cortex underneath the plate and may predispose the bone to delayed healing, refracture, or infection [35–37]. To minimize damage to the bone, bone plates have progressively evolved to limit the contact between the plate and the bone [e.g., Limited Contact Dynamic Compression Plate (LC-DCP™), DePuy Synthes, West Chester, PA, USA], while still optimizing stability. This evolution has led to the recent development of the locking plate [35].

Locking Plates

The search for a bone plate that minimizes the biological impact while providing superior stability has led to the development of locking plate systems. These plates provide a mechanism to lock the screws within the plate, providing an angle-stable construct, in ways similar to external fixators or pin and PMMA constructs. Unlike traditional plates, locking plates do not require intimate contact with the bone and the screws do not need to generate compression to provide stability. In contrast with traditional screws designed to resist pull-out forces, locking screws are mostly loaded in shear and bending and are designed to better fulfil this role (see Figure 2.11). The thread has become symmetrical to equally resist pull-out or push-in forces. The core diameter of the screw has become relatively larger, along with a smaller thread to resist bending and shear forces, which are now the predominant forces acting upon them [32].

Two broad categories of locking plates exist: *fixed-angle* and *variable-angle* locking plates [32]. In most veterinary implants, locking of the screws is achieved when the threaded screw head engages and locks into a corresponding thread cut into the plate hole (Figure 2.12). In contrast, some systems achieve locking when the smooth conical screw head is press fitted into a softer bushing.

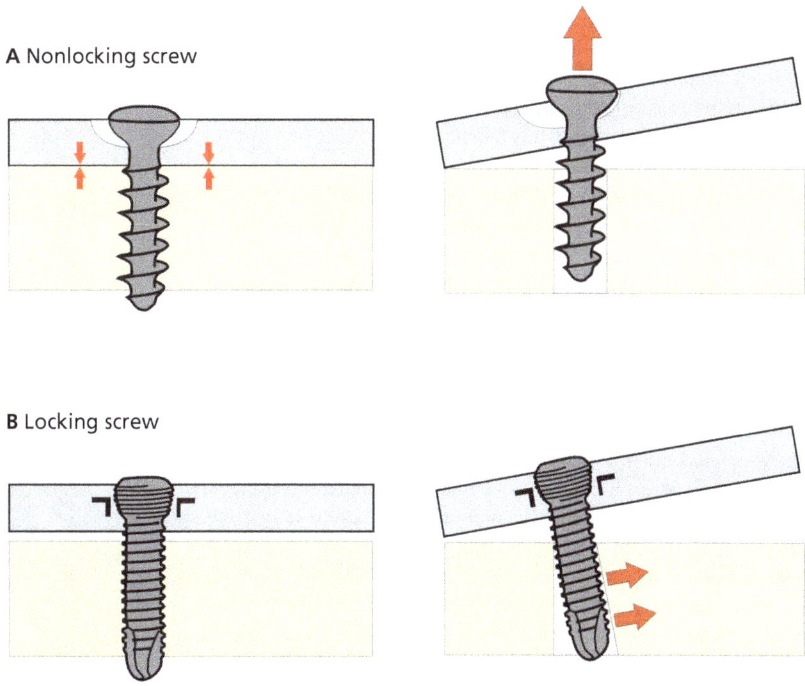

Figure 2.11 Regular nonlocking plate screws (A) work by compressing the plate against the bone and the friction generated provides stability (small red arrows). Once the friction is lost or exceeded, stability is lost. As the plate pulls away from the bone, the screw reorients itself within the plate and pull-out occurs (large red arrow). Locking screws (B) are locked into the plate and into the bone and do not require intimate contact between the plate and the bone to provide stability. If the plate is pulled away from the bone, because of the fixed angle between the plate and the screw, the screw is loaded in bending and compressive stresses develop in the cortex (red arrows). If failure occurs, locking constructs generally fail by fracturing a large segment of bone.

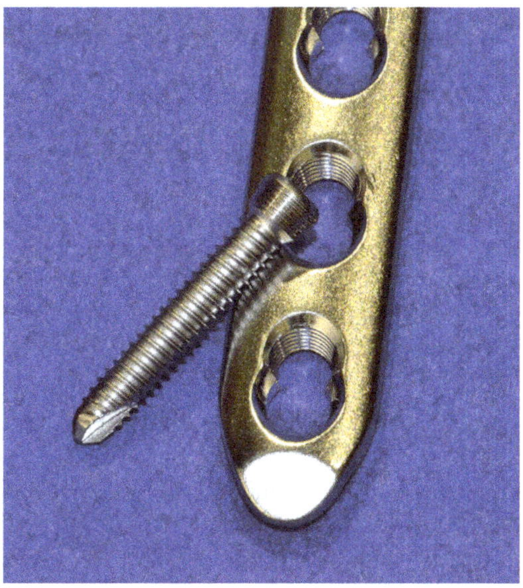

Figure 2.12 Detail of the screw and plate hole of the LC-DCP™ system (DePuy Synthes). In this fixed-angle locking system, the thread of the screw head fully engages the thread of the hole in the plate. Note that in this system, the plate holes are designed to be used either with a locking screw (in the threaded portion of the hole) or a regular screw (in the nonthreaded portion of the hole).

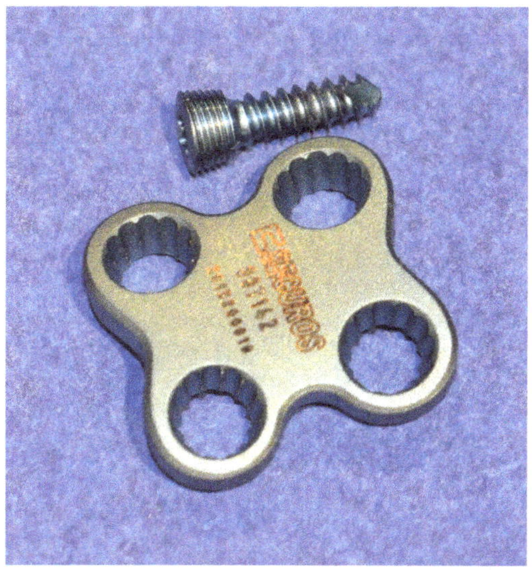

Figure 2.13 Detail of a variable-angle locking system (Pax System™; Securos, Fiskdale, MA, USA). In this system, the thread of the screw head carves its own thread into the ridges of the plate hole, allowing a narrow choice of orientation during insertion. *Source*: Courtesy of Securos Surgical.

In fixed-angle locking plates, the direction of the screw is dictated by the orientation of the hole in the plate. The only options for changing the screw orientation are to contour the plate in order to change the orientation of the hole or to use a nonlocking screw instead of a locking screw. In variable-angle locking plates, the screw can be oriented and locked within a narrow cone of possibilities (generally ±10°). The locking mechanism of variable-angle plates is created by either purposefully cross-threading the head of the screw into a specially designed plate hole or, in some systems, by cutting a new thread into the softer material of the bone plate (Figure 2.13).

Locking plates have several proven and theoretical advantages over conventional plates. Because stability of the construct does not rely on plate compression against the bone, the plate does not need to be in direct contact with the bone and there is therefore no need for extensive plate contouring [33]. The space between the bone and the plate allows for preservation of the periosteum and for greater vascularization of the bone underneath the plate. Greater vascularization may lead to faster callus production and improved resistance against infection [35]. Arguably, one of the greatest advantages of the locking plate is its ability to provide superior fixation in poor-quality bone [32,33,38]. This characteristic may be of great benefit in neurosurgery where the vertebral cortices are thin, the bone is mostly cancellous, and sufficient bone stock for traditional fixation is frequently lacking.

In human long bone fractures, it has been suggested that, because of the fixed angle, sufficient stability could be achieved with the exclusive use of monocortical locking screws. In dogs and cats, even diaphyseal bones have thinner cortices than those of humans and the exclusive use of monocortical locking screws must be considered carefully. Additionally, results obtained in long bone research may not be directly applicable to vertebral bone in which cancellous bone predominates. In human and canine spinal fixation the use of bicortical implants has been shown to provide superior stability compared with monocortical implants [14,39]. In dogs, however, accurate placement of bicortical implants in the spine can be challenging and carries a high risk of spinal canal penetration [40,41]. For this reason, the use of monocortical locking screws may be beneficial and has recently been investigated and used effectively to stabilize spinal segments in vivo and ex vivo [41–47]. When using monocortical locking screws, the longest screw possible should be used to maximize bone purchase into the cancellous bone [13,39].

Although locking plates have significant advantages over traditional plating in neurosurgery, there are also disadvantages that are worth noting. When using locking plates, there is limited to no ability to orient the screws and therefore appropriate plate design and contouring is necessary for appropriate fixation. Contouring of small and complex plates could be a difficult task and may result in inappropriate screw placement. Because of the extreme variability in body shape and size of our veterinary patients, custom-designed plates that would fit all breeds is not a realistic concept and plates appropriate for one animal may not be appropriate for another. Some plates of the variable-angle design provide more freedom when it comes to screw orientation; however, the insertion angles remain limited and the screw–plate interface has been shown to be significantly weaker than that of fixed-angle plates [48]. Another disadvantage is that although locking plates provide superior holding in poor-quality bone, if they fail they generally do so catastrophically by cutting through the bone or by fracturing a large segment of bone [32,49]. This could be highly problematic in neurosurgery and may significantly complicate any eventual revision surgery.

String of Pearls™

String of Pearls™ (SOP; Orthomed UK Ltd, Halifax, West Yorkshire, UK) is a specific type of locking plate composed of a series of spherical nodes, linked together by thick cylindrical internode sections. What makes the SOP different from other locking plates is that the nodes accommodate and provide locking capabilities for regular cortical bone screws as opposed to specifically designed locking screws. The plate can be cut to length and can easily be contoured in multiple planes at the level of the internodes, giving great freedom to orient the screws in multiple directions in order to match complex bone surfaces. Biomechanically, the SOP compares favorably to several other locking systems [50,51]. The regular bone screws, with their smaller core diameter than typical locking screws, appear to be the weakest point of this system and may explain why the SOP does not outperform other locking systems [50,51] despite being a stronger implant in itself [52]. The SOP has been used successfully in neurosurgery for stabilization of vertebral fractures and spinal instability [53] (Figure 2.14).

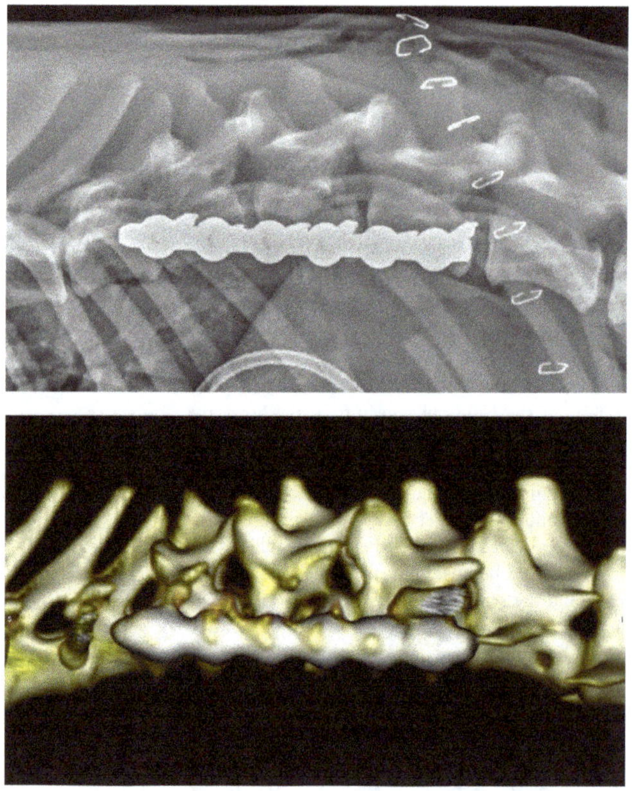

Figure 2.14 Lateral radiographs and CT reconstruction of String of Pearls (SOP) plate system used for stabilization of a vertebral fracture in a dog. *Source*: Courtesy of Dr. Laurent Guiot.

Summary

The recent years have seen the development of new surgical implants and surgical techniques. Each implant comes with its own intricacies and technical requirements that makes each of them unique. A sound understanding of each implant's capabilities and shortcomings will allow the surgeon to successfully adapt and design their fixation to fit each specific situation, even if the implant may not have been originally designed for that purpose. Great attention to detail is paramount in neurosurgery as the fixations are often technically difficult due to the unique nature of the axial skeleton. Small technical errors in implant selection or their application can easily jeopardize the final outcome. Many of these errors can go unnoticed during surgery and are difficult to detect on postoperative radiographs. Familiarity with each implant system and a sound knowledge of their unique capabilities is essential to ensure consistent, positive results.

Video clips to accompany this book can be found on the companion website at:
www.wiley.com/go/shores/neurosurgery

References

1 Bennett RA, Egger EL, Histand M, Ellis AB. Comparison of the strength and holding power of 4 pin designs for use with half pin (type I) external skeletal fixation. *Vet Surg* 1987;16:207–211.

2 Palmer RH, Aron DN. Ellis pin complications in seven dogs. *Vet Surg* 1990;19: 440–445.

3 Lewis DD, Cross AR, Carmichael S, Anderson MA. Recent advances in external skeletal fixation. *J Small Anim Pract* 2001;42:103–112.
4 Eriksson A, Albrektsson T, Grane B, McQueen D. Thermal injury to bone. *Int J Oral Surg* 1982;11:115–121.
5 Egger EL, Histand MB, Blass CE, Powers BE. Effect of fixation pin insertion on the bone–pin interface. *Vet Surg* 1986;15:246–252.
6 Gumbs JM, Brinker WO, DeCamp CE, Schaeffer R, Kaneene JB, Soutas-Little RW. Comparison of acute and chronic pull-out resistance of pins used with the external fixator (Kirschner splint). *J Am Anim Hosp Assoc* 1988;24:231–234.
7 Matthews LS, Green CA, Goldstein SA. The thermal effects of skeletal fixation-pin insertion in bone. *J Bone Joint Surg Am* 1984;66:1077–1083.
8 Clary EM, Roe SC. In vitro biomechanical and histological assessment of pilot hole diameter for positive-profile external skeletal fixation pins in canine tibiae. *Vet Surg* 1996;25:453–462.
9 Dernell WS, Harari J, Blackketter DM. A comparison of acute pull-out strength between two-way and one-way transfixation pin insertion for external skeletal fixation in canine bone. *Vet Surg* 1993;22:110–114.
10 Oliphant BW, Kim H, Osgood GM et al. Predrilling does not improve the pullout strength of external fixator pins: a biomechanical study. *J Orthop Trauma* 2013;27:e25–e30.
11 Sener BC, Dergin G, Gursoy B, Kelesoglu E, Slih I. Effects of irrigation temperature on heat control in vitro at different drilling depths. *Clin Oral Implants Res* 2009;20:294–298.
12 Erikssons AR, Albrektsson T, Albrektsson B. Heat caused by drilling cortical bone: temperature measured in vivo in patients and animals. *Acta Orthop Scand* 1984;55:629–631.
13 Hitchon PW, Brenton MD, Coppes JK, From AM, Torner JC. Factors affecting the pullout strength of self-drilling and self-tapping anterior cervical screws. *Spine* 2003;28:9–13.
14 Blass CE, Seim III HB. Spinal fixation in dogs using Steinmann pins and methylmethacrylate. *Vet Surg* 1984;13:203–210.
15 Beaver DP, MacPhersont GC, Muir P, Johnson KA. Methyl-methacrylate and bone screw repair of seventh lumbar vertebral fracture-luxations in dogs. *J Small Anim Pract* 1996;37:381–386.
16 Garcia JN, Milthorpe BK, Russell D, Johnson KA. Biomechanical study of canine spinal fracture fixation using pins or bone screws with polymethylmethacrylate. *Vet Surg* 1994;23:322–329.
17 Ahmed AM, Raab S, Miller JE, Miller E. Metal/cement interface strength in cemented stem fixation. *J Orthopaed Res* 1984;2:105–118.
18 Stone MH, Wilkinson R, Stother IG. Some factors affecting the strength of the cement–metal interface. *J Bone Joint Surg Br* 1989;71:217–221.
19 Collinge C, Hartigan B, Lautenschlager EP. Effects of surgical errors on small fragment screw fixation. *J Orthop Trauma* 2006;20:410–413.
20 Pitzen T, Franta F, Barbier D, Steudel W-I. Insertion torque and pullout force of rescue screws for anterior cervical plate fixation in a fatigued initial pilot hole. *J Neurosurg Spine* 2004;1:198–201.
21 Wall SJ, Soin SP, Knight TA, Mears SC, Belkoff SM. Mechanical evaluation of a 4-mm cancellous "rescue" screw in osteoporotic cortical bone: a cadaveric study. *J Orthop Trauma* 2010;24:379–382.
22 Griffon DJ, Stoller A, Schaeffer DJ, Seddighi MR, Johnson AL, Kurath P. Evaluation of 2 cement techniques for augmentation of stripped 1.5 mm screw sites in the distal metaphysis of feline radii. *Vet Surg* 2005;34:223–230.
23 Sarzier JS, Evans AJ, Cahill DW. Increased pedicle screw pullout strength with vertebroplasty augmentation in osteoporotic spines. *J Neurosurg* 2002;96(3 Suppl):309–312.
24 Hearn T, Surowiak J, Schatzker J, Hearn T, Surowiak J, Schatzker J. Effects of tapping on the holding strength of cancellous bone screws. *Vet Comp Orthop Traumatol* 1992;5:14–16.
25 Chapman JR, Harrington RM, Lee KM, Anderson PA, Tencer AF, Kowalski D. Factors affecting the pullout strength of cancellous bone screws. *J Biomech Eng* 1996;118:391–398.
26 Baumgart FW, Cordey J, Morikawa K et al. AO/ASIF self-tapping screws (STS). *Injury* 1993;24(Suppl 1):S1–S17.
27 Andrea CR, Stover SM, Galuppo LD, Taylor KT, Rakestraw PC. Comparison of insertion time and pullout strength between self-tapping and non-self-tapping AO 4.5-mm cortical bone screws in adult equine third metacarpal bone. *Vet Surg* 2002;31:189–194.
28 Murphy TP, Hill CM, Kapatkin AS, Radin A, Shofer FS, Smith GK. Pullout properties of 3.5-mm AO/ASIF self-tapping and cortex screws in a uniform synthetic material and in canine bone. *Vet Surg* 2001;30:253–260.
29 Battula S, Schoenfeld A, Vrabec G, Njus GO. Experimental evaluation of the holding power/stiffness of the self-tapping bone screws in normal and osteoporotic bone material. *Clin Biomech* 2006;21:533–537.
30 Heidemann W, Terheyden H, Gerlach KL. Analysis of the osseous/metal interface of drill free screws and self-tapping screws. *J Maxillofac Surg* 2001;29:69–74.
31 Sowden D, Schmitz JP. AO self-drilling and self-tapping screws in rat calvarial bone: an ultrastructural study of the implant interface. *J Oral Maxillofac Surg* 2002;60:294–299.
32 Cronier P, Pietu G, Dujardin C, Bigorre N, Ducellier F, Gerard R. The concept of locking plates. *Orthop Traumatol Surg Res* 2010;96(4):S17–S36.
33 Miller DL, Goswami T. A review of locking compression plate biomechanics and their advantages as internal fixators in fracture healing. *Clin Biomech* 2007;22:1049–1062.
34 Matthews SJE, Nikolaou VS, Giannoudis PV. Innovations in osteosynthesis and fracture care. *Injury* 2008;39:827–838.
35 Perren SM. Evolution of the internal fixation of long bone fractures. The scientific basis of biological internal fixation: choosing a new balance between stability and biology. *J Bone Joint Surg Br* 2002;84:1093–1110.
36 Roush JK, Wilson JW. Effects of plate luting on cortical vascularity and development of cortical porosity in canine femurs. *Vet Surg* 1990;19:208–214.
37 Wilson JW. Blood supply to developing, mature, and healing bone. In: Sumner-Smith G (ed.) *Bone in Clinical Orthopedics*, 2nd edn. Stuttgart: Thieme, AO Publishing, 2002: 23–116.
38 Miranda MA. Locking plate technology and its role in osteoporotic fractures. *Injury* 2007;38(Suppl 3):S35–S39.
39 Zindrick MR, Wiltse LL, Widell EH et al. A biomechanical study of intrapeduncular screw fixation in the lumbosacral spine. *Clin Orthop Related Res* 1986;203:99–112.
40 Corlazzoli D. Bicortical implant insertion in caudal cervical spondylomyelopathy: a computed tomography simulation in affected Doberman Pinschers. *Vet Surg* 2008;37:178–185.
41 Hettlich BF, Allen MJ, Pascetta D, Fosgate GT, Litsky AS. Biomechanical comparison between bicortical pin and monocortical screw/polymethylmethacrylate constructs in the cadaveric canine cervical vertebral column. *Vet Surg* 2013;42:693–700.
42 Agnello KA, Kapatkin AS, Garcia TC, Hayashi K, Welihozkiy AT, Stover SM. Intervertebral biomechanics of locking compression plate monocortical fixation of the canine cervical spine. *Vet Surg* 2010;39:991–1000.
43 Bergman RL, Levine JM, Coates JR, Bahr A, Hettlich BF, Kerwin SC. Cervical spinal locking plate in combination with cortical ring allograft for a one level fusion in dogs with cervical spondylotic myelopathy. *Vet Surg* 2008;37:530–536.
44 Dickomeit M, Alves L, Pekarkova M, Gorgas D, Forterre F. Use of a 1.5 mm butterfly locking plate for stabilization of atlantoaxial pathology in three toy breed dogs. *Vet Comp Orthop Traumatol* 2011;24:246–251.
45 Steffen F, Voss K, Morgan JP. Distraction-fusion for caudal cervical spondylomyelopathy using an intervertebral cage and locking plates in 14 dogs. *Vet Surg* 2011;40:743–752.
46 Trotter EJ. Cervical spine locking plate fixation for treatment of cervical spondylotic myelopathy in large breed dogs. *Vet Surg* 2009;38:705–718.
47 Voss K, Steffen F, Montavon PM. Use of the ComPact UniLock System for ventral stabilization procedures of the cervical spine: a retrospective study. *Vet Comp Orthop Traumatol* 2006;19:21–28.
48 Boudreau B, Benamou J, von Pfeil DJF, Guillou RP, Beckett C, Déjardin LM. Effect of screw insertion torque on mechanical properties of four locking systems. *Vet Surg* 2013;42:535–543.
49 Rose SA, Bruecker KA, Petersen SW, Uddin N. Use of locking plate and screws for triple pelvic osteotomy. *Vet Surg* 2012;41:114–120.
50 Blake CA, Boudrieau RJ, Torrance BS et al. Single cycle to failure in bending of three standard and five locking plates and plate constructs. *Vet Comp Orthop Traumatol* 2011;24:408–417.
51 Cabassu JB, Kowaleski MP, Shorinko JK, Blake CA, Gaudette GR, Boudrieau RJ. Single cycle to failure in torsion of three standard and five locking plate constructs. *Vet Comp Orthop Traumatol* 2011;24:418–425.
52 DeTora M, Kraus K. Mechanical testing of 3.5 mm locking and non-locking bone plates. *Vet Comp Orthop Traumatol* 2008;21:318–322.
53 McKee WM, Downes CJ. Vertebral stabilisation and selective decompression for the management of triple thoracolumbar disc protrusions. *J Small Anim Pract* 2008;49:536–539.

3 Minimum Database for Intracranial Surgery

Theresa E. Pancotto

Introduction

The more common indications for intracranial surgery in the veterinary population include tumor resection or biopsy, biopsy of other brain disorders (inflammatory, metabolic, genetic), foramen magnum decompression for patients with caudal occipital malformation and syringohydromyelia, ventriculoperitoneal shunt placement for patients with hydrocephalus, decompression of traumatic brain injury, and drainage of intracranial abscesses. Patient characteristics such as age and concurrent disease as well as the nature of the inciting cause will influence the specific tests that are selected as part of the minimum database. The veterinary literature is insufficiently rigorous to allow for complete assessment of the utility of a general panel of preoperative laboratory testing. Therefore, recommendations for minimum database tests required prior to intracranial surgery are often based on the results of physical examination identifying comorbid conditions, anticipation and avoidance of specific surgical complications, and severity of existing neurological signs. Selective preoperative testing also helps reduce medical costs. In North American human hospitals, estimates show that $30–40 billion per year is spent on preoperative testing of which about half may be unnecessary [1]. The following is an overview of how concurrent diseases and surgical procedure will influence minimum database testing.

Preanesthetic

It is important not to overlook the value of the initial medical history and neurological and physical examinations in identifying concurrent disorders that may have an important bearing on selection of diagnostics and patient management.

Medical History

A conversation with clients about spectrum of clinical signs and duration may help identify extraneural systemic disorders and will guide formulation and ranking of differential diagnoses. A list of current medications and knowledge of their side effects will guide testing. For example, patients on phenobarbital for seizures associated with a cerebral mass should have accurate serum concentrations available as well as recent evaluation of liver function. In canines, heartworm status should be known for all patients undergoing anesthesia as heartworm disease can contribute to cardiovascular problems and complicate anesthesia. For felines, feline leukemia virus (FeLV)/feline immunodeficiency virus (FIV) status should be determined. Occasionally, environmental factors will impact selection of testing (e.g., the patient lives in a smoking household or tick exposure has been documented).

Neurological Assessment

A neuroanatomical diagnosis is established prior to surgery based on the findings of a complete neurological examination. A list of differentials is subsequently generated based on signalment, history, and clinical signs. In patients presented for intracranial emergencies, an abbreviated examination may be performed and imaging and surgery may follow promptly. The Small Animal Coma Scale (SACS)/Modified Glasgow Coma Scale (MGCS) provides the attending veterinarian with rapid assessment of neurological function and allows detection of signs associated with elevated intracranial pressure (ICP) [2,3]. The SACS includes evaluation of level of consciousness, motor function, and select brainstem reflexes. Patients with depressed sensorium are at increased risk of aspiration pneumonia [4]. Anisocoria, weakness, or absence of pupillary light and/or oculocephalic reflexes indicates intracranial

Current Techniques in Canine and Feline Neurosurgery, First Edition. Edited by Andy Shores and Brigitte A. Brisson.
© 2017 John Wiley & Sons, Inc. Published 2017 by John Wiley & Sons, Inc.
Companion website: www.wiley.com/go/shores/neurosurgery

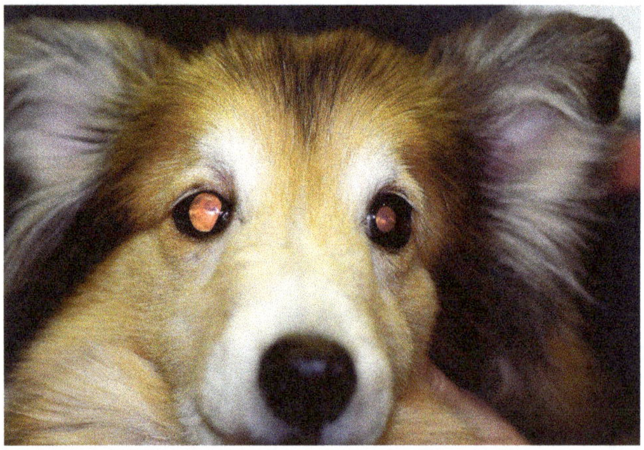

Figure 3.1 Sheltie with anisocoria and absent pupillary light reflexes as a result of transtentorial herniation.

hypertension; brain herniation and death may be imminent if appropriate therapy is not instituted (Figure 3.1).

Identification and treatment of increased ICP is extremely important prior to anesthesia to avoid neurological decompensation. Although not directly a part of the neurological evaluation, noninvasive blood pressure evaluation is indicated in patients who have suspected increased ICP to identify a Cushing's reflex. A Cushing's reflex occurs when the brain is receiving too little oxygen and glucose as a result of life-threatening increases in ICP and cerebral vascular compromise. In an effort to maintain cerebral blood flow, the sympathetic centers discharge to increase blood pressure and drive up cerebral perfusion pressure. This increase in blood pressure is usually obvious (>180 mmHg). The carotid and aortic body baroreceptors respond to this by triggering a reflex bradycardia [5].

If neuroimaging is done under a separate anesthetic episode to allow for surgical planning, a complete neurological examination should be performed and documented prior to induction of anesthesia for the intended neurosurgical procedure. Ideally the examination is done the morning of the procedure. This will allow for assessment of any changes that have occurred since imaging or previous evaluation, as well as provide a baseline for postoperative comparison.

Physical Examination and Extraneural Systems Functions

Respiratory System

Basic respiratory evaluation includes resting respiratory effort, rate and rhythm, auscultation of lung quadrants, evaluation of mucous membrane color, and palpation of the trachea. Patients with primary lesions in the medulla or craniocervical junction may develop respiratory ataxia, particularly after trauma or surgery. More severe injury to the brainstem respiratory centers could result in either respiratory arrest or the need for mechanical ventilation or death. Concurrent diseases of the lower cervical spine may interfere with phrenic nerve integrity and decrease chest expansion through paresis or paralysis of the diaphragm. Arterial blood gas evaluation will provide the best assessment of ventilation. If hypoventilation from neurological disease is diagnosed [$Pao_2 < 60$ mmHg, $Paco_2 > 60$ mmHg, normal alveolar–arterial (AA) gradient], mechanical ventilation is indicated. An AA gradient below 5 mmHg or greater than 10 mmHg is indicative of mismatch in ventilation and perfusion (V/Q mismatch) and further diagnostics including thoracic radiographs are warranted.

Lesions of the glossopharyngeal and vagus nuclei or nerves can depress the swallowing reflex (gag reflex) and result in movement of contents from the oral cavity into the lungs. This can lead to pneumonitis or pneumonia. Risks for aspiration pneumonia are compounded in patients with depressed levels of consciousness with intracranial disease [4]. Intracranial lesions may lead to abnormal sensorium through direct involvement of the ascending reticular activating system (ARAS) or indirect involvement of the ARAS associated with prosencephalic lesions, intracranial hypertension, and secondary brainstem compression. Careful attention should be paid to auscultation when evaluating the mentally altered patient.

Further respiratory evaluation is considered in patients with abnormal respiratory rates or effort, a cough of unknown etiology, or abnormal lung sounds on auscultation. Cyanotic mucous membranes may be indicative of poor gas exchange at the alveolar level and should be investigated prior to any anesthetic event. Cough during tracheal palpation is most commonly associated with tracheal collapse or tracheitis. Significant respiratory signs reported by the owner such as a honking cough that interferes with daily activities may prompt the need for cervicothoracic radiographs to evaluate the intrathoracic and extrathoracic trachea for collapse. Tracheal collapse may be made transiently worse by intubation and respiratory depression. If infectious tracheitis is suspected other diagnostics may be indicated. In people with pulmonary disease, both an abnormal chest radiograph and spirometry are risk factors for anesthetic complications. However, the strongest predictor of anesthetic outcome in humans with pulmonary disease is serum albumin concentration less than 3.5 g/dL [6].

Cardiovascular System

Cardiovascular disease can be a significant risk factor for anesthesia. In patients undergoing anesthesia for intracranial surgery, hemodynamic stability is critical. Additionally, intracranial disease may lead to arrhythmias via an ischemic phenomenon known as brain-heart or cerebro-cardiac syndrome; these arrhythmias may be fatal [5].

Initial cardiac evaluation includes assessment of cardiac rate and rhythm, pulse quality, and capillary refill time. Presence of a murmur not previously documented or one that has recently changed in quality or character should prompt cardiac consultation and echocardiography. ECG, electrolyte panel, and packed cell volume (PCV) should be performed in patients with arrhythmias. Cardiac evaluation including ECG and thoracic radiographs should be performed in all patients over 7 years of age and in recumbent patients, trauma victims, and patients with suspected neoplasms [7]. The presence of abnormalities on any of these tests may need additional evaluation of the patient by a cardiologist. In breeds at risk for developing life-threatening cardiac diseases, such as dilated cardiomyopathy in Doberman Pinschers and arrhythmogenic right ventricular cardiomyopathy in Boxers, Holter monitoring prior to surgical admission may identify abnormal rhythms and determine risk category [8,9]. Cavalier King Charles Spaniels are the most frequent patients undergoing surgery for Chiari-like malformation and also have a very high incidence of genetically influenced mitral valve disease. In patients with stable cardiac disease, current thoracic radiographs may be valuable in evaluating cardiac size and pulmonary changes but are not always indicated.

In people, specific indices have been developed that predict mortality rates of cardiac patients undergoing noncardiac procedures.

Among the risk factors associated with mortality are high-risk surgery, history of ischemic heart disease, history of congestive heart failure, history of cerebrovascular disease, preoperative treatment with insulin, and preoperative serum creatinine concentration greater than 2.0 mg/dL [1]. It is unknown if any of these risk factors apply to the veterinary population.

Gastrointestinal System

Although vomiting, regurgitation, diarrhea, and abdominal pain are all signs usually referable to gastrointestinal tract abnormalities, vomiting is occasionally a manifestation of intracranial disease. Patients with full stomachs or megaesophagus are at risk for aspiration pneumonia. Presence of megaesophagus should prompt concern for paraneoplastic syndromes [10] or endocrinopathies manifesting with motor unit signs, e.g., hypothyroidism [11–14]. All patients are fasted at least 12 hours prior to surgery and kept nil by mouth for 24 hours postoperatively to minimize risk of aspiration pneumonia. If mentation is not improved by 24 hours postoperatively, food should continue to be withheld and alternative nutrition considered.

Routine blood chemistry provides basic liver parameters. Hepatomegaly, jaundice, ascites and/or ecchymoses should cause alarm regarding adequate liver function. Decreased albumin and blood urea nitrogen (BUN) are biochemical changes often associated with liver failure. Liver function tests such as preprandial and postprandial bile acid concentration and prothrombin time (PT)/partial thromboplastin time (PTT) may be advisable in some patients. Abdominal ultrasound may distinguish between a focal liver abnormality and a diffuse one. Aspirates or biopsies are done accordingly and clotting times are typically recommended prior to performing a liver biopsy.

Oral cavity inspection may identify a source of bacteria that could contribute to postoperative infections. Effectively dealing with dental disease prior to intracranial surgery is often dangerous to the patient and impractical. Intraoperative antibiotics are warranted.

Renal System

Advanced imaging of the brain with MRI or CT often necessitates the use of intravenous contrast (gadolinium or iodine based respectively). Because these agents undergo renal excretion, renal parameters and hydration status should be assessed in all patients prior to contrast administration. At the very least, BUN reagent strip, PCV, and urine specific gravity should be performed. This rapid and abbreviated assessment is most useful in young healthy animals or emergent situations. A more complete evaluation would include a complete blood count (CBC), full chemistry, and urinalysis. Renal complications associated with contrast agents include contrast-induced nephropathy and worsening of existing renal disease. Hypovolemia may predispose to contrast-associated or postanesthetic renal complications and should be corrected prior to anesthesia.

Azotemia can be prerenal, renal, or postrenal and should be addressed prior to surgical consideration. Chronic renal failure is typically due to primary kidney disease and poses significant anesthetic challenges. Patients with chronic renal disease may develop electrolyte abnormalities, encephalopathy, metabolic acidosis, gastrointestinal bleeding, nonregenerative anemia, hypertension, and fluid imbalances. A complete chemistry panel, urinalysis, CBC, and blood pressure are indicated in patients with known or suspected renal disease. The ECG should be reviewed if electrolyte abnormalities are present that could cause arrhythmias (hyperkalemia, hypocalcemia).

Appropriate correction of fluid and electrolyte imbalances is necessary prior to anesthesia, and electrolytes and volume status should be monitored to avoid rapid fluid shifts and iatrogenic brain edema, hemorrhage, or encephalopathy. Acidosis from intraoperative hypercapnea along with existing metabolic acidosis from renal disease could lead to significant respiratory depression [1]. Blood pressure may be elevated in patients with renal disease and could impact short-term outcomes by influencing cerebral perfusion pressure and surgical bleeding [7]. Anemia, depending on severity, may require preoperative or postoperative transfusion. Mannitol is contraindicated in volume-depleted or anuric patients.

Urinary culture may be justified based on the presence of active sediment seen on preliminary urinalysis. Patients with a history of urinary tract infection should also have a presurgical urine culture. Early identification and treatment of urinary tract infection is important to prevent hematogenous seeding of the surgical site.

Hematological System

Intraoperative or postoperative intracranial hemorrhage has the potential to be catastrophic with devastating clinical effects. Depending on the procedure the risk for hemorrhage varies. Minimally, CBC including a platelet count, blood type (for dogs), and blood type and cross-match (for cats) are recommended prior to most intracranial surgeries. Dogs that have previously undergone blood transfusion will need to be cross-matched in addition to blood typing. The supervising surgeon should confirm that an appropriate blood product is available should the need arise.

Endocrine System

Medical history of patients with endocrinopathies may include unintentional weight gain or loss, abnormal hair growth/loss, polydipsia/polyuria, poor vision, and lethargy. On physical examination one may find the coat sparse with abnormal pigmentation, skin pigmentation, redistribution of fat to the face and abdomen, hepatomegaly, cataracts, and occasionally motor unit signs [11–14]. Abnormalities present on routine chemistry analysis can also provide evidence of concurrent endocrine diseases. Some endocrine diseases such as hyperadrenocorticism and diabetes mellitus can predispose to development of urinary tract infections, skin infections or cutaneous ulceration, and delayed wound healing. Hyperadrenocorticism can be confirmed with either an adrenocorticotropic hormone (ACTH) stimulation test and/or low-dose dexamethasone suppression test. Levels of serum thyroxine and thyroid-stimulating hormone (TSH), with or without free thyroxine, should be evaluated in patients demonstrating clinical signs and/or clinicopathological abnormalities consistent with hypothyroidism. Hypothyroidism can impair both central and peripheral nervous system function as well as contribute to myopathic changes [12], all of which may complicate patient management.

Integument

Skin infections should be identified and treated prior to surgery. Surgery should be postponed, if at all possible, if infection is present at the expected incision site. Hematogenous spread of dermal infections is one of the most common sources of bacteria contributing to catheter infections and surgical site infections, which may be devastating with intracranial procedures.

Intracranial Imaging

Based on advanced imaging a presumptive diagnosis is made and consideration for surgery begins. Characteristics of the skull shape and brain lesion will influence patient positioning, surgical approach, and need for additional medical intervention.

Specific Neurosurgery Considerations

General Considerations

Most commonly, CBC, serum chemistry, and urinalysis have been performed prior to surgery; in most cases this has been done in association with presurgical neuroimaging. However, additional testing is recommended in some situations based on examination findings (see above) or surgical approach. In situations where surgical bleeding is anticipated, preoperative PCV and total solids (TS) is helpful for postoperative comparisons because it requires less blood than that needed for a CBC. If there is a significant time lapse (1 week or more) between previous blood work and the date of the surgical procedure, abbreviated hematological and biochemical assessment should be done including PCV/TS, blood glucose, and rapid azotemia assessment. The most common protocols are summarized in Table 3.1.

Increases in ICP and surgical bleeding can be lethal complications of intracranial surgery. All blood from the cranial vault eventually leaves via the jugular veins. Venipuncture of the jugular veins and jugular catheters should be avoided when possible and blood is preferably collected from a peripheral vessel. Neck collars, wraps, and e-collars should be avoided as well. When elevating the head, an angle of 30° is appropriate and support should be ramp-like with padding extending from under the shoulder to the mid-mandible to avoid kinking of the cervical spine and vasculature. Elevated ICP should be addressed medically as soon as detected. During surgery maintenance of physiological mean arterial blood pressure is critical. Autoregulatory mechanisms to maintain cerebral blood flow at a rate of 50 mL per 100 g [1] are effective when systemic blood pressure is kept between 50 and 150 mmHg. Outside of this range or within injured areas, autoregulatory mechanisms fail. With hypotension there is risk for decreased perfusion and ischemic injury, and with hypertension ICP may rise and surgical bleeding may worsen.

Table 3.1 The most common protocols for neurosurgical assessment.

Diagnostic test	Tumor resection	FMD	VP shunt	Trauma
Abdominal ultrasound	√			+/–
Resting blood pressure	√		+/–	√
Blood type	√		+/–	+/–
CBC	√	+/–	+/–	√
Chemistry	√	+/–	+/–	√
Electrolytes	+/–	√	√	+/–
ECG	√			+/–
PCV	√			+/–
Thoracic radiographs	√			+/–
Urinalysis	√	+/–*	+/–*	√

*In otherwise healthy patients, PCV, TS, blood glucose, BUN, and urine specific gravity may suffice.
FMD, foramen magnum decompression; VP, ventriculoperitoneal.

Tumor Resection/Biopsy

Intracranial neoplasms, even when aggressive, rarely metastasize. However, 23% of patients diagnosed with primary brain neoplasms have primary neoplasms in other locations [15]. For this reason, imaging of the thoracic cavity and abdomen are recommended prior to surgery. Thoracic radiographs and abdominal ultrasound are most commonly performed. Bicavitary CT may be done at some institutions and is likely more sensitive, particularly in the detection of pulmonary nodules (Figure 3.2) [16].

Any nodules, masses, or otherwise abnormal-appearing organs should be aspirated at the clinician's discretion to rule out significant pathology. The presence of extracranial malignancies may preclude intracranial surgery for some patients or clients and certainly can worsen the overall long-term prognosis. It may be difficult to obtain a definitive diagnosis by fine-needle aspirate. Splenic and hepatic nodules are not uncommon in older dogs and adrenal masses may be incidental in up to 57% of dogs (Figure 3.3) [17]. In these situations, the risks and benefits of surgical or percutaneous

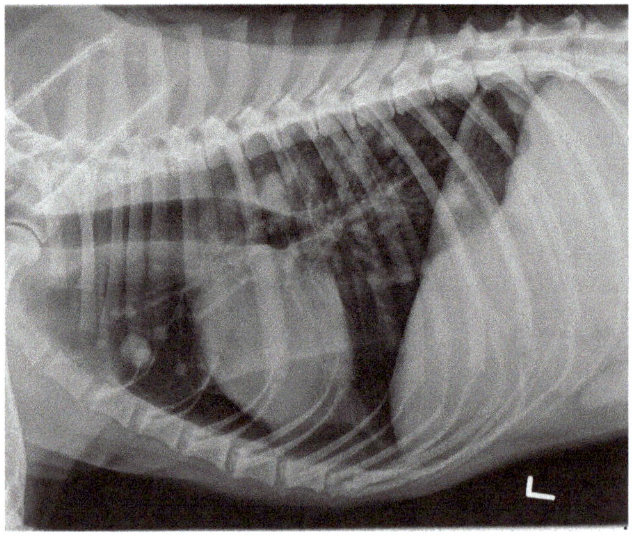

Figure 3.2 Left lateral radiograph demonstrating diffuse pulmonary nodules consistent with metastatic disease.

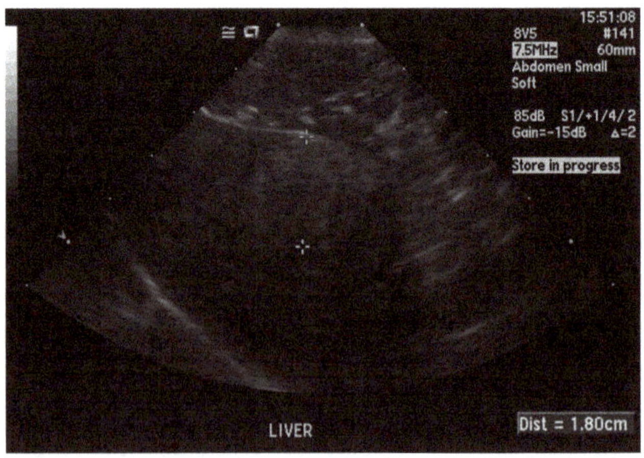

Figure 3.3 Still image from an abdominal ultrasound of a patient with a glioblastoma. Aspirates of the nodule were nondiagnostic and surgical treatment was performed.

biopsy before neurosurgical intervention must be weighed and discussed with the client (Figure 3.4).

Preprandial and postprandial bile acid concentrations are indicated when liver abnormalities are identified ultrasonographically or when liver function is questionable based on abnormalities in the chemistry profile. If liver function is abnormal, a clotting profile is warranted and surgery may be postponed. A coagulation profile is indicated in patients with known or suspected clotting disorder. Dobermans that have not been evaluated for von Willebrand's disease should be tested and a buccal mucosal bleeding time should always be performed prior to surgery (Figures 3.5 and 3.6). If coagulation abnormalities are identified, appropriate blood products should be available for transfusion if needed.

Bleeding is a significant concern associated with removal of tumors located near the venous sinuses (e.g., meningiomas). All these patients should be blood typed and/or cross-matched prior to surgery.

In addition to documenting primary or metastatic pulmonary diseases, thoracic radiographs are useful as a baseline for detection and monitoring of aspiration pneumonia (Figure 3.7). Craniotomy/craniectomy patients are at high risk of aspiration pneumonia in the perioperative period. Thoracic radiographs also allow estimation of heart size and shape and pulmonary changes associated with cardiac disease. Since cardiovascular disease may increase anesthetic morbidity, this additional information is helpful in patients with cardiac abnormalities undergoing intracranial surgery (Figures 3.8 and 3.9).

Recent serum concentrations should be available for any patient with a seizure disorder, as dose adjustments are required. The anticonvulsant medications phenobarbital and levetiracetam may have

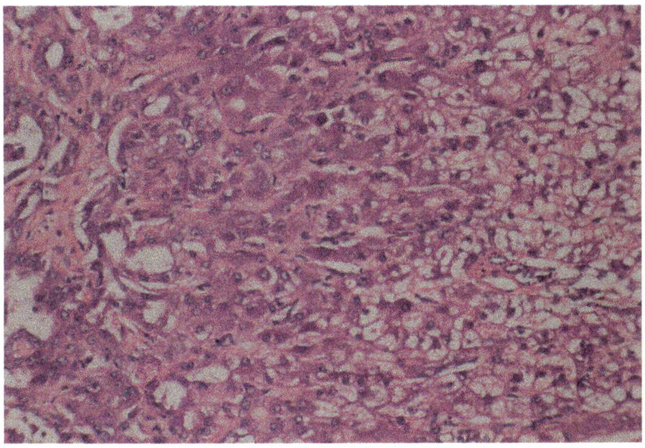

Figure 3.4 Four months later when the patient in Figure 3.3 was euthanized from complications associated with radiation therapy, histopathology revealed hepatocellular adenocarcinoma.

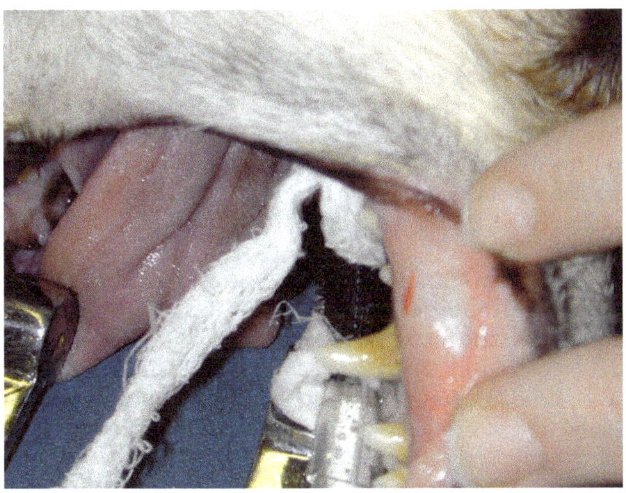

Figure 3.5 Two small incisions (5 × 1 mm) created by a spring-loaded lancet placed on the mucosa of the upper lip.

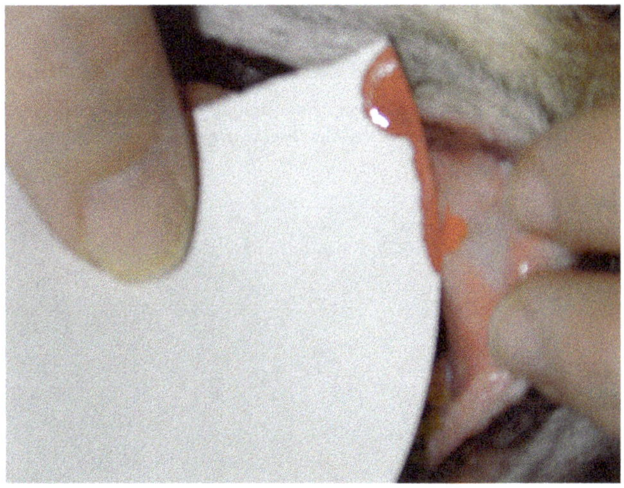

Figure 3.6 Blood is blotted with filter paper without touching the incisions until a clot is formed. Normal time for platelet plug formation and cessation of bleeding should be less than 4 min.

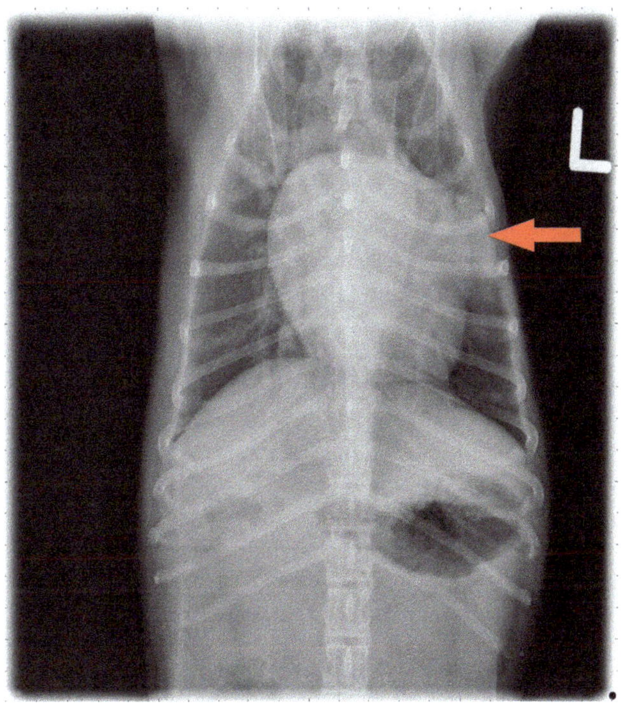

Figure 3.7 This ventrodorsal radiograph shows a diffuse interstitial pattern with consolidation of the left middle lung lobe most consistent with aspiration pneumonia.

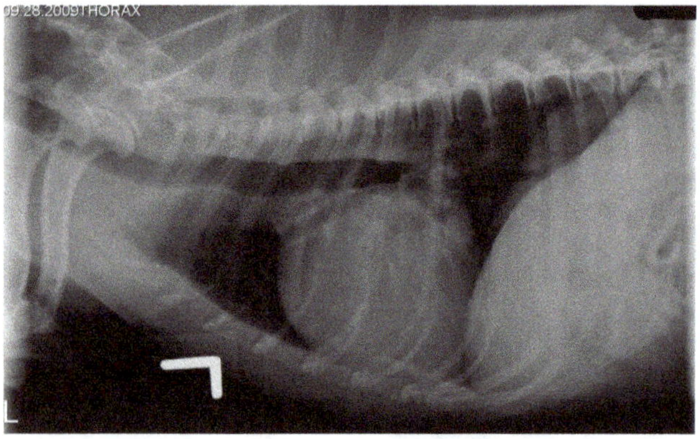

Figure 3.8 Left lateral projection demonstrating left-sided heart enlargement associated with chronic valvular disease in a geriatric Chihuahua.

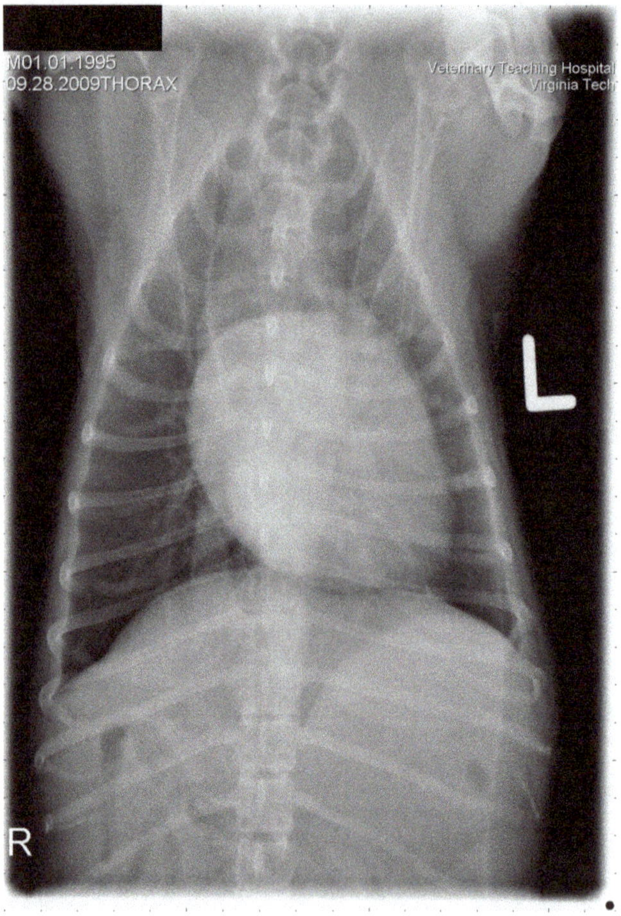

Figure 3.9 Ventrodorsal view of the patient shown in Figure 3.8.

neuroprotective properties [18] and some individuals advocate their use in the perioperative period for patients undergoing surgery for prosencephalic lesions even in absence of clinical seizure activity.

Foramen Magnum Decompression

Many of the patients presenting for consideration of foramen magnum decompression (FMD) have been medically managed for a period of time with corticosteroids, furosemide, and/or proton pump inhibitors after initial imaging diagnosis. The latter has few systemic side effects but furosemide can contribute to electrolyte abnormalities, and long-term prednisone therapy may cause iatrogenic Cushing's disease. Routine blood chemistry is evaluated prior to surgery and should include an electrolyte panel. Electrolyte abnormalities should be corrected prior to anesthesia and surgical decompression.

Many candidates for FMD are healthy juveniles or young adults, most commonly of the Cavalier King Charles Spaniel (CKCS) and Brussels Griffon breeds [19]. The CKCS breed also has a high incidence of mitral valve disease and prolapse, although Rusbridge and Knowler [20] found that dogs with earlier onset of clinical signs associated with caudal occipital malformation and syringohydromyelia often have a later onset of cardiac disease and vice versa. This was theorized to be a result of modifications of breeding protocols when mitral valve disease was being documented in the young CKCS population. For this reason, it may be prudent to evaluate cardiac function more extensively prior to surgery in CKCS. That being said, the operative complication rate associated with FMD is extremely low and most often related to transient worsening of existing clinical neurological signs after recovery [21–23].

Ventriculoperitoneal Shunt Placement

Ventriculoperitoneal shunt placement for the treatment of hydrocephalus is pursued in patients with progressive signs of obstructive ventricular disease and resultant cerebrospinal fluid (CSF) accumulation. Hydrocephalus may be congenital or acquired and causes clinical signs related to forebrain dysfunction. The most common congenital cause of obstructive hydrocephalus is atresia of the mesencephalic aqueduct associated with fusion of the rostral colliculi [24].

Elevated ICP is a concern in these patients and clinical parameters that reflect intracranial hypertension should be evaluated as previously stated. For patients with malignant causes of obstructive hydrocephalus (neoplasia, inflammatory disease), minimum database testing is dictated based on clinical examination as described above. Ruling out metastatic disease, extraneural primary tumors, and infectious diseases is warranted. Some clients will choose to pursue shunt placement for relief of clinical signs, irrespective of findings with malignant characteristics. Skin, abdominal, or systemic infections are contraindications for shunt placement and should be identified and resolved prior to surgery [24].

Over-shunting is uncommon but can lead to cortical collapse and tearing of the meninges. Rupture of meningeal vessels can result in significant bleeding. Current PCV and blood typing prior to surgery may be indicated.

Like patients undergoing FMD, patients with hydrocephalus may have been medically managed prior to surgery. At a minimum, electrolytes should be evaluated preoperatively. It is not uncommon for patients with hydrocephalus to have seizures and recent serum concentrations of antiepileptic drugs should be available.

Posttraumatic Decompression and Intracranial Abscess Drainage

In emergent situations rapid hematological assessment (PCV, TS, blood glucose, BUN) may be necessary but complete blood work should be performed when possible, even if after surgery. Blood pressure monitoring should be undertaken in these patients to assess hemodynamic stability. If excessive bleeding occurred at the time of injury, blood transfusion prior to surgery and further hematological evaluation may be indicated. Colloids and hypertonic saline are advantageous in acute resuscitation of

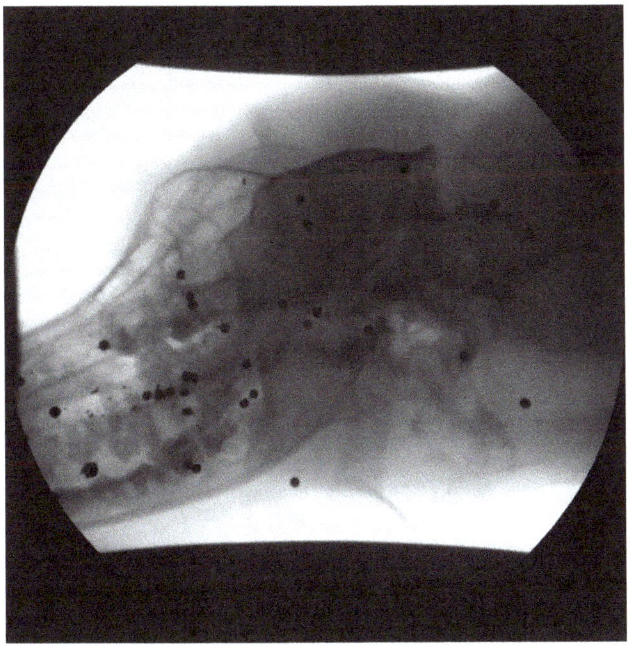

Figure 3.10 Lateral static fluoroscopic image of a dog shot in the craniocervical area with a BB gun.

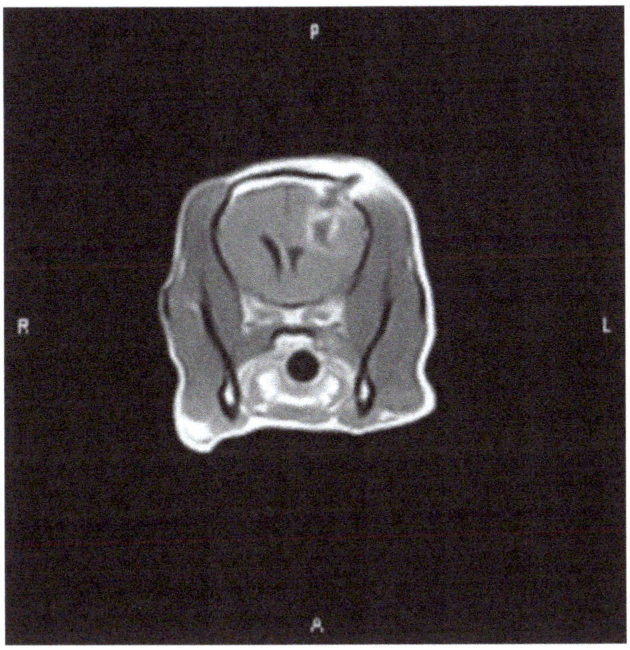

Figure 3.11 Post-contrast T1-weighted MRI of a patient who was bitten on the head 4 days earlier demonstrating intraaxial abscess with ring enhancement. The skull defect is visible.

these patients to avoid increases in ICP associated with excessive crystalloid administration.

It is vitally important to identify concurrent life-threatening injuries such as cervical trauma, airway compromise, other orthopedic injuries, gastrointestinal issues, or diaphragmatic hernias (Figure 3.10). A full-body CT scan may be the fastest way to make a complete assessment. However, it is prudent and more cost-effective to use the neurological and physical examinations to guide selection of appropriate body cavities for imaging.

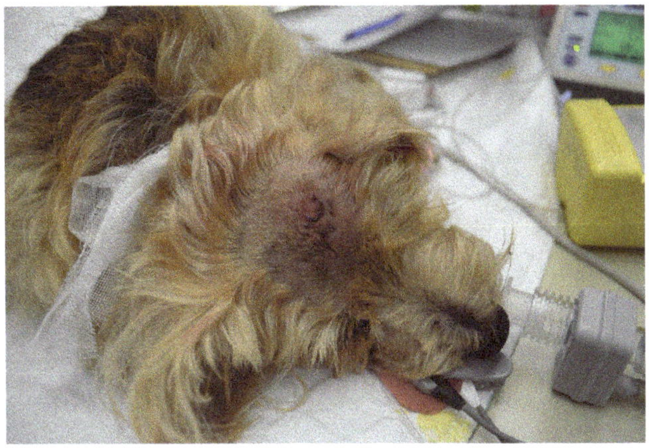

Figure 3.12 This is the penetrating bite wound shown in Figure 3.11. The wound was cleaned by the initial treating veterinarian on the day of the injury but no radiographs were taken. Intracranial abscess formation leading to marked neurological deterioration occurred 72 hours later and the patient was referred.

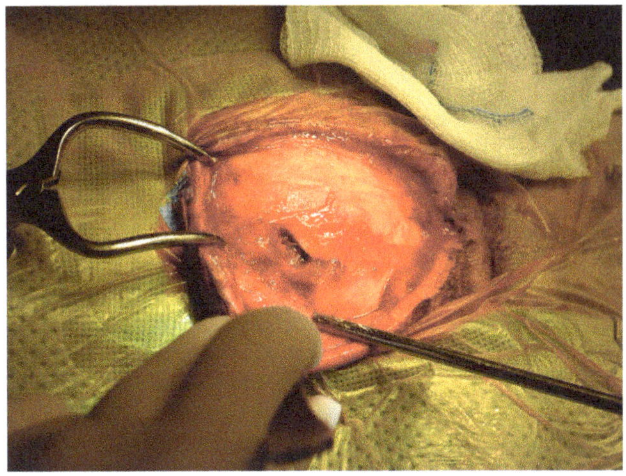

Figure 3.13 This is the wound from the same patient presented in Figures 3.11 and 3.12. The skull defect is visible in the center of the surgical field. Hair and fibrous tissue can be seen overlying the defect.

For the general practitioner, skull radiographs may be of great value in determining the presence of foreign material or depressed skull fragments. Although these may be difficult to obtain or interpret, detection of these abnormalities on survey radiographs should encourage prompt referral after patient stabilization. Immediate surgical resolution of these wounds will prevent adhesions and abscess formation. Surgical drainage is recommended for intracranial abscesses (Figures 3.11, 3.12 and 3.13). Cultures of the wound are best collected at the time of surgery and multiple samples (including deep tissue samples rather than superficial wound swabs) should be obtained. Perioperative antibiotics should be avoided until samples have been collected. Betadyne preps are preferred as chlorhexidine carries a precaution of CNS toxicity.

Indications for intracranial surgery after traumatic head injury include removal of penetrating foreign body, decompression of depressed skull fracture fragments, or removal of a compressive hematoma. The nature of the initial injury and the clinical and neurological status of the patient may dictate the imaging modality selected (CT vs. MRI). Extraneural imaging is indicated in victims of polytrauma to identify concurrent pulmonary, bladder, and spinal injury.

Video clips to accompany this book can be found on the companion website at:
www.wiley.com/go/shores/neurosurgery

References

1 Deepak S, Lam AM. Neuroanesthesia: preoperative evaluation. In: Winn HR (ed.) *Youmans Neurological Surgery*, 6th edn. Philadelphia, PA: Saunders Elsevier, 2011: 395–407.

2 Shores A. Craniocerebral trauma. In: Kirk RW (ed.) *Current Veterinary Therapy X*. Philadelphia, PA: WB Saunders, 1983: 847–854.

3 Platt SR, Radaelli ST, McDonnell JT. The prognostic value of the modified Glasgow coma scale in head trauma in dogs. *J Vet Intern Med* 2001;15:581–584.

4 Fransson BA, Bagley RS, Gay JM, Gavin PR. Pneumonia after intracranial surgery in dogs. *Vet Surg* 2001;30:432–439.

5 Bagley RS. Intracranial disease: pathophysiologic sequelae of intracranial disease. *Vet Clin North Am Small Anim Pract* 1996;26:711–734.

6 Smetana GW, Lawrence VA, Cornell JE. Preoperative pulmonary risk stratification for noncardiothoracic surgery: systematic review for the American College of Physicians. *Ann Intern Med* 2006;144:581–595.

7 Sharp NJH, Wheeler SJ. *Small Animal Spinal Disorders: Diagnosis and Surgery*, 2nd edn. Edinburgh: Elsevier Mosby, 2005.

8 Calvert CA, Jacobs GJ, Smith DD, Pickus CW. Association between results of ambulatory electrocardiography and development of cardiomyopathy during long-term follow-up of Doberman pinschers. *J Am Vet Med Assoc* 2000;216:34–39.

9 Hariu CD, Carpenter DH Jr. Arrhythmogenic right ventricular cardiomyopathy in boxers. *Compend Contin Educ Vet* 2010;32(12):E1–E7.

10 Day MJ. Review of thymic pathology in 30 cats and 36 dogs. *J Small Anim Pract* 1997;38:111–117.

11 Fracassi F, Tamborini A. Reversible megaoesophagus associated with primary hypothyroidism in a dog. *Vet Rec* 2011;168(12):329b

12 Panciera DL. Conditions associated with canine hypothyroidism. *Vet Clin North Am Small Anim Pract* 2001;31:935–950.

13 Burgener IA, Gerold A, Tomek A, Konar M. Empty sella syndrome, hyperadrenocorticism and megaoesophagus in a dachshund. *J Small Anim Pract* 2007;48:584–587.

14 Whitley NT. Megaoesophagus and glucocorticoid-deficient hypoadrenocorticism in a dog. *J Small Anim Pract* 1995;36:132–135.

15 Snyder JM, Shofer FS, Van Winkle TJ, Massicotte C. Canine intracranial primary neoplasia: 173 cases (1986–2003). *J Vet Intern Med* 2006;20: 669–675.

16 Nemanic S, London CA, Wisner ER. Comparison of thoracic radiographs and single breath-hold helical CT for detection of pulmonary nodules in dogs with metastatic neoplasia. *J Vet Intern Med* 2006;20:508–515.

17 Barthez PY, Marks SL, Woo J, Feldman EC, Matteucci M. Pheochromocytoma in dogs: 61 cases (1984–1995). *J Vet Intern Med* 1997;11:272–278.

18 Willmore LJ. Antiepileptic drugs and neuroprotection: current status and future roles. *Epilepsy Behav* 2005;7(Suppl 3):S25–S28.

19 Rusbridge C. Syringomyelia and Chiari-like malformation. In: Tilley LP, Smith FWK (eds) *Blackwell's Five Minute Veterinary Consult: Canine and Feline*, 4th edn. Ames, IA: Blackwell Publishing, 2007: 1321.

20 Rusbridge C, Knowler SP. Inheritance of occipital bone hypoplasia (Chiari type I malformation) in Cavalier King Charles spaniels. *J Vet Intern Med* 2004; 18:673–678.

21 Dewey CW, Berg JM, Barone G, Marino DJ, Stefanacci JD. Foramen magnum decompression for treatment of caudal occipital malformation syndrome in dogs. *J Am Vet Med Assoc* 2005;227:1270–1275.

22 Dewey CW, Marino DJ, Bailey KS et al. Foramen magnum decompression with cranioplasty for treatment of caudal occipital malformation syndrome in dogs. *Vet Surg* 2007;36:406–415.

23 Takagi S, Kadosawa T, Ohsaki T, Hoshino Y, Okumura M, Fujinaga T. Hindbrain decompression in a dog with scoliosis associated with syringomyelia. *J Am Vet Med Assoc* 2005;226:1359–1363.

24 Thomas WB. Diseases of the brain: hydrocephalus in dogs and cats. *Vet Clin North Am Small Anim Pract* 2010;40:143–159.

4 Advanced Imaging: Intracranial Surgery

Simon Platt and J. Fraser McConnell

Introduction

Diagnostic imaging is important in the characterization and identification of gross structural abnormalities affecting the nervous system. All imaging studies in the neurological patient should be preceded by clinical assessment aiming at ruling out nonneurological causes of signs or systemic disease, determining the lesion localization within the nervous system, and identifying possible concurrent injuries. As with anatomical imaging elsewhere in the body, functional disorders and diseases that do not result in a gross structural change in an organ may not be visible on images. Such imaging is only useful if interpreted along with the patient's signalment and history and with the information provided by a comprehensive neurological examination.

The choice of imaging modality depends upon multiple factors, not least expense. Advanced neuroimaging is expensive and interpretation is dependent on correlation of the neurological examination with the imaging findings. Magnetic resonance imaging (MRI) or computed tomography (CT) should not be used as substitutes for a thorough neurological evaluation. MRI requires general anesthesia and imaging may need to be delayed until the animal is stable. If the neurological examination indicates a central lesion, advanced imaging will be required to confirm or exclude a gross structural lesion. Other than in cases of known or suspect trauma, MRI is the preferred imaging modality because it provides excellent soft tissue contrast. In the majority of cases of intracranial disease, radiography is of limited or no value.

When considering using imaging during an intracranial surgical procedure, the aims of imaging and the type of surgery will help determine the technique that should be chosen. However, the availability of intraoperative imaging at an individual center will limit the choices that can be made as will the user's experience in interpretation, which can be quite different from more standard intracranial imaging. This chapter addresses the use of radiography, ultrasound, CT, and MRI for intracranial imaging both prior to and during surgery. Additionally, from the perspective of what is currently done in human medicine, we discuss what may be possible in veterinary patients in the future.

Overview of Intracranial Imaging Techniques

Survey Radiography

Survey radiography of the cranium provides information largely limited to the osseous component of the skull. Nonetheless plain radiographs are quick to obtain and relatively inexpensive but often in neurological emergencies have a low diagnostic yield. The correlation between radiological abnormalities and neurological status is poor and fractures are often missed [1].

Radiography has a very low diagnostic yield for the diagnosis of intracranial pathology (Figure 4.1) and survey radiographs are not usually indicated unless there is external swelling or known history of severe head trauma. Even with skull fractures, radiography will not provide information on severity of brain injury and many skull fractures may be missed. Depressed fractures or swellings will only be visible if the X-ray beam is tangential to the lesion. A specific lesion-orientated oblique view may be required. This is obtained by angling the X-ray beam so it skylines the swelling or depression.

Skull radiographs can be used in the investigation of peripheral vestibular syndromes and facial nerve paresis due to otitis media-interna (albeit with relatively low accuracy) but have limited value in the investigation of most cranial nerve or peripheral nerve lesions. Survey radiography to assess the bullae in cases of peripheral vestibular disease involves a rostro-caudal open mouth oblique or lateral oblique views and a dorsoventral view. The sensitivity of radiography for the diagnosis of otitis media compared with CT was only 0.85 in one study, with a specificity of 0.68 [2]. Bullae radiographs are more difficult to interpret in large dogs because of the large amounts of overlying soft tissue and radiographs provide no information about the intracranial extension of otitis media (Figure 4.2). Soft tissue/fluid opacity within the bullae may also be nonsignificant as primary secretory otitis media is a common, apparently incidental finding in brachycephalic dogs.

Current Techniques in Canine and Feline Neurosurgery, First Edition. Edited by Andy Shores and Brigitte A. Brisson.
© 2017 John Wiley & Sons, Inc. Published 2017 by John Wiley & Sons, Inc.
Companion website: www.wiley.com/go/shores/neurosurgery

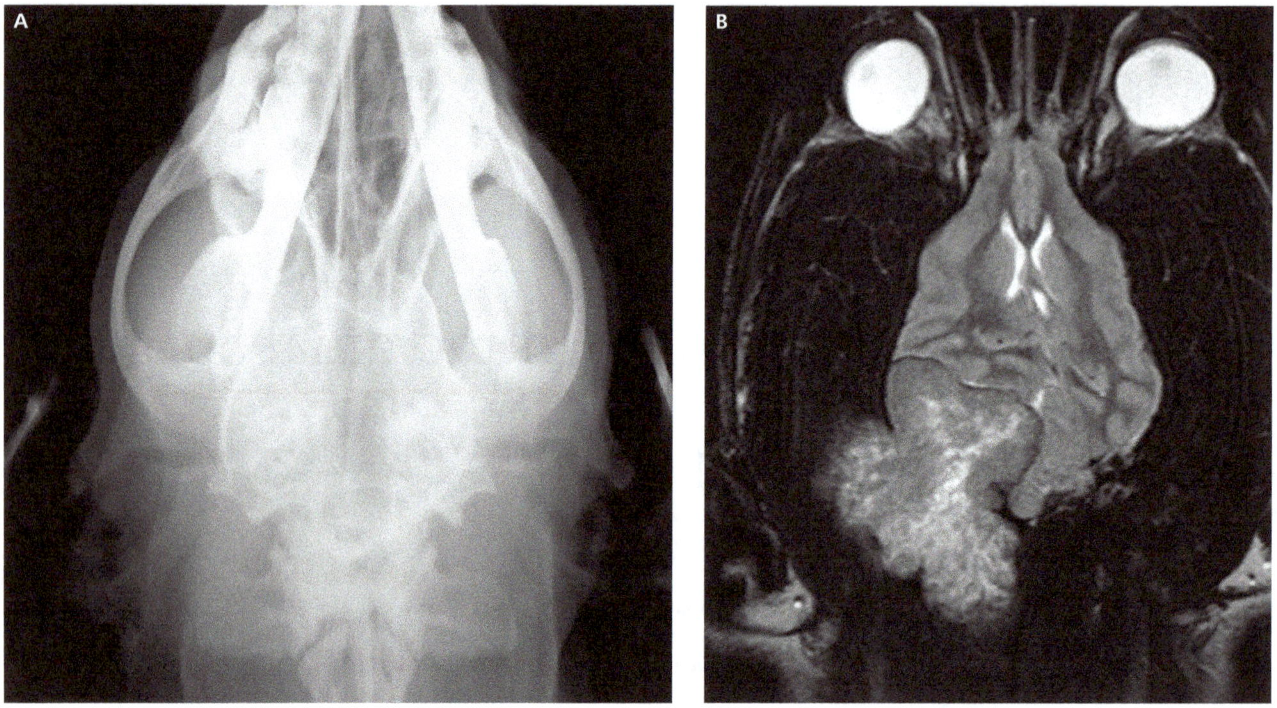

Figure 4.1 (A) Dorsoventral radiograph of a dog which had a palpable cranial swelling due to a primary bone tumor arising from the right occipital bone. Despite the large size of the mass, the focal area of bone lysis is difficult to recognize due to superimposition and inherent low contrast of radiographs. (B) Dorsal plane T2-weighted MRI of the same dog. Due to the better soft tissue contrast of MRI and lack of superimposition, the mass is easily recognized and the degree of intracranial extension and compression of the brain can be accurately determined.

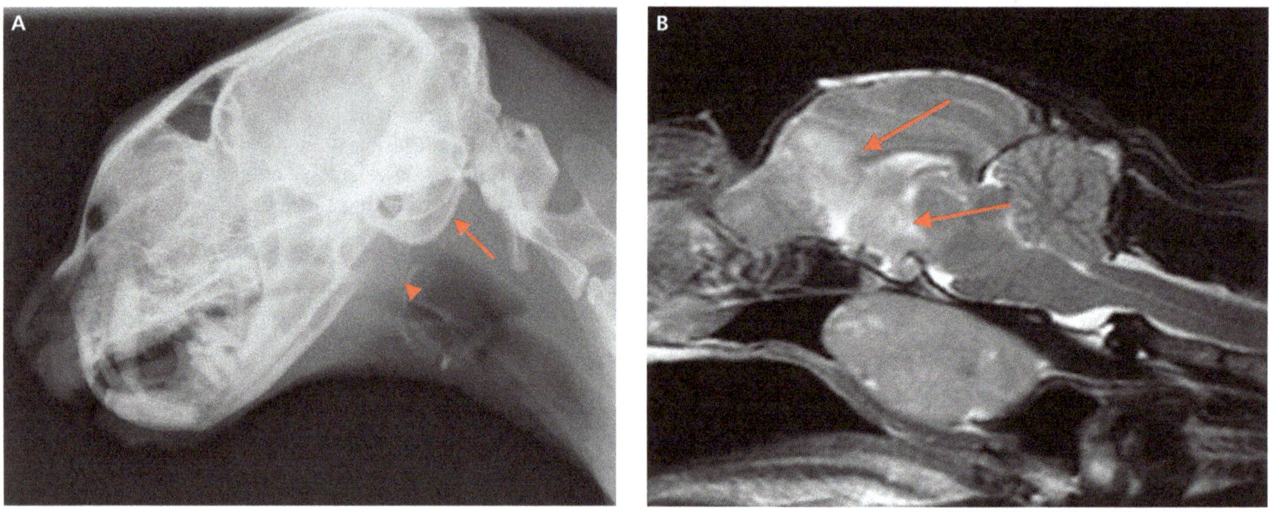

Figure 4.2 (A) Lateral radiograph of a cat's skull that shows thickening of the tympanic bulla wall (arrow) and increased opacity of the lumen suggestive of otitis media. Additionally, a soft tissue mass is visible within the nasopharynx (arrowhead). The combination of middle ear disease and nasopharyngeal mass is commonly seen with nasopharyngeal polyps. In this case the radiograph does not show the full extent of the pathology present and does not demonstrate intracranial extension seen on MRI. (B) Sagittal T2-weighted MRI of the same cat. The image shows the full extent of the nasopharyngeal mass but additionally shows intracranial extension of pathology (arrows). Biopsy of the mass confirmed lymphoma.

Ultrasound

Ultrasound is a noninvasive and accessible modality, but is of limited use in the presurgical evaluation of the nervous system because of sound attenuation by surrounding bone. However, there are specific indications for sonographic evaluation of the nervous system [3,4]. These include (i) assessment of the brain to identify hydrocephalus (Figure 4.3) and other congenital anomalies [5–8]; (ii) examination of soft tissue masses, for example within the brachial plexus, to aid in biopsy (Figure 4.4) [9]; and (iii) intraoperative assessment of the brain to identify and aid in the biopsy of intraparenchymal lesions [10], as well as for stereotaxis [11]. A skilled ultrasonographer is needed to address these indications adequately.

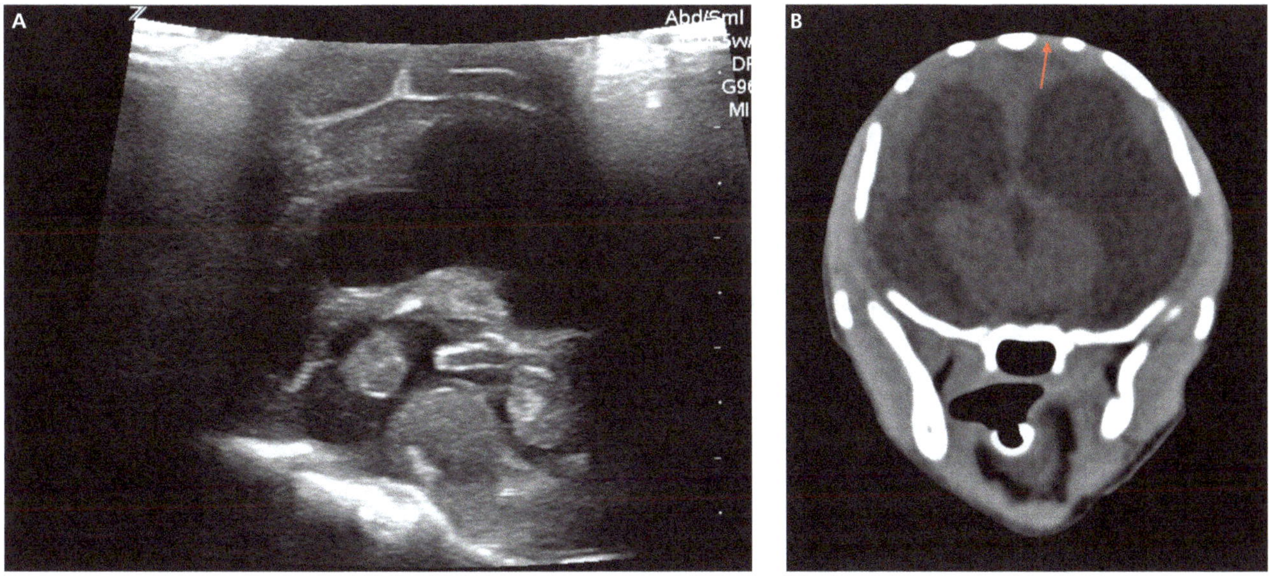

Figure 4.3 (A) Sagittal plane ultrasound of the brain of a 5-month-old Chihuahua presented with episodic depression and progressive ataxia. Transcranial ultrasound is easily performed in young or small animals if the fontanelle is open, as in this case. Due to high contrast between soft tissue and fluid it is easy to assess the ventricular system within the brain provided a suitable acoustic window is available. The ultrasound study in this case allowed clear visualization of the entire ventricular system and confirmed the presence of hydrocephalus. (B) Transverse plane CT of the same dog showing moderately severe hydrocephalus and open fontanelles (arrow). In this case the hydrocephalus was possibly an incidental finding as the dog also had atlanto-axial subluxation.

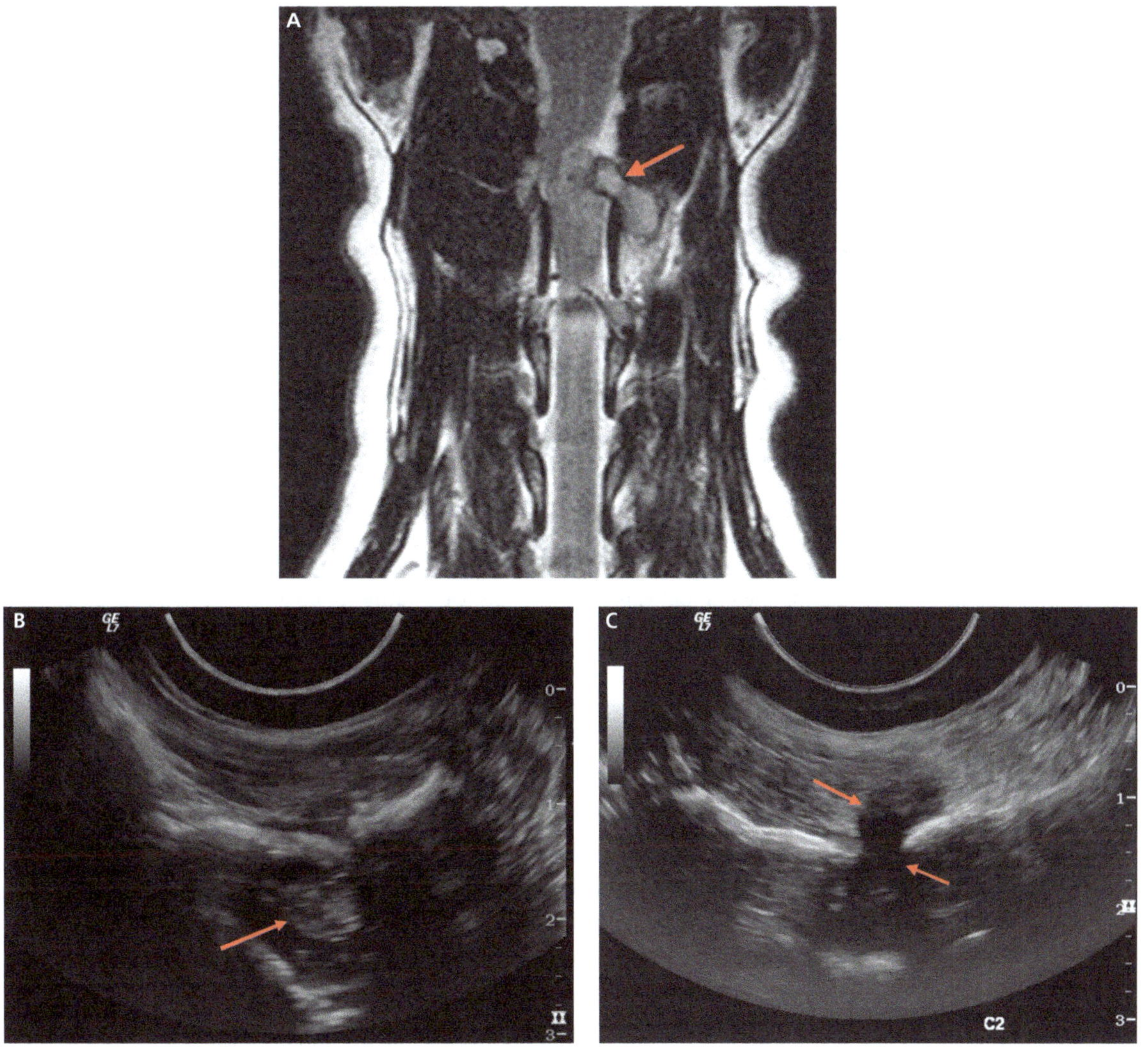

Figure 4.4 (A) Dorsal plane T2-weighted MRI of a 10-year-old Fox Terrier presented with progressive hemiparesis. The image shows a large intradural–extramedullary mass (arrow) at C1–2 and presumed to represent a malignant peripheral nerve tumour. (B, C) Ultrasound images of the left side of C1 and C2 clearly show the mass as an irregular hypoechoic mass (arrows) extending through the intervertebral foramen and into the vertebral canal. It was possible to perform ultrasound-guided fine-needle aspiration of the mass.

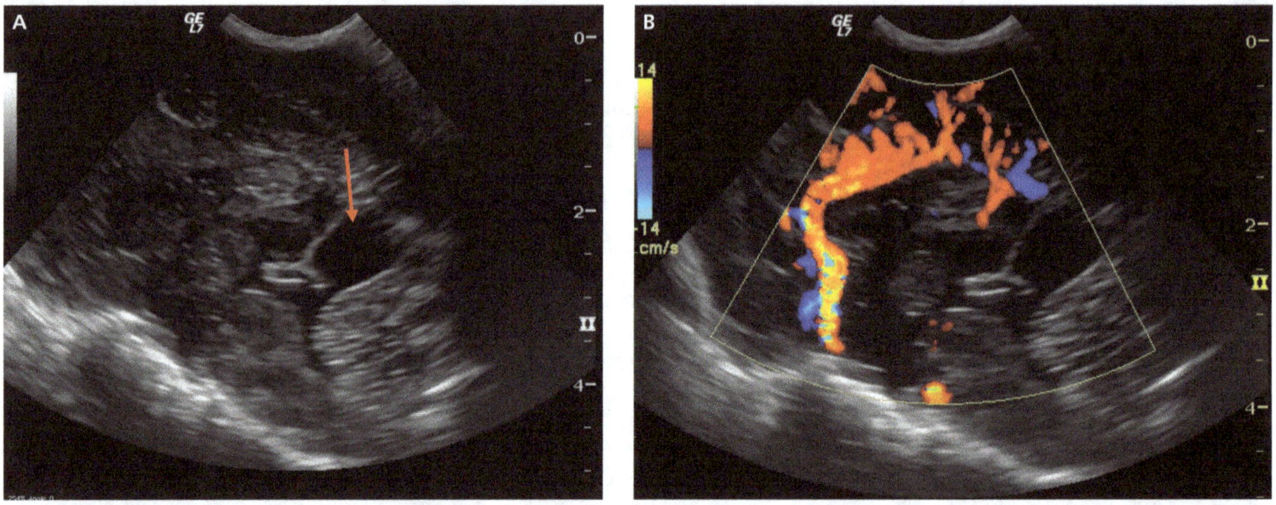

Figure 4.5 Sagittal B-mode (A) and color flow Doppler (B) ultrasound images of the brain of a 5-month-old Shih Tzu presented with seizures and poor growth (due to congenital dwarfism). Because of an open fontanelle, ultrasonography allowed assessment of the brain and in this case shows the presence of a small quadrigeminal cistern cyst (arrow). Color flow Doppler shows the direction and some assessment of blood flow velocity. The color flow Doppler study shows blood flow within the rostral cerebral and callosal arteries. To obtain resistive index measurements, pulsed wave Doppler is used to allow measurement of diastolic and systolic velocities within a blood vessel.

Recently, work has been published on coregistering ultrasound with MRI to aid tissue identification and this may have a future in veterinary neurosurgery [12].

Ultrasonography can be useful in animals with thin calvaria or open fontanelles that allow an acoustic window. The ultrasonographic anatomy of the brain has been described, and its utility for identifying hydrocephalus and other congenital malformations, such as arachnoid cysts, Dandy–Walker syndrome, and cerebellar herniation associated with Chiari-like malformation, has been reported [5,13–15].

Doppler ultrasonography is also useful for evaluating blood flow in the CNS [16–18]. Transcranial Doppler ultrasound can be used to evaluate the blood flow in the basilar artery via the foramen magnum in most patients, and the cerebral arteries can be evaluated in animals with a persistent fontanelle (Figure 4.5). The resistance index, a measure of resistance to blood flow, can be calculated for the basilar artery and has been shown to be related to intracranial pressure (ICP) and neurological status in dogs [19,20]. The current literature describes Doppler sonographic findings in inflammatory disease, abscessation, ischemia, hemorrhage, and neoplasia of the brain in dogs [21–26].

Ultrasonography was adapted for imaging the brain in experimental dogs in one study [27]. A transducer originally designed for transesophageal echocardiography was adapted for real-time volumetric endoscopic imaging of the brain. The purpose of the study was to evaluate the clinical feasibility of real-time three-dimensional intracranial ultrasound. A transcalvarial acoustic window was created under general anesthesia by placing a 10-mm burr hole in the parietal calvaria of a 50-kg dog. The burr-hole was placed in a left parasagittal location to avoid the sagittal sinus, and the transducer was placed against the intact dura mater for ultrasound imaging. Images of the lateral ventricles were produced, including real-time three-dimensional guidance of a needle puncture of one ventricle. In a second canine subject, contrast-enhanced three-dimensional Doppler color flow images were made of the cerebral vessels, including the complete circle of Willis. Clinical applications may include real-time three-dimensional guidance of cerebrospinal fluid (CSF) extraction from the lateral ventricles and bedside evaluation of critically ill patients where CT and MRI techniques are unavailable.

Computed Tomography

CT can be performed in various planes depending on patient position and the CT gantry angle within its limited arc. Historically, direct coronal-plane CT imaging of the paranasal sinuses or brain was performed with the patient in a supine "hanging-head" position with the head of the patient literally hanging over the edge of the CT scanner table or with the patient in the prone position and the neck hyperextended. CT imaging of the brain and spine is now usually performed in the axial plane with the patient in a prone or supine position on the scanner table and the head and neck in a neutral position. The need for a direct coronal patient position has been made redundant since the advent of high-resolution multiplanar reconstruction capabilities on newer multislice CT scanners. These reconstruction capabilities can generate axial images in 0.5–0.6 mm increments, which can then be reformatted into the sagittal, coronal, and oblique planes with image quality nearly identical to that obtained from direct scanning [28].

A typical routine brain CT scan consists of 3–4 mm axial images through the entire brain from the skull base to the vertex without the intravenous injection of iodinated contrast material. With multislice CT scanners the brain is usually imaged in helical mode with at least 50% slice overlap. This is usually followed by another set of axial images through the brain after the intravenous administration of a contrast agent, typically iodinated contrast material (600 mg iodine/kg) injected through an 18- or 20-gauge intravenous catheter. Scanning intervals can be and are adjusted for clinical need and indications such as patient age and size, need for higher-resolution images of specific anatomy such as the orbits, temporal bone, and skull base, or for CT angiography. With the multidetector CT scanners, images can be reconstructed into submillimeter axial images that can be used to generate two-dimensional and three-dimensional reformatted sagittal and coronal images and thus better delineate parenchymal, vascular, and osseous anatomy.

In humans, CT is usually the first study of choice for evaluation of a patient with suspected acute intracranial pathology because of its availability, ease of use, short acquisition time, and high sensitivity for detection of acute hemorrhage and fractures. It can provide a wealth of information about the brain, including ventricular size, presence of brain edema, mass effect, presence and location of hemorrhage or masses, midline shift, evolving ischemic injuries, fractures, benign and malignant osseous pathology, and the paranasal sinuses [29–32]. Its availability and short acquisition time also allow frequent repeat scanning of the brain that can contribute to the management and follow-up of patients in the acute, subacute, and chronic phases in both inpatient and outpatient settings. In veterinary patients, CT of the brain is often less useful than in human patients due to differences in anatomy and image quality.

In neurosurgery, CT of the head is used for preoperative and postoperative evaluation of patients for hemorrhage, infarction, inflammation [33], hydrocephalus, mass effect, fracture, and post-surgical assessment [30–32,34–45]. CT was historically the study of choice when evaluating for acute hemorrhage because it had higher sensitivity and specificity than MRI. With developments in MRI pulse sequences, MRI currently has similar or greater accuracy for the detection of intracranial hemorrhage than CT (Figure 4.6) [46], but usually requires anesthesia in veterinary patients. Intracranial hemorrhage is typically described in terms of its location within the head, such as epidural, subdural, subarachnoid, intraventricular, and parenchymal, with each type of hemorrhage having sufficiently distinct appearance and location. Epidural hemorrhage has a biconvex contour of its borders in relation to the cranial vault and adjacent brain parenchyma and is usually the result of acute trauma associated with an acute fracture across branches of meningeal arteries that hemorrhage into the epidural space.

Magnetic Resonance Imaging

The physics of magnetic resonance image generation is highly complex and specific details are beyond the scope of this chapter. The combination of magnetic fields and radiofrequency pulses used to create a magnetic resonance image is called a pulse sequence Spin-echo pulse sequences are designed to emphasize various types of proton relaxation. Images generated using spin-echo pulse sequences are either T1-weighted or T2-weighted depending on whether T1 or T2 relaxation controls tissue contrast [47].

T1 relaxation relates to the spins of protons in the patient that are perturbed by a radiofrequency pulse realigning into their normal position parallel with the main magnetic field. T2 relaxation relates to the rate of dephasing of the protons immediately after being perturbed by the radiofrequency pulse. Most important is that the difference in these relaxation times can be used to influence tissue contrast [47]. For example, fluid has very long T1 and T2 relaxation times and will create low signal (dark gray/black) in a T1-weighted image but will create high signal (white) in a T2-weighted image. Thus, because most CNS lesions have increased fluid associated with edema, they will be conspicuous as regions of increased signal in a T2-weighted image. However, some substances, such as proteinaceous exudates and methemoglobin, have short T1 relaxation times and will have high signal in a T1-weighted image. Thus, the signal characteristics of a lesion in T1- versus T2-weighted images can be used to estimate its composition.

As a general rule, T2-weighted images are often the most useful for neuroimaging as they provide the best soft tissue contrast. On a T2-weighted image, fluid and fat are hyperintense. As most pathology results in an increase in water content, pathology is often hyperintense (bright) on a T2-weighted image [47]. A routine brain protocol in veterinary medicine includes transverse precontrast and postcontrast T1-weighted, T2-weighted, T2W-FLAIR (fluid attenuated inversion recovery), and sagittal and dorsal T2-weighted images. In some cases T1-weighted (postcontrast) images may be useful in the sagittal and dorsal planes (e.g., assessment of the pituitary gland and extraaxial masses). The T2W-FLAIR sequence suppresses the signal from CSF and allows assessment of periventricular changes difficult to see on T2-weighted images. This sequence has high sensitivity for inflammatory CNS disease. FLAIR images are particularly useful if there is hydrocephalus or an intracranial cyst. T2* gradient-echo (GRE) images are very useful for evaluation of hemorrhage or bony changes. In some cases, diffusion-weighted imaging (DWI) may be helpful in aging infarcts and in the identification of small infarcts in the peracute stage [47]. Images acquired with fat suppression (short-tau inversion recovery, or postcontrast T1-weighted with fat saturation) are useful for showing pathology in the extracranial soft tissues, particularly orbital disease and pathology affecting the bone marrow. In unstable patients, the sequences most likely to give a diagnosis and assess secondary effects of increased ICP should be obtained first (transverse and sagittal T2-weighted images), in case the MRI study needs to be aborted.

Like CT, MRI provides cross-sectional images, but unlike CT these can be acquired in any anatomical plane without repositioning the patient. This means that multiplanar reformatting of images is not necessary; reformatted CT images can be of very high quality but primary image acquisitions have the best detail. The effects of radiofrequency currents and magnetic fields on protons generate magnetic resonance images. The strength of magnets available for clinical use in veterinary medicine range from 0.2 to 7 Tesla (T) [48–51]. Low-field magnets are less expensive but image quality is affected by lower signal to noise and scan times can be prolonged [52].

As with CT, patterns of contrast enhancement are an important feature of MRI. However, the mechanism of action of contrast media in CT compared with MRI is quite different. CT contrast media are iodinated and alter X-ray attenuation within the patient, with the iodine atoms directly visualized on the image. MRI contrast media are paramagnetic and function by changing the relaxation rate of protons. In MRI the contrast media is not seen directly on the image, as the mechanism of enhancement is indirect. In MRI, increased concentration of contrast medium changes the relaxation time of protons in the immediate area leading to a signal change in the image. In both CT and MRI, contrast media accumulate in regions of hypervascularity or altered vascular permeability. Most MRI contrast studies are based on changes in T1 relaxation, where increased relaxation leads to increased signal coming from regions of increased contrast medium.

Specialized imaging sequences other than spin-echo pulse sequences are often helpful for CNS imaging. It is possible to suppress the signal from fat; this is beneficial due to the high signal emitted from fat in many pulse sequences. This high signal from fat can hide smaller, adjacent lesions or may also be misinterpreted as disease [53]. The signal from fat can be suppressed in a spin-echo pulse sequence by the addition of a radiofrequency saturation pulse that nulls the signal from fat within the image. The high signal of fat may also be reduced using a type of pulse sequence called short-tau inversion recovery (STIR) sequence.

Certain types of hemorrhage have paramagnetic effects that can be imaged with MRI [54]. A very effective way of detecting these

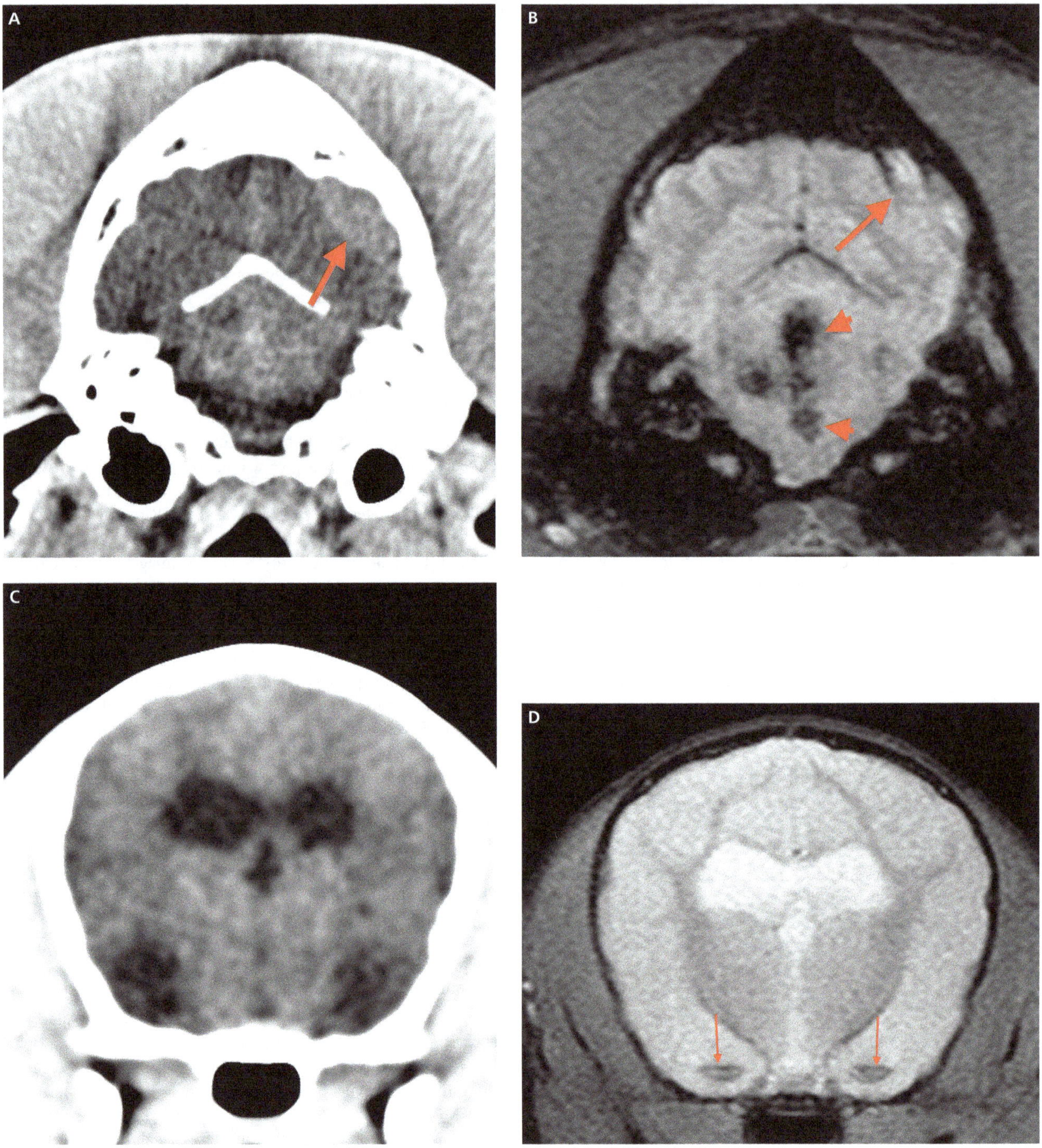

Figure 4.6 Transverse plane CT (A) and T2* GRE MRI (B) of a Labrador Retriever with subdural hematoma and intraparenchymal hemorrhage due to coagulopathy secondary to *Angiostrongylus vasorum* infection. The subdural hematoma (arrow in A, B) is seen clearly on both the CT and MRI but the bleeding within the cerebellum and brainstem (arrowheads) is seen much better on the MRI. Transverse CT (C) and T2* GRE MRI (D) of a Cavalier King Charles Spaniel with head trauma. The MRI shows intraventricular hemorrhage with blood products ventrally (arrows in D) within both lateral ventricles. No abnormalities are visible on the corresponding CT.

paramagnetic effects is with a GRE pulse sequence. In this sequence, magnetic gradients are used in a critical step of proton rephasing needed for image formation; this is very different from the more commonly used spin-echo pulse sequence where refocusing magnetic gradients are not used. Because the paramagnetic effects of hemorrhage, especially those of hemosiderin, interfere with the magnetic gradient used for proton rephasing and image formation, a conspicuous artifact, called a magnetic susceptibility artifact, is created [54]. The artifact essentially destroys the image in the region of hemorrhage and creates a region of signal void [55]. Inclusion of a GRE pulse sequence can be very useful for confirming or excluding hemorrhage. A newer form of GRE imaging called susceptibility weighted imaging (SWI) using phase and magnitude information from the magnetic resonance signal can be used to create images with exquisite sensitivity for hemorrhage. SWI has been shown to be significantly more sensitive than conventional T2* GRE images in showing cerebral hemorrhage [56]. The MRI effects of hemorrhage are quite complex, being dependent on the age of the hemorrhage and the pulse sequence used.

Magnetic Resonance Spectroscopy

Nuclear magnetic resonance spectroscopy (MRS) is an analytical technique that employs the magnetic resonance hardware used in chemistry for many years and more recently with in vitro research and clinically to determine the structure of compounds and composition of mixtures of compounds. In vivo this technique allows examination of the biochemical status of living tissue in a noninvasive manner. Most research with, and clinical applications of, MRS have involved the human brain. Examples include research into human brain tumors and brain abscesses, which typically require invasive surgical biopsies or ultrasound-guided aspirates for diagnoses. Research over the past few decades has elucidated that the use of MRS in these disease processes may aid in diagnosis and monitoring of treatment, without the use of invasive techniques. Until recently, MRS in animals has typically been in the context of models for human neurological diseases but the utility of MRS in clinical veterinary medicine is now being investigated (Figure 4.7) [57,58]. Hydrogen is the most frequently used nucleus in MRS, referred to as proton MRS or H-MRS. Hydrogen has a high sensitivity because of its high gyro-magnetic ratio, high natural abundance and favorable relaxation time and because it can be analyzed using conventional MRI hardware and radiofrequency coils [59,60]. The latter two reasons for selecting hydrogen for MRS are because the magnetic resonance signal of hydrogen nuclei within fat and water are obtained to produce images. Using specialized equipment, other nuclei can be used for in vivo MRS. These include carbon-13, nitrogen-15, and phosphorus-31. These nuclei have lower sensitivity and lower natural abundance. Therefore, their use results in lower resolution, longer scan times, and increased cost due to the different equipment needed for analysis [59,61]. As mentioned, hydrogen nuclei have the highest sensitivity and thus yield the largest signal, but other factors including temperature and, most significantly, magnetic field strength, have an impact on the signal produced. Numerous studies have used MRS for the diagnosis of brain tumors, differentiating types of brain tumor, grading tumors, determining brain tumor margins, and monitoring response to treatment in humans [60,62–81]. In a study by Fountas et al. [66], MRS was successful in establishing a correct diagnosis of tumor type in 85.6% of the population, whereas standard MRI was correct in only 78% of the cases. A study using MRS imaging in conjunction with perfusion MRI enabled the differentiation between metastatic lesions, lymphoma, and glioblastoma multiforme, the most aggressive glial cell tumor in humans, with high specificity [63]. Differentiation of tumor types, without the use of biopsy, can allow diagnosis, treatment, and follow-up of brain tumors without the use of invasive biopsy techniques. This would be especially useful in the veterinary community, where brain biopsy is performed less commonly.

Numerous studies using MRS have shown that brain tumors exhibit decreased levels of *N*-acetylaspartate (NAA) and increased levels of choline (Cho), causing a decrease in the NAA/Cho ratio [69,82]. These findings are thought to be associated with the absence of normal neuronal tissue and increased membrane turnover [59]. Other changes such as increased lactate and lipid may be evident, with alterations in metabolism (anaerobic glycolysis) or necrosis or ischemia associated with tissue damage and areas of decreased blood supply [82]. Occasionally, increased levels of myoinositol are detected when a short echo time is used. This is thought to be associated with increased number of glial cells, which contain myoinositol, especially in tumors such as high-grade gliomas [70,83]. High-grade brain tumors in children have a 60% lower NAA/Cho ratio, a 50% higher Cho to creatine (Cr) ratio (Cho/Cr), and a 43% lower NAA/Cr ratio than nonneoplastic lesions; low-grade tumors have a 50% higher Cho/Cr ratio than nonneoplastic lesions [70]. Other studies have demonstrated similar findings suggesting high-grade tumors will have higher Cho levels and therefore lower NAA/Cho levels than low-grade tumors [70,73]. In addition, high-grade tumors have higher lactate and lipid levels than low-grade tumors [73,80]. Another study using preoperative, high

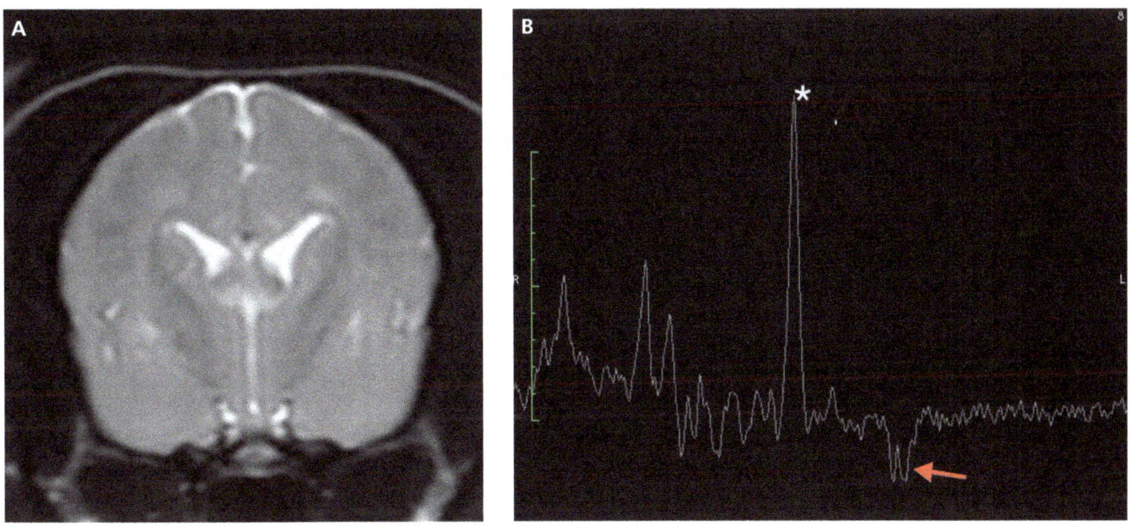

Figure 4.7 Transverse T2-weighted MRI (A) and MRS spectra (TE = 144 ms) (B) of an English Springer Spaniel with confirmed fucosidosis. The T2-weighted image shows symmetrical T2 hyperintensity within the white matter, which is a nonspecific finding. On MRS there is an abnormal lactate peak (inverted doublet, arrow) and elevated NAA peak (asterisk), which in dogs appear to be characteristic of fucosidosis.

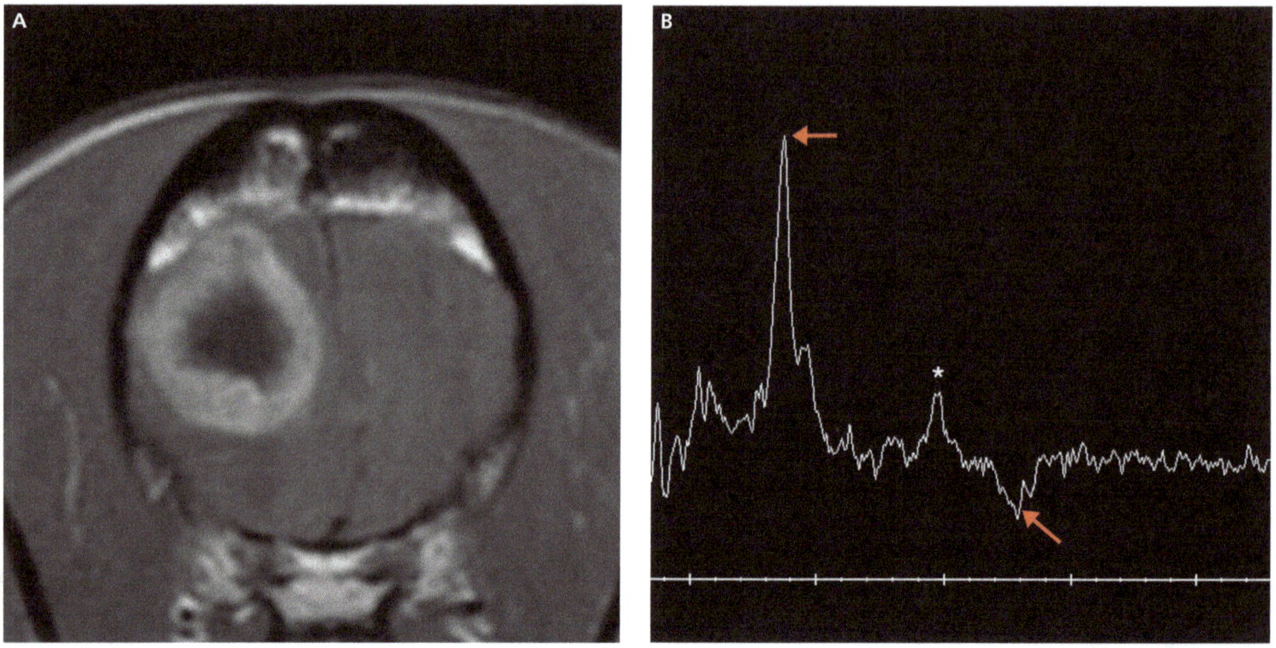

Figure 4.8 Transverse T1-weighted postcontrast MRI (A) and MRS spectra (TE = 144 ms) (B) of a crossbred dog with presumed glioma in the right frontal lobe. The spectra was obtained within the intraaxial mass, clearly seen on the postcontrast image. The spectrum shows an abnormal lactate peak (upper arrow), markedly reduced NAA peak (asterisk), and elevation of the choline peak (lower arrow), all typical of a high-grade glioma.

spatial resolution (nominal voxel size, 0.45 cm^3) MRS imaging to grade gliomas determined that there were significantly higher total NAA values, lower Cho values, and lower Cho/NAA ratios for grade II gliomas compared with grade III tumors [74]. This study also determined that chemical shift imaging (CSI) spectra from grade III astrocytomas had significantly higher maximum Cr values compared with grade III oligodendrogliomas and grade III oligoastrocytomas in human patients. This higher maximum Cr concentration in grade III astrocytomas compared with grade II oligodendrogliomas is theorized as a result of the increased energy metabolism and increased growth rate of the high-grade tumors [74]. The Cho/PCr-Cr (phosphocreatine–creatine) ratio is also a reliable marker for tumor grade identification. The Cho/PCr-Cr ratio was 2.05 ± 0.18 in low-grade astrocytomas, 2.58 ± 0.11 in grade III, and 5.1 ± 0.89 in grade IV [66]. These are typical examples, where MRS studies have used the ratios of NAA, Cho and Cr to diagnose and differentiate brain lesions. A study by Vuori et al. [84] showed that the total Cho and Cr values helped differentiate astrocytomas from oligodendrogliomas and oligoastrocytomas, but that none of the metabolite ratios (NAA/Cho, NAA/Cr, Cho/Cr) helped differentiate the tumor type. The use of metabolite ratios can result in loss of metabolic information, since a ratio does not change when neither the numerator nor the denominator change, and the ratio does not reveal the direction of change. Furthermore, the ratios may not take into account regional and age-dependent differences in metabolite signals. A study by McKnight et al. [85] used three-dimensional CSI to establish a linear model of total Cho versus NAA, in the form of a Gaussian *z*-score, the Cho to NAA index (CNI) indicating the number of standard deviations of difference between amount of Cho and NAA at a voxel location and mean values of control spectra. Spectra from normal, edematous, and necrotic regions will have CNIs close to zero, whereas those recorded from tumor are elevated. A CNI of 2.0 was used as a threshold to determine tumor versus peritumoral tissue [85]. This technique may help to increase the likelihood of a biopsy targeting the tissue with the highest probability of being malignant, and in aiding inclusion of all neoplastic tissue while sparing normal tissue during tumor resection. This same laboratory performed a follow-up experiment using CNI to compare contrast-enhancing versus noncontrast-enhancing areas associated with gliomas that were hyperintense on T2-weighted images [86]. This study confirmed the original data in that the CNIs of biopsy samples not containing tumors were significantly different from those obtained within tumors; tumors were distinguished from nontumor with 0.96 sensitivity but only 0.57 specificity. When a CNI of 2.5 was used, the sensitivity and specificity were 0.9 and 0.86, respectively [86]. Half of the 42 biopsy specimens from contrast-enhancing tumors that were positively identified as tumor with histopathology came from nonenhancing portions of the lesions. Additionally, 36–45% of the hyperintense lesions that did not enhance on contrast-enhanced T1-weighted MRI were suspicious for tumor cells, based on the CSI spectra and CNI of greater than 2.5 [86]. Unfortunately, histopathology was not available for confirmation. This robust tool for differentiating tumor versus peritumoral edema, necrosis, and normal tissue is valuable when using MRS with brain lesions, because of the high sensitivity to metabolic changes.

Only a few reports have studied the use of MRS in canine brain tumors [62,87,88]. NAA and Cr were decreased and lactate was increased in brain tumors (Figure 4.8) compared with the internal control (normal contralateral side), but Cho exhibited no significant difference between neoplastic and normal tissues [62,87].

General Assessment of Images from CT and MRI

Once images have been evaluated for positioning and diagnostic quality, they can be critically assessed. Interpretation of images from CT and MRI is similar to that for radiography and based on classical Röentgen signs (size, shape, number, alignment, margination) plus signal intensity or tissue attenuation [47]. The comparison of signal intensity on different pulse sequences allows identification of properties of the tissue (e.g., fatty, cystic). With CT, tissue contrast is largely due to differences in tissue density. Suspected lesions should be cross-referenced with different imaging planes and sequences as most genuine lesions are visible on more than one plane. Partial volume averaging is common and can be mistaken for pathology (e.g., apparent defects of skull bones).

Assessment of brain images on CT and MRI is mainly based on changes in symmetry (mass effect, loss of parenchyma), changes in the ventricular system, and shape and size of the cerebellum and cranial spinal cord. CT may be of limited value for evaluation of caudal fossa lesions, especially in larger dogs because of beam hardening artifact resulting in hypoattenuating streaks, which can obscure pathology. It is important to recognize MRI alterations in signal intensity (gray matter, white matter). CT images should be evaluated for alterations in attenuation of tissues.

The extracranial soft tissues should be evaluated for:

- muscle volume;
- muscle signal;
- nasal or orbital lesions;
- lymph nodes;
- changes in skull bones (loss of signal, erosion).

Following administration of MRI contrast media (gadolinium chelates), the images should be assessed to ensure that normal contrast enhancement has occurred. With CT, the normal contrast enhancement pattern is similar to that seen on MRI, with contrast evident in larger blood vessels and in tissues outside the blood–brain barrier. The choroid plexuses, large veins, pituitary gland, nasal mucosa, salivary glands, and trigeminal nerve ganglia/periganglionic vascular plexuses should all enhance in a normal animal [47]. Failure of enhancement of a lesion may be due to lack of blood supply or intact blood-brain barrier but may also be due to failure of administration of contrast media (e.g., contrast still in catheter, leakage from catheter). The mechanism of contrast enhancement is different on CT and MRI. CT contrast enhancement is the result of direct visualization of the contrast agent, whereas with MRI the contrast agent is not directly visualized; enhancement occurs due to the effect of the contrast agent on the immediately adjacent tissues. The acquisition times of the images following contrast can affect interpretation of the underlying lesions but contrast enhancement cannot be consistently relied upon to detect similar pathologies [89,90]. A technique described as dynamic contrast-enhanced MRI has been useful in more specifically detecting histopathological abnormalities but it is still in its early assessment period [91,92].

Brain Masses

Most brain masses are readily identified on MRI or CT images [23,45,93,94]. They are often hyperintense on T2-weighted MRI, and are associated with a mass effect: midline shift, and compression of ventricles and adjacent parenchyma [95]. Much of the mass effect is often due to perilesional edema [94]. The presence of edema is easier to appreciate on MRI than CT. On CT, edema results in reduced attenuation of the brain tissue. On MRI, edema is hyperintense on T2-weighted images, poorly marginated, usually most severe within the white matter, and tends to follow the white matter tracts (especially the corona radiata) (Figure 4.9) [96].

Differential diagnosis of brain masses is based on classification into extraaxial or intraaxial locations. Extraaxial masses arise from outside the neuraxis (e.g., meninges, skull bone). Intraaxial masses arise from within the neuraxis (e.g., glial cell tumors). Intraventricular masses are classified as extraaxial. The imaging features of masses are nonspecific. A mass lesion is not necessarily neoplastic and other causes (e.g., granuloma, hematoma) should be

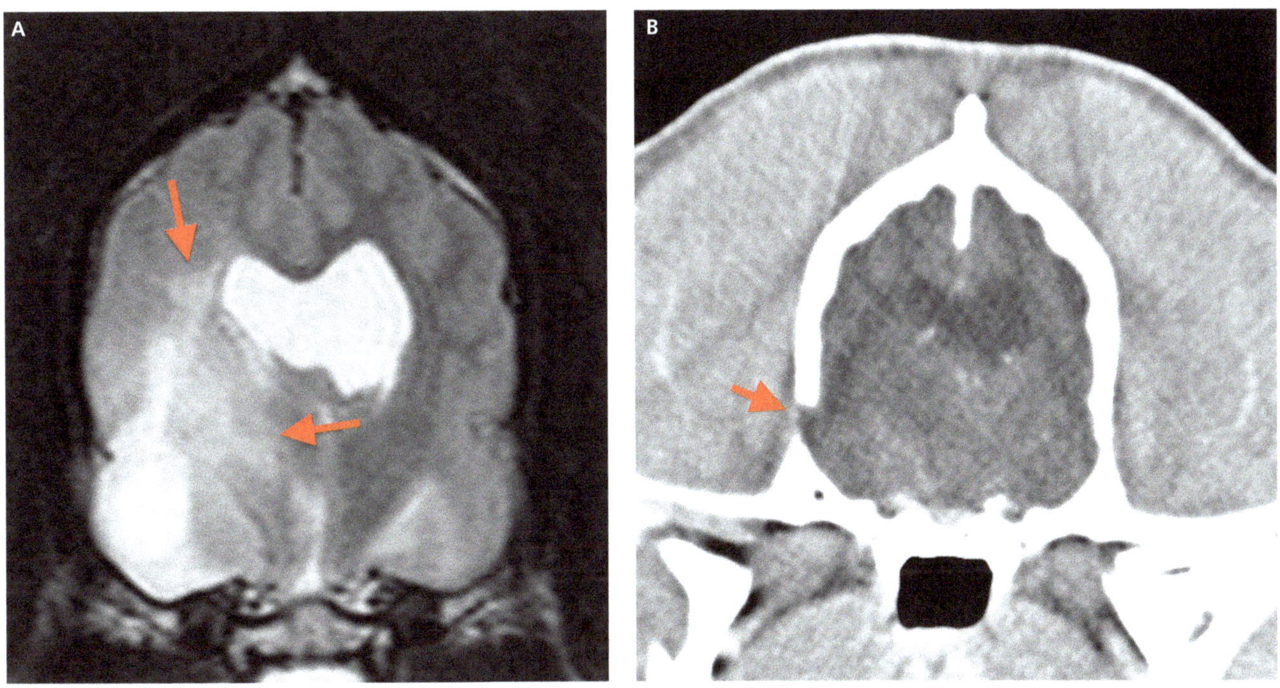

Figure 4.9 Transverse plane T2-weighted MRI (A) and postcontrast CT (B) of the brain of a Boxer with presumed glioma. While a mass effect is seen on CT, the boundaries of the mass and the extent of the perilesional edema (arrows in A) are seen much better on MRI. The mass has resulted in a small focal defect in the bone adjacent to the mass that is seen more clearly on CT (arrow in B).

considered. Definitive diagnosis requires tissue biopsy (stereotaxis, free-hand or open surgical biopsy).

The diagnosis of a brain tumor relies on diagnostic imaging. The aim of imaging an animal with a suspect brain tumor is to confirm the diagnosis, screen for metastases either to or from the brain, and to aid therapeutic planning. MRI also allows identification of the secondary pathological effects of intracranial masses and inflammation (e.g., hydrocephalus, vasogenic edema, bleeding, or brain herniation) [93,97,98].

Most primary brain tumors in dogs result in no changes to the skull and are not visible on plain radiography. Meningiomas in cats can be associated with hyperostosis of the calvaria (Figure 4.10), which can occasionally be visualized on radiographs, as can areas of mineralization of the tumor. As with any animal with a suspected tumor, it is advisable to obtain thoracic radiographs to screen for pulmonary metastases. While primary brain tumors rarely spread to the lungs, metastasis does occur and this has consequences for treatment and prognosis. It is more common for tumors to metastasize to the brain than vice versa. Metastases to the brain are less common than primary brain tumors. When they do occur, they are usually multiple, small, located at the junction between gray and white matter (i.e., watershed zone), and surrounded by marked edema (Figure 4.11).

Most intraaxial tumors (and other types of brain pathology) result in an increase in water content, which appears hyperintense on T2-weighted images and hypointense on T1-weighted images [93,95,99]. Extraaxial masses are variable in appearance depending on cellularity and mineralization [94]. Most extraaxial masses are associated with marked contrast enhancement (Figures 4.10 and 4.12). The contrast uptake by intraaxial masses is variable, from none to marked [100]. While the mass effect produced by brain tumors is obvious, delineating the mass is not always easy. In some cases of diffuse neoplasia (e.g., lymphoma or gliomatosis cerebri) the changes may mimic inflammatory disease. Definitive diagnosis may require brain biopsy.

In addition to identifying the primary lesion, the brain should also be evaluated for secondary pathological effects. Hydrocephalus is commonly seen with masses within the caudal fossa (e.g., brainstem masses) due to compression of the CSF pathways or due to increased CSF production and protein concentrations seen with choroid plexus masses. With certain tumors (e.g., choroid plexus tumors), treatment may need to be directed to the secondary pathological effects. Any disease that increases ICP may result in brain herniation. This is easiest to see on T2-weighted sagittal images,

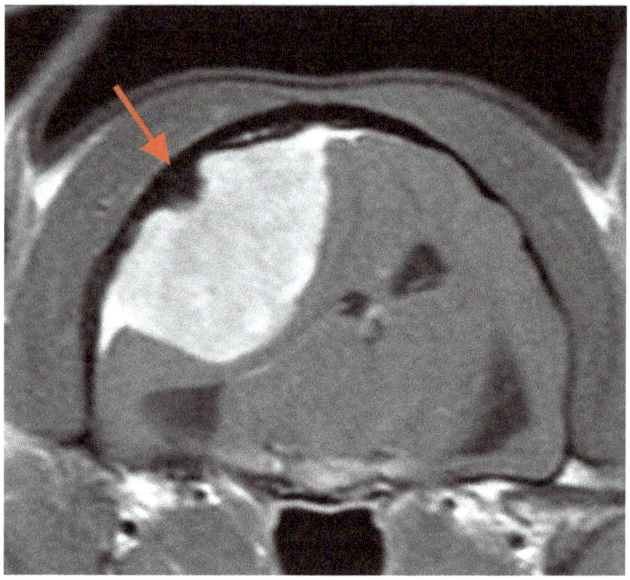

Figure 4.10 Transverse plane T1-weighted postcontrast MRI of a cat with a meningioma. Note the thickening and reduced signal of the calvarium overlying the mass due to hyperostosis (arrow). The dense homogeneous contrast enhancement is common with meningiomas and other extraaxial masses.

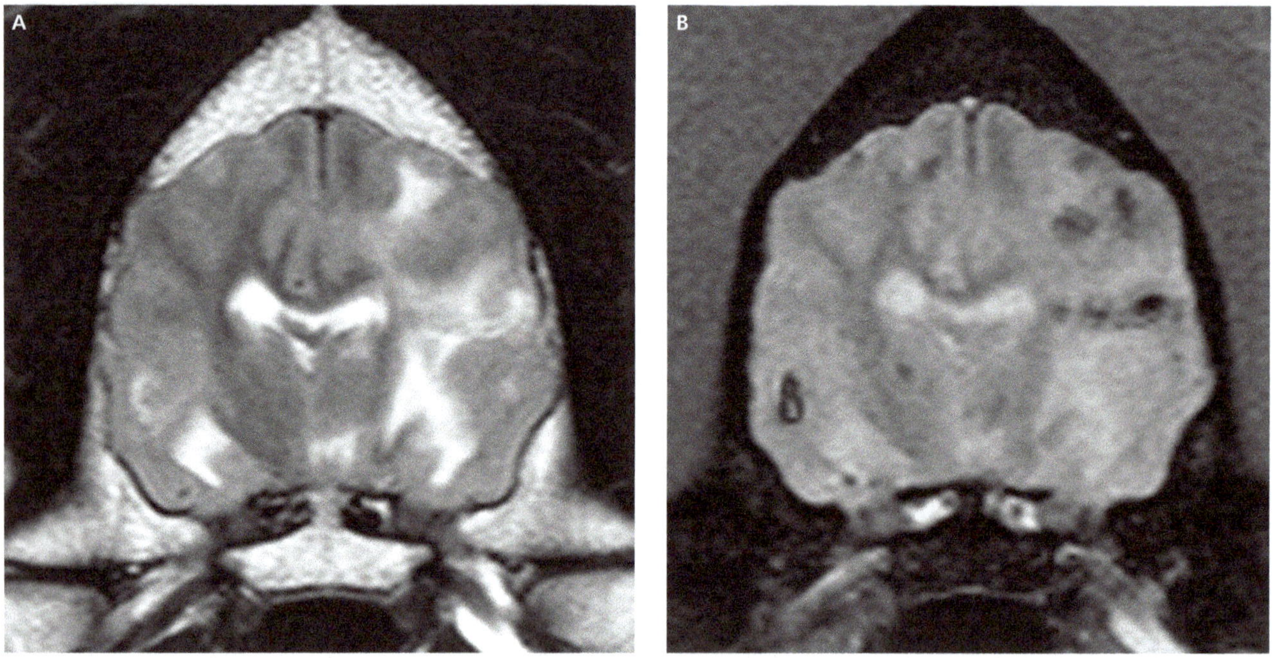

Figure 4.11 Transverse plane T2-weighted (A) and T2* GRE (B) MRI of a dog with cerebral metastases from hemangiosarcoma. Note the multiple small hemorrhagic nodules (best seen on the T2* GRE image) with extensive perilesional edema.

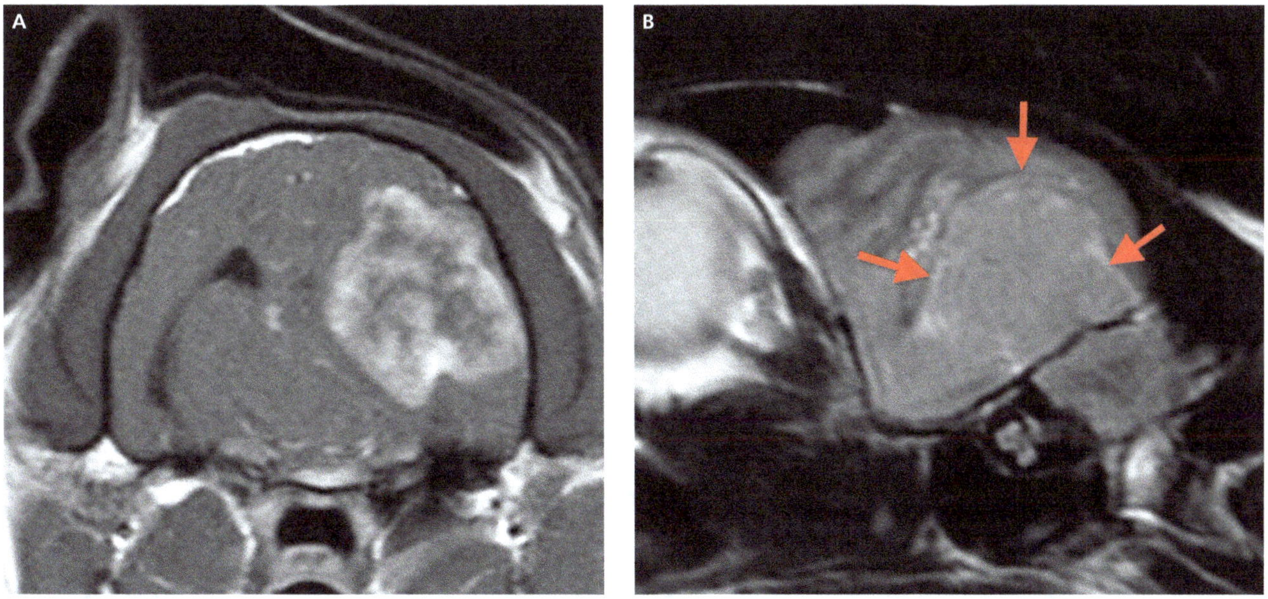

Figure 4.12 Transverse T1-weighted postcontrast (A) and sagittal T2-weighted (B) MRI of a cat with a meningioma (arrows) rising from the meninges overlying the osseous tentorium cerebelli. The superficial location of the mass with displacement of the overlying brain parenchyma away from the osseous tentorium is best seen on the sagittal plane images. On the transverse plane images the extraaxial location cannot be determined but the mass shows marked contrast enhancement typical of an extraaxial mass. Brain masses need to be evaluated on multiple imaging planes to allow correct anatomical localization.

where displacement of the occipital lobes under the osseous tentorium or caudal displacement of the cerebellum through the foramen magnum may be seen (Figure 4.13). There are many treatments for intracranial neoplasia and CT or MRI is required in most for accurate treatment planning. The postradiation MRI appearance of brain tumors has been described, including the necrosis that can be associated with this treatment modality [101].

Intracranial Hemorrhage

CT is exquisitely sensitive at detecting acute hemorrhage, which is evident as increased density due to attenuation of X-rays by the globin portion of blood [32,41]. The attenuation gradually decreases until the hematoma is isodense at about 1 month after the onset. The periphery of the hematoma enhances with contrast at 6 days to 6 weeks due to revascularization. Until recently, CT was the preferred imaging modality in human patients for determining the presence of hemorrhage in early stroke. Recent developments in MRI mean that CT now offers little advantage apart from time of acquisition in the diagnosis of stroke [102].

The appearance of hemorrhage on MRI is variable and depends on the age of the hemorrhage, pH, oxygenation, size of bleed, and magnetic field strength. T2* GRE sequences are the most sensitive for visualizing hemorrhage, which always appears as a signal void (black) (see Figures 4.6 and 4.11). On spin-echo sequences, the appearance depends on the degree of conversion of hemoglobin (Table 4.1).

In small animals the main causes of intraparenchymal hemorrhage are coagulopathy, neoplasia, and trauma [54,55]. Subdural and subarachnoid hematomas are rare in small animals in comparison with humans. Most brain hemorrhage seen in dogs and cats is intraparenchymal [103]. Hemorrhage is commonly seen associated with tumors but the MRI appearance is predominantly of a solid mass rather than a hematoma. Hemorrhagic tumors are often complex masses with solid contrast-enhancing parts (Figure 4.14). Lack of a distinct, complex hypointense rim and bleeding of different durations within the lesion is suggestive of neoplasia. In some cases, repeat MRI to monitor progression of the lesion is required. The presence of edema at a later stage, regression in size of the lesion, and failure to follow the expected evolution of a hematoma are indicative of neoplasia.

Large hematomas may show distinct fluid lines; if there is intraventricular bleeding, then alterations in signal intensity (decreased signal on T2W and increased on T1W and FLAIR images) and layered fluid–fluid levels within ventricular CSF will be seen (see Figure 4.6). The presence of high signal on a T1-weighted image within the brain and very low signal on a T2-weighted image are suggestive of recent hemorrhage. T2* GRE images are the most sensitive for showing small hemorrhages (which are hypointense) [54]. Hyperintensity on a T1-weighted image is not 100% specific for hemorrhage and may be seen with melanin, high protein, flow artifacts, and paramagnetic effects (e.g., due to manganese) [104].

Cerebral Infarction

Infarcts in the CNS of dogs are usually ischemic with little or no hemorrhage. They are usually arterial and have characteristic imaging findings [105]. CT images are frequently normal during the acute phase of ischemia; therefore the diagnosis of ischemic stroke using CT relies on the exclusion of "mimics" of stroke. Early CT signs of ischemia can be subtle (Figure 4.15) and difficult to detect even by experienced readers and include parenchymal hypodensity, loss of gray–white matter differentiation, subtle effacement of the cortical sulci, and local mass effect [39].

MRI lesions are most obvious on T2-weighted and FLAIR images where they are usually hyperintense. They have minimal or no mass effect and are usually homogeneous, and sharply marginated with clear demarcation from adjacent parenchyma [106,107]. Gray matter is most severely affected and lesions are usually confined to one vascular territory (Figure 4.16) [108].

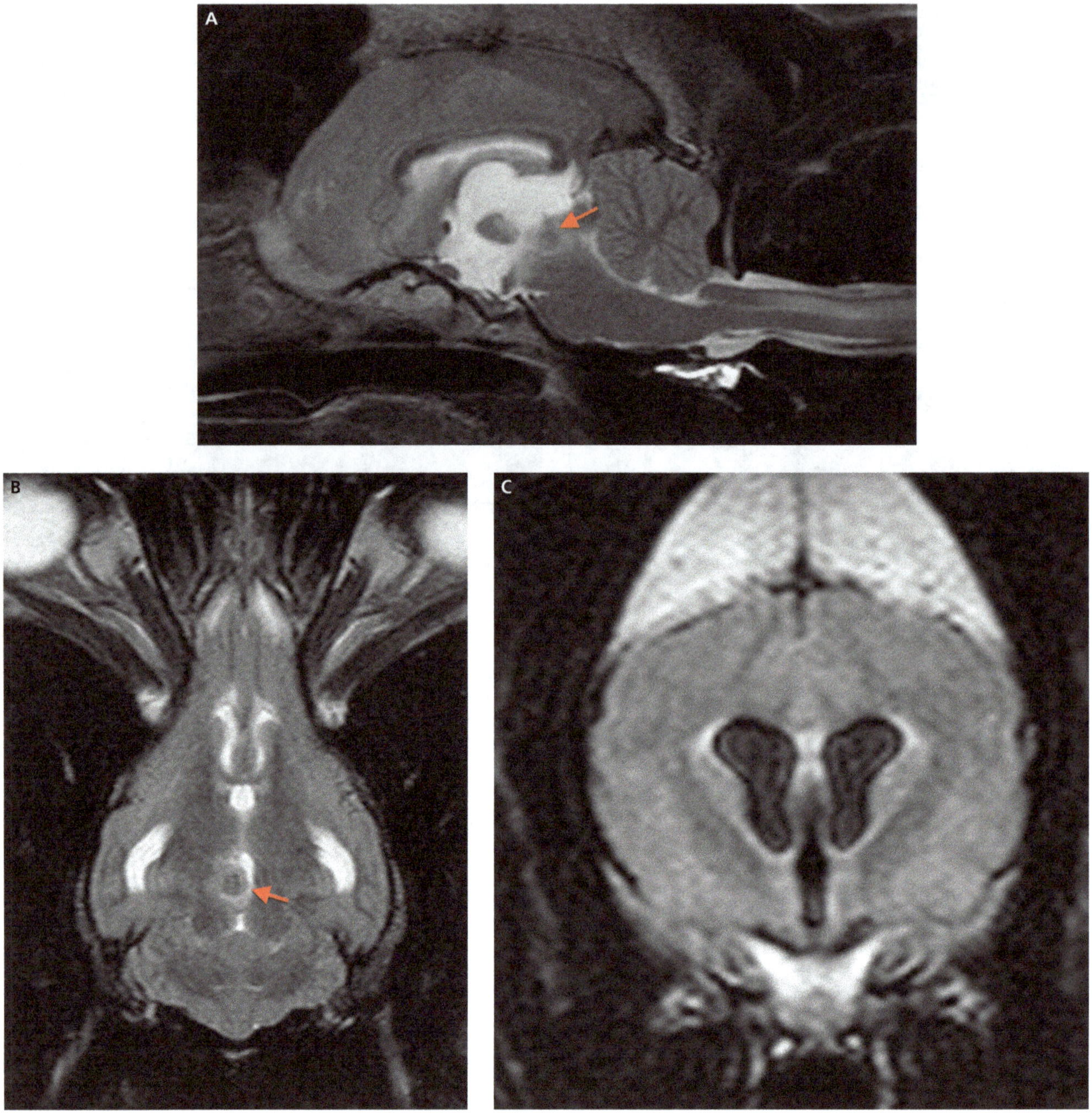

Figure 4.13 Sagittal (A), dorsal (B), and T2-weighted and transverse FLAIR (C) MRI of a dog with obstructive hydrocephalus due to a small mass (arrows in A, B) compressing the mesencephalic aqueduct. Rostral to the mass there is severe dilation of the third ventricle. The FLAIR images show dilated, rounded lateral ventricles and T2 hyperintensity in the periventricular region consistent with interstitial edema due to increased intraventricular pressure.

Table 4.1 T1 and T2 appearances of the five stages of parenchymal brain hemorrhage.

Phase	Time (days)	Hemoglobin	Location	T1	T2
Hyperacute	<1	Oxyhemoglobin	Intracellular	Isointense or hyperintense	Hyperintense
Acute	1–3	Deoxyhemoglobin	Intracellular	Hypointense	Hypointense
Early subacute	>3	Methemoglobin	Intracellular	Hyperintense	Hypointense
Late subacute	>7	Methemoglobin	Extracellular	Hyperintense	Hyperintense
Chronic	>14	Ferritin/hemosiderin	Extracellular	Hypointense	Hypointense

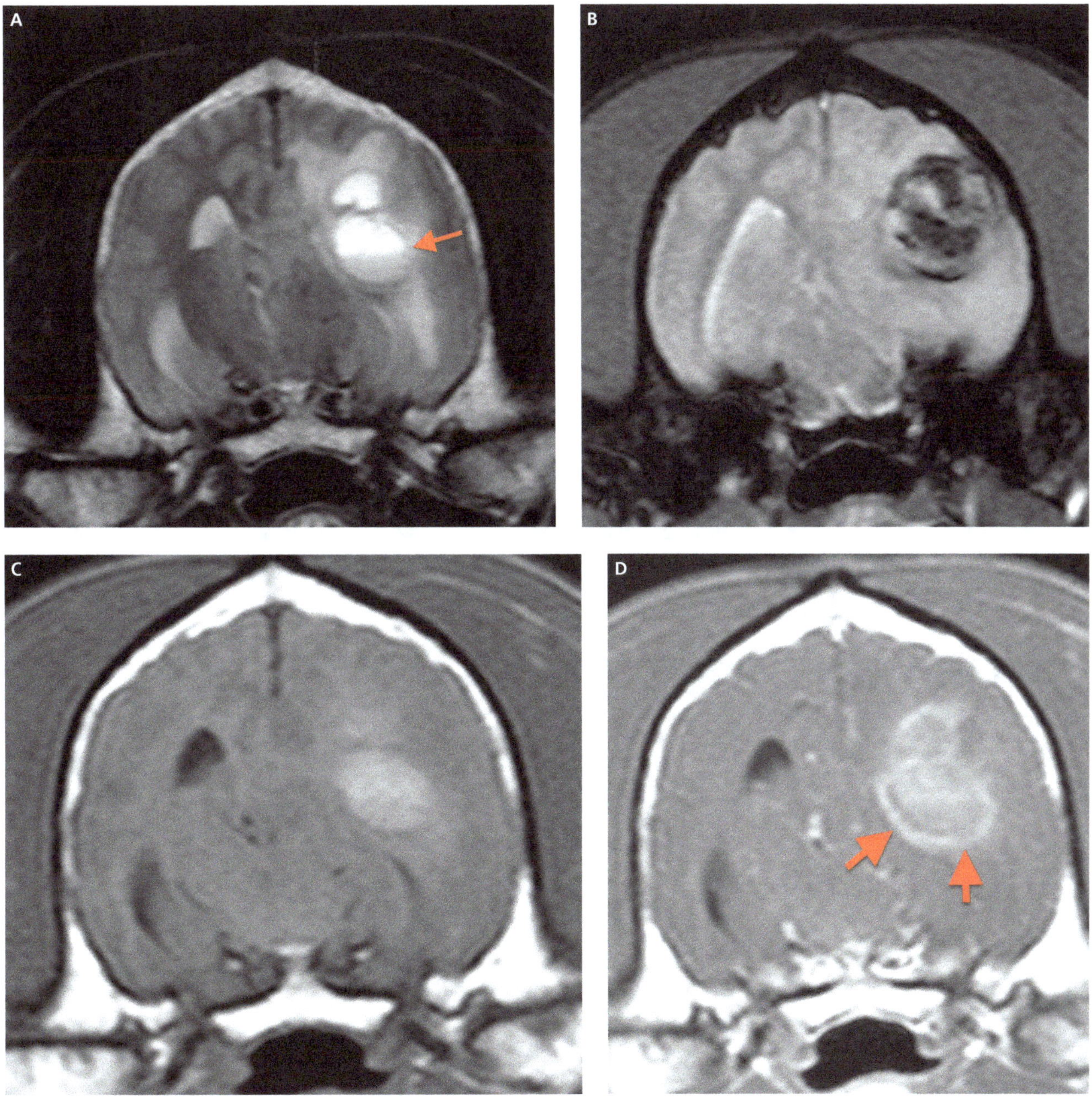

Figure 4.14 Transverse T2-weighted (A), T2* GRE (B), T1-weighted (C), and T1-weighted postcontrast (D) MRI of a 12-year-old English Springer Spaniel presented with acute-onset progressive obtundation. The mass is complex with fluid–fluid levels (arrow in A) and evidence of hemorrhage (susceptibility artifact on the T2* GRE images and high signal on the T1W images). The complex nature of the mass, lack of distinct rim, extensive perilesional edema, and enhancement (arrows in D) of the solid components of the mass are suggestive of a hemorrhagic neoplasm rather than benign hematoma.

Territorial infarcts occur with large artery disease and result in large rectangular/wedge-shaped lesions. They are most commonly seen in the cerebellum (small breeds, with Cavalier King Charles Spaniels being predisposed) [109]. Large territorial infarcts in the vascular territory of the middle or rostral cerebral arteries are occasionally seen in sight-hounds among other breeds.

Lacunar infarcts are small infarcts affecting end arteries within deep gray matter structures (e.g., thalamus and caudate nucleus) (Figure 4.17) [108]. They are most commonly seen in larger dogs and may be multiple. Chronic lacunar infarcts are sometimes seen as an incidental finding.

DWI is useful in determining the age of the infarct, with acute (<9 days old) infarcts appearing hyperintense on DWI and hypointense on the apparent diffusion coefficient (ADC) map [110–113]. After 7–9 days the DWI pseudonormalizes. DWI may be helpful in giving some prognostic information if there are multiple infarcts by showing if they are occurring at different time periods. MRI and CT angiography of intracranial arteries is usually of limited or no value for the diagnosis of canine and feline brain infarcts due to the small size of the blood vessels affected, which are often not visible even in normal animals [48,114]. However, recent work has suggested that MRS

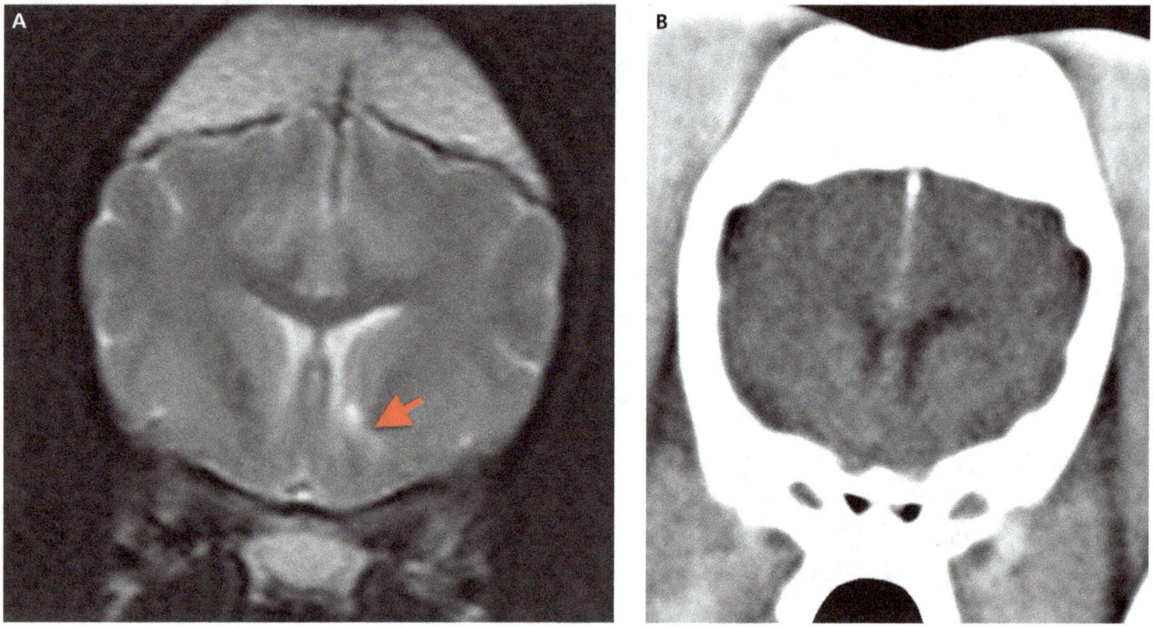

Figure 4.15 Transverse plane T2-weighted MRI (A) and postcontrast CT (B) of a dog with a small lacunar infarct (arrow in A) within the rostroventral part of the left caudate nucleus and adjacent white matter. The lesion is clearly seen on MRI but is not visible on the CT image. CT is relatively insensitive for detection of small infarcts, and metabolic and inflammatory disease.

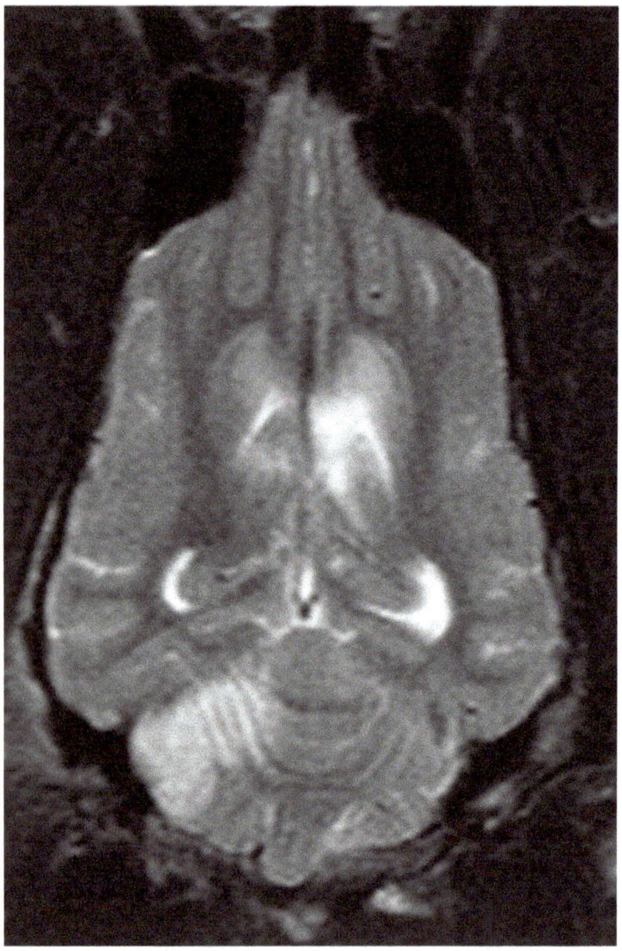

Figure 4.16 Dorsal T2-weighted MRI of a greyhound with an acute ischemic cerebellar infarct within the territory of the right rostral cerebellar artery. Note the sharp margination, wedge/angular shape, homogeneous T2 hyperintensity, and lack of mass effect, which are all characteristics of infarction.

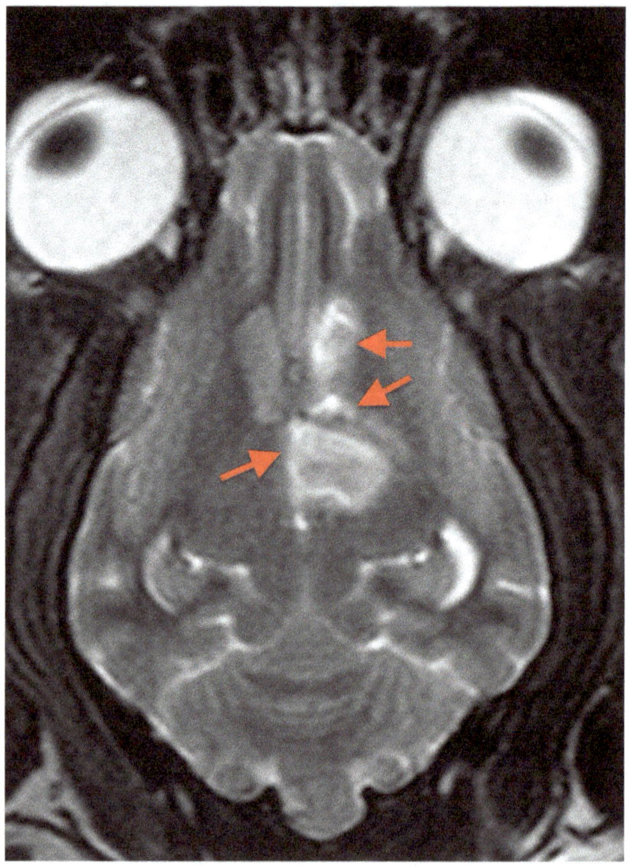

Figure 4.17 Dorsal T2-weighted MRI of a dog with multiple lacunar infarcts (arrows) within the left thalamus and caudate nucleus. Note the classic appearance of infarction with sharp margination, gray matter predilection, and minimal/absence of mass effect.

may offer some diagnostic benefit for ischemic stroke, especially in cases that could be confused with inflammatory lesions [115].

Radiography and ultrasonography are useful in looking for the underlying systemic causes of strokes (renal disease and adrenal disease most commonly) [112].

Head Trauma

Even mild neurological signs following head trauma exhibit a high incidence of lesions detectable on CT [116]. Most cases of head trauma resulting in neurological signs will show changes on MRI and the imaging study needs to determine if there is significant brain compression due to fracture fragments or hematoma formation or mass effect. CT examination will clearly show the presence of skull fractures and allow detection of depressed fractures that may need surgical decompression. MRI, while not showing such clear bone detail, provides more information on the extent of brain injury and allows identification of shearing or contusive injuries (Figure 4.18). Imaging of the patient's head is often indicated, especially in animals that fail to respond to aggressive medical therapy or which deteriorate after initially responding. Lesions of intracranial structures which may benefit from surgical therapy such as hematomas and pneumocephalus (Figures 4.19 and 4.20) can be accurately identified using advanced imaging [117].

Hydrocephalus

In severe cases the diagnosis of hydrocephalus is straightforward on MRI, with marked dilation of the lateral ventricles, and thinning of the overlying cortex in congenital cases, being obvious (Figure 4.21) [6,102,118]. The fontanelle is usually open in toy breed dogs with congenital hydrocephalus and this allows ultrasonography of the brain to identify the enlarged lateral anechoic ventricles [5,6]. However, this is not always the case especially if the hydrocephalus is not a congenital lesion. Although the diagnosis may be made with ultrasound in some cases, MRI is indicated to confirm the diagnosis and identify any underlying cause for the hydrocephalus. In most cases of congenital hydrocephalus, only the lateral ventricles, with or without the third ventricle, is affected. Dilation of the mesencephalic aqueduct and fourth ventricle often indicates obstruction to CSF flow at the lateral apertures of the fourth ventricle or the foramen magnum. Mild hydrocephalus is commonly seen in association with occipital malformation (Chiari-like malformation) but intracranial signs are not usually seen. In older animals, hydrocephalus is often secondary to inflammatory or neoplastic disease. In such cases, it is essential that FLAIR images be obtained to identify periventricular lesions. In dogs with choroid plexus tumors and cats with feline infectious peritonitis (FIP) (Figure 4.22), there may be intraventricular masses arising from the choroid plexuses. Seeding along the CSF pathways with lesions in multiple parts of the ventricular system may be seen with choroid plexus carcinomas and FIP. Choroid plexus masses normally exhibit marked contrast enhancement. Dilation of the olfactory recesses of the lateral ventricle and a periventricular halo of increased signal (seen on FLAIR images) is suggestive of increased intraventricular pressure.

Compensatory hydrocephalus (hydrocephalus ex vacuo) is seen secondary to loss of brain parenchyma with widening of the sulci in addition to the ventriculomegaly. This is most commonly due to chronic inflammatory/vascular disorders and degenerative

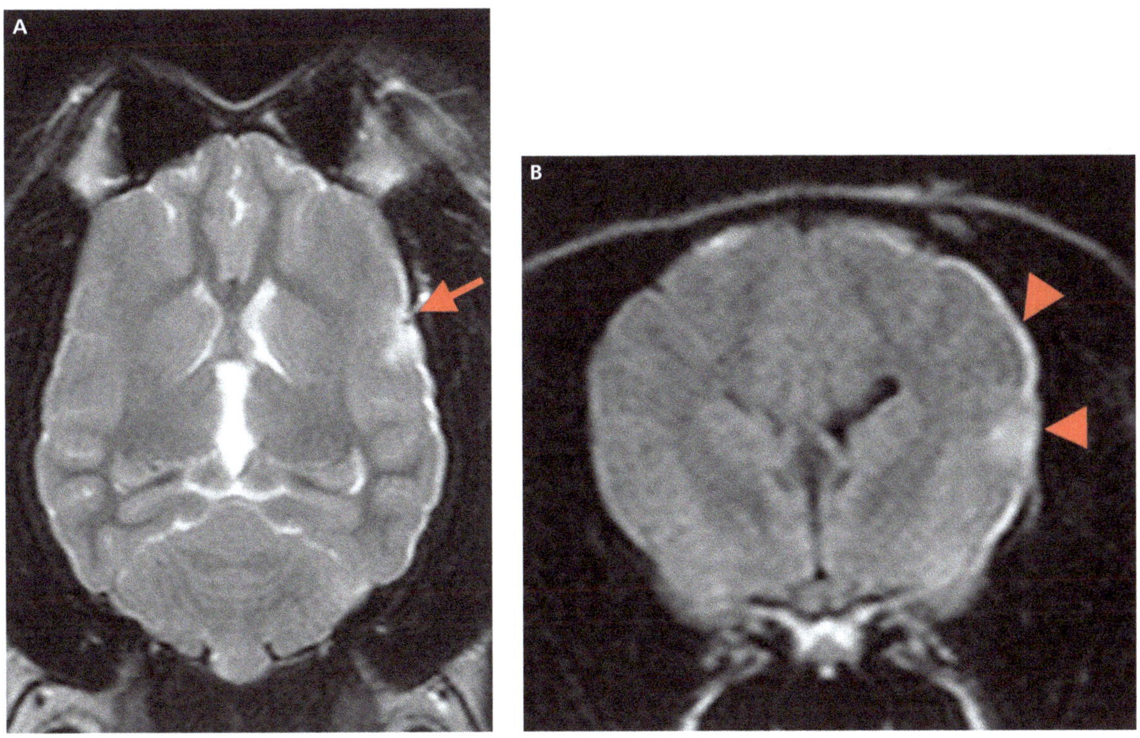

Figure 4.18 Dorsal T2-weighted (A) and transverse plane FLAIR (B) MRI of a Cavalier King Charles Spaniel 4 days post cranial trauma. There is a small depressed cranial fracture (arrow), which is difficult to visualize, but MRI shows clearly the cerebral concussion and subarachnoid hemorrhage (arrowheads), best seen on the FLAIR images.

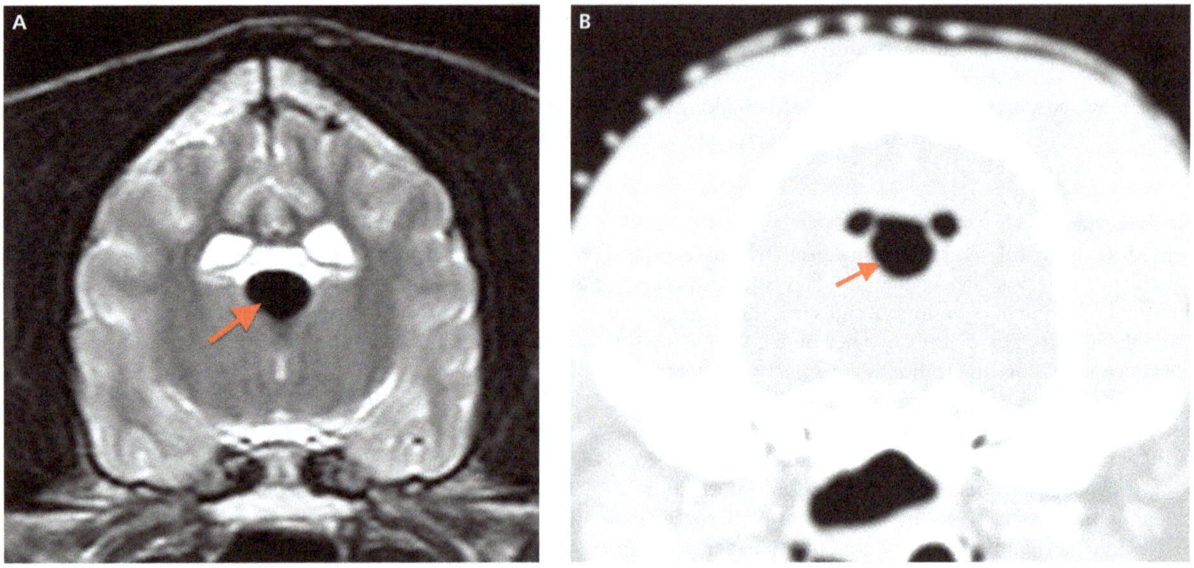

Figure 4.19 Transverse T2-weighted MRI (A) and CT with lung window and level (B) of a dog with pneumocephalus. Note the presence of intraventricular gas (arrow in A, B) that in this case was secondary to surgery for a frontal meningioma. Air appears as a signal void on MRI and in this case the air bubble is seen surrounded by CSF. Differentiation of signal voids can be difficult on MRI but is easy in CT where gas is hypoattenuating and easily differentiated from bone, ligaments, or metal.

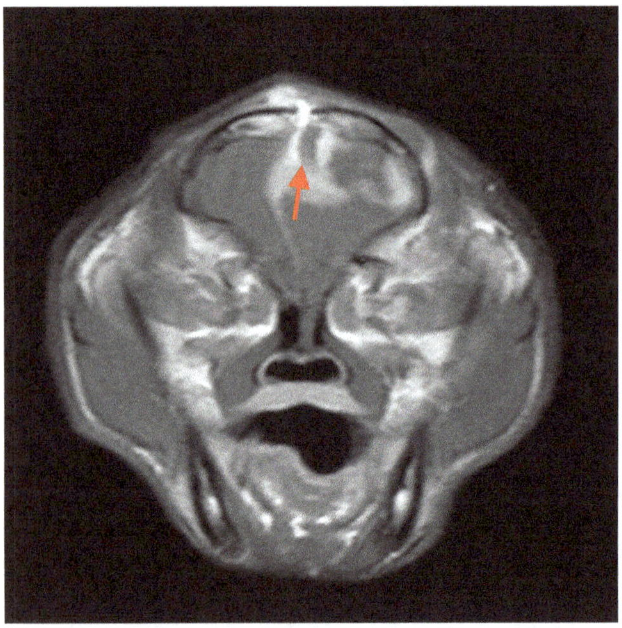

Figure 4.20 Transverse T1-weighted postcontrast MRI of a cat that presented with progressive obtundation following a bite to the head 2 weeks previously. The MRI shows a defect within the frontal bone, meningitis, cellulitis, and subdural empyema (arrow).

disease. It is often seen in older animals and is not associated with thinning of the calvaria (Figure 4.23) [119,120].

Inflammatory Diseases

Inflammatory CNS disease may be associated with a normal MRI. In one study, 6 of 25 dogs with inflammatory CSF had a normal MRI examination [121]. Investigation of suspected inflammatory/infectious disease therefore requires CSF analysis.

Intraoperative Imaging

Image-guided procedures have recently been introduced into the neurosurgical armamentarium and have provided major advances in neurosurgery. In essence, these promising technologies have emerged from the need to acquire data that is more accurate than that obtained from routine preoperative imaging. Classic surgical planning relies on preoperative imaging and indirect localization methods. Although current neuroimaging techniques can elegantly define anatomy and pathology in most clinical settings, preoperative images have significant limitations, for example distortion between the image space and the physical space, which may result in less-than-optimal localization of the lesion [122]. In addition, intraoperative alterations in the anatomical characteristics of the surgical field may be visualized only with the use of intraoperative imaging modalities. These techniques may also be beneficial in determining the extent of surgical resection during brain tumor surgery. This section presents several techniques that may provide intraoperative image guidance during brain surgery.

Rationale for Intraoperative Image Guidance

Problems related to the accuracy of localization in neurosurgery are mainly caused by anatomical and physiological properties of the brain that prevent wide surgical exposures and, in most cases, direct visualization of surrounding structures; however, a safe neurosurgical approach to a mass lesion requires precise spatial knowledge of the relevant pathology as it relates to surrounding bone and vascular structures and the localization of the lesion with respect to normal tissue. Although conventional neurosurgery training and subsequent experience enable the surgeon to navigate safely within the brain parenchyma, additional intraoperative anatomical information is still valuable, especially in situations in which individual anatomical variations or prior treatment complicate the anatomy [123]. Mass lesions, together with their surrounding edema, often distort normal anatomical relationships, thus posing a significant challenge to the neurosurgeon trying to navigate using conventional landmarks. The effect of such anatomical alterations may be

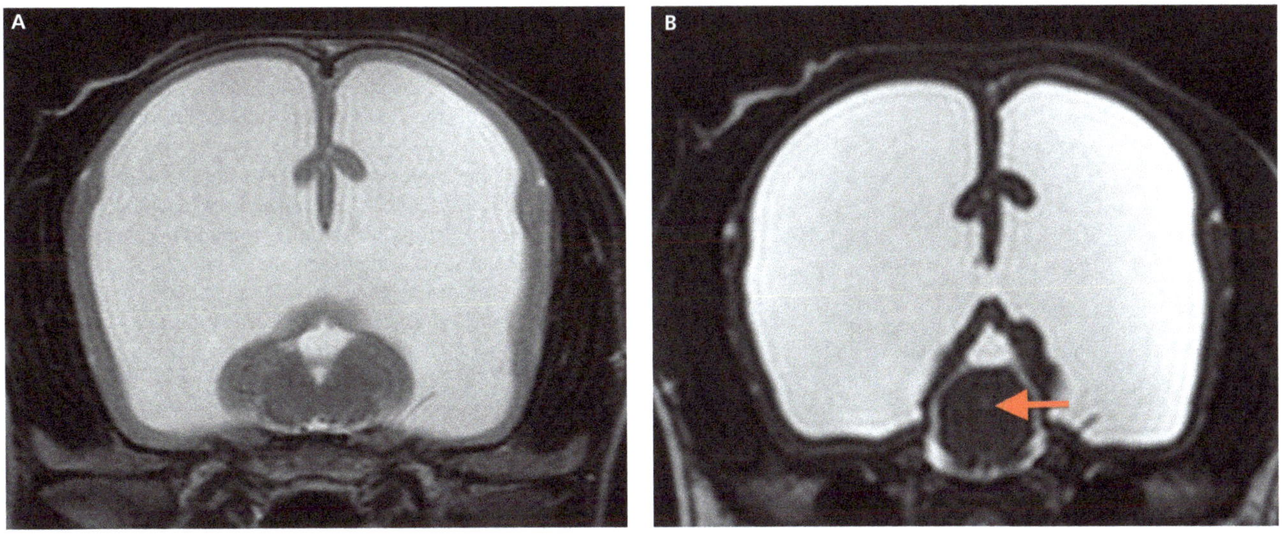

Figure 4.21 Transverse T2-weighted (A) and constructive interference in steady state, or CISS (B) MRI of a 5-month-old dog with severe congenital hydrocephalus. The cortical thinning and massive dilation of the ventricles and thin dome-shaped calvarium may be seen in congenital hydrocephalus but are not seen with acquired hydrocephalus in older dogs. The hydrocephalus was due to stenosis (arrow) of the mesencephalic aqueduct with reduced size and axial displacement of the caudal colliculi visible on the CISS image.

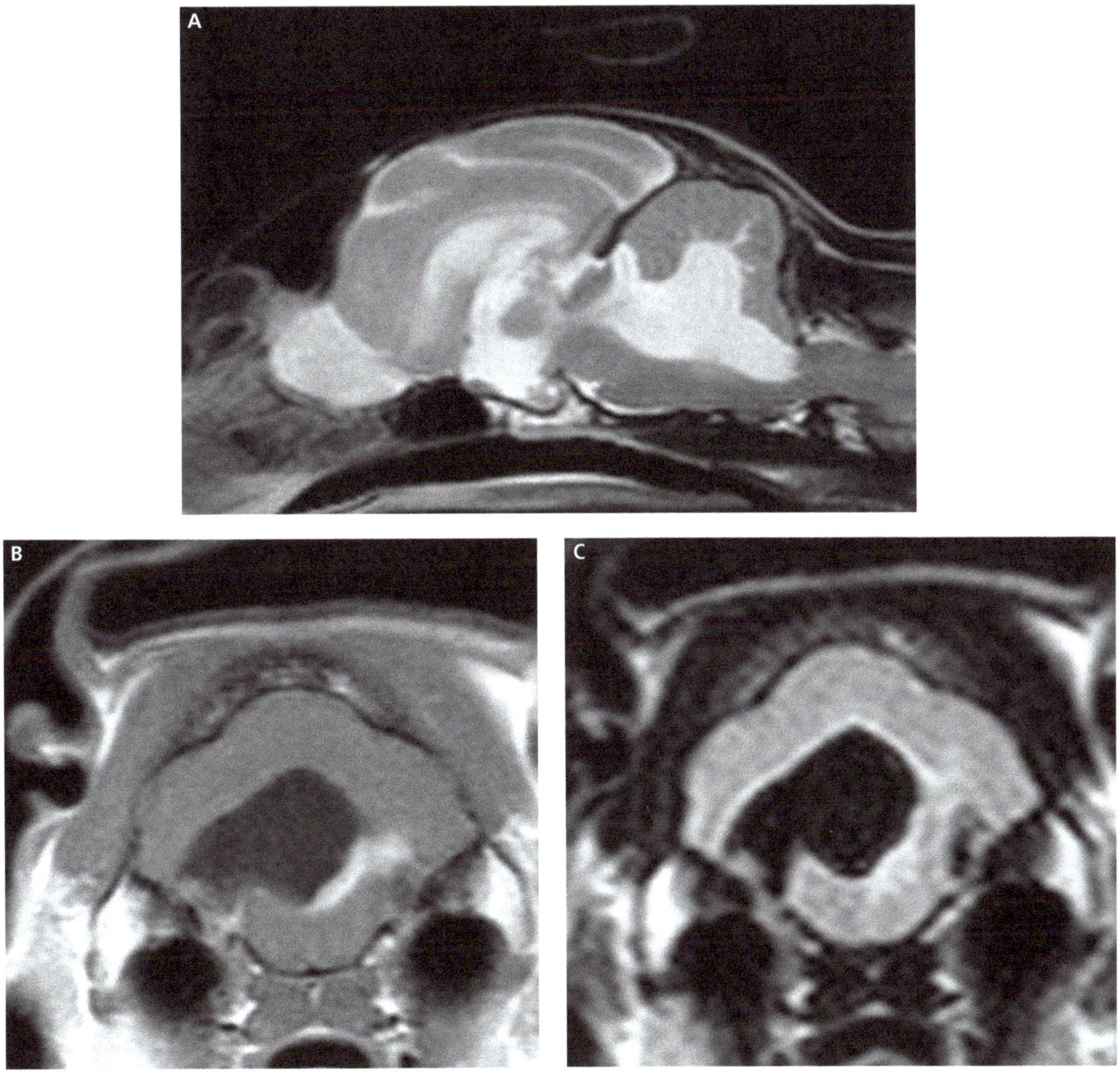

Figure 4.22 Sagittal T2-weighted (A), transverse FLAIR (B), and transverse T1-weighted postcontrast (C) MRI of a cat with obstructive hydrocephalus due to feline infectious peritonitis. Note the dilation of all parts of the ventricular system rostral to the foramen magnum, indicating that the obstruction to CSF flow is likely to be at the lateral apertures of the fourth ventricle or at the foramen magnum. The FLAIR and postcontrast images show abnormal T2 hyperintensity and enhancement of the ependyma within the fourth ventricle and irregular enhancement of the choroid plexi commonly seen with FIP. On the sagittal T2-weighted images the low signal of the CSF within the mesencephalic aqueduct was due to a flow artifact.

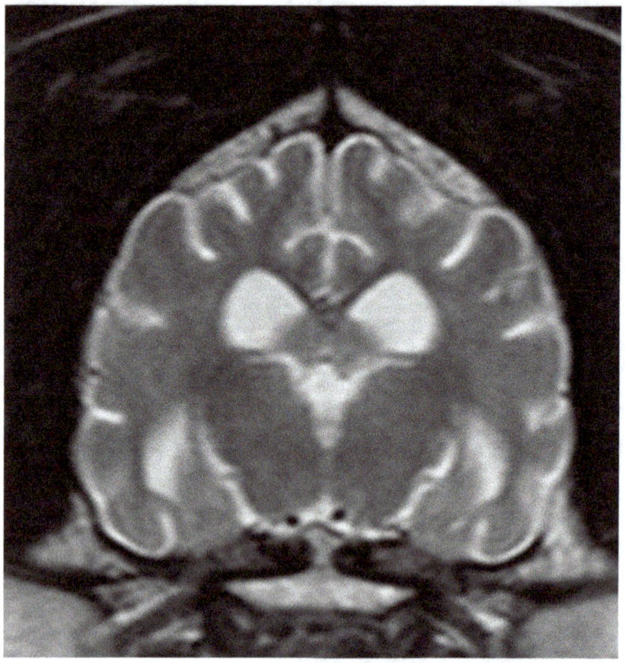

Figure 4.23 Transverse T2-weighted MRI of an aged dog with cortical atrophy due to senile changes. Note the sulcal widening and mild ventriculomegaly. Increased intraventricular pressure in obstructive hydrocephalus may result in reduced or absent CSF signal within the sulci.

minimized with real-time information obtained by real-time imaging techniques [122]. Intraoperative image guidance may also provide critical information during resection of tumors with a consistency similar to normal brain tissue by delineating T2-weighted imaging margins. This information, coupled with intraoperative stimulation mapping data for lesions involving functionally eloquent cortical and subcortical areas, enables the surgeon to maximize resection without causing additional neurological morbidity. In addition, intraoperative anatomical information is helpful by visualizing any brain displacement that may occur intraoperatively as a result of resection cavity, brain retraction, or CSF leakage, causing significant discrepancy between preoperative imaging data and the surgical field [124].

Intraoperative imaging is more powerful than direct visualization in detecting diseased tissue from normal brain parenchyma because it permits one to see beyond the exposed surgical field. Following resection, intraoperative imaging techniques may be used to determine the extent of resection and to check for any residual disease. Overall, intraoperative image guidance techniques help the neurosurgeon to plan surgery, approach and resect the tumor, and evaluate the extent of resection.

Intraoperative Ultrasonography

Intraoperative ultrasonography provides a method for obtaining real-time imaging of the intracranial contents during surgical procedures for precise localization of a lesion within the surgical field. The craniotomy used for the surgery provides the acoustic window necessary to image the CNS tissue. The portability, low cost, safety, and real-time evaluation capability of intraoperative ultrasound make this technology an important adjunct in the treatment of neurosurgical disease [123]. It has been shown to be useful in the management of intracranial tumors (Figure 4.24), cysts, abscesses, vascular malformations, and hematomas. Recent studies reveal that cranial ultrasound is diagnostically accurate when compared with MRI and useful for determining initial clinical management [125,126].

The size of the craniotomy determines the size of the transducer used. Subcortical lesions can be insonated at a frequency of 7.5 to 15 MHz or more, which provides a high-resolution image [127]. For superficial lesions, small-footprint linear transducers can be used which have little near-field artifact. Deeper lesions may require a lower-frequency transducer because attenuation is less with lower-frequency sound. The selected probe is draped in a sterile cover filled with sterile jelly and all air bubbles should be eliminated. Sterile irrigation with saline is employed during the procedure to ensure optimal coupling. The probe frequency is adjusted (with a variable frequency probe) to suitably insonate both superficial and deep structures as required [128].

Several investigators have described the benefits of using intraoperative ultrasonography [129–138]. In a study of 186 patients, Rubin and Dohrmann [139] found intraoperative ultrasonography to be more useful for small subcortical lesions. The literature describes a number of novel uses of intraoperative ultrasonography, ranging from the more traditional localization of subcortical lesions to the localization of contusions in trauma and monitoring of ventricular catheter placement [140,141]. The efficacy of ultrasound in localizing the lesion, especially for metastases and high-grade tumors, is good [132,133,142]. Even with low-grade diffuse gliomas, ultrasound has been shown to be better able to demarcate the hyperechoic tumor, which may not be discernible on CT [143,144] and difficult to localize with the naked eye at surgery. However, there remain concerns regarding the ability of ultrasound to resolve differences between peritumoral edema, infiltrative margin, and normal parenchyma [145]. Interestingly, in a study where histological correlation was attempted, ultrasound showed a good positive predictive value for tumor-infiltrated margin [146]. However, it was less reliable in cases followed after treatment, where diffuse changes related to the treatment effect could not be differentiated from recurrence of tumor [147]. It is also unable to provide histological characterization of lesions [131,132] but is an excellent tool for differentiating solid and cystic lesions. Attempts have even been made to perform volumetric studies using intraoperative ultrasound. However, its efficacy vis-á-vis MRI remains to be proven [135,147–149]. With advances in image resolution and use of contrast ultrasound, there could be better scope in the future [150–152]. Another recent application of intraoperative ultrasound in cranial neurosurgery has been to correct for the effect of brain shift after craniotomy or stereotactic localization of lesions [153].

The use of intraoperative micro-Doppler sonography has become invaluable to vascular neurosurgeons in human medicine. With current technology, vessels less than 1 mm in diameter can be discretely insolated to assess for patency. Although crude compared with transcranial Doppler or duplex sonography, micro-Doppler can determine vessel patency, direction of flow, and the presence of laminar versus turbulent flow. With this technology, anastomotic sites can easily be evaluated in bypass surgery, and the patency of parent vessels and their branches can be assessed during aneurysm clipping.

Recently, a report described 25 dogs which underwent craniotomy or craniectomy procedures for removal/debulking of an intracranial mass using intraoperative ultrasound-guided visualization of the mass. Mass removal was accomplished using an ultrasonic aspirator. Of the 25 patients, 24 survived surgery and 17 were eventually discharged to the owners' care. In all patients, the intracranial mass

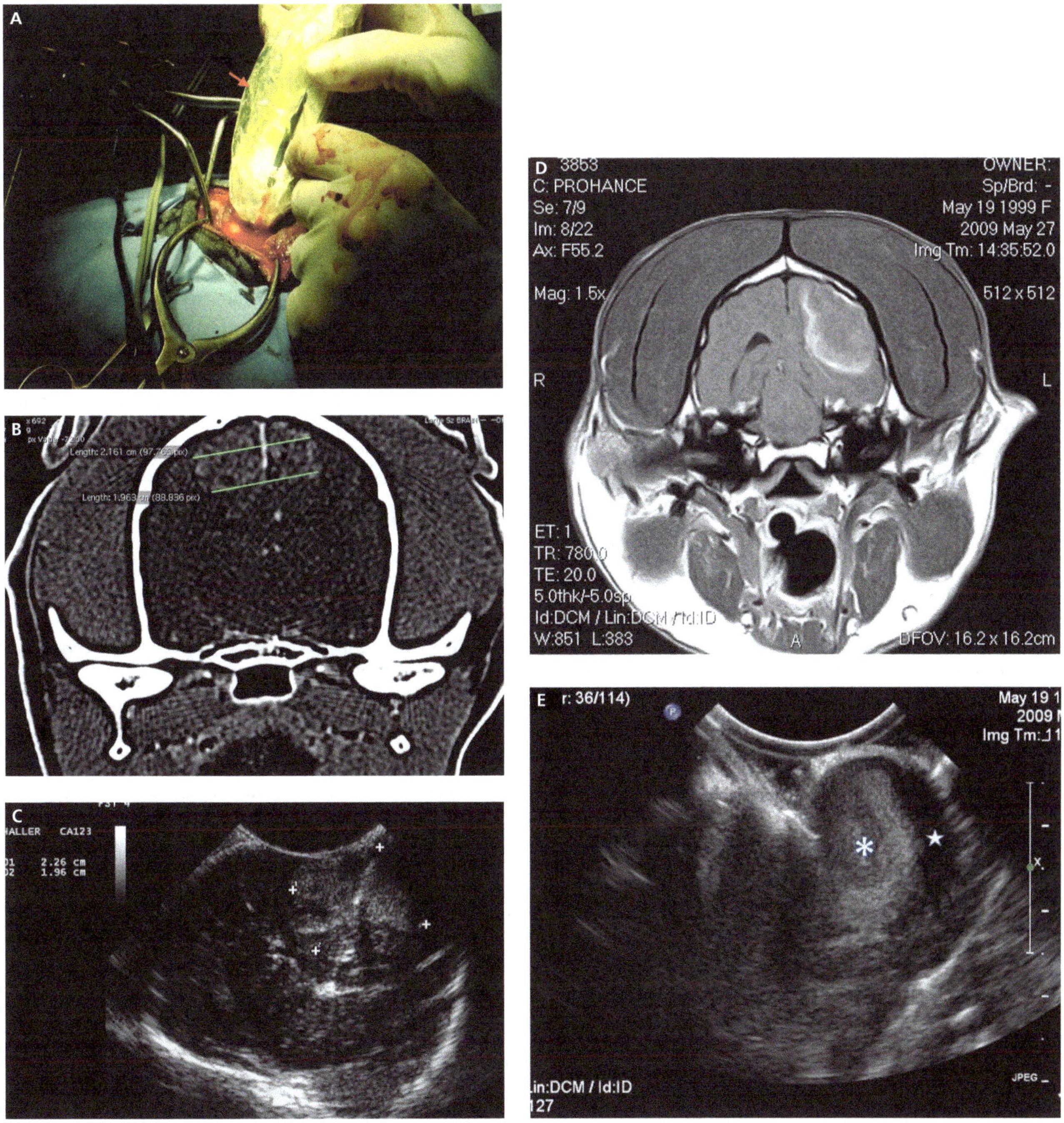

Figure 4.24 Intraoperative ultrasound. (A) The ultrasound probe (arrow) is covered with a sterile sleeve, the opening in the calvarium is flooded with warm saline, and the probe is placed directly on the brain parenchyma. Sterile ultrasound gel is placed inside the sleeve. (B, C) A transfalcine meningioma on CT and intraoperatively using ultrasound. (D, E) A left cortical high-grade glioma on transverse MRI and on intraoperative ultrasound imaging. In (E), the asterisk denotes the hyperechoic mass and the star a hypoechoic region where some of the mass has been removed using an ultrasonic surgical aspirator (CUSA).

was identified intraoperatively after craniectomy and durotomy using a 5–8 MHz probe enveloped in a sterile sleeve containing sterile ultrasound lubricant. The covered probe was placed directly on the cerebral, cerebellar, or brainstem tissue to visualize the mass after flooding the craniectomy site with sterile saline. The intracranial lesions were imaged in both sagittal and transverse planes. Most of each intracranial neoplasm appeared distinctly hyperechoic. The distinct imaging characteristics of the ventricles, falx cerebri, gray matter, and white matter were easily differentiated from the generally more heterogeneous hyperechoic intracranial tumors. Cystic areas of the tumors and the one cystic mass in this study were contrasted from surrounding structures by their hypoechogenicity. Size and shape of the masses approximated the same parameters identified on advanced imaging (MRI, CT). Noncystic portions of the meningiomas appeared most hyperechoic. The gliomas often were less heterogeneously hyperechoic than the meningiomas. Vascular supply to the intracranial tumors was detected by color Doppler and aided in directing the approach to the masses using the ultrasonic aspirator [154].

Correlating the preoperative MRI or CT images with the intraoperative ultrasound images was very valuable to the surgeons in gaining a perspective of the size of the mass, the proximity of ventricles, the eloquent areas of the brain, and the location of larger blood vessels. In addition, the serial images consistently gave the surgeons a definitive perspective on the completeness of the resection and helped differentiate grossly abnormal from grossly normal structures. Postoperative imaging correlated well with ultrasound imaging at the conclusion of the surgeries. The authors conclude that the use of intraoperative ultrasound imaging is a valuable adjunct and correlates well with both preoperative and postoperative advanced imaging. Intraoperative ultrasound should be a standard imaging modality for intracranial procedures. Additional development of this technique, including the use of three-dimensional ultrasound, is warranted. Intraoperative ultrasonography is helpful in localizing and defining the margins of intracranial masses and accurately determines the extent of resection, as confirmed by postoperative MRI or CT [154].

Image-guided Brain Biopsy in Veterinary Patients

Needle biopsy may be performed either "freehand," usually to access very superficial lesions through a burr-hole created following imaging and localization (with or without the assistance of ultrasonography), or using a stereotactic frame to guide the needle, again following imaging and localization. Freehand fine-needle aspiration may also be performed on superficial lesions.

Stereotactic biopsy is generally performed using a side-cutting brain cannula. The cannula is a blunt-ended needle with an inner and outer sheath, both of which contain a lateral window. Once the cannula is introduced into the region to be sampled, tissue is drawn into the inner sheath using gentle suction applied via a syringe attached to the end of the cannula. The inner sheath is then rotated through 180° in relation to the outer sheath; the sharp edges of the lateral window of the inner sheath excise the brain fragment within the inner sheath using a guillotine action. The sample is then collected by withdrawing the inner sheath from the outer sheath. Stereotactic needle biopsy has been used in human neurosurgical institutions extensively over the past two decades, and stereotactic frames and biopsy systems have now been developed for use with dogs and cats, although they are not yet widely available [10,40,155–161].

Frameless stereotactic systems have also been developed which utilize cameras and fiducial markers placed on the skin to triangulate the position of the tip of the biopsy needle in three-dimensional space and reference this to previously acquired CT or MRI images in real time.

CT-assisted Biopsy

The most well-documented CT-guided brain biopsy system in veterinary use is a modification of the Pelorus Mark III Stereotactic System, which is a commercially available device for CT-guided stereotactic brain biopsy in humans [159,160]. This device has been used to safely and accurately perform CT-guided stereotactic brain biopsies in dogs with intracranial lesions. Modifications were necessary to accommodate a 90° shift in orientation of the canine head compared with the human head during the imaging phase of the procedure, and to facilitate other phases of the biopsy procedure that are affected by the uneven and variable topography of the canine skull. A description of a typical CT-guided brain biopsy procedure in dogs using the modified Pelorus Mark III Stereotactic System has been published [159,160]. Accuracy of biopsy needle placement was determined by comparing the *x*, *y*, and *z* coordinates of the biopsy target site with the actual coordinates of the needle tip on CT images. Mean needle placement error was 3.5 ± 1.6 mm. Needle placement error was not significantly related to operator experience, dog size (body weight), or needle path length, although needle placement error was significantly affected by lesion location [160]. CT-guided stereotactic brain biopsies were performed on 50 consecutive dogs using this system [159]. Based on available histopathological samples (stereotactic biopsy, $n = 50$; surgery, $n = 17$; necropsy, $n = 9$) the patient population consisted of 34 dogs with primary brain tumors, two with invasive nasal adenocarcinomas, and 13 with nonneoplastic brain lesions. Brain tissue was not obtained from one dog. In 22 dogs a final diagnosis was made from tissue subsequently obtained from surgical resection or at necropsy. The final diagnosis was in agreement with the stereotactic biopsy diagnosis in 20 of these 22 dogs. In 17 other dogs without follow-up, stereotactic biopsy provided a diagnosis of a specific primary brain tumor subtype.

Postoperative complications associated with the biopsy procedure were assessed in 41 dogs. The other nine dogs either went directly to surgery ($n = 7$) or were euthanized ($n = 2$) immediately after the biopsy procedure; 36 dogs recovered without apparent clinical complications. Postoperative clinical complications in the remaining five dogs included transient epistaxis (one dog), transient exacerbation of cerebellar signs (one dog), obtundation progressing to coma (one dog), and medically uncontrollable seizures (two dogs). The latter three dogs with severe neurological complications all had large primary brain tumors and had been receiving high doses of phenobarbital and glucocorticoids to control seizures at the time of biopsy. These results suggest that this CT-guided biopsy procedure can provide an accurate pathological diagnosis of brain lesions detected by CT and MRI neuroimaging [159].

A more recent study evaluated a Kopf stereotactic system, a commercially available patient restraint system that does not require additional modification for use in small animals [40]. The accuracy of biopsy needle placement was determined by injecting dilute iohexol into cadaver brains and comparing the three-dimensional coordinates of the desired target location to the actual needle tract observed on postcontrast CT images. Overall mean error in needle placement in a dorsoventral trajectory was 0.9 ± 0.9 mm ($n = 80$ injections) for dogs and 1.0 ± 1.1 mm ($n = 30$ injections) for cats. The overall mean error in needle placement via an oblique trajectory in five dogs was 1.7 ± 1.6 mm ($n = 12$ injections). Another study assessing a different device evaluated its accuracy on 23 client-owned dogs which presented with a brain lesion [157]. Biopsy of the lesion was achieved in 95% of cases. The target tissue was not sampled in one dog. Complications were observed in six dogs. Two dogs with highly vascularized brainstem tumors died after CT-guided stereotactic brain biopsy. Minor complications (slight variation in the neurological status) were observed in a further four cases. A diagnosis was reached in 16 dogs after cytological examination and in 21 dogs after histological evaluation.

MRI-assisted Biopsy

The Brainsight™ system is an example of a frameless stereotactic MRI device developed for use in animals, and has the advantage of allowing both needle biopsy and intraoperative navigation to be performed during open craniectomy (Figure 4.25) [161]. A recent

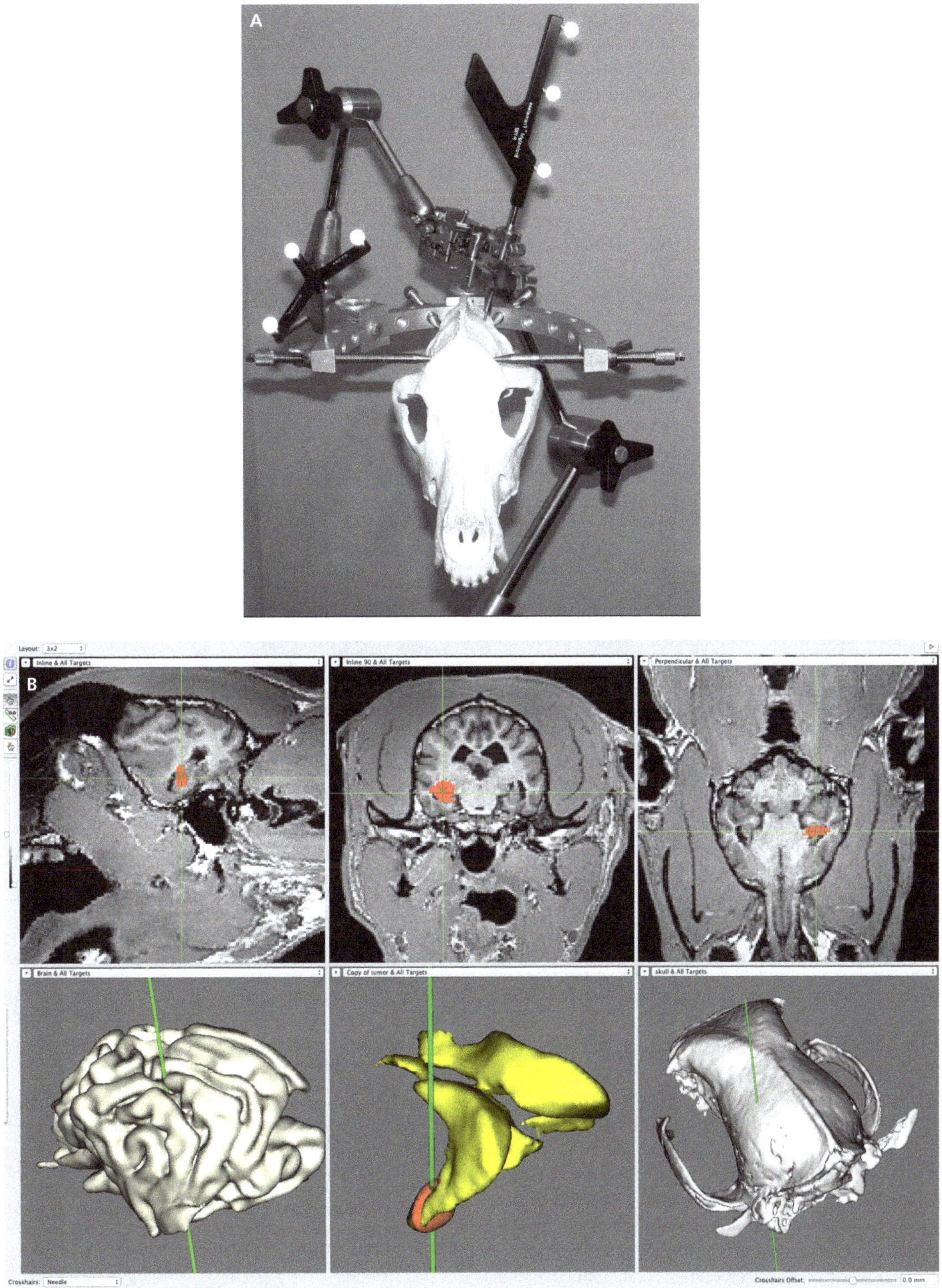

Figure 4.25 Brainsight™ stereotactic MRI-based biopsy device. (A) During surgery, the head of the animal is held rigidly in place using a c-clamp and skull screws, which press against the animal's skull. The c-clamp is attached to a standard operating table using a large adjustable arm. An articulated surgical arm is attached the c-clamp to guide tools to the target. In conjunction with the neuronavigation software and the position sensor, a path is set to target the brain of the animal. (B) Brainsight™ software enables the three-dimensional reconstruction of clinical data, which is then used to target a tumor with a biopsy needle. Reconstructions of the skin, skull, and brain are generated from the magnetic resonance images. A lesion or tumor is identified as a target (red) in the right temporal region using MRI of the dog and the Brainsight™ software. The center of the target is visualized in three dimensions and the most appropriate trajectory to the tumor, avoiding key structures such as the ventricular system (yellow), is saved by the software. Coregistration of the animal to the magnetic resonance images is performed by identifying homologous points between the images and the subject with the help of fiducial markers that are rigidly fixed to the animal's head. Once registered, neuronavigation is performed in real time with the aid of a position sensor in the operating suite to precisely target the tumor. *Sources*: (A) Courtesy of Rogue Research Inc.; (B) Courtesy of Stephen Frey.

study aimed to determine the mean needle placement error in the caudate nucleus, thalamus, and midbrain of a canine cadaver brain using the modified Brainsight stereotactic system. Relocatable fiducial markers were attached to a cadaver head using a dental bite block. A T1-weighted GRE three-dimensional sequence was acquired using set parameters. Fiducial markers were used to register the head to the acquired images in reference to a three-dimensional position sensor. This allowed the planning of trajectory path to brain targets in real time. Coordinates (x, y, z) were established for each target and 0.5 µL of diluted gadolinium was injected at each target using a 26 G needle to create a lesion. The center of the gadolinium deposition was identified on the postoperative images and coordinates (x', y', z') were established. The precision of this system in bringing the needle to target (needle placement error) was calculated. Seventeen sites were targeted in the brain. The mean needle placement error for all target sites was 1.79 ± 0.87 mm. The upper bound of error for this stereotactic system was 3.31 mm. There was no statistically significant relationship between needle placement error and target depth ($P = 0.23$). The ease of use and precision of this stereotactic system support its development for clinical use in dogs with brain lesions larger than 3.31 mm [161].

Summary

The decision regarding which method to use is dictated primarily by the facilities available to the neurosurgeon. Other factors that need to be considered include the appearance of the lesion on CT and/or MRI, the location of the lesion (intraaxial vs. extraaxial), and the neurological status of the patient. If the neurological status of the patient is poor and raised ICP is suspected, a craniectomy and biopsy may be performed to allow decompression and alleviation of the clinical signs, in addition to providing tissue for diagnosis. However, lesions in deep structures may be difficult to biopsy via an open craniectomy. This particularly applies to lesions in the deep gray matter of the forebrain (e.g., thalamus and hypothalamus) or brainstem (e.g., medulla oblongata). In this situation, stereotactic needle biopsy may be preferable, if available, as it causes less damage to vital structures. With lesions that are thought to be very vascular, based on their imaging characteristics, conventional biopsy obtained via a craniectomy may be more desirable than a needle biopsy as hemorrhage can be controlled intraoperatively.

Stereotactic biopsy is also associated with complications, although these are generally rare. The most common problem is hemorrhage caused by the biopsy procedure; this may lead to significant neurological deficits and can be life-threatening. To prevent this, the trajectory of the biopsy needle must be planned carefully in order to avoid major blood vessels and care should be taken if imaging findings suggest the lesion is highly vascular (e.g., choroid plexus papilloma). In addition, it is important to maintain normal systemic blood pressure during surgery, as hypertension in humans has been reported to increase the risk of hemorrhage following biopsy. As with conventional craniectomy, postoperative imaging is recommended following needle biopsy to detect hemorrhage. Close monitoring of the patient's neurological status should also be performed for 48 hours following the procedure and scanning should be repeated if any deterioration in the level of consciousness occurs. In rare cases, a craniectomy may be required to alleviate raised ICP or to adequately control hemorrhage.

A rare complication reported in humans is "seeding" of a tumor along the needle tract. Morbidity and mortality rates associated with brain biopsy in dogs and cats are 12–26% and 7–8%, respectively, and are higher than in humans (morbidity 3.5%, mortality <1%) [157–160]. In addition, it should be remembered that due to the small volume of tissue yielded during needle biopsy procedures, it is fairly common to obtain a nondiagnostic sample, especially if a nonrepresentative part of the tumor is targeted. It is therefore extremely helpful to perform cytology or to preserve frozen sections during the procedure to ensure that a representative sample has been obtained.

Video clips to accompany this book can be found on the companion website at:
www.wiley.com/go/shores/neurosurgery

References

1 Bar-Am Y, Pollard RE, Kass PH, Verstraete FJ. The diagnostic yield of conventional radiographs and computed tomography in dogs and cats with maxillofacial trauma. *Vet Surg* 2008;37:294–299.

2 Doust R, King A, Hammond G et al. Assessment of middle ear disease in the dog: a comparison of diagnostic imaging modalities. *J Small Anim Pract* 2007;48: 188–192.

3 Smith CW, Marshall AE, Knecht CD. Detection of artificially produced intracranial midline shifts of the brain in the dog with A-mode echoencephalography. *Am J Vet Res* 1972;33:2423–2427.

4 Smith CW, Marshall AE, Knecht CD. Use of A-mode echoencephalography in the dog. *Am J Vet Res* 1972;33:2415–2421.

5 Hudson JA, Finn-Bodner ST, Steiss JE. Neurosonography. *Vet Clin North Am Small Anim Pract* 1998;28:943–972.

6 Harrington ML, Bagley RS, Moore MP. Hydrocephalus. *Vet Clin North Am Small Anim Pract* 1996;26:843–856.

7 Tucker RL, Gavin PR. Brain imaging. *Vet Clin North Am Small Anim Pract* 1996;26:735–758.

8 Brown JA, Rachlin J, Rubin JM, Wollmann RL. Ultrasound evaluation of experimental hydrocephalus in dogs. *Surg Neurol* 1984;22:273–276.

9 Platt SR, Graham J, Chrisman CL et al. Magnetic resonance imaging and ultrasonography in the diagnosis of a malignant peripheral nerve sheath tumor in a dog. *Vet Radiol Ultrasound* 1999;40:367–371.

10 Thomas WB, Sorjonen DC, Hudson JA, Cox NR. Ultrasound-guided brain biopsy in dogs. *Am J Vet Res* 1993;54:1942–1947.

11 Brown FD, Rachlin JR, Rubin JM, Fessler RG, Smith LJ, Schaible KL. Ultrasound-guided periventricular stereotaxis. *Neurosurgery* 1984;15:162–164.

12 Chandrana C, Bevan P, Hudson J et al. Development of a platform for co-registered ultrasound and MR contrast imaging in vivo. *Physics Med Biol* 2011;56:861–877.

13 Noureddine C, Harder R, Olby NJ, Spaulding K, Brown T. Ultrasonographic appearance of Dandy Walker-like syndrome in a Boston Terrier. *Vet Radiol Ultrasound.* 2004;45:336–339.

14 Saito M, Olby NJ, Spaulding K. Identification of arachnoid cysts in the quadrigeminal cistern using ultrasonography. *Vet Radiol Ultrasound.* 2001;42:435–439.

15 Gallagher JG, Penninck D, Boudrieau RJ, Schelling SH, Berg J. Ultrasonography of the brain and vertebral canal in dogs and cats: 15 cases (1988–1993). *J Am Vet Med Assoc* 1995;207:1320–1324.

16 Werner C, Hoffman WE, Kochs E, Albrecht RF, Schulte am Esch J. Transcranial Doppler sonography indicates critical brain perfusion during hemorrhagic hypotension in dogs. *Anesth Analg* 1995;81:1203–1207.

17 Rim SJ, Leong-Poi H, Lindner JR et al. Quantification of cerebral perfusion with "real-time" contrast-enhanced ultrasound. *Circulation* 2001;104:2582–2587.

18 Hudson JA, Buxton DF, Cox NR et al. Color flow Doppler imaging and Doppler spectral analysis of the brain of neonatal dogs. *Vet Radiol Ultrasound* 1997; 38:313–322.

19 Saito M, Olby NJ, Spaulding K, Munana K, Sharp NJ. Relationship among basilar artery resistance index, degree of ventriculomegaly, and clinical signs in hydrocephalic dogs. *Vet Radiol Ultrasound* 2003;44:687–694.

20 Fukushima U, Miyashita K, Okano S, Higuchi S, Takase K, Hagio M. Evaluation of intracranial pressure by transcranial Doppler ultrasonography in dogs with intracranial hypertension. *J Vet Med Sci* 2000;62:353–355.

21 Carvalho CF, Perez RB, Chamas MC, Maiorka PC. Transcranial Doppler sonographic findings in granulomatous meningoencephalitis in small breed dogs. *Can Vet J* 2012;53:855–859.

22 Fukushima U, Sasaki S, Okano S et al. Non-invasive diagnosis of ischemic brain damage after cardiopulmonary resuscitation in dogs by using transcranial Doppler ultrasonography. *Vet Radiol Ultrasound* 2000;41:172–177.

23 Britt RH, Lyons BE, Enzmann DR, Saxer EL, Bigner SH, Bigner DD. Correlation of neuropathologic findings, computerized tomographic and high-resolution ultrasound scans of canine avian sarcoma virus-induced brain tumors. *J Neurooncol* 1987;4:243–268.

24 Lillehei KO, Chandler WF, Knake JE. Real time ultrasound characteristics of the acute intracerebral hemorrhage as studied in the canine model. *Neurosurgery* 1984;14:48–51.
25 Enzmann DR, Britt RH, Lyons B, Carroll B, Wilson DA, Buxton J. High-resolution ultrasound evaluation of experimental brain abscess evolution: comparison with computed tomography and neuropathology. *Radiology* 1982;142:95–102.
26 Enzmann DR, Lyons BE, Carroll B et al. Experimental brain abscess: enhanced sonography and pathologic correlation. *AJNR Am J Neuroradiol* 1982;3:41–45.
27 Light ED, Mukundan S, Wolf PD, Smith SW. Real-time 3-D intracranial ultrasound with an endoscopic matrix array transducer. *Ultrasound Med Biol* 2007;33: 1277–1284.
28 Mahesh M. Search for isotropic resolution in CT from conventional through multiple-row detector. *Radiographics* 2002;22:949–962.
29 De Rycke LM, Gielen IM, Van Meervenne SA, Simoens PJ, van Bree HJ. Computed tomography and cross-sectional anatomy of the brain in clinically normal dogs. *Am J Vet Res* 2005;66:1743–1756.
30 Naidich TP, Lin JP, Leeds NE, Pudlowski RM, Naidich JB. Primary tumors and other masses of the cerebellum and fourth ventricle: differential diagnosis by computed tomography. *Neuroradiology* 1977;14:153–174.
31 Koo AH, LaRoque RL. Evaluation of head trauma by computed tomography. *Radiology* 1977;123:345–350.
32 Liliequist B, Lindqvist M, Valdimarsson E. Computed tomography and subarachnoid hemorrhage. *Neuroradiology* 1977;14:21–26.
33 Ducote JM, Johnson KE, Dewey CW, Walker MA, Coates JR, Berridge BR. Computed tomography of necrotizing meningoencephalitis in 3 Yorkshire Terriers. *Vet Radiol Ultrasound* 1999;40:617–621.
34 Lin JP, Pay N, Naidich TP, Kricheff, II, Wiggli U. Computed tomography in the postoperative care of neurosurgical patients. *Neuroradiology* 1977;12:185–189.
35 Hryshko FG, Deeb ZL. Computed tomography in acute head injuries. *J Comput Tomogr* 1983;7:331–344.
36 Merino-deVillasante J, Taveras JM. Computerized tomography (CT) in acute head trauma. *AJR Am J Roentgenol* 1976;126:765–778.
37 Fitz CR, Harwood-Nash DC. Computed tomography in hydrocephalus. *J Comput Tomogr* 1978;2:91–108.
38 Harden SP, Dey C, Gawne-Cain ML. Cranial CT of the unconscious adult patient. *Clin Radiol* 2007;62:404–415.
39 Paul AE, Lenard Z, Mansfield CS. Computed tomography diagnosis of eight dogs with brain infarction. *Aust Vet J* 2010;88:374–380.
40 Troxel MT, Vite CH. CT-guided stereotactic brain biopsy using the Kopf stereotactic system. *Vet Radiol Ultrasound* 2008;49:438–443.
41 Thomas WB. Nonneoplastic disorders of the brain. *Clin Tech Small Animal Pract* 1999;14:125–147.
42 Tidwell AS, Jones JC. Advanced imaging concepts: a pictorial glossary of CT and MRI technology. *Clin Tech Small Animal Pract* 1999;14:65–111.
43 Vernau KM, Kortz GD, Koblik PD, LeCouteur RA, Bailey CS, Pedroia V. Magnetic resonance imaging and computed tomography characteristics of intracranial intra-arachnoid cysts in 6 dogs. *Vet Radiol Ultrasound* 1997;38:171–176.
44 Iwamoto KS, Norman A, Freshwater DB, Ingram M, Skillen RG. Diagnosis and treatment of spontaneous canine brain tumors with a CT scanner. *Radiother Oncol* 1993;26:76–78.
45 Whelan HT, Clanton JA, Wilson RE, Tulipan NB. Comparison of CT and MRI brain tumor imaging using a canine glioma model. *Pediatr Neurol* 1988;4:279–283.
46 Kidwell CS, Chalela JA, Saver JL et al. Comparison of MRI and CT for detection of acute intracerebral hemorrhage. *JAMA* 2004;292:1823–1830.
47 Hecht S, Adams WH. MRI of brain disease in veterinary patients. Part 1: Basic principles and congenital brain disorders. *Vet Clin North Am Small Anim Pract* 2010;40:21–38.
48 Martin-Vaquero P, da Costa RC, Echandi RL, Tosti CL, Knopp MV, Sammet S. Time-of-flight magnetic resonance angiography of the canine brain at 3.0 Tesla and 7.0 Tesla. *Am J Vet Res* 2011;72:350–356.
49 Martin-Vaquero P, Da Costa RC, Echandi RL, Tosti CL, Knopp MV, Sammet S. Magnetic resonance imaging of the canine brain at 3 and 7 T. *Vet Radiol Ultrasound* 2011;52:25–32.
50 Kang BT, Ko KJ, Jang DP et al. Magnetic resonance imaging of the canine brain at 7 T. *Vet Radiol Ultrasound* 2009;50:615–621.
51 Kang MH, Lim CY, Park C, Yoo JH, Kim DY, Park HM. 7.0-Tesla Tesla magnetic resonance imaging of granulomatous meningoencephalitis in a Maltese dog: a comparison with 0.2 and 1.5-Tesla. *J Vet Med Sci* 2009;71:1545–1548.
52 Konar M, Lang J. Pros and cons of low-field magnetic resonance imaging in veterinary practice. *Vet Radiol Ultrasound* 2011;52(1 Suppl 1):S5–S14.
53 D'Anjou MA, Carmel EN, Blond L, Beauchamp G, Parent J. Effect of acquisition time and chemical fat suppression on meningeal enhancement on MR imaging in dogs. *Vet Radiol Ultrasound* 2012;53:11–20.
54 Lowrie M, De Risio L, Dennis R, Llabres-Diaz F, Garosi L. Concurrent medical conditions and long-term outcome in dogs with nontraumatic intracranial hemorrhage. *Vet Radiol Ultrasound* 2012;53:381–388.
55 Fulkerson CV, Young BD, Jackson ND, Porter B, Levine JM. MRI characteristics of cerebral microbleeds in four dogs. *Vet Radiol Ultrasound* 2012;53:389–393.
56 de Souza JM, Domingues RC, Cruz LC Jr, Domingues FS, Iasbeck T, Gasparetto EL. Susceptibility-weighted imaging for the evaluation of patients with familial cerebral cavernous malformations: a comparison with T2-weighted fast spin-echo and gradient-echo sequences. *AJNR Am J Neuroradiol* 2008;29:154–158.
57 Ober CP, Warrington CD, Feeney DA, Jessen CR, Steward S. Optimizing a protocol for (1)H-magnetic resonance spectroscopy of the canine brain at 3T. *Vet Radiol Ultrasound* 2013;54:149–158.
58 Martin-Vaquero P, da Costa RC, Echandi RL, Sammet CL, Knopp MV, Sammet S. Magnetic resonance spectroscopy of the canine brain at 3.0 T and 7.0 T. *Res Vet Sci* 2012;93:427–429.
59 Barker PB, Bizzi A, Stefano ND, Gullapalli R, Lin DDM (eds) *Clinical MR Spectroscopy: Techniques and Applications.* Cambridge: Cambridge University Press, 2010.
60 van der Graaf M. In vivo magnetic resonance spectroscopy: basic methodology and clinical applications. *Eur Biophys J* 2010;39:527–540.
61 Brown MA, Semelka RC. *MRI: Basic Principles and Applications*, 4th edn. Hoboken, NJ: Wiley-Blackwell, 2010.
62 Anderson JH, Strandberg JD, Wong DF et al. Multimodality correlative study of canine brain tumors. Proton magnetic resonance spectroscopy, positron emission tomography, and histology. *Invest Radiol* 1994;29:597–605.
63 Bendini M, Marton E, Feletti A et al. Primary and metastatic intraaxial brain tumors: prospective comparison of multivoxel 2D chemical-shift imaging (CSI) proton MR spectroscopy, perfusion MRI, and histopathological findings in a group of 159 patients. *Acta Neurochir (Wien)* 2011;153:403–412.
64 Buhl R, Stark AM, Hugo HH, Rohr A, Mehdorn HM. Gliosarcoma: clinical experiences and additional information with MR spectroscopy. *Neurol Res* 2009;31: 873–877.
65 Castillo M, Kwock L, Scatliff J, Mukherji SK. Proton MR spectroscopy in neoplastic and non-neoplastic brain disorders. *Magn Reson Imaging Clin North Am* 1998;6: 1–20.
66 Fountas KN, Kapsalaki EZ, Gotsis SD et al. In vivo proton magnetic resonance spectroscopy of brain tumors. *Stereotact Funct Neurosurg* 2000;74:83–94.
67 Gillies RJ, Bhujwalla ZM, Evelhoch J et al. Applications of magnetic resonance in model systems: tumor biology and physiology. *Neoplasia* 2000;2:139–151.
68 Gillies RJ, Raghunand N, Karczmar GS, Bhujwalla ZM. MRI of the tumor microenvironment. *J Magn Reson Imaging* 2002;16:430–450.
69 Horska A, Barker PB. Imaging of brain tumors: MR spectroscopy and metabolic imaging. *Neuroimaging Clin North Am* 2010;20:293–310.
70 Hourani R, Horska A, Albayram S et al. Proton magnetic resonance spectroscopic imaging to differentiate between nonneoplastic lesions and brain tumors in children. *J Magn Reson Imaging* 2006;23:99–107.
71 Kinoshita Y, Yokota A. Absolute concentrations of metabolites in human brain tumors using in vitro proton magnetic resonance spectroscopy. *NMR Biomed* 1997;10:2–12.
72 Lehnhardt FG, Röhn G, Ernestus RI, Grüne M, Hoehn M. ^{1}H- and ^{31}P-MR spectroscopy of primary and recurrent human brain tumors in vitro: malignancy-characteristic profiles of water soluble and lipophilic spectral components. *NMR Biomed* 2001;14:307–317.
73 Meyerand ME, Pipas JM, Mamourian A, Tosteson TD, Dunn JF. Classification of biopsy-confirmed brain tumors using single-voxel MR spectroscopy. *AJNR Am J Neuroradiol* 1999;20:117–123.
74 Stadlbauer A, Gruber S, Nimsky C et al. Preoperative grading of gliomas by using metabolite quantification with high-spatial-resolution proton MR spectroscopic imaging. *Radiology* 2006;238:958–969.
75 Sundgren PC, Nagesh V, Elias A et al. Metabolic alterations: a biomarker for radiation-induced normal brain injury. An MR spectroscopy study. *J Magn Reson Imaging* 2009;29:291–297.
76 Terpstra M, High WB, Luo Y, de Graaf RA, Merkle H, Garwood M. Relationships among lactate concentration, blood flow and histopathologic profiles in rat C6 glioma. *NMR Biomed* 1996;9:185–194.
77 Tong Z, Yamaki T, Harada K, Houkin K. In vivo quantification of the metabolites in normal brain and brain tumors by proton MR spectroscopy using water as an internal standard. *Magn Reson Imaging* 2004;22:1017–1024.
78 Whelan HT, Clanton JA, Moore PM, Tolner DJ, Kessler RM, Whetsell WO Jr. Magnetic resonance brain tumor imaging in canine glioma. *Neurology* 1987;37: 1235–1239.
79 Wilken B, Dechent P, Herms J et al. Quantitative proton magnetic resonance spectroscopy of focal brain lesions. *Pediatr Neurol* 2000;23:22–31.
80 Yamasaki F, Takaba J, Ohtaki M et al. Detection and differentiation of lactate and lipids by single-voxel proton MR spectroscopy. *Neurosurg Rev* 2005;28:267–277.
81 Zonari P, Baraldi P, Crisi G. Multimodal MRI in the characterization of glial neoplasms: the combined role of single-voxel MR spectroscopy, diffusion imaging and echo-planar perfusion imaging. *Neuroradiology* 2007;49:795–803.

82 Bruhn H, Michaelis T, Merboldt KD et al. On the interpretation of proton NMR spectra from brain tumours in vivo and in vitro. *NMR Biomed* 1992;5:253–258.

83 Teresi LM. *A Practicing Radiologist Guide to MR Spectroscopy of the Brain.* Bloomington, IN: Xlibris, 2007.

84 Vuori K, Kankaanranta L, Hakkinen AM et al. Low-grade gliomas and focal cortical developmental malformations: differentiation with proton MR spectroscopy. *Radiology* 2004;230:703–708.

85 McKnight TR, Noworolski SM, Vigneron DB, Nelson SJ. An automated technique for the quantitative assessment of 3D-MRSI data from patients with glioma. *J Magn Reson Imaging* 2001;13:167–177.

86 McKnight TR, von dem Bussche MH, Vigneron DB et al. Histopathological validation of a three-dimensional magnetic resonance spectroscopy index as a predictor of tumor presence. *J Neurosurg* 2002;97:794–802.

87 Barker PB, Blackband SJ, Chatham JC et al. Quantitative proton spectroscopy and histology of a canine brain tumor model. *Magn Reson Med* 1993;30:458–464.

88 Gambino JM, Shores A, Haller J et al. In vivo noninvasive single voxel ^{1}H magnetic resonance spectroscopy at 3T for the evaluation of intracranial neoplasms in the dog [Abstract]. In: Procedings of the American College of Veterinary Radiology, Savannah, GA, 2013: 42. Available at https://www.acvr.org/sites/default/files/2013-acvr-proceedings.pdf

89 Joslyn S, Sullivan M, Novellas R, Brennan N, Cameron G, Hammond G. Effect of delayed acquisition times on gadolinium-enhanced magnetic resonance imaging of the presumably normal canine brain. *Vet Radiol Ultrasound* 2011;52:611–618.

90 Singh JB, Oevermann A, Lang J et al. Contrast media enhancement of intracranial lesions in magnetic resonance imaging does not reflect histopathologic findings consistently. *Vet Radiol Ultrasound* 2011;52:619–626.

91 Lee J, Platt S, Kent M, Zhao Q. An analysis of the pharmacokinetic parameter ratios in DCE-MRI using the reference region model. *Magn Reson Imaging* 2012;30:26–35.

92 Zhao Q, Lee S, Kent M, Schatzberg S, Platt S. Dynamic contrast-enhanced magnetic resonance imaging of canine brain tumors. *Vet Radiol Ultrasound* 2010;51:122–129.

93 Wolff CA, Holmes SP, Young BD et al. Magnetic resonance imaging for the differentiation of neoplastic, inflammatory, and cerebrovascular brain disease in dogs. *J Vet Intern Med* 2012;26:589–597.

94 Sturges BK, Dickinson PJ, Bollen AW et al. Magnetic resonance imaging and histological classification of intracranial meningiomas in 112 dogs. *J Vet Intern Med* 2008;22:586–595.

95 James FM, da Costa RC, Fauber A et al. Clinical and MRI findings in three dogs with polycystic meningiomas. *J Am Anim Hosp Assoc* 2012;48:331–338.

96 Cha S. Update on brain tumor imaging: from anatomy to physiology. *AJNR Am J Neuroradiol* 2006;27:475–487.

97 Wisner ER, Dickinson PJ, Higgins RJ. Magnetic resonance imaging features of canine intracranial neoplasia. *Vet Radiol Ultrasound* 2011;52(1 Suppl 1): S52–S61.

98 Freeman AC, Platt SR, Kent M, Hofmeister E. What is the evidence? Diagnosis of an intracranial lesion as a meningioma on the basis of MRI characteristics. *J Am Vet Med Assoc* 2011;239:60–62.

99 Cervera V, Mai W, Vite CH, Johnson V, Dayrell-Hart B, Seiler GS. Comparative magnetic resonance imaging findings between gliomas and presumed cerebrovascular accidents in dogs. *Vet Radiol Ultrasound* 2011;52:33–40.

100 Rodenas S, Pumarola M, Gaitero L, Zamora A, Anor S. Magnetic resonance imaging findings in 40 dogs with histologically confirmed intracranial tumours. *Vet J* 2011;187:85–91.

101 Kumar AJ, Leeds NE, Fuller GN et al. Malignant gliomas: MR imaging spectrum of radiation therapy- and chemotherapy-induced necrosis of the brain after treatment. *Radiology* 2000;217:377–384.

102 Hecht S, Adams WH. MRI of brain disease in veterinary patients. Part 2: Acquired brain disorders. *Vet Clin North Am Small Anim Pract* 2010;40:39–63.

103 Garosi LS, Platt SR, McConnell JF, Wrayt JD, Smith KC. Intracranial haemorrhage associated with *Angiostrongylus vasorum* infection in three dogs. *J Small Anim Pract* 2005;46:93–99.

104 Cooper JJ, Young BD, Hoffman A et al. Intracranial magnetic resonance imaging artifacts and pseudolesions in dogs and cats. *Vet Radiol Ultrasound* 2010;51:587–595.

105 Garosi LS. Cerebrovascular disease in dogs and cats. *Vet Clin North Am Small Anim Pract* 2010;40:65–79.

106 Kang BT, Jang DP, Gu SH et al. MRI features in a canine model of ischemic stroke: correlation between lesion volume and neurobehavioral status during the subacute stage. *Comp Med* 2009;59:459–464.

107 Platt SR, Garosi L. Canine cerebrovascular disease: do dogs have strokes? *J Am Anim Hosp Assoc* 2003;39:337–342.

108 Goncalves R, Carrera I, Garosi L, Smith PM, Fraser McConnell J, Penderis J. Clinical and topographic magnetic resonance imaging characteristics of suspected thalamic infarcts in 16 dogs. *Vet J* 2011;188:39–43.

109 McConnell JF, Garosi L, Platt SR. Magnetic resonance imaging findings of presumed cerebellar cerebrovascular accident in twelve dogs. *Vet Radiol Ultrasound* 2005;46:1–10.

110 Garosi L, McConnell JF, Platt SR et al. Clinical and topographic magnetic resonance characteristics of suspected brain infarction in 40 dogs. *J Vet Intern Med* 2006;20:311–321.

111 Garosi LS, McConnell JF. Ischaemic stroke in dogs and humans: a comparative review. *J Small Anim Pract* 2005;46:521–529.

112 Garosi L, McConnell JE, Platt SR et al. Results of diagnostic investigations and long-term outcome of 33 dogs with brain infarction (2000–2004). *J Vet Intern Med* 2005;19:725–731.

113 Sutherland-Smith J, King R, Faissler D, Ruthazer R, Sato A. Magnetic resonance imaging apparent diffusion coefficients for histologically confirmed intracranial lesions in dogs. *Vet Radiol Ultrasound* 2011;52:142–148.

114 Kang BT, Jang DP, Gu SH et al. Three-dimensional time-of-flight magnetic resonance angiography of intracranial vessels in a canine model of ischemic stroke with permanent occlusion of the middle cerebral artery. *Comp Med* 2009;59:72–77.

115 Kang BT, Jang DP, Lee JH et al. Detection of cerebral metabolites in a canine model of ischemic stroke using ^{1}H magnetic resonance spectroscopy. *Res Vet Sci* 2009;87:300–306.

116 Platt SR, Radaelli ST, McDonnell JJ. Computed tomography after mild head trauma in dogs. *Vet Rec* 2002;151:243.

117 Haley AC, Abramson C. Traumatic pneumocephalus in a dog. *J Am Vet Med Assoc* 2009;234:1295–1298.

118 MacKillop E. Magnetic resonance imaging of intracranial malformations in dogs and cats. *Vet Radiol Ultrasound* 2011;52(1 Suppl 1):S42–S51.

119 Davies ES, Volk HA, Behr S et al. Porencephaly and hydranencephaly in six dogs. *Vet Rec* 2012;170:179.

120 Schmidt MJ, Klumpp S, Amort K, Jawinski S, Kramer M. Porencephaly in dogs and cats: magnetic resonance imaging findings and clinical signs. *Vet Radiol Ultrasound* 2012;53:142–149.

121 Lamb CR, Croson PJ, Cappello, JCherubini GB. Magnetic resonance imaging findings in 25 dogs with inflammatory cerebrospinal fluid. *Vet Radiol Ultrasound* 2005;46(1):17–22. Epub 2005/02/08.

122 Zakhary R, Keles GE, Berger MS. Intraoperative imaging techniques in the treatment of brain tumors. *Curr Opin Oncol* 1999;11:152–156.

123 Lowe LH, Bailey Z. State-of-the-art cranial sonography: Part 1, modern techniques and image interpretation. *AJR Am J Roentgenol* 2011;196:1028–1033.

124 Roberts DW, Hartov A, Kennedy FE, Miga MI, Paulsen KD. Intraoperative brain shift and deformation: a quantitative analysis of cortical displacement in 28 cases. *Neurosurgery* 1998;43:749–758; discussion 758–760.

125 Daneman A, Epelman M, Blaser S, Jarrin JR. Imaging of the brain in full-term neonates: does sonography still play a role? *Pediatr Radiol* 2006;36:636–646.

126 Epelman M, Daneman A, Kellenberger CJ et al. Neonatal encephalopathy: a prospective comparison of head US and MRI. *Pediatr Radiol* 2010;40:1640–1650.

127 Kane RA, Kruskal JB. Intraoperative ultrasonography of the brain and spine. *Ultrasound Q* 2007;23:23–39.

128 Moiyadi A, Shetty P. Objective assessment of utility of intraoperative ultrasound in resection of central nervous system tumors: a cost-effective tool for intraoperative navigation in neurosurgery. *J Neurosci Rural Pract* 2011;2:4–11.

129 Dohrmann GJ, Rubin JM. Use of ultrasound in neurosurgical operations: a preliminary report. *Surg Neurol* 1981;16:362–366.

130 Dohrmann GJ, Rubin JM. Dynamic intraoperative imaging and instrumentation of brain and spinal cord using ultrasound. *Neurol Clin* 1985;3:425–437.

131 Cengiz C, Keramettin A. Intraoperative ultrasonographic characteristics of malignant intracranial lesions. *Neurol India* 2005;53:208–211; discussion 212.

132 Machi J, Sigel B, Jafar JJ et al. Criteria for using imaging ultrasound during brain and spinal cord surgery. *J Ultrasound Med* 1984;3:155–161.

133 Sun H, Zhao JZ. Application of intraoperative ultrasound in neurological surgery. *Minim Invasive Neurosurg* 2007;50:155–159.

134 Erdogan N, Tucer B, Mavili E, Menku A, Kurtsoy A. Ultrasound guidance in intracranial tumor resection: correlation with postoperative magnetic resonance findings. *Acta Radiol* 2005;46:743–749.

135 Renner C, Lindner D, Schneider JP, Meixensberger J. Evaluation of intra-operative ultrasound imaging in brain tumor resection: a prospective study. *Neurol Res* 2005;27:351–357.

136 Ray WZ, Barua M, Ryken TC. Anatomic visualization with ultrasound-assisted intracranial image guidance in neurosurgery: a report of 30 patients. *J Am Coll Surg* 2004;199:338–343.

137 Unsgaard G, Gronningsaeter A, Ommedal S, Nagelhus Hernes TA. Brain operations guided by real-time two-dimensional ultrasound: new possibilities as a result of improved image quality. *Neurosurgery* 2002;51:402–411; discussion 411–412.

138 Unsgaard G, Ommedal S, Muller T, Gronningsaeter A, Nagelhus Hernes TA. Neuronavigation by intraoperative three-dimensional ultrasound: initial experience during brain tumor resection. *Neurosurgery* 2002;50:804–812; discussion 812.
139 Rubin JM, Dohrmann GJ. Efficacy of intraoperative US for evaluating intracranial masses. *Radiology* 1985;157:509–511.
140 Rubin JM, Dohrmann GJ. Use of ultrasonically guided probes and catheters in neurosurgery. *Surg Neurol* 1982;18:143–148.
141 Andrews BT, Bederson JB, Pitts LH. Use of intraoperative ultrasonography to improve the diagnostic accuracy of exploratory burr holes in patients with traumatic tentorial herniation. *Neurosurgery* 1989;24:345–347.
142 Kumar P, Sukthankar R, Damany BJ, Mishra J, Jha AN. Evaluation of intraoperative ultrasound in neurosurgery. *Ann Acad Med Singapore* 1993;22(3 Suppl):422–427.
143 Hatfield MK, Rubin JM, Gebarski SS, Silbergleit R. Intraoperative sonography in low-grade gliomas. *J Ultrasound Med* 1989;8:131–134.
144 Le Roux PD, Berger MS, Wang K, Mack LA, Ojemann GA. Low grade gliomas: comparison of intraoperative ultrasound characteristics with preoperative imaging studies. *J Neurooncol* 1992;13:189–198.
145 van Velthoven V. Intraoperative ultrasound imaging: comparison of pathomorphological findings in US versus CT, MRI and intraoperative findings. *Acta Neurochir Suppl* 2003;85:95–99.
146 Chacko AG, Kumar NK, Chacko G, Athyal R, Rajshekhar V. Intraoperative ultrasound in determining the extent of resection of parenchymal brain tumours: a comparative study with computed tomography and histopathology. *Acta Neurochir* 2003;145:743–748; discussion 748.
147 Hammoud MA, Ligon BL, el Souki R, Shi WM, Schomer DF, Sawaya R. Use of intraoperative ultrasound for localizing tumors and determining the extent of resection: a comparative study with magnetic resonance imaging. *J Neurosurg* 1996;84:737–741.
148 LeRoux PD, Berger MS, Ojemann GA, Wang K, Mack LA. Correlation of intraoperative ultrasound tumor volumes and margins with preoperative computerized tomography scans. An intraoperative method to enhance tumor resection. *J Neurosurg* 1989;71:691–698.
149 LeRoux PD, Winter TC, Berger MS, Mack LA, Wang K, Elliott JP. A comparison between preoperative magnetic resonance and intraoperative ultrasound tumor volumes and margins. *J Clin Ultrasound* 1994;22:29–36.
150 Engelhardt M, Hansen C, Eyding J et al. Feasibility of contrast-enhanced sonography during resection of cerebral tumours: initial results of a prospective study. *Ultrasound Med Biol* 2007;33:571–575.
151 He W, Jiang XQ, Wang S et al. Intraoperative contrast-enhanced ultrasound for brain tumors. *Clin Imaging* 2008;32:419–424.
152 Kanno H, Ozawa Y, Sakata K et al. Intraoperative power Doppler ultrasonography with a contrast-enhancing agent for intracranial tumors. *J Neurosurg* 2005;102:295–301.
153 Letteboer MM, Willems PW, Viergever MA, Niessen WJ. Brain shift estimation in image-guided neurosurgery using 3-D ultrasound. *IEEE Trans Biomed Eng* 2005;52:268–276.
154 Shores A, Holland M, Hudson J et al. Intraoperative ultrasound for intracranial surgery. In: Proceedings of the American College of Veterinary Internal Medicine Forum 2012. Available at http://www.vin.com/acvim/2012/Default.htm
155 Flegel T, Podell M, March PA, Chakeres DW. Use of a disposable real-time CT stereotactic navigator device for minimally invasive dog brain biopsy through a mini-burr hole. *AJNR Am J Neuroradiol* 2002;23:1160–1163.
156 Giroux A, Jones JC, Bohn JH, Duncan RB, Waldron DR, Inzana KR. A new device for stereotactic CT-guided biopsy of the canine brain: design, construction, and needle placement accuracy. *Vet Radiol Ultrasound* 2002;43:229–236.
157 Moissonnier P, Blot S, Devauchelle P et al. Stereotactic CT-guided brain biopsy in the dog. *J Small Anim Pract* 2002;43:115–123.
158 Moissonnier P, Bordeau W, Delisle F, Devauchelle P. Accuracy testing of a new stereotactic CT-guided brain biopsy device in the dog. *Res Vet Sci* 2000;68:243–247.
159 Koblik PD, LeCouteur RA, Higgins RJ et al. CT-guided brain biopsy using a modified Pelorus Mark III stereotactic system: experience with 50 dogs. *Vet Radiol Ultrasound* 1999;40:434–440.
160 Koblik PD, LeCouteur RA, Higgins RJ et al. Modification and application of a Pelorus Mark III stereotactic system for CT-guided brain biopsy in 50 dogs. *Vet Radiol Ultrasound* 1999;40:424–433.
161 Chen AV, Wininger FA, Frey S et al. Description and validation of a magnetic resonance imaging-guided stereotactic brain biopsy device in the dog. *Vet Radiol Ultrasound* 2012;53:150–156.

5 Cisterneal Cerebrospinal Fluid Taps

Nora Ortinau

Introduction

Cerebrospinal fluid (CSF) analysis is an important part of a complete neurological work-up. However, while it is useful for limiting the differential diagnosis list when evaluated in conjunction with imaging results, it rarely yields a definitive diagnosis [1]. The clinician should be familiar with the clinical indications for performing a CSF tap and the risks involved. In the appropriate patient, cisterna magna puncture is a relatively straightforward procedure for obtaining a sample of adequate size and quality to help form a complete clinical picture. Cisternal taps are also coupled with injections of nonionic iodinated contrast agents for myelography. Only approved agents for intrathecal are used for this purpose.

Clinician familiarity with anatomical landmarks, sample handling, and the supplies necessary to perform the tap is essential. The cisterna magna is located dorsal to the caudal brainstem between the foramen magnum and C1 [2]. Important anatomical landmarks include the external occipital protuberance, the widest points of the wings of the atlas, and the spinous process of C2 (Figure 5.1) [1,3]. In large or obese dogs, the spinous process of C2 may be very difficult to palpate.

The cells in the fluid begin to degenerate within 30 min [1], and therefore it is also important to know where the samples will be submitted and when they will be analyzed, as this will determine the type of sample tube needed. The necessary supplies include sterile gloves, spinal needles, and sample tubes. Typically, a 22G 1.5-inch (3.8 cm) spinal needle with stylet is sufficient for most small animal patients (Figure 5.2) [1]. In only the very large patient, a longer spinal needle (2.5 inch, 6.35 cm) may be necessary; however, the longer needles are more likely to deflect laterally and there may be some loss of digital perception when performing the puncture.

Patient Preparation and Positioning

The patient is intubated and in a surgical plane of anesthesia for sample acquisition. Anesthetic protocol is based on clinician preference and patient status, but should be chosen to have a minimum effect on intracranial pressure. The patient is placed on a flat stable surface in lateral recumbency. The same procedure can be performed in sternal recumbency; however, this positioning usually requires the sample to be drawn by suction into a syringe, necessitating additional manipulation of the needle while in the medullary cistern and may enhance the possibility of blood contamination. Typically the patient is placed in right lateral recumbency for right-handed collectors, and left lateral if the collector is left-handed. The hair on the dorsal midline from approximately the external occipital protuberance to the spinous process of C2 is clipped and the area aseptically prepared.

Proper patient position is of upmost importance in facilitating the acquisition of CSF from the cisterna magna, and thus staff should be familiar with how to position the patient. The patient's dorsum is positioned so it is even with the edge of the table. The positioner should grasp the nose, extend the head and neck forward, and then flex the nose toward the chest, perpendicular to the axis of the spine (Figure 5.1). In large dogs it is often helpful if the positioner makes a fist, places it at the angle of the jaw, and then flexes the head around the fist (Figure 5.3), thus affording maximum opening of the cisternal space. The ears, if floppy, are held or taped out of the way; often it is easiest to have the positioner hold the ears against the head. When the head is flexed, an imaginary line is drawn sagittally along the midline and parallel to the table (Figure 5.1B). At this juncture, the anesthetist makes sure the endotracheal tube is not kinked and the airway is maintained.

Sample Acquisition

Once the patient has been properly prepared and positioned, the collector evaluates the positioning and is ready to obtain a CSF sample. Sterile gloves are donned and the collector uses the thumb and second finger of the left hand (if right-handed) to palpate and identify the widest point of the wings of the atlas. The dorsal midline is identified by palpating the spinous process of C2 and the occipital protuberance with the index finger of the left hand (Figure 5.4). The spinal needle is held like a dart and slowly inserted through the skin at a point just cranial to the intersection of an

Current Techniques in Canine and Feline Neurosurgery, First Edition. Edited by Andy Shores and Brigitte A. Brisson.
© 2017 John Wiley & Sons, Inc. Published 2017 by John Wiley & Sons, Inc.
Companion website: www.wiley.com/go/shores/neurosurgery

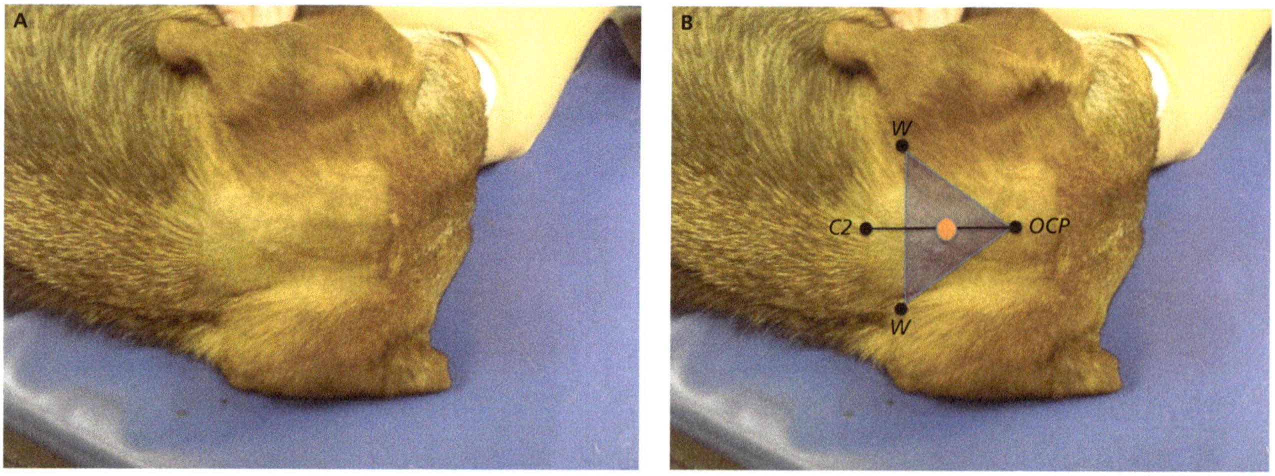

Figure 5.1 Positioning and landmarks for cisternal CSF tap. (A) Patient is in left lateral recumbency with the head flexed and the nose parallel to the plane of the table. (B) Landmarks: W, widest point of the wings of the atlas (C1); OCP, occipital protuberance; C2, cranial tip of the C2 spinous process. Note the OCP and C2 are in alignment and represent the mid-sagittal plane of the patient.

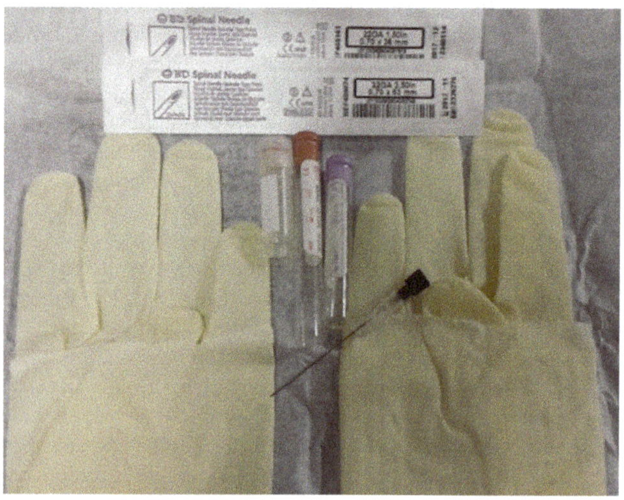

Figure 5.2 Supplies for a cisternal CSF tap: sterile gloves, spinal needle (Quincke point), collection tubes.

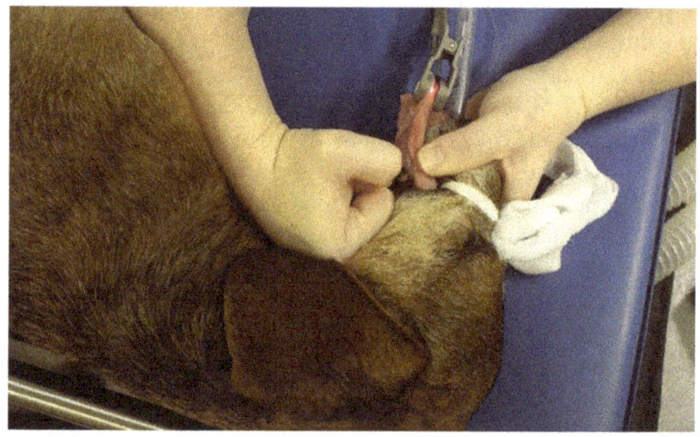

Figure 5.3 Technique for flexion of the head and extension of the neck for cisternal CSF tap positioning.

imaginary line drawn transversely between the widest points of the wings of the atlas and a line drawn sagittally along the midline from the external occipital protuberance to the spinous process of C2 (Figure 5.1). The needle is slowly advanced further, making sure that it remains on the midline and parallel to the table. The stylet is periodically removed if necessary to check for CSF flow. The spinal needle is stabilized while removing and reinserting the stylet to avoid needle movement. In some patients, particularly those with domed heads, it is helpful to angle the needle at a more caudal angle, maintaining the needle on the midline. As the needle is advanced the collector often notes changes in resistance as the needle passes through the fascial planes of the muscle and finally through the dorsal atlanto-occipital membrane and dura into the subarachnoid space [3].

If the occipital bone is encountered, the needle is redirected caudally along the sagittal (midline) plane [2]. If CSF is not obtained after two redirection attempts, then the needle is completely withdrawn, landmarks reestablished and sample collection attempted again. If free-flowing blood is observed in the needle, it is likely the needle was directed just lateral to the cisterna magna. The needle should be withdrawn and a new needle used for another attempt at sample collection [2].

Once CSF flow is visualized, an assistant catches the drops in the sample tube(s) (Figure 5.5 and Video 5.1). Sometimes there is a small amount of blood associated with minor iatrogenic trauma to a small meningeal or muscle vessel in the first couple of drops [2]. These first few drops can be collected in a separate tube, and then a second tube used to collect the clearer CSF.

If the CSF flow is slow, an assistant can *carefully* occlude the jugular veins without changing position of the patient to help increase flow. It is important that the position of the head and/or needle is not changed. Aspiration of the fluid with a syringe is not recommended. Approximately 1 mL of CSF can be safely removed per 5 kg of body weight [3]; however, most routine sampling only requires a total volume of 1 mL for any patient.

Once the sample is obtained, the needle is carefully removed before the holder relaxes the head. It is not necessary to replace the stylet prior to removing the needle. In cases where only a small amount of CSF was obtained in the sample tube, the residual volume in the needle is also collected in the tube.

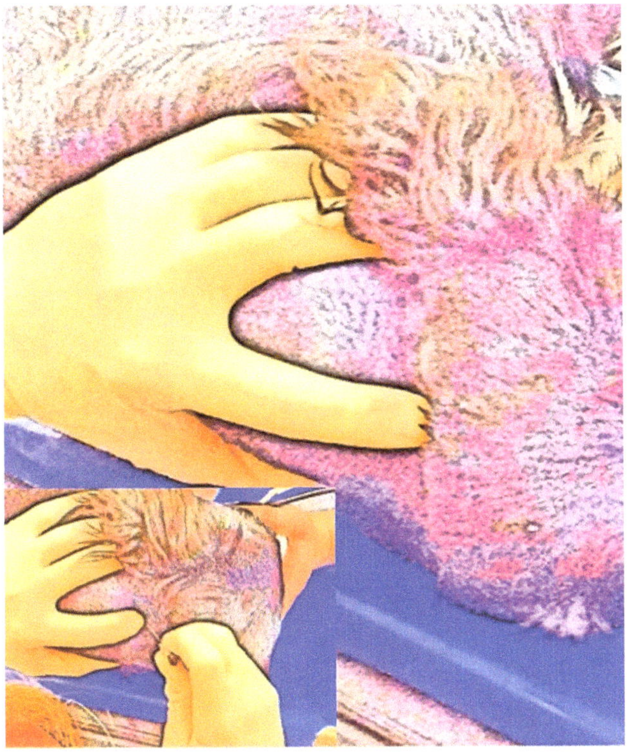

Figure 5.4 Palpating landmarks for cisternal CSF tap. The gloved left hand is used to grasp the wings of the atlas and identify the occipital protuberance to visualize the insertion point for the spinal needle (*inset*).

Possible Complications

As with any procedure, complications can occur secondary to CSF sample acquisition. Most complications are minor and self-limiting, while others can be life-threatening. Minor hemorrhage due to trauma to a minor vessel can be a relatively common complication and is generally self-limiting. Hemorrhage can be severe if the patient is thrombocytopenic or has a coagulopathy [2]. Other, more severe, complications can include herniation associated with markedly increased intracranial pressure (i.e., intracranial neoplasia) and iatrogenic brainstem trauma (pithing) [2,3].

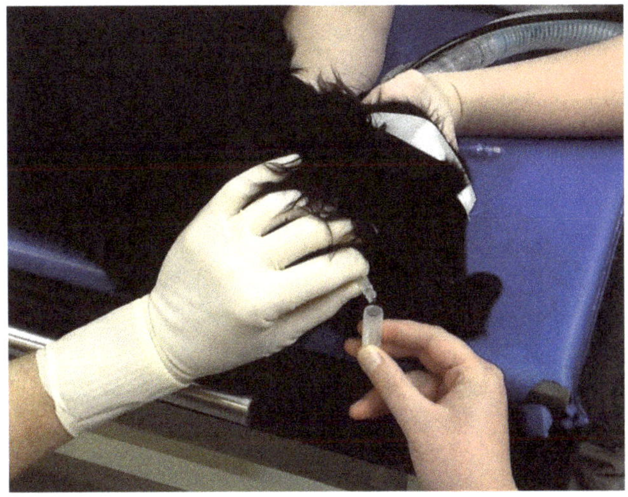

Figure 5.5 Collection of the CSF sample. An assistant collects the CSF into the sample tube as it drips from the needle.

Interpretation

Optimally, cell counts and cytological preparations should be performed within 20 min of sample acquisition. Protein analysis and PCR, antigen or antibody tests can be performed later. The samples are submitted to a qualified laboratory and routine analyses should include color, clarity, red cell and white cell counts, cytology, and protein quantity.

Video clips to accompany this book can be found on the companion website at:
www.wiley.com/go/shores/neurosurgery

References

1 Lorenz MD, Coates JR, Kent M. *Handbook of Veterinary Neurology*, 5th edn. St Louis, MO: Elsevier, 2011: 81–85.

2 Bagley RS. *Fundamentals of Veterinary Clinical Neurology*. Ames, IA: Wiley-Blackwell, 2005: 217–219.

3 Dewey CW. *A Practical Guide to Canine and Feline Neurology*, 2nd edn. Ames, IA: Wiley-Blackwell, 2008: 75–78.

6 Minimum Database: Spinal Surgery

Luis Gaitero and Brigitte A. Brisson

Introduction

Therapeutic options for spinal neurological diseases often include both medical and surgical procedures. Neurosurgical treatment is selected when the procedure has proven to be significantly more effective than the conservative approach, the disease does not respond to medical therapy, the clinical signs are severe or rapidly progressive, or when there is spinal instability [1]. Some of the most common indications for spinal surgery are intervertebral disc herniation, cervical spondylomyelopathy, degenerative lumbosacral stenosis, and vertebral fracture/luxation. The main complications include iatrogenic injury to neural structures, severe intraoperative hemorrhage, spinal vascular compromise, vertebral column instability, and excessive scar tissue formation [1].

The specific surgical risk for each patient varies depending on the primary condition and other preexisting abnormalities that affect the general health of the patient [2]. Evaluation of the surgical risk will allow the neurosurgeon to weigh the potential benefits of a spinal neurosurgical procedure against the potential complications and prognosis. A comprehensive presurgical evaluation allows the surgeon to detect risk factors that could affect outcome and guides the surgeon to anticipate and, where possible, limit complications. Furthermore, it provides valuable information on the presurgical status to establish a patient's baseline values so that changes during and after surgery can be adequately interpreted.

Diagnostic tests are performed to screen asymptomatic patients and identify risk factors for occult disease. These are extremely valuable in evaluating anesthetic risk, particularly considering that neurosurgical patients almost invariably require initial general anesthesia for extensive diagnostic imaging investigations or cerebrospinal fluid collection. The information obtained contributes to planning the most appropriate anesthetic strategy. Although economic considerations should be taken into account, a thorough presurgical examination can avoid more expensive complications. The extent of the presurgical screening is typically adjusted according to the animal's unique circumstances such as age and the emergent nature of the procedure; however, obtaining a standard minimum database (MDB) is always recommended, even if in some cases the results will only be available postoperatively.

Laboratory testing is not a substitute for complete physical examination and the value of a detailed history should not be underestimated. Orthopedic conditions such as bilateral cruciate rupture can also easily be misinterpreted as neurological disorders. Equally, accurate lesion localization based on a neurological examination is very important for identifying the significance of any identified spinal lesions, since asymptomatic lesions are commonly detected on advanced diagnostic imaging.

The presurgical MDB for a neurosurgical patient includes complete history, physical examination, neurological and orthopedic examinations, complete blood count (CBC), comprehensive serum biochemistry profile, and urinalysis. In cats, assessment of feline leukemia virus (FeLV)/feline immunodeficiency virus (FIV) status before spinal surgery is strongly advised, particularly when spinal lymphoma is suspected due to its association with FeLV-positive results in more than 50% of cases [3]. Thoracic radiographs and abdominal ultrasound are recommended as part of the MDB in dogs and cats with a spinal cord disorder. This is especially important in patients aged 6 years and older, in those where cardiovascular or respiratory abnormalities are suspected, and in those with an accompanying history, clinical signs or MDB abnormalities that increase suspicion for spinal neoplasia (primary, secondary or metastatic), infectious disease, trauma, or other complicating medical conditions such as cardiac, hepatic, or renal disease. Diagnostic tests directed toward identification of extraneural neoplasia, infectious conditions, or concomitant disease have diagnostic value for the final diagnosis, but can also provide prognostic value to the owner. Further diagnostic tests can be selected for investigation of disorders suspected on the basis of the initial screening tests or based on the planned surgical procedure.

In people, spinal procedures have historically been associated with higher rates of infection in comparison to other orthopedic procedures, with rates ranging between 0.3 and 9% compared with 1–2% for primary total joint arthroplasty [4]. Although intraoperative factors play a significant role in the risk of developing infection,

Current Techniques in Canine and Feline Neurosurgery, First Edition. Edited by Andy Shores and Brigitte A. Brisson.
© 2017 John Wiley & Sons, Inc. Published 2017 by John Wiley & Sons, Inc.
Companion website: www.wiley.com/go/shores/neurosurgery

this risk is also affected by the presence of patient comorbidities and various individual factors. Consequently, recognition of a patient's individual risk factors is an important step towards optimization and can lead to modified protocols in order to reduce risk. Numerous factors have been associated with postoperative infection of surgical wounds in humans and animals. Some patient-based risk factors for infection associated with spinal surgery that have been identified in people include anemia, coronary artery disease, coagulopathy, bone and tissue neoplasia, malnutrition, diabetes mellitus, smoking, immunocompromised hosts, obesity, alcohol abuse, advanced age (>60 years), surgical duration, and previous surgical infection [5,6]. In dogs, contamination of the surgical field due to either a break in asepsis or traumatic wound is an obvious risk factor for infection [7]. Other suspected or proven factors which are not specific to neurosurgery include length of anesthesia and length of surgery, number of people in the operating room, postoperative wound drainage, increasing body weight, intraoperative hypothermia, increasing age (>8 years), severe blood loss, shock or hypotension, presence of a distant infection, prior irradiation of the surgical site, systemic disease (e.g., uremia), endocrinopathies, excessive use of electrocautery, use of propofol in the anesthetic protocol, use of high doses of corticosteroids, postoperative admission to an intensive care unit (increases with increased duration of stay), antimicrobial prophylaxis, contaminated suction tips, and use of braided multifilament suture material [7–10]. Although not reported specifically, tissue trauma resulting in poor tissue perfusion, poor tissue apposition resulting in dead space and seroma formation, and poor hemostasis resulting in hematoma also appear to increase the risk of postoperative inflammation, dehiscence and/or infection. Seromas and hematomas provide a good medium for small numbers of contaminating bacteria to thrive since therapeutic antibiotic levels cannot be reached in previously formed tissue exudate and blood clots.

Complete Blood Count

Although some neoplasias such as multiple myeloma and lymphoma (which can be associated with hyperglobulinemia and abnormal circulating lymphocytes respectively) can cause spinal and hematological abnormalities, this is rarely the case for conditions restricted to the vertebral column [3,11]. Regardless, a CBC is still useful for detecting systemic diseases that may have neurological manifestations, such as spinal infectious pathologies, and is recommended in all cases. At a minimum, packed cell volume (hematocrit) and total serum protein are recommended for all surgical candidates as they provide baseline data for monitoring hemorrhage and fluid balance. A platelet count is also important for detecting thrombocytopenia and possible bleeding tendencies.

Abnormalities [12,13]

Erythrocytes

Morphology

Poikilocytes

Red blood cells with different and abnormal shapes. The most common types include:

- echinocytes (associated with dehydration, inherited erythrocyte defect or snake bite);
- acanthocytes (seen with concurrent hepatic or renal disease, hemangiosarcoma, iron deficiency, and disseminated intravascular coagulation [DIC] syndrome);
- eccentrocytes (associated with onion toxicity and some drugs; Figure 6.1);
- schistocytes (fragmented erythrocytes seen in DIC, iron deficiency, hemangiosarcoma or valvular stenosis);
- spherocytes (associated with hemolytic anemia, DIC, and iron deficiency; Figure 6.2).

Inclusions

- Heinz bodies (acetaminophen, propylene glycol, propofol, zinc and copper toxicities, diabetes mellitus, renal disease, lymphoma, and hyperthyroidism);
- Howell–Jolly bodies (accelerated erythropoiesis, and secondary to splenectomy, increased circulating corticosteroids, septicemia/endotoxemia, and hypoxia);
- basophilic stippling (associated with lead poisoning);
- infectious (canine distemper virus, *Babesia* spp., *Cytauxzoon felis*, *Mycoplasma* spp.).

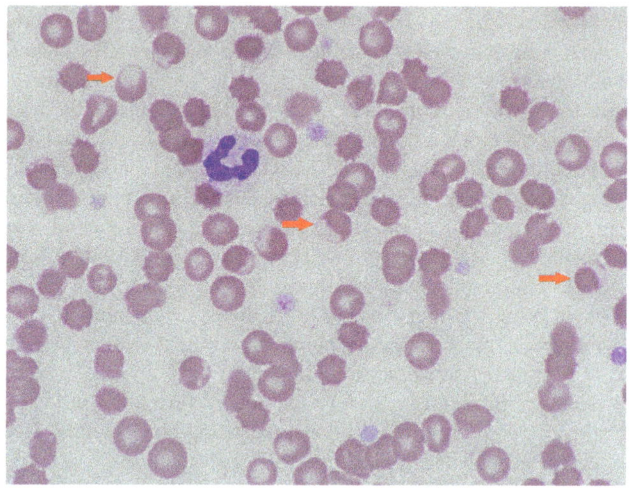

Figure 6.1 Blood smear from a dog presenting with oxidative damage to erythrocytes causing eccentrocyte formation (erythrocytes in which the hemoglobin is localized to part of the cell, leaving a portion with little hemoglobin; arrows). *Source*: Courtesy of Dr. Darren Wood.

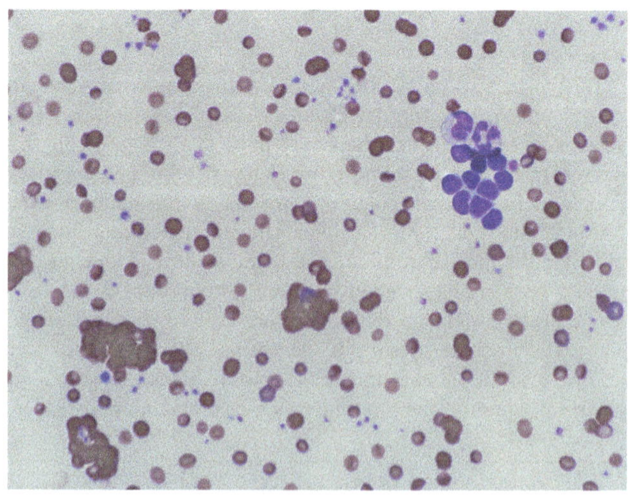

Figure 6.2 Blood smear from a dog with immune-mediated hemolytic anemia exhibiting autoagglutination. *Source*: Courtesy of Dr. Darren Wood.

Size Alterations

- Microcytosis can be caused by congenital portosystemic shunt or iron deficiency, or be a normal finding in some canine breeds (Shiba Inu, Akita, Chow Chow).
- Macrocytosis can be the result of regenerative anemias or myeloproliferative diseases.

Anemia

- Regenerative: with evidence of bone marrow response to a decreased hematocrit, that typically is based on the presence of reticulocytes in circulation. Associated with acute blood loss or hemolysis (immune-mediated hemolytic anemia, toxicity, erythroparasites, hereditary diseases).
- Nonregenerative: with no evidence of bone marrow response, usually normocytic/normochromic. Associated with underlying conditions that affect bone marrow erythrocyte production such as neoplasia (leukemia or metastatic), aplastic anemia, infectious disease, toxin-induced, iron deficiency, immune-mediated, or due to chronic systemic disease.

Polycythemia (Erythrocytosis)

- Relative: hemoconcentration due to dehydration, splenic contraction.
- Absolute: primary polycythemia vera, or secondary in response to chronic generalized hypoxia, focal renal hypoxia, or secondary to a paraneoplastic syndrome.

Leukocytes

Leukocytosis or Leukopenia

Classified based on the differentiated cell type (Table 6.1).

Atypical Circulating Leukocytes

Usually indicate neoplasia, although some hereditary disorders can result in abnormal circulating leukocytes. One such disorder seen in Australian Shepherd dogs is the Pelger–Huët anomaly which is associated with hyposegmented neutrophils and eosinophils [14] (Figure 6.3).

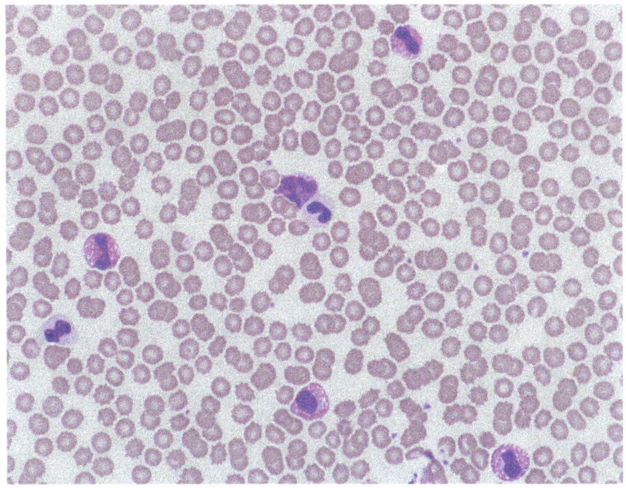

Figure 6.3 Blood smear from an Australian shepherd dog with Pelger-Huët anomaly showing hyposegmentation of granulocyte nuclei. *Source*: Courtesy of Dr. Darren Wood.

Inclusions or Granules

Associated with infectious (canine distemper virus) or hereditary (lysosomal) diseases.

Platelets

Thrombocytosis

- Reactive: acute hemorrhage, increased granulopoiesis due to chronic inflammation, increased erythropoiesis.
- Storage site release: splenic contraction, drugs (corticosteroids, epinephrine), hyperadrenocorticism, post splenectomy.

Table 6.1 The most common diseases associated with leukocytosis or leukopenia by cell type.

Type of leukocyte	Abnormality	Associated diseases
Neutrophil	Neutrophilia	Inflammation: infection, necrosis. Left-shift when presence of immature neutrophils (bands; inflammatory leukogram). Toxic neutrophils most often in septic process Stress Corticosteroid-induced: associated with lymphopenia and monocytosis Excitement (epinephrine-induced): associated with lymphocytosis in cats
	Neutropenia	Severe inflammation: usually with left-shift and toxic changes Bone marrow injury: infection, chemotherapy, estrogens, neoplasia, idiopathic
Lymphocyte	Lymphocytosis	Excitement (epinephrine-induced in cats) Vaccination (1–2 weeks after) Lymphoid leukemia Ehrlichiosis Hypoadrenocorticism
	Lymphopenia	Stress Chylothorax, lymphangiectasia Viral disease Hereditary immune-deficiency diseases
Monocyte	Monocytosis	Chronic inflammation, necrosis
Eosinophil	Eosinophlia	Hypersensitivity, allergy Parasitism Eosinophilic enteritis Hypereosinophilic syndrome Fungal disease Mast cell tumor Hypoadrenocorticism

Source: Data from Marioni-Henry et al. [10] and Dewey [11].

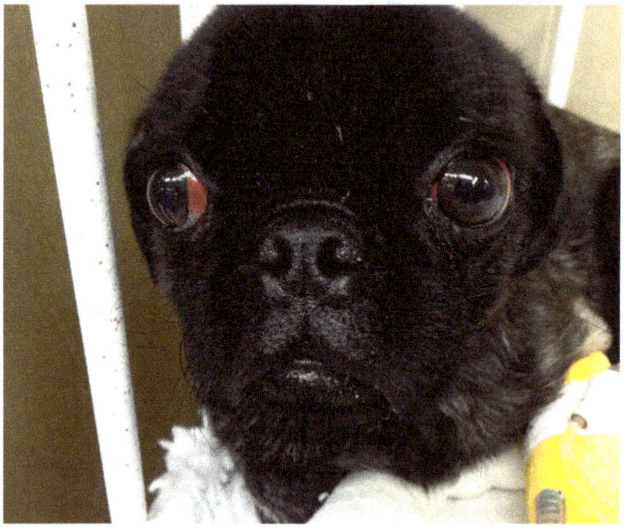

Figure 6.4 Dog with scleral hemorrhage due to immune-mediated thrombocytopenia. *Source*: Courtesy of Dr. Shauna Blois.

- Increased production: drugs (vincristine), myeloproliferative syndrome.
- Mixed or idiosyncratic: neoplasia, iron deficiency.

Thrombocytopenia

- Increased destruction: immune-mediated (Figure 6.4).
- Accelerated utilization: DIC, major vessel thrombosis, acute severe hemorrhage.
- Increased storage site sequestration: splenic disease/neoplasia, anaphylaxis, endotoxemia, drugs (barbiturates), hypoadrenocorticism.
- Decreased production: pancytopenic syndrome, bone marrow infiltration, chemotherapy.
- Mixed or idiosyncratic: infectious (rickettsial, FeLV, histoplasmosis), nonleukemic neoplasia, bacterial septicemia or endotoxemia, severe inflammation or necrosis, uremia.

Although automated platelet counts may be accurate, it is always indicated to review a peripheral blood smear, as platelet clumping or changes in mean platelet volume can result in erroneous values, especially in cats. In a blood smear, each platelet observed on a 100× high-power field represents approximately $20 \times 10^3/\mu L$ circulating platelets [15].

In the absence of other concurrent hemostatic defects, excessive surgical bleeding is uncommon if the platelet count is greater than $50 \times 10^3/\mu L$ and spontaneous bleeding is unlikely with counts above $30 \times 10^3/\mu L$ [15,16]. However, no specific values have been shown to be predictive of surgical bleeding, despite data proving that human critical care patients with counts below $100 \times 10^3/\mu L$ present a 10-fold increased risk of bleeding compared with those with counts of $100–150 \times 10^3/\mu L$ [17–19].

Serum Biochemistry

A comprehensive serum biochemistry panel is necessary to look for metabolic diseases that could be associated with the spinal neurosurgical condition or could increase the anesthetic and surgical risks. Review of all serum biochemical tests and possible alterations is beyond the scope of this chapter and the reader is referred to comprehensive internal medicine or clinical biochemistry texts. Considerations for some common serum biochemical clinical findings are as follows [13,20].

Alterations in Glucose Levels

- Hypoglycemia: associated with hepatic disease, insulinoma, hypoadrenocorticism, sepsis/toxemia, neonatal.
- Hyperglycemia: associated with diabetes mellitus, stress in cats.

Alterations in Blood Urea Nitrogen (BUN) and Creatinine Levels

- Azotemia: prerenal, renal, or postrenal causes (evaluation of urine specific gravity before fluid therapy is necessary to differentiate prerenal from renal causes).
- Low BUN: due to hepatic insufficiency or low-protein diet.

Increased Alkaline Phosphatase Activity

- Due to hepatic disease, steroid or anticonvulsant therapy, extrahepatic biliary obstruction, neoplasia, and normal increases related to osteoblastic bone activity in growing animals.

Increased Alanine Aminotransferase Activity

- Associated with hepatic disease and severe muscle injury.
- Alanine aminotransferase levels may be normal in some animals with severe hepatic disease.

Decreased Albumin Concentration

- Associated with hepatic disease, protein-losing nephropathy or enteropathy, severe exudative cutaneous lesions.

Alterations in Calcium Levels

- Hypercalcemia: paraneoplastic syndrome (lymphoma, anal sac adenocarcinoma), primary hyperparathyroidism, hypervitaminosis D, hypoadrenocorticism, chronic renal failure.
- Hypocalcemia: renal disease, pregnancy (eclampsia), hypovitaminosis D, hypoparathyroidism.

Hypernatremia

- Associated with vomiting, diarrhea, renal failure, diabetes insipidus, inappropriate fluid therapy, adipsia.

Alterations in Potassium Levels

- Hyperkalemia: acute or chronic renal failure, urinary tract obstruction or uroabdomen, rhabdomyolysis, hypoadrenocorticism, diabetes mellitus with ketoacidosis, excessive supplementation and secondary to administration of some diuretics and cardiac drugs. Pseudohyperkalemia has been reported in certain breeds such as the Shar-pei, Akita and Shiba Inu [21,22].
- Hypokalemia: vomiting, diarrhea, diuretic therapy, chronic renal failure, inappropriate fluid therapy.

Other frequently performed but more specific serum biochemical tests include, but are not limited to:

- blood gases;
- bile acids (preprandial and postprandial) and ammonia level (to evaluate hepatic function);
- endocrine assays such as thyroid, parathyroid hormone, adrenocorticotropic hormone, and cortisol levels;
- anticonvulsant serum concentration;
- serum osmolality and osmolal gap;
- serum protein electrophoresis;

- genetic disease testing;
- specific assays for infectious agents or immune-mediated diseases (serology, PCR).

Urinalysis

Although not routinely included in the MDB for most surgical candidates, urinalysis is an essential component of the initial evaluation as an easy and inexpensive diagnostic and monitoring test. There are many parameters on the biochemistry profile that cannot be interpreted without a urinalysis, especially when evaluating renal, hepatic and endocrine functions, as well as the acid-base status. Urine is preferably collected by cystocentesis and is submitted fresh along with the blood samples. The complete urinalysis includes the evaluation of the physical, chemical, and formed element characteristics of urine. More specifically, the routine urinalysis consists of a visual inspection to determine color and clarity/turbidity, measurement of urine specific gravity, chemical evaluation using a urine reagent strip (routine) or a chemical analyzer, and microscopic analysis of the sediment to assess mostly for the presence of cells and crystalluria [13]. Additional tests can be performed on urine to evaluate changes in glomerular filtration (determination of microalbumin level and urine protein/creatinine ratio), endocrine abnormalities (urine cortisol/creatinine ratio), presence of Bence Jones proteinuria (associated with multiple myeloma), urate crystals (seen with portosystemic shunts), urine organic acids levels, or fungal hyphae (associated with systemic aspergillosis).

Visual Inspection

Normal urine is clear with a light yellow to amber color. Possible alterations include the following [13].

- Yellow–orange discoloration: presence of bilirubin, fluorescein, concentrated urine.
- Brown–black discoloration: bile pigments, myoglobin, methemoglobin.
- Green–blue discoloration: presence of biliverdin, methylene blue.
- Red: blood, myoglobin.
- Milky: pyuria, lipiduria, phosphate crystalluria.

Urine Specific Gravity

Normal gravity should be greater than 1.030 in dogs and greater than 1.035 in cats with normal renal function and normally hydrated or dehydrated. Urine specific gravity is an essential value for determination of the underlying cause of azotemia and for differentiating prerenal from renal azotemia. A decreased urine specific gravity (isosthenuria, hyposthenuria) suggests an inability of the kidneys to concentrate urine. Hyposthenuria (gravity <1.007) can occur secondary to increased fluid intake, or renal or endocrine diseases (hypoadrenocorticism, hyperadrenocorticism). Hyposthenuria is usually associated with a lack of response to antidiuretic hormone (ADH; nephrogenic diabetes insipidus), absence of ADH (central diabetes insipidus), or excessive water consumption.

Chemical Evaluation

Chemical evaluation is routinely performed with a urine reagent strip (dipstick) specifically designed for this purpose or by using a chemical analyzer if sent to a laboratory. Urine reagent strips allow the semi-quantitative assessment of pH, proteinuria, glucosuria, ketonuria, bilirubinuria, hematuria, and several other parameters.

- Proteinuria: suggests urinary tract hemorrhage or inflammation, or renal disease due to glomerular or tubular dysfunction. Transient proteinuria can be associated with strenuous exercise or fever.
- Glucosuria: usually due to diabetes mellitus or stress-associated hyperglycemia (in cats), although can also be the result of acute renal failure or Fanconi syndrome.
- Ketonuria: associated diabetic ketoacidosis, starvation, or fasting.
- Bilirubinuria: caused by hepatic disease, posthepatic bile duct obstruction, or hemolysis.
- Hematuria: suggests urinary tract infection (UTI), urolithiasis, coagulopathies, trauma, or neoplasia.

Sediment Evaluation

To assess for the presence of erythrocytes, white blood cells, epithelial cells, casts, crystals, and microorganisms (bacteria, fungi, parasites).

- Pyuria: suggests UTI. Discospondylitis, prostatic disease, and pyometra are frequently associated with UTI.
- Hematuria: UTI, urolithiasis, coagulopathies, trauma, or neoplasia.
- Microorganisms: support UTI or pyelonephritis in the presence of pyuria.
- Crystalluria: ammonium biurate crystals are indicative of high serum ammonia levels, frequently associated with portosystemic shunting, but can also develop secondary to severe primary hepatic disease and naturally in Dalmatians.
- Casts: can suggest chronic renal disease or renal tubular necrosis.

Hemostasis Assays

Spinal surgery complications due to excessive bleeding are not uncommon. Surgical bleeding can be exacerbated by acquired or congenital hemostatic disorders as a result of a defect in one or more of the three major components of hemostasis: (i) vascular wall integrity, (ii) platelets (numbers or function), and (iii) coagulation cascade. The necessity for a presurgical hemostatic assessment is indicated by patient-associated and procedure-associated factors [18]. The potential risk of the presence of a hemostatic disorder in a specific patient together with the expected risks of bleeding for the specific surgical procedure should be taken into account. Patient-associated risk factors are evaluated based on medical history, physical examination (for any evidence of bleeding), the underlying disease, current and past medications, and previous abnormal results. Regarding procedure-associated factors, hemostatic assessment is recommended in spinal surgeries where massive noncompressible bleeding is possible, such as with extensive cervical dorsal approaches in large and giant breed dogs.

A minimum hemostatic screening has to include a platelet count, coagulation times (prothrombin time, PT and activated partial thromboplastin time, aPTT), and a buccal mucosal bleeding time. While a platelet count identifies a quantitative deficit in platelets, a bleeding time evaluates the qualitative function of the platelets. The mucosal bleeding time assesses platelet function in animals with normal platelet counts through the penetration of the buccal mucosa with a sharp blade (usually a standardized disposable lancet) and assessment of the time required for clotting to occur. Normal bleeding time should be less than 4 min in healthy dogs and 3 min in cats [15].

Two frequently used tests to evaluate the coagulation cascade are PT and aPTT. PT assesses the extrinsic coagulation pathway (factors I, II, V, VII, X) while aPTT evaluates the intrinsic pathway (factors I, II, V, VIII, IX, X, XI, XII) and both tests evaluate the common coagulation pathway. The activated clotting time (ACT), which can be performed easily at the patient's bedside, evaluates the intrinsic and common coagulation pathways.

Hemostatic deficiencies can be acquired or congenital. Inherited deficiencies of coagulation factors are reported in dogs and cats, and those factors can be quantitatively measured in blood. Hemophilia A is a sex-linked recessive disorder manifesting in males that results in low levels of coagulation factor VIII, while hemophilia B causes a deficiency of factor IX; both are associated with prolonged aPTT. Abnormal bleeding is usually intraarticular, intramuscular, retroperitoneal, or from the gastrointestinal or genitourinary tracts.

Another common congenital bleeding disorder is von Willebrand disease, an autosomal dominant condition, where patients suffer from low levels of von Willebrand factor (vWF). vWF is a glycoprotein produced by endothelial cells and is necessary for normal platelet aggregation and adhesion to the subendothelium. Patients with severe vWF deficits typically present with abnormal bruising, mucosal bleeding, prolonged bleeding after trauma, and have an increased mucosal bleeding time. Inherited vWF deficiency has been reported in several dog breeds but is most commonly seen in Doberman Pinschers [15]. This factor can be quantified in plasma prior to surgery and reported as a percentage of control mean. Dogs with vWF antigen less than 50% are considered positive and dogs with greater than 70% are considered negative, with intermediate values being unclassified [15]. Pretreating with desmopressin acetate (DDAVP) or administration of preoperative and/or intraoperative DDAVP-boosted fresh frozen plasma may be recommended in these patients.

In addition to congenital deficiencies there are many acquired bleeding disorders. Warfarin inhibits the formation of vitamin K-dependent factors (prothrombin, factors VII, IX, and X, and proteins C and S) and therefore intoxicated patients suffer from prolonged PT and slightly increased aPTT. Hepatic failure can also cause prolonged bleeding since the liver produces all coagulation factors except factor VIII. Aspirin prolongs bleeding time by irreversibly inhibiting the cyclooxygenase enzyme and consequently decreasing platelet adhesion. Like von Willebrand's disease, platelet function disorders related to administration of aspirin can be treated by administration of DDAVP 30 min prior to surgery [23]. Other platelet function or quantitative disorders can be treated with platelet-rich concentrate.

These standard hemostatic screening tests (platelet count, coagulation times, and mucosal bleeding time) have limitations and no

A

R	K	Angle	MA	G	CI	LY30	CL60	LY60	CL30
min	min	deg	mm	d/sc		%	%	%	%
2.0	0.8	78.0	70.4	11.9K	4.3	0.0	99.4	0.0	100.0
2–12	1–6	37–78	44–62	3.7K–7.6K	0–3	0–5	85–100	0–15	92–100

B

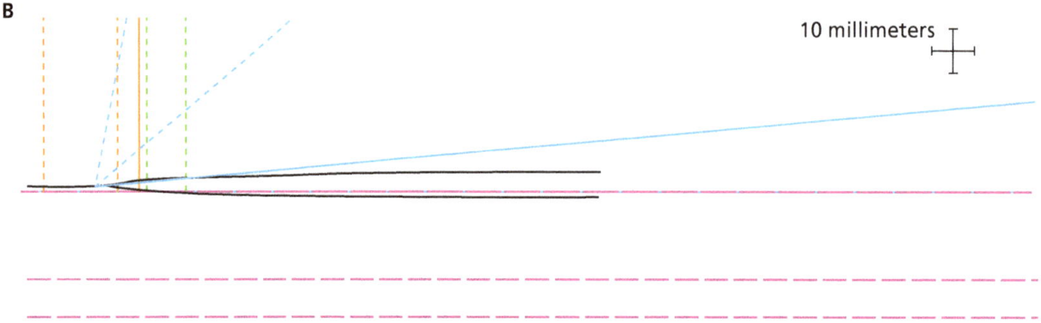

R	K	Angle	MA	G	CI	LY30	CL60	LY60	CL30
min	min	deg	mm	d/sc		%	%	%	%
14.9	N\A	4.6	2.9	0.1K		0.0	100.0	0.0	100.0
2–12	1–6	37–78	44–62	3.7K–7.6K		0–5	85–100	0–15	92–100

Figure 6.5 Thromboelastography traces: (A) mild hypercoagulable state in a dog; (B) hypocoagulable state in a dog with coagulopathy. *Source*: Courtesy of Dr. Shauna Blois.

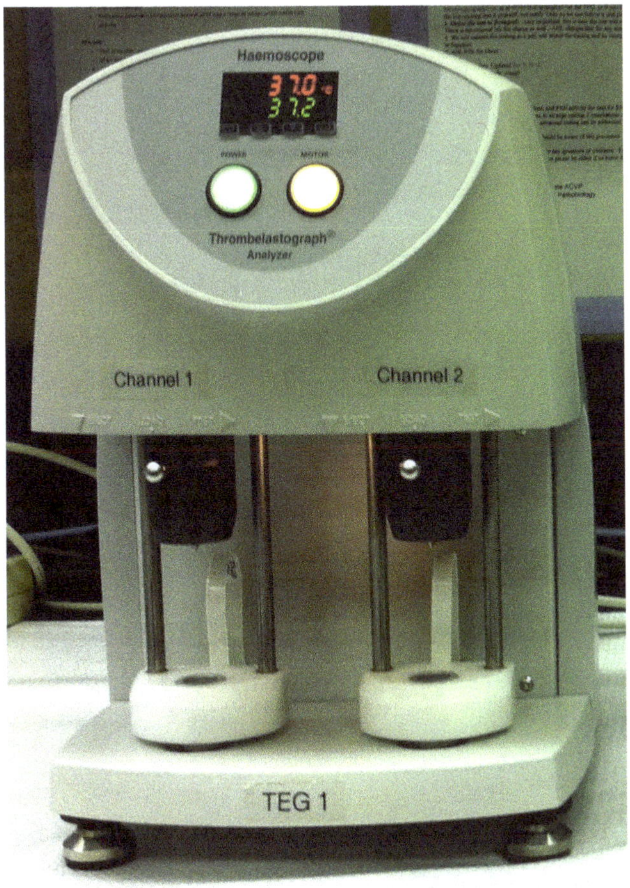

Figure 6.6 Thromboelastograph analyzer. *Source*: Courtesy of Dr. Shauna Blois.

specific values have been shown to be predictive of surgical bleeding [17,18]. More elaborate platelet function testing such as thromboelastography (TEG) have been described and used in animals in research and the clinical setting. TEG is able to detect and continuously display changes in viscoelastic properties of the blood as it clots, providing a more global evaluation of hemostasis in vivo than occurs when components of coagulation are studied independently. TEG traces can suggest the presence of normocoagulable, hypocoagulable, hypercoagulable, and secondary fibrinolytic states (Figure 6.5) and are thought to be more predictive of surgical bleeding [24] (Figure 6.6).

Other tests, such as fibrin–fibrinogen degradation products (FDPs) and D-dimer assays, can provide evidence of fibrinolysis and fibrinogenolysis, which are indicative of DIC, but those tests can also be positive in dogs with other conditions including neoplasia, immune-mediated hemolytic anemia, pancreatitis, and sepsis [15,20].

Thoracic Radiographs

Thoracic radiographs are one of the most commonly performed radiographic examinations in small animal practice. Ideally, they should be obtained as part of the MDB in all animals with spinal cord disorder, particularly in those older than 6 years and those with cardiovascular and/or respiratory abnormalities. Any animal with an increased suspicion for neoplasia, infectious disease, trauma, or comorbidities that could increase the anesthetic or surgical risk should also have thoracic radiographs performed as part of the work-up (Figure 6.7).

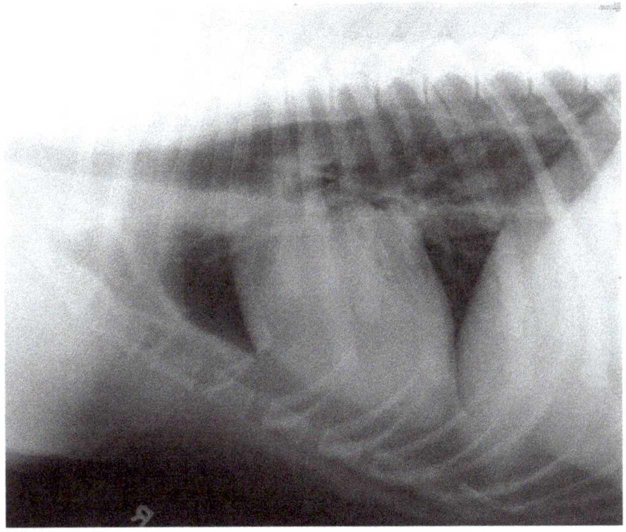

Figure 6.7 Lateral radiograph of the thorax in a 1-year-old male Newfoundland dog presented for progressive generalized weakness showing evidence of megaesophagus.

Some diseases such as multifocal or metastatic tumours, trauma, or infectious diseases can affect the thorax and the spine concurrently. Thoracic radiographs are indicated in trauma patients to rule out conditions such as pulmonary contusions, pneumothorax, hemothorax, and diaphragmatic hernia. Thoracic radiographs are often indicated even when the clinical signs are confined to the neurological system (Figure 6.8).

Thoracic computed tomography (CT) is more sensitive than thoracic radiography in the screening and detection of pulmonary nodules in dogs with malignant neoplasia [25] (Figure 6.9). However, radiographs are still considered the standard of care due to CT's limited availability, higher cost, and requirement for general anesthesia. In addition, there is evidence that CT's high sensitivity could lead to a possible over-interpretation and diagnosis of metastatic disease [26].

Thoracic radiographic examination must include a minimum of two orthogonal views, although a three-view thoracic examination is becoming routine standard of care (Figure 6.10). Recognition of radiographic abnormalities is based on a thorough understanding of normal radiographic appearance. Evaluation of each of the four basic anatomical regions is the basis for interpretation: (i) extrathoracic region including thoracic skeleton and soft tissues of the thoracic wall and diaphragm; (ii) pleural space; (iii) pulmonary parenchyma; and (iv) mediastinum including heart and great vessels [27]. Many radiographic abnormalities are nonspecific and it can be difficult to differentiate between normal and abnormal. Interpretation by an experienced radiologist is extremely valuable.

Abdominal Ultrasound

Similar to thoracic radiographs, evaluation of the abdomen is recommended when assessing for systemic conditions such as neoplasia, trauma, and infectious diseases that affect the spine

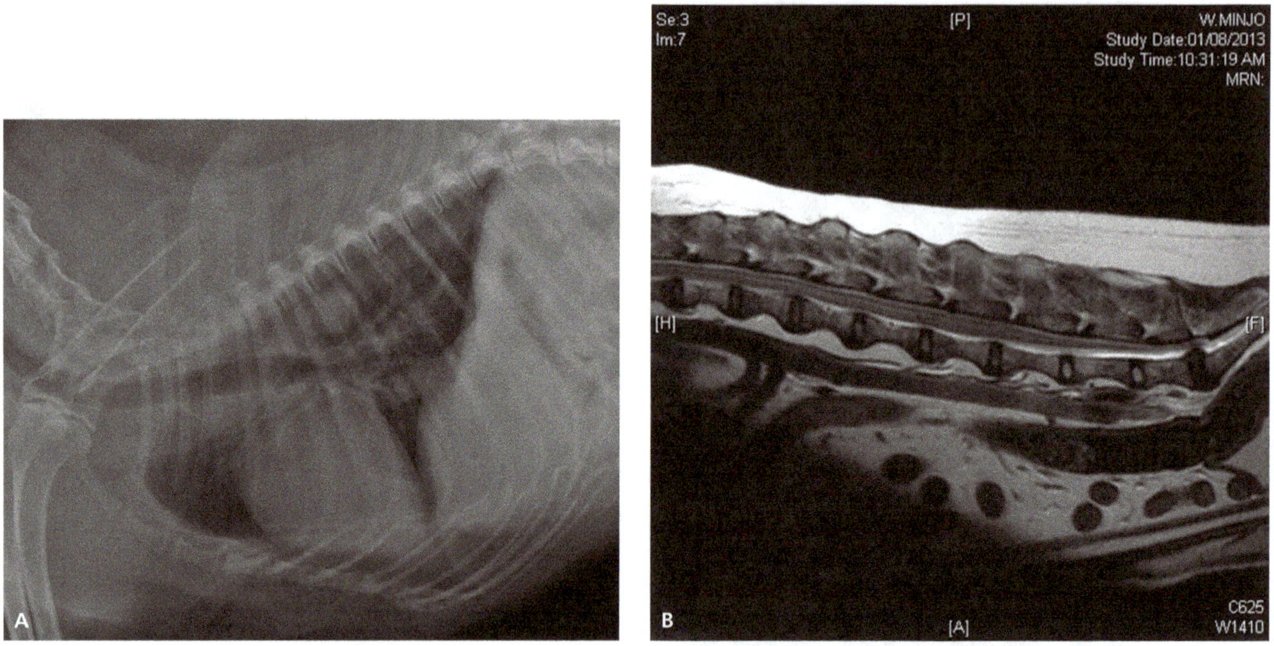

Figure 6.8 A 13-year-old male Shetland sheepdog presented for severe lumbosacral pain. (A) Left lateral thoracic radiograph exhibiting an incidental focal thoracic nodule dorsal to the carina. (B) Sagittal T2-weighted MRI of the caudal vertebral column showing moderate intervertebral disc protrusion and decreased disc signal intensity at L7–S1.

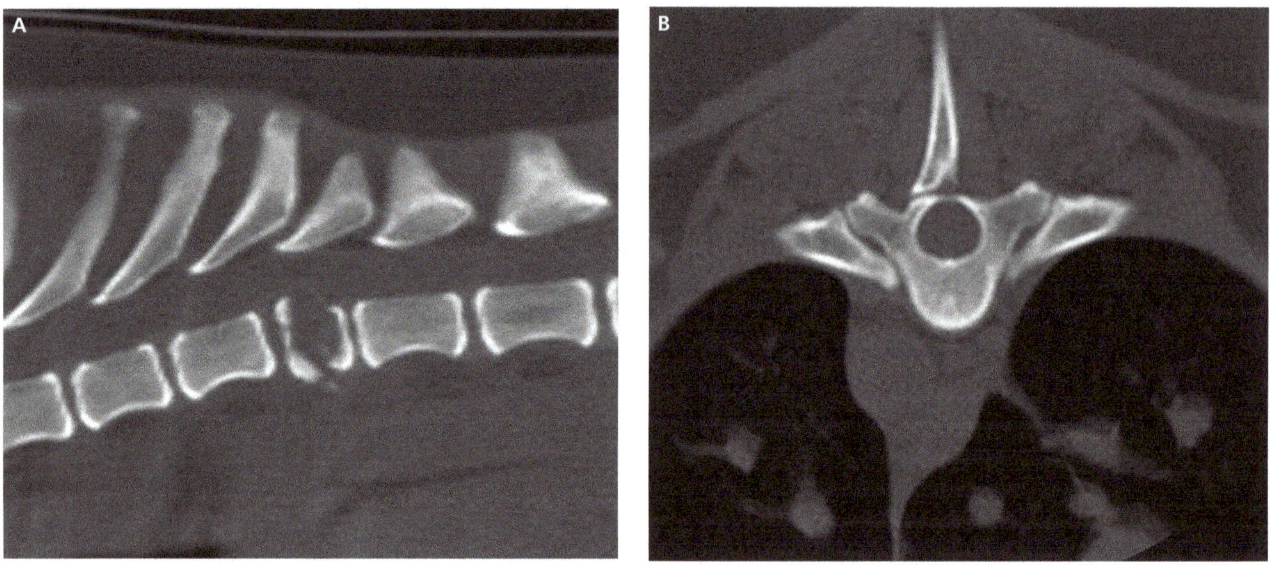

Figure 6.9 CT of the thoracolumbar region in a 12-year-old female Jack Russell Terrier dog presenting acute paraplegia. (A) Sagittal reformatted image showing severe bone lysis of the T10 vertebra, shortening of the vertebral body length, and minimally displaced compression fracture. (B) Transverse image showing multifocal pulmonary nodules. Final histopathological diagnosis was primary vertebral osteosarcoma with vertebral pathological fracture and pulmonary metastasis.

concurrently, and for assessing the patient's general health status for surgical and anesthetic risk evaluation purposes. Accordingly, abdominal ultrasound is strongly recommended in animals older than 6 years, and those with suspected spinal neoplasia, trauma, infectious disease, or other comorbidities (Figures 6.11 and 6.12). Metastatic carcinomas, particularly those arising from the mammary gland, prostate and urinary bladder, have a predilection to metastasize to the vertebral column with lumbar and thoracic vertebrae predominantly affected [28].

Although abdominal ultrasound can be complementary to radiography, since the combination of both imaging modalities results in more information relating to size, shape, and position of organs, ultrasound alone provides accurate information regarding the outline and architecture of tissues [29]. Ultrasonography can be performed anywhere along the abdominal wall, the only impediment being bone and gas-filled structures, which should be avoided. If a general examination is to be performed, a systematic approach is required. Possible abnormalities include the presence of abdominal masses (from enlargement of one or more of the intraabdominal

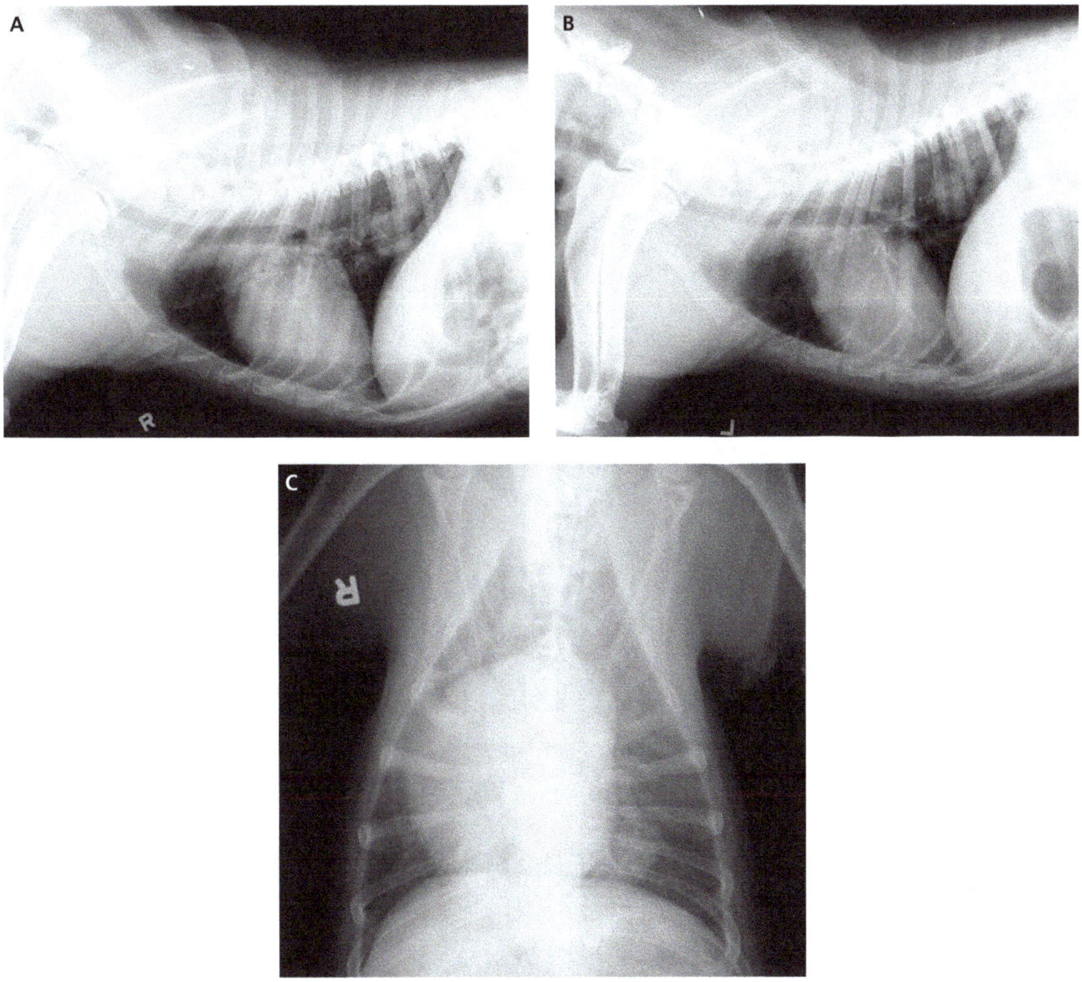

Figure 6.10 Three-view radiographic study of the thorax in an 8-year-old female Boxer dog presented for chronic cervical myelopathy. Multifocal pulmonary masses were detected in the caudal/accessory lung lobes. (A) Right lateral view; (B) left lateral view; (C) ventrodorsal view.

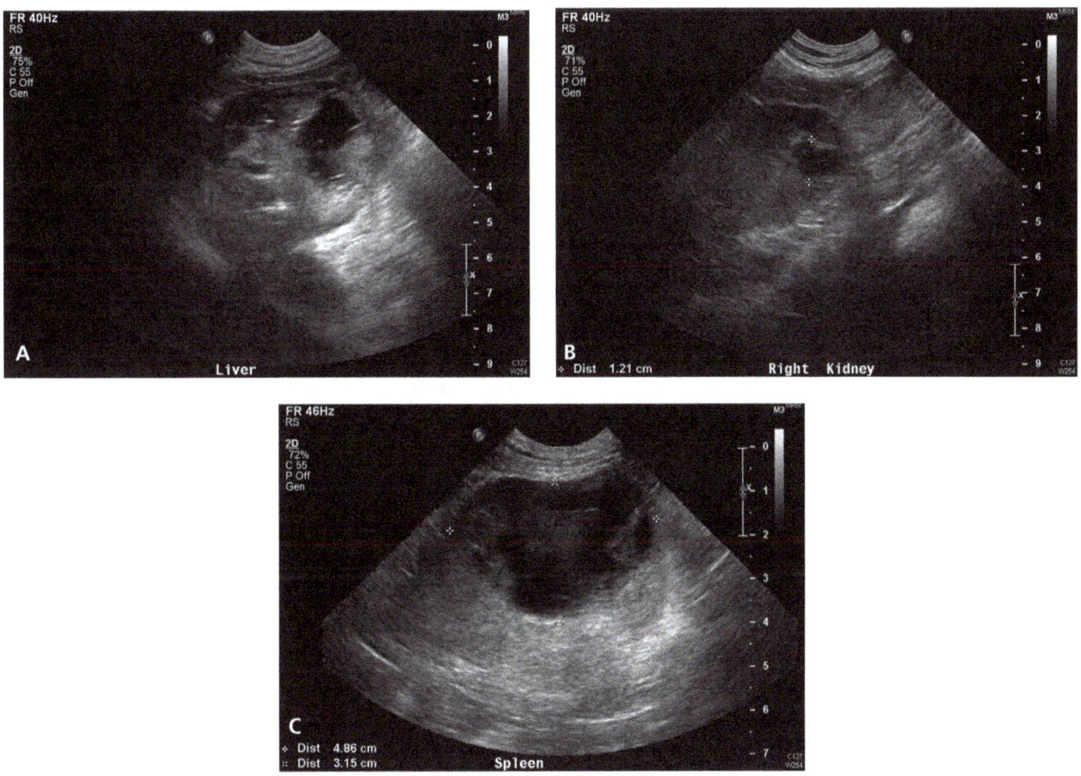

Figure 6.11 Abdominal ultrasound study in a 13-year-old female Labrador Retriever dog presented for cervical myelopathy and nonregenerative anemia with findings suggesting abdominal metastatic neoplasia. (A) Focal mixed echogenic and cavitated mass in the liver. (B) Focal hypoechoic nodule in the right kidney. (C) Mixed echogenic nodule in the spleen.

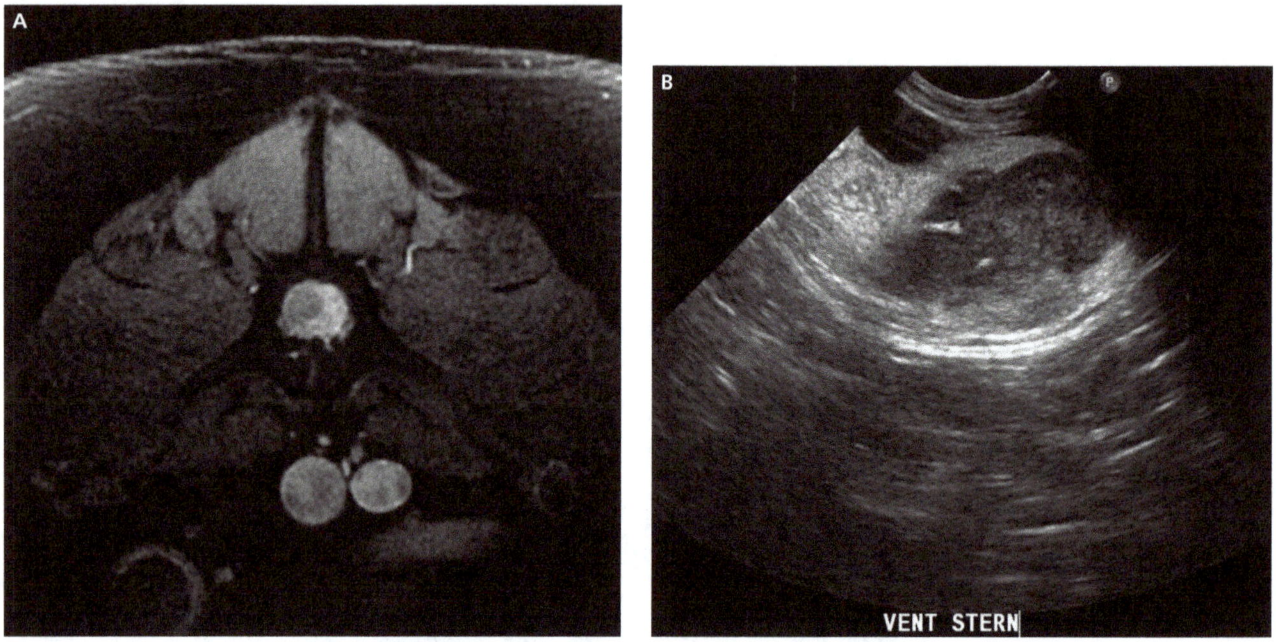

Figure 6.12 A 13-year-old male mixed-breed dog with progressive paraparesis and urinary and fecal incontinence. (A) Transverse postcontrast T1-weighted MRI at L4–L5 showing a right-sided, contrast-enhanced, intradural mass diagnosed as meningioma. (B) Ultrasound of a focal multilobulated mixed echogenicsubcutaneous mass along the sternum which was incidentally detected during the physical examination and later diagnosed as sarcoma.

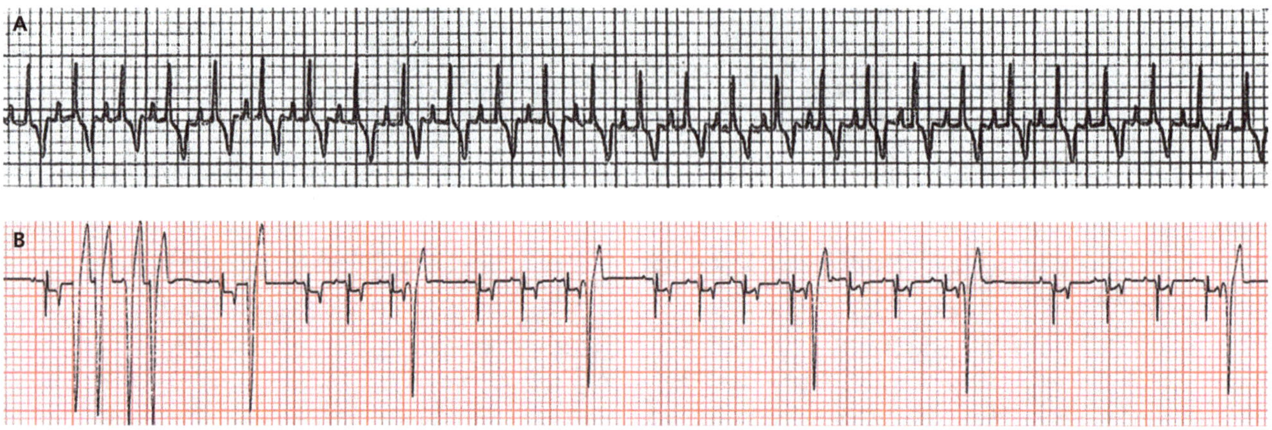

Figure 6.13 Electrocardiogram traces (lead II, 12.5 mm/s, 0.5 cm/mV). (A) Sinus tachycardia due to severe spinal pain as a result of acute intervertebral disc extrusion in a dog. Heart rate is about 170 bpm but it has the features of normal sinus rhythm with P for every QRS complex, P–QRS relationship constant, and positive P in lead II. (B) Ventricular premature complexes (VPCs) in a dog. These are commonly detected in polytraumatized patients associated with pain, hypotension, and hypovolemia/hypoperfusion. The sinus beats show evidence of myocardial ischemia in the form of ST-segment depression, which could be the result of acute myocardial necrosis/neurogenic cardiomyopathy syndrome. *Source*: Courtesy of Dr. Lynne O'Sullivan.

organs due to physiological or pathological processes such as neoplasia, torsion, or hematoma), peritoneal effusion, localized or generalized peritonitis, and free gas in the abdomen.

Electrocardiogram

Electrocardiography is a valuable diagnostic test and is the initial diagnostic test of choice to confirm and diagnose arrhythmias in dogs and cats. It should be recorded when an arrhythmia (bradycardia, tachycardia, or irregularity of rhythm not secondary to respiratory sinus arrhythmia) is detected during physical examination, in patients with a history of syncope or episodic weakness, and in those with suspected heart disease [30] (Figure 6.13A). Moreover, it can provide clues to cardiac chamber enlargement and hypertrophy, electrolyte imbalance (hyperkalemia, hyponatremia, hypercalcemia, hypocalcemia), myocardial ischemia/hypoxemia, drug intoxication, and thoracic and pericardial effusion. Significant arrhythmias may occur in patients with systemic diseases such as those suffering from electrolyte imbalances, neoplasia (particularly splenic neoplasia), and sepsis.

Although relatively rare, acute spinal cord trauma, spinal cord compression related to intervertebral disc herniation or other space-occupying lesions and infection can result in acute myocardial necrosis (neurogenic cardiomyopathy), probably as a result of increased sympathetic tone and release of catecholamines [31,32]. Myocardial necrosis typically presents clinically as cardiac arrhythmias with ST segment depression, prolonged QT interval, and even T-wave abnormalities (Figure 6.13B).

Video clips to accompany this book can be found on the companion website at:
www.wiley.com/go/shores/neurosurgery

References

1 Sturges BK, Dickinson PJ. Principles of neurosurgery. In: Platt SR, Olby NJ (eds) *BSAVA Manual of Canine and Feline Neurology*, 3rd edn. Gloucester, UK: British Small Animal Veterinary Association, 2004: 355–367.

2 Shmon C. Assessment and preparation of the surgical patient and the operating team. In: Slatter D (ed.) *Textbook of Small Animal Surgery*, 3rd edn. Philadelphia, PA: Elsevier Saunders, 2003: 162–178.

3 Marioni-Henry K, Van Winkle TJ, Smith SH, Vite CH. Tumors affecting the spinal cord of cats: 85 cases (1980–2005). *J Am Vet Med Assoc* 2008;232:237–243.

4 Fang A, Hu SS, Endres N, Bradford DS. Risk factors for infection after spinal surgery. *Spine* 2005;30:1460–1465.

5 Abdul-Jabbar A, Takemoto S, Weber MH, Hu SS, Mummaneni PV, Deviren V, Ames CP, Chou D, Weinstein PR, Burch S, Berven SH. Surgical site infection in spinal surgery: description of surgical and patient postoperative infection using administrative claims data. *Spine* 2012;37:1340–1345.

6 Dubory A, Giorgi H, Walter A et al. Surgical-site infection in spinal injury: incidental and risk factors in a prospective cohort of 518 patients. *Eur Spine J* 2015;24:543–554.

7 Eugster S, Schawalder P, Gaschen F, Boerlin P. A prospective study of postoperative surgical site infections in dogs and cats. *Vet Surg* 2004;33:542–550.

8 Heldmann E, Brown DC, Shofer F. The association of propofol usage with postoperative wound infection rate in clean wounds: a retrospective study. *Vet Surg* 1999;28:256–259.

9 Nazarali A, Singh A, Weese JS. Perioperative administration of antimicrobials during tibial plateau leveling osteotomy. *Vet Surg* 2014;43:966–971.

10 Yap FW, Calvo I, Smith KD, Parkin T. Perioperative risk factors for surgical site infection in tibial tuberosity advancement: 224 stifles. *Vet Comp Orthop Traumatol* 2015;28:199–206.

11 Dewey CW. Myelopathies: disorders of the spinal cord. In: Dewey CW (ed.) *A Practical Guide to Canine and Feline Neurology*, 2nd edn. Ames, IA: Wiley-Blackwell, 2008: 323–388.

12 Walker D. Peripheral blood smears. In: Cowell RT, Tyler RD, Meinkoth JH, DeNicola DB (eds) *Diagnostic Cytology and Hematology of the Dog and Cat*, 3rd edn. St Louis, MO: Elsevier Health Sciences, 2007: 390–421.

13 Willard MD, Tvedten H. *Small Animal Diagnosis by Laboratory Methods*, 5th edn. St Louis, MO: Elsevier Saunders, 2012.

14 Latimer KS, Campagnoli RP, Danilenko DM. Pelger-Huët anomaly in Australian shepherds: 87 cases (1991–1997). *Comp Haematol Int* 2000;10:9–13.

15 Harvey JW. Evaluation of hemostasis: coagulation and platelet disorders. In: Harvey JW (ed.) *Veterinary Hematology: A Diagnostic Guide and Color Atlas*. St Louis, MO: Elsevier Saunders, 2012: 192–233.

16 Brainard BM, Brown AJ. Defects of coagulation encountered in small animal critical care. *Vet Clin North Am Small Anim Pract* 2011;41:783–803.

17 Chee YL, Crawford JC, Watson HG, Greaves M. Guidelines on the assessment of bleeding risk prior to surgery or invasive procedures. British Committee for Standards in Haematology. *Br J Haematol* 2008;140:496–504.

18 Hackner SG, Carrie RW. Bleeding and hemostasis. In: Tobias KM, Johnston SA (eds) *Veterinary Surgery: Small Animal*. St Louis, MO: Elsevier Saunders, 2012: 94–120.

19 Vanderschueren S, De Weerdt A, Malbrain M, Vankersschaever D, Frans E, Wilmer A, Bobbaers H. Thrombocytopenia and prognosis in intensive care. *Crit Care Med* 2000;28:1871–1876.

20 Kaneko JJ, Harvey JW, Bruss ML. *Clinical Biochemistry of Domestic Animals*, 6th edn. Burlington, MA: Academic Press, 2008.

21 Battison A. Apparent pseudohyperkalemia in a Chinese Shar Pei dog. *Vet Clin Pathol* 2007;36:89–93.

22 Degen M. Pseudohyperkalemia in Akitas. *J Am Vet Med Assoc* 1987;190: 541–543.

23 Di Mauro FM, Holowaychuk MK. Intravenous administration of desmopressin acetate to reverse acetylsalicylic acid-induced coagulopathy in three dogs. *J Vet Emerg Crit Care* 2013;23:455–458.

24 Kheirabadi, BS, Crissey, JM, Deguzman, R, Holcomb JB. In vivo bleeding time and in vitro thromboelastography are better indicators of dilutional hypothermic coagulopathy than prothrombin time. *J Trauma* 2007;62:1352–1359.

25 Eberle N, Fork M, von Babo V, Nolte I, Simon D. Comparison of examination of thoracic radiographs and thoracic computed tomography in dogs with appendicular osteosarcoma. *Vet Comp Oncol* 2011;9:131–140.

26 Oblak ML, Boston SE, Woods JP, Nykamp S. Comparison of concurrent imaging modalities for staging of dogs with appendicular primary bone tumours. *Vet Comp Oncol* 2015;13:28–39.

27 Berry CR, Graham JP, Thrall JP. Interpretation paradigms for the small animal thorax. In: Thrall DE (ed.) *Textbook of Veterinary Diagnostic Radiology*, 5th edn. St Louis, MO: Saunders Elsevier, 2007: 462–485.

28 Cooley DM, Waters DJ. Skeletal metastasis as the initial clinical manifestation of metastatic carcinoma in 19 dogs. *J Vet Intern Med* 1998;12:288–293.

29 Kealy JK, McAllister H, Graham JP. The abdomen. In: *Diagnostic Radiology and Ultrasonography of the Dog and Cat*, 5th edn. St Louis, MO: Saunders Elsevier, 2011: 23–198.

30 Tilley LP, Smith Jr FWK. Electrocardiography. In: Tilley LP, Smith Jr FWK, Oyama MA, Sleeper MM (eds) *Manual of Canine and Feline Cardiology*, 4th edn. St Louis, MO: Saunders Elsevier, 2007: 49–77.

31 Smith Jr FWK, Schrope DP, Sammarco CD. Cardiovascular effects of systemic disease. In: Tilley LP, Smith Jr FWK, Oyama MA, Sleeper MM (eds) *Manual of Canine and Feline Cardiology*, 4th edn. St Louis, MO: Saunders Elsevier, 2007: 240–276.

32 King JM, Roth L, Haschek WM. Myocardial necrosis secondary to neural lesions in domestic animals. *J Am Vet Med Assoc* 1982;180:144–148.

7 Advanced Imaging: Spinal Surgery

Stephanie Nykamp

Myelography

Although computed tomography (CT) and magnetic resonance imaging (MRI) have replaced myelography in many institutions, myelography remains an excellent modality for localizing spinal cord disease when other modalities are unavailable. Orthogonal survey and post-myelogram images of the entire region of interest should be performed. Postcontrast ventrodorsal oblique views are frequently advantageous for the circumferential localization of extradural lesions [1,2].

Myelography is performed by injection of a nonionic iodinated contrast medium (0.3–0.45 mL/kg) into the subarachnoid space. Iohexol (which contains 240 mg iodine per milliliter) and iopamidol (200 mg of iodine per milliliter) are commonly used, safe, and effective contrast agents [3–5]. The ideal iodine concentration has been reported to be 200 mg/mL but higher concentrations (up to 350 mg/mL) have been used with no increase in complication rate [6,7]. Myelography can be performed at either the cerebellomedullary cistern or in the caudal lumbar region. Myelography is always performed under general anesthesia using aseptic technique. A 22G spinal needle is commonly used and a spinal needle is preferred because the short bevel minimizes concurrent injection into the epidural space.

Cervical Technique

The technique for performing puncture of the cerebellomedullary cistern has been well described previously [8]. Briefly, the head should be flexed and the needle placed on the midline between the occipital protuberance and the wings of the atlas. The bevel should be directed caudally and the needle advanced slowly with the myelographer stopping frequently, withdrawing the stylet, and checking for cerebrospinal fluid (CSF) flow as a distinctive "pop" when entering the dura is not always encountered [3]. Once flow of CSF is established contrast medium should be injected slowly. Raising the head will aid the caudal flow of contrast medium. Once the injection is complete this can be achieved by tilting the radiographic table or by placing the patient in sternal recumbency with the head elevated [9]. It should be noted that cervical injection of contrast medium has been associated with a higher risk of post-myelographic seizures [10,11]. When fluoroscopy is unavailable or myelography is performed in the CT suite, the cervical technique is often used as it is easier to perform than lumbar injection [12].

In cases of severe spinal cord swelling, as is seen in most acute intervertebral disc extrusions, cervical injection frequently fails to fully outline the lesion because contrast medium will not flow caudal to the affected spinal cord. Raising the head and neck can encourage contrast medium to flow caudally but if unsuccessful a lumbar puncture may be needed to outline the lesion [12].

Lumbar Technique

This technique is often preferred because it is associated with a lower risk and it provides higher-quality myelograms for thoracolumbar lesions [13]. Because the dural sac ends blindly in the lumbar region it is possible to pressurize the injection, forcing contrast medium past the swollen area of spinal cord and helping to outline the entire lesion and aid accurate localization. Although fluoroscopy is not required, it is useful for aiding needle placement. Lumbar injection is most commonly performed between L4–L5 and L6–L7 with L5–L6 being the preferred site. Previous work has shown that it can be performed at any lumbar site without increased risk of complication but is not typically recommended [14]. If fluoroscopy is not available, a radiograph should be obtained after initial placement of the needle but prior to entering the vertebral canal to confirm the site of injection. Once the needle has been placed in the vertebral canal a small test injection (0.5–1.0 mL) can be made to confirm appropriate placement prior to injecting the full contrast dose.

Needle placement can be achieved by a paramedian or median approach (Figure 7.1) using a 22G spinal needle of appropriate length. For the paramedian approach the needle is placed lateral to the spinous process and angled craniomedially, entering the subarachnoid space at an oblique angle (approximately 45°). The skin is entered at the level of the spinous process with the needle directed ventral until it rests on the lamina and then walked off the lamina in a craniomedial direction into the vertebral canal. On fluoroscopy or

Current Techniques in Canine and Feline Neurosurgery, First Edition. Edited by Andy Shores and Brigitte A. Brisson.
© 2017 John Wiley & Sons, Inc. Published 2017 by John Wiley & Sons, Inc.
Companion website: www.wiley.com/go/shores/neurosurgery

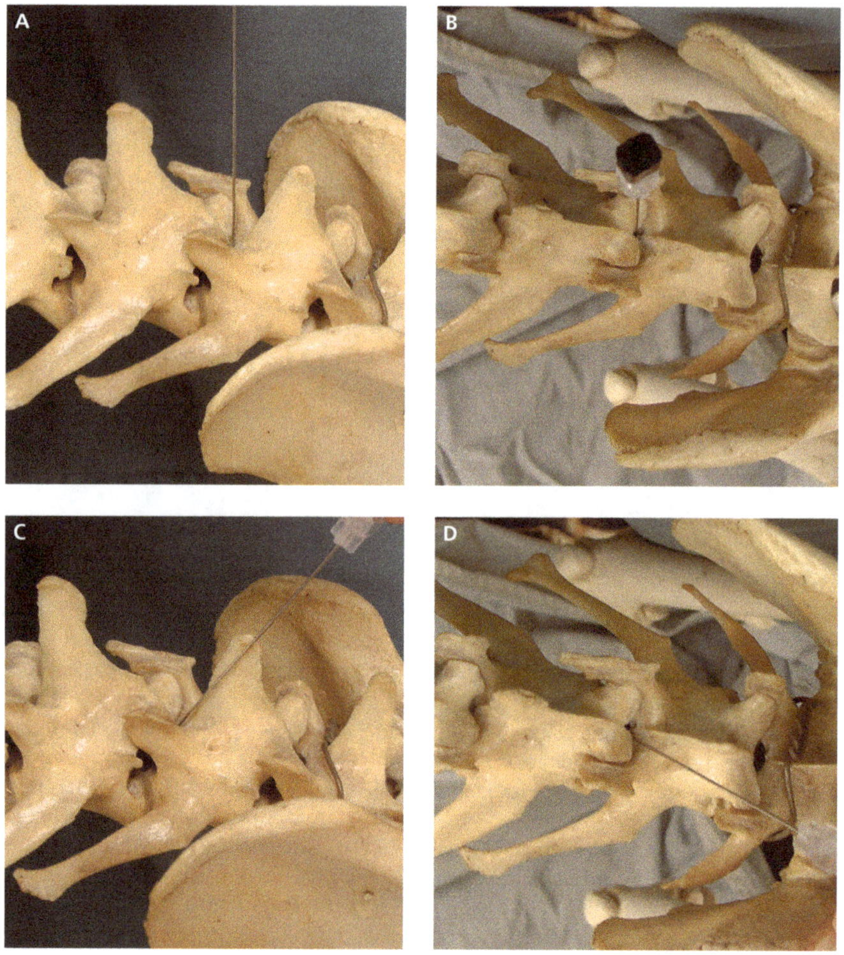

Figure 7.1 Technique for lumbar puncture. For the median approach (A, B) the needle is placed perpendicular to the spine along the midline, cranial to the spinous process of L6. For the paramedian approach (C, D) the needle is placed to the left or right of the spinous process and directed cranially approximately 45°.

survey radiographs the angle of the needle typically parallels the angle of the spinal articulation. The median approach involves placement of the needle immediately cranial to the spinous process on the midline and directing the needle ventrally (perpendicular to the vertebral canal).

For each approach the contrast medium can be injected into either the dorsal or the ventral subarachnoid space. Injecting into the ventral subarachnoid space is technically easier and decreases the risk of intramedullary injection but results in the needle traversing the spinal cord or nerve roots with the potential to cause damage [3]. In a study by Tilmant et al. [15] injection into the dorsal subarachnoid space results in compression of the spinal cord by 1–2 mm as the dura is indented prior to needle penetration and this resulted in needle penetration of the spinal cord once the dura was punctured. Therefore regardless of technique some spinal cord penetration is inevitable. Although clinical signs are often not evident, spinal cord puncture can be associated with hemorrhage, gliosis, and axonal degeneration [16]. Multiple needle punctures should be avoided to reduce the risk of epidural leakage.

Artifacts

Artifacts, including air in the subarachnoid space and epidural injections, can negatively affect the interpretation of the myelogram and care should be taken to avoid these occurring. Epidural leakage is more common when multiple punctures are made through the dura and in obese animals where the landmarks are not easily palpable [9]. Epidural contrast can mimic the signs of an extradural lesion so proper identification of this artifact is critical (Figure 7.2). Epidural contrast medium is absorbed faster than contrast medium in the subarachnoid space. Repeating the radiographs 10–15 min after the injection may allow for sufficient clearing of epidural contrast medium to facilitate interpretation. Air bubbles in the subarachnoid space frequently change position between images so careful evaluation should prevent misinterpretation of air as a lesion [3].

Normal Variations

The dorsal subarachnoid space is widest at C2. The ventral subarachnoid space at C2–C3 is narrow and slightly dorsally deviated [9]. In the caudal cervical region the ventral subarachnoid space is often wide, creating the false impression of spinal cord displacement [3]. Focal attenuation and slight undulation of the ventral contrast column is common over the intervertebral disc spaces.

Opacification of the central canal can occur if the bevel of the needle is placed in the central canal, the central canal communicates with the subarachnoid space at the conus medullaris, or if there is disruption of the spinal cord parenchyma from neoplasia or severe trauma [17]. In normal dogs opacification of the central canal is more likely to occur if the injection is cranial to L5–L6 and

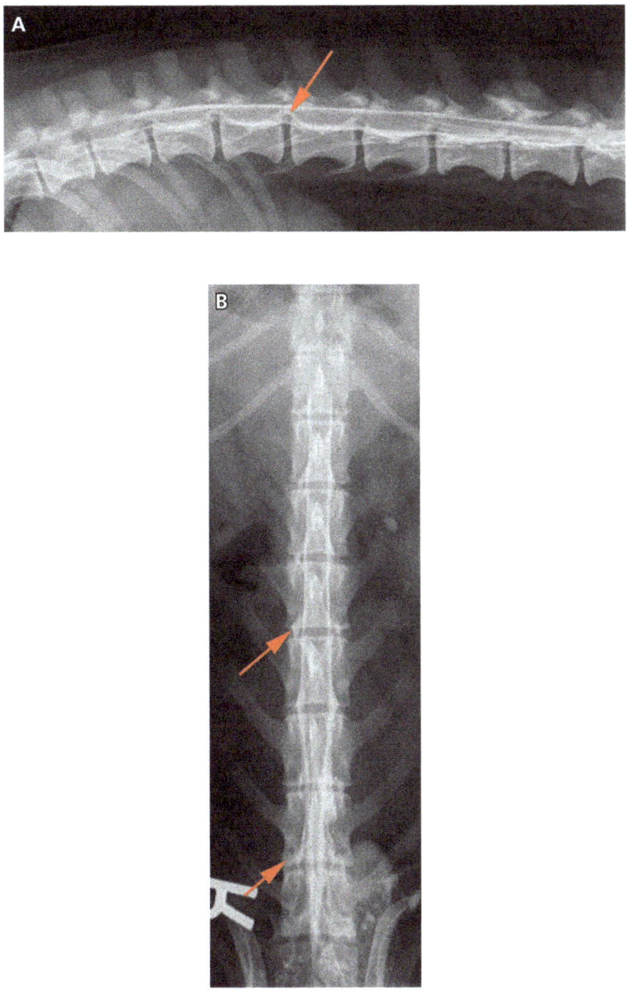

Figure 7.2 The presence of contrast in the epidural space (arrows in A,B) creates an undulating margin that can be confused with an extradural compression on the lateral view (A) but can be seen extending out the intervertebral foramen on the ventrodorsal view (B).

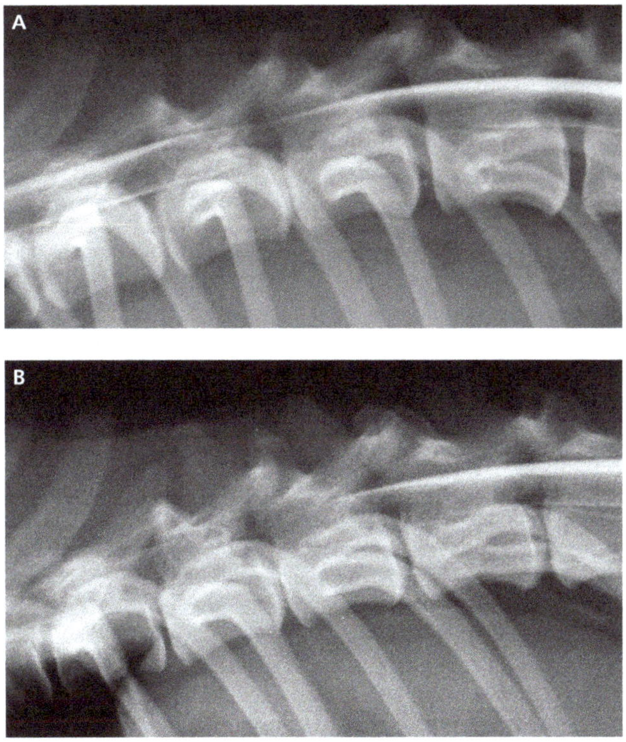

Figure 7.3 Obtaining an image while injecting contrast medium into the subarachnoid space (A) can result in better definition of the lesion when there is spinal cord swelling. When images are obtained after the injection is made (B) the contrast medium dissipates from the lesion site and accurate localization is more difficult.

made rapidly [17]. The normal central canal should be small (<1 mm) and uniform in size. Slight iatrogenic hydromyelia can occur if the injection is made under high pressure [9]. If preferential opacification of the central canal is identified during the injection, the procedure should be stopped and repeated from an alternative site or with the needle in the dorsal subarachnoid space.

Side Effects

The primary disadvantage of myelography is that it is an invasive technique. Reported side effects include worsening of the myelopathy, apnea, cardiac arrhythmias, and seizures [10,11,18,19]. The incidence of side effects is significantly reduced with newer contrast agents such as iohexol. Seizures remain the most common complication of myelography, with an incidence of 3–21% in dogs. Factors that significantly impacted post-myelographic seizures include iohexol dose (total volume), size of dog (large breeds are at higher risk), and injection site [10,11]. Many of these factors are interrelated and it was concluded that dogs receiving a higher total volume of contrast medium (despite the same mg/kg dose) and having a cervical injection were more likely to have a seizure upon recovery. Subsequent work suggested a maximum total volume of 8 mL of contrast medium for cervical injection in large breed dogs [11].

Tips

Contrast medium is hyperosmolar relative to CSF and is subject to redistribution with gravity. On the ventrodorsal view of the cervical vertebral column the contrast medium tends to accumulate cranially, resulting in poor opacification of the caudal cervical region. Obtaining a dorsoventral view in these cases redistributes the contrast medium to the caudal cervical region, thus facilitating a diagnosis [20]. Similar phenomena can be seen on the lateral views. Elevating the front or hind end (or both) can help to redistribute the contrast medium to the area of interest [9,12]. Rarely do we consider the patient's state of recumbency during myelography but this gravity effect can influence whether lesions are detected. One case report indicates that a lateralized lesion was not evident when the images were acquired in right lateral recumbency but was clearly defined when the images were acquired in left lateral recumbency [21]. This lesion was also noted on the oblique ventrodorsal views but, if these are not routinely obtained, consideration should be given to obtaining both lateral views when a lesion is not clearly defined.

Inadequate characterization of the lesion can occur when there is severe attenuation of the subarachnoid space. In some cases this can be overcome by obtaining an image while injecting so the subarachnoid space is maximally distended (Figure 7.3). This is particularly true in cats [22].

Advantages

- Requires no special equipment so is readily available.
- Typically is less expensive than CT and MRI.

Disadvantages
- Invasive.
- Mild risk of side effects.
- Cannot always provide circumferential lesion localization.

Computed Tomography

CT examination is noninvasive and relatively rapid. To maximize the information the CT scan can provide requires optimization of the scanning protocol. Consideration should be given to the algorithm, mode of acquisition (axial vs. helical), slice thickness, pitch or interval (slice overlap), field of view, and slice orientation. Commonly used imaging parameters are included in Table 7.1 [23]. Post acquisition, appropriate window and level of the images and use of reformatted images can add to the diagnostic ability of CT [24].

It is important to review images in more than one window/level setting to obtain all the necessary information (Table 7.2). When performed without myelography, a soft tissue window is useful for evaluating the epidural fat and spinal cord while a bone window is better for evaluation of the vertebrae (Figure 7.4). When combined with myelography a bone window is most useful for reducing the blooming artifact from the contrast medium.

The ability to acquire thin slices and reformat CT images provides an advantage over MRI in evaluating the intervertebral foramen for stenosis and nerve root compression. Intravenous contrast administration can also improve the assessment of nerve roots for neuritis and neoplasia.

When performing unenhanced CT a decision must be made whether to scan the entire region of the neuroanatomical localization (e.g., T3–L3) or a more limited area (T9–L3). The advantage of a more limited scan is shorter scan times with smaller slice thicknesses (reducing partial volume averaging artifacts) and less wear on the X-ray tube [25]. However, this approach should only be used if the probability of intervertebral disc herniation is very high as other lesions may be missed [26]. An alternative approach is a survey of the entire region of neuroanatomical localization with a larger slice thickness and a smaller group of thin sections through the lesions identified. This is less of a concern as the availability of multislice scanners is increasing.

Although CT is very good for detecting bony lesions, the lower contrast resolution of CT compared with MRI makes it less sensitive to intramedullary spinal cord lesions. Epidural fat is hypoattenuating (darker) relative to soft tissue and provides contrast to the spinal cord and nerve roots. Inability to see the epidural fat occurs with spinal cord enlargement (swelling, neoplasia, etc.) or when the fat is displaced by intervertebral disc or a soft tissue mass. Evaluating the CT images in both a soft tissue and a bone window may improve the ability to localize lesions [26].

Table 7.1 Commonly used imaging parameters for spine CT.

Positioning	Dorsal recumbency
kVp	100–120
mAs	200
Slice thickness	1–2 mm (up to 5 mm for entire spine survey)
Reconstruction algorithm (kernel)	Soft tissue (medium frequency) Bone (high frequency)

Table 7.2 Typical window width and level settings for bone and soft tissue.

	Window width	Window level
Soft tissue	300	100
Bone	3000	500

Nonenhanced CT, Contrast-enhanced CT, and CT Myelography

Numerous authors have compared the use of unenhanced CT, contrast-enhanced CT (intravenous contrast), and CT myelography for spinal cord disease [25–32]. The ability to detect pathology on unenhanced CT is dependent on the presence of epidural fat and changes in density of the pathological tissue (e.g., mineralized disc material, acute hemorrhage, contrast enhancement). When minimal epidural fat is present and the lesion is of soft tissue density, contrast medium (either intravenous or intrathecal) may be required to characterize the lesion.

The intravenous contrast medium used for CT is iodinated contrast (ionic or nonionic) administered intravenously at a dose of 600 mg iodine per kilogram. Nonionic contrast medium is typically more expensive but has a lower risk of complications. Contraindications to intravenous contrast administration include previous contrast reactions and dehydration. The rate of serious contrast reactions in veterinary patients is unknown but likely similar to that in humans (2–4%) [33]. Minor reactions such as vomiting, nausea, and a burning sensation at the injection site are not typically noted as most of our patients are under anesthesia when iodinated contrast medium is administered. Hemodynamic changes including hypertension, tachycardia, and bradycardia can also occur [34–36]. The serious contrast reactions that have been described are anaphylaxis and contrast-induced nephropathy. Anaphylaxis should be treated in the routine manner. Contrast-induced nephropathy can only be treated supportively. Patients with preexisting renal disease, diabetes mellitus, and multiple myeloma may have an increased risk of contrast-induced nephropathy [37].

Advantages
- Noninvasive (survey or contrast-enhanced CT).
- Typically lower cost than MRI.
- Often more readily available than MRI.

Disadvantages
- Intrathecal contrast medium may be required to identify some lesions.
- Little information regarding the integrity of the spinal cord and spinal cord pathology.

Magnetic Resonance Imaging

MRI is generally considered to be the best imaging modality for spinal disease because of the high tissue contrast. Because MRI is highly sensitive it is imperative that a careful clinical examination be performed to localize the lesion to avoid false-positive results from subclinical disease.

Both high- and low-field strength magnets can be used to obtain diagnostic images of the spine. Low-field magnets typically require more time for each imaging sequence but are also less prone to artifacts and have lower operating and purchase costs.

The physics of MRI will not be discussed but image acquisition requires the use of a radiofrequency coil to receive or send and receive the radiofrequency pulse from which magnetic resonance

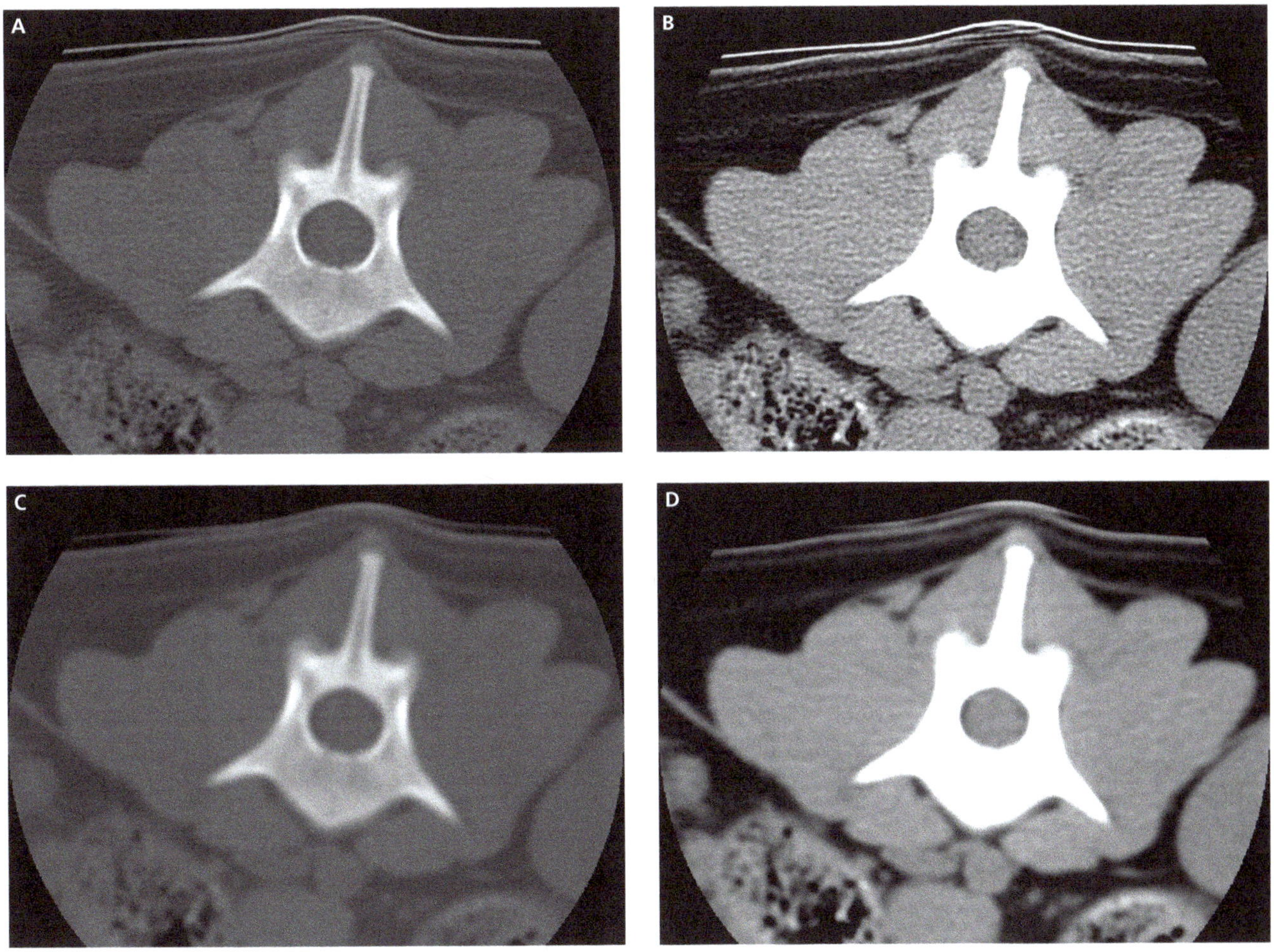

Figure 7.4 These CT images were obtained in a bone algorithm (A, B) and a soft tissue algorithm (C, D) and are displayed in a bone window (A, C) and a soft tissue window (B, D). Bony detail is best evaluated with a bone algorithm in a bone window (A) while soft tissue is best evaluated with a soft tissue algorithm in a soft tissue window (C).

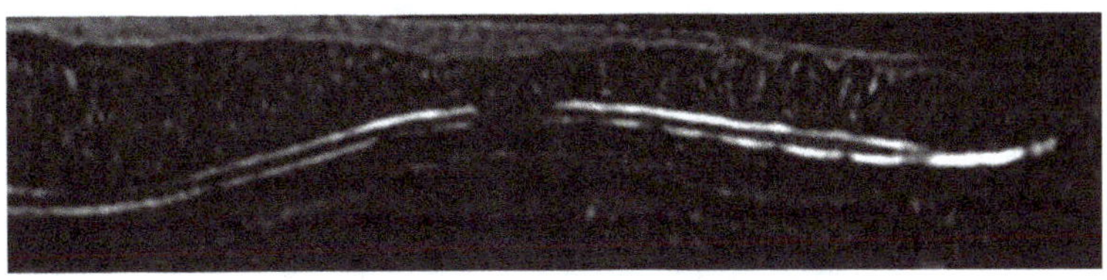

Figure 7.5 T2 myelogram image of the thoracic and lumbar vertebral column demonstrating attenuation of the subarachnoid space at the thoracolumbar junction.

images are generated. Choice and placement of the radiofrequency coil can have a dramatic effect on image quality. The signal intensity drops off with increasing distance from the coil so it should always be placed as close to the spine as possible. For medium to large breed dogs a phased array spine coil is ideal [38]. These coils have multiple adjacent individual coils with a small field of view that when combined provide large anatomical coverage with maximum signal-to-noise ratio. For small dogs and cats a phased array cardiac or knee coil can also be used. Positioning the patient in dorsal recumbency locates the spine closest to the coil and minimizes respiratory motion.

Many possible pulse sequences are available and their names may vary depending on the scanner. The ideal spine protocol would include sufficient pulse sequences in varied anatomical planes to diagnose or rule out all possible spinal diseases unless interpretation and adaptation of the protocol is possible while the scan is being performed. However, there is a balance to be achieved between total acquisition time and diagnostic information facilitating the customization of the scan protocol for the primary diagnostic questions. Any lesion should be evaluated in three planes to provide maximum anatomical information but these do not need to be all in the same pulse sequence. The following is a reasonable minimum protocol [38–40].

- Sagittal T2 myelogram (heavily T2-weighted images) (Figure 7.5).
- Sagittal T2-weighted images.
- Dorsal T2-weighted images.
- Transverse T2-weighted images through any suspected lesions (or through each intervertebral disc if no lesion is identified).
- Transverse T1-weighted images before and after contrast administration (post contrast with fat suppression).

In cases of suspected intervertebral disc herniation there may be a temptation to omit the T1-weighted images, but hydrated disc material has a similar signal intensity to epidural fat on T2-weighted images and noncompressive material (type III intervertebral disc herniation) may be overlooked if T1 images are not obtained (Figure 7.6). T2 images with fat suppression (T2 Fat Sat or STIR) are useful for evaluation of the vertebral canal for infection or neoplasia. T2* images are useful for assessing for hemorrhage [41].

Signal characteristics of tissues vary with pulse sequences. Relative signal intensities are given in Table 7.3. The majority of tumors and inflammatory lesions have relatively high T2 signal intensity and intermediate to low T1 signal intensity with variable degrees of contrast enhancement. Degenerative discs have low signal intensity on both T1 and T2 sequences. Hemorrhage has different imaging characteristics depending on the age of the hemorrhage and the imaging sequence [41].

Advantages

- Superior soft tissue resolution provides information on spinal cord integrity.

Disadvantages

- Cost.
- Availability.
- Contraindicated in dogs with pacemakers or with metallic implants near the area of interest.

Interpretation

The general principles of interpretation apply to projection and cross-sectional imaging modalities. Normally, the contrast columns or subarachnoid space should be thin, sharply margined, and parallel to the vertebral canal on all projections (Figure 7.7A). The ventral subarachnoid space can undulate and thin over the intervertebral disc spaces. Spinal disease is classified as extradural, intramedullary, and intradural–extramedullary based on changes in the size (attenuation or enlargement of) and displacement of the subarachnoid space and spinal cord. Some diseases, such as ischemic myelopathy, degenerative myelopathy, myelitis, and meningitis, can have normal imaging.

Signs of an extradural lesion include attenuation and deviation of the subarachnoid space toward the center of the vertebral canal (Figure 7.7B). Differentiating normal undulation of the ventral subarachnoid space from clinically important lesions is dependent on attenuation of the dorsal subarachnoid space. With myelography, if a lesion is directly ventral or lateral, deviation of the contrast column centrally will be noted on one view and the orthogonal projection will show signs of an intramedullary lesion (deviation of the contrast columns toward the vertebral canal). With MRI, intervertebral disc protrusions can often be differentiated from extrusions by their broad-based contact with the intervertebral disc and a fusiform shape, while extrusions tend to have less contact with the intervertebral disc, are longer dorsally compared to ventrally, and a have a rounded shape (Figure 7.8).

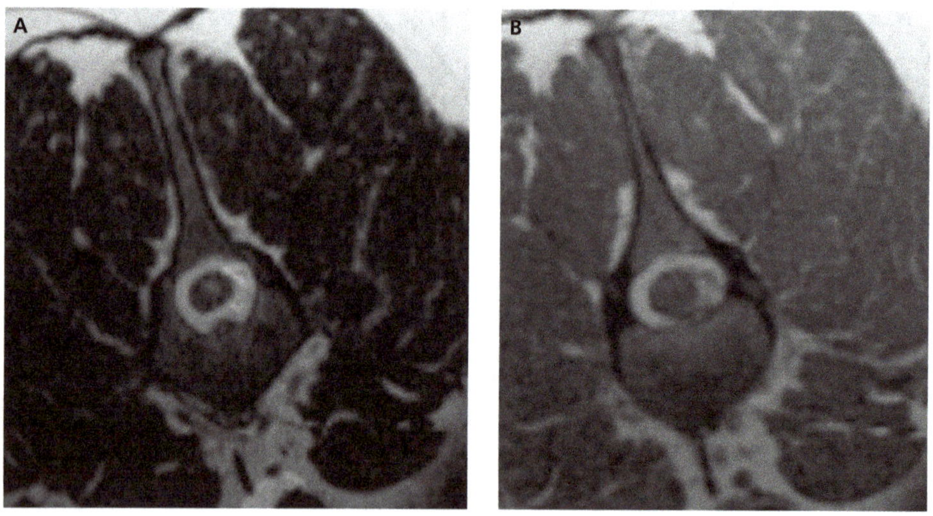

Figure 7.6 Transverse T2-weighted (A) and T1-weighted (B) MRI of herniation of hydrated intervertebral disc material into the left ventral vertebral canal. Although slight displacement of the spinal cord is evident on the T2-weighted images, the disc material is best identified on the T1-weighted images.

Table 7.3 Relative signal intensities of vertebral column tissues for the common pulse sequences.

	T1	T2	STIR
Nucleus of the intervertebral disc	Intermediate	High	High
Annulus of the intervertebral disc	Low	Low	Low
Cortical bone	Low	Low	Low
Cancellous bone	Intermediate to high	Intermediate to high	Low
Spinal cord	Intermediate	Intermediate	Intermediate
Subarachnoid space	Low	High	High
Muscle	Intermediate	Intermediate	Intermediate
Fat	High	High	Low

The differential diagnosis for extradural lesions includes intervertebral disc herniation, ligamentous hypertrophy, hemorrhage, neoplasia (vertebral or soft tissue), abscess, and vertebral fracture or luxation.

Intramedullary lesions are characterized by enlargement of the spinal cord and deviation of the subarachnoid space toward the vertebral canal on all projections (outward deviation) (Figure 7.7C). With myelography and CT, enlargement may be the only finding unless there is a tear in the dura resulting in contrast diffusion into the spinal cord. With MRI, a change in signal intensity due to the primary lesion or from edema secondary to the primary lesion is often evident. Intravenous contrast enhancement may be present with CT or MRI if there is breakdown of the blood–spinal cord barrier. The differential diagnosis for intramedullary lesion includes spinal cord edema, ischemic myelopathy, neoplasia, and inflammatory disease. Neoplasia and ischemia tend to be focal lesions while inflammatory disease is more commonly multifocal.

Intradural–extramedullary lesions (Figure 7.7D) are most evident when there is contrast medium in the subarachnoid space or on heavily T2-weighted MRI (myelogram-like images).

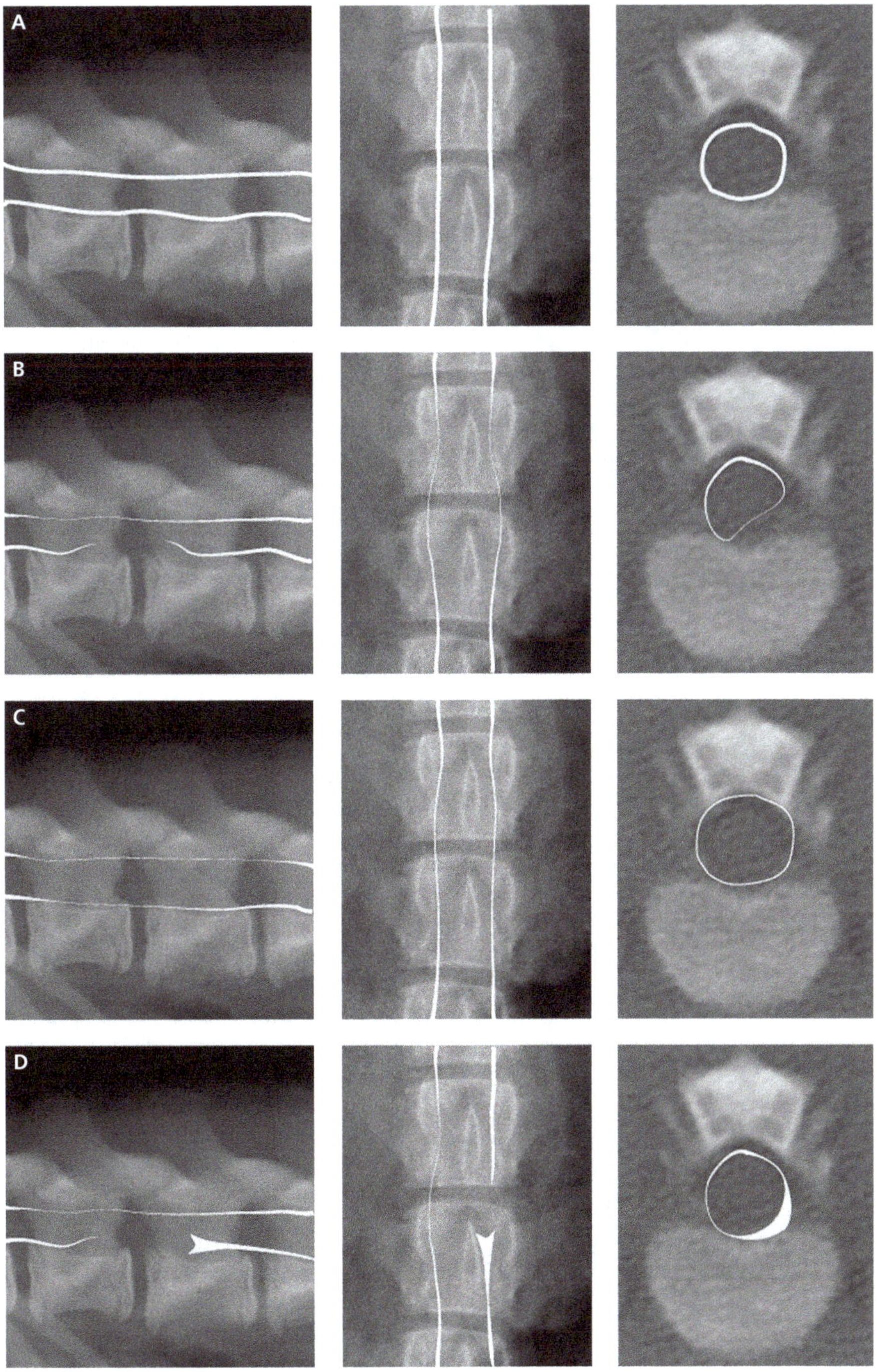

Figure 7.7 Lateral (sagittal), ventrodorsal (dorsal), and transverse representations of the subarachnoid space in normal (A), extradural (B), intramedullary (C), and intradural–extramedullary (D) spinal cord lesions.

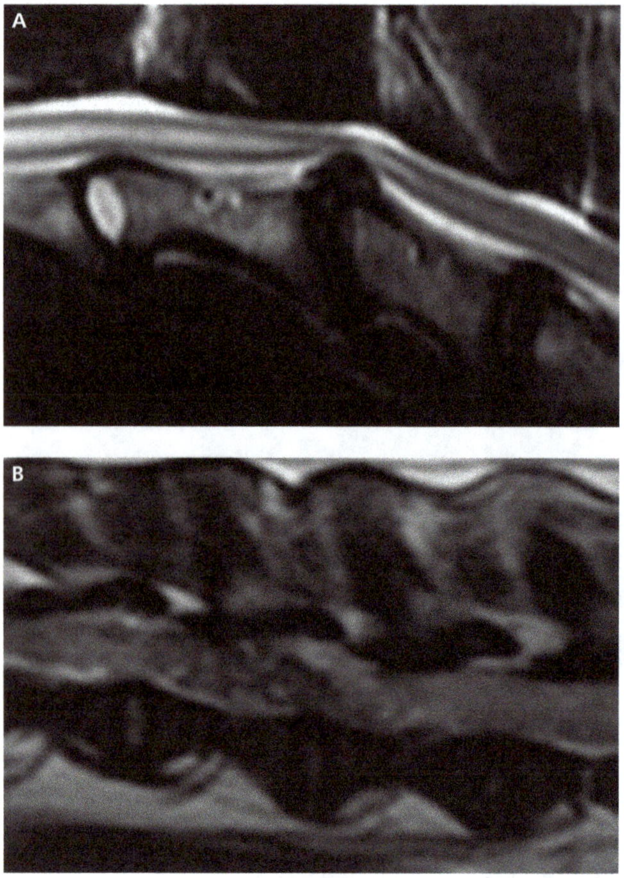

Figure 7.8 Sagittal MRI of an intervertebral disc protrusion (A) compared with an intervertebral disc extrusion (B). The protrusion has a broad base along the dorsal aspect of the intervertebral disc and a fusiform shape while the extrusion has a narrow base along the intervertebral disc and a rounded shape.

An intradural–extramedullary lesion will cause a filling defect in the subarachnoid space on at least one projection. This is classically described as a "golf-tee" sign where there is focal widening of the subarachnoid space with a convex margin adjacent to the filling defect. On the orthogonal view the appearance is similar to that seen with an intramedullary lesion. The primary differential diagnosis for an intradural–extramedullary lesion is neoplasia, such as peripheral nerve sheath neoplasms and meningiomas. A focal round dilation of the subarachnoid space can also be seen (golf ball sign) and is associated with a subarachnoid cyst/diverticulum (Figure 7.9).

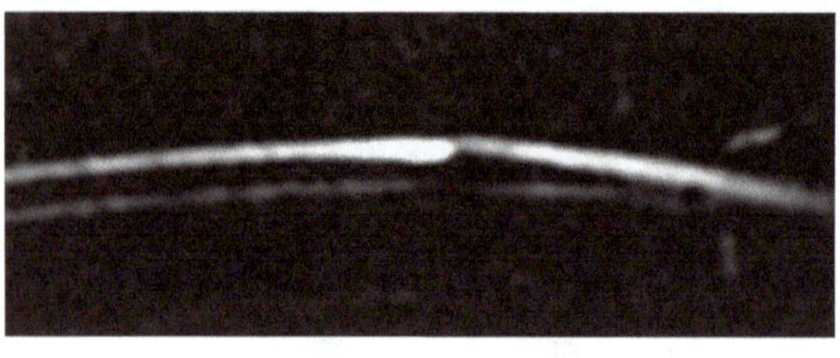

Figure 7.9 MRI T2 myelogram image showing focal dilation of the subarachnoid space with a rounded margin (golf ball sign). This is consistent with a subarachnoid cyst.

Intervertebral Disc Disease

The decision to use myelography to assess spinal cord disease is now dependent on the availability of CT or MRI and the suspected clinical problem [42]. Although CT and MRI are frequently preferred, myelography remains a viable method of assessing spinal cord disease in dogs and cats, with an accuracy of 86–97% and the choice of imaging modality does not affect patient outcome [13,43–45].

Intervertebral disc herniation can present with either an extradural or intramedullary pattern depending on the degree of spinal cord swelling. In the face of severe spinal cord swelling adequate localization of the lesion can be difficult. Careful evaluation for any deviation of the subarachnoid space is critical. Radiographs made during or immediately following the contrast injection frequently allow for improved localization as the contrast medium disperses from the swollen area over time [13,22,46]. Circumferential localization of herniated disc material is important if hemilaminectomy or pediculectomy are planned. Clinical lateralization is not always consistent with lateralization on imaging and cannot be relied upon to plan surgery [2].

The accuracy of myelography for circumferential localization ranges from 41 to 100% depending on whether or not oblique views were obtained [1,2,13]. Ventrodorsal views alone resulted in accurate lateralization in 41–70% of patients [1,2]. Various techniques used to improve the accuracy of myelography in the circumferential localization of extradural material include the paradoxical contrast obstruction sign and oblique radiographs [1,2,47]. If deviation of the contrast column is not seen on the ventrodorsal view, the paradoxical contrast obstruction sign can be used to determine the circumferential localization of the extradural lesion. When a lateralized extradural lesion is present, the spinal cord and subarachnoid space will be displaced away from the side of the lesion. The vertebral canal is a rigid structure and when the spinal cord is pushed against the canal the attenuation of the subarachnoid space will occur over a longer distance on the side opposite the extradural material (Figure 7.10). This sign has been shown to allow for lateralization of the extradural compression in 83% of dogs that had no clear deviation of the contrast column on the ventrodorsal view [47]. Many authors advise that ventral 45° left-dorsal right and ventral 45° right-dorsal left oblique radiographs should be obtained in all cases where the ventrodorsal view does not provide adequate lateralization as oblique radiographs facilitate the lateralization of lesions in 94–100% of cases (Figure 7.11) [1,2,13]. Oblique projections facilitate the imaging of the extradural lesion tangentially, allowing for detection of the medial deviation of the contrast column.

Splitting of the contrast column (double myelographic line sign) occurs because the spinal cord is draped over the extradural material. This was originally reported to be associated with lateralization of the extradural material but has subsequently been shown to also occur with ventral extradural lesions and bilateral ventrolateral extradural lesions, resulting in this sign only being useful in confirming that a lesion is extradural in location [48,49].

For extradural lesions CT allows more accurate circumferential localization compared with myelography [28]. The major question about spinal CT is whether or not to combine it with myelography. The advantage of not performing a myelogram prior to CT is that it is a less invasive study that requires less time to acquire. For the evaluation of all spinal cord disease the sensitivities of myelography, CT, and CT myelography are 79%, 66%, and 97%, respectively [29]. Noncontrast CT can be used to diagnose intervertebral disc when there is mineralization or hemorrhage associated with the disc

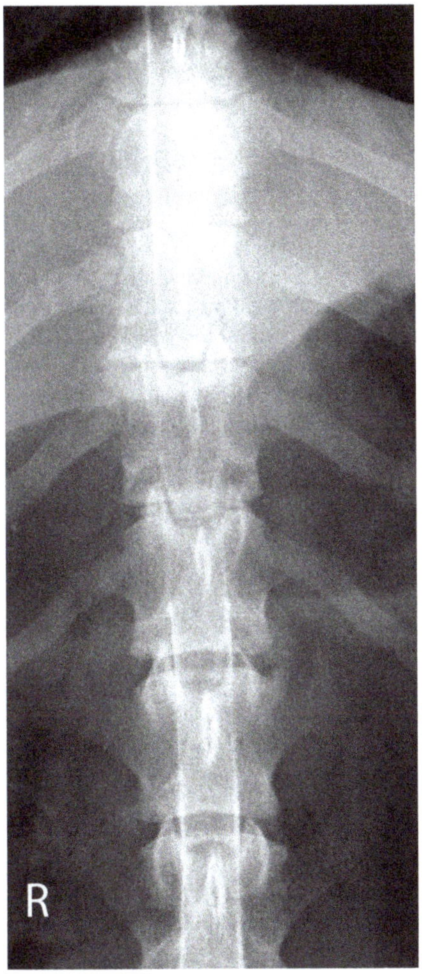

Figure 7.10 A ventrodorsal post-myelogram radiograph shows attenuation of the right contrast column over a greater length than the left contrast column. Based on the paradoxical contrast obstruction, this indicates that the extradural lesion (confirmed extradural on the lateral view) is on the left side. This finding was confirmed at surgery.

material (which is hyperdense to the spinal cord) (Figure 7.12). CT is very sensitive to small amounts of mineralization but if the herniated material is not mineralized it may not be detected. Additionally, if there is little epidural fat (high spinal cord to vertebral canal ratio), as seen in small breed dogs, there may be insufficient contrast to detect nonmineralized material (Figure 7.13).

Another confounding issue is when there are multiple herniated discs, as it may not be possible to determine which is the active lesion when there is no contrast ring. Attenuation of the contrast ring indicates spinal cord swelling that can point to the acute lesion. As spinal cord swelling can also be related to prognosis, this additional information may justify the use of CT myelography over unenhanced CT [30,50].

Several studies have concluded that plain CT is as effective as myelography in detecting intervertebral disc herniation, with a sensitivity of 81–97% [25,26,31,51,52]. Unfortunately, although

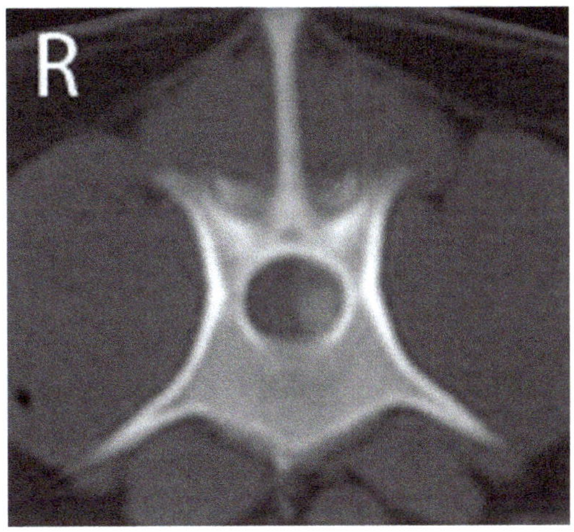

Figure 7.12 Transverse CT at the cranial aspect of L2 shows hyperdense (mineralized) intervertebral disc material in the left vertebral canal causing compression of the spinal cord. This lesion is clearly evident without the need for intravenous or intrathecal contrast medium.

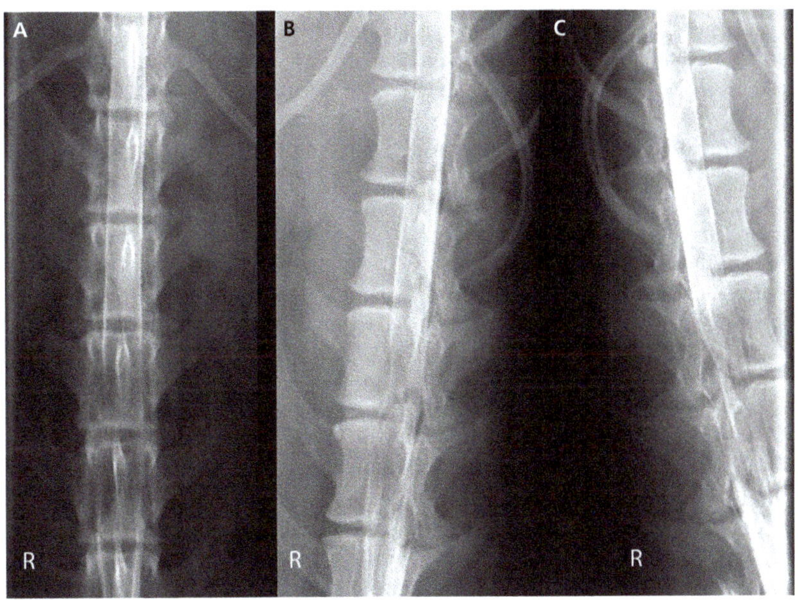

Figure 7.11 Ventrodorsal (A), left ventral–right dorsal oblique (B), and right ventral–left dorsal oblique (C) radiographs of a lumbar myelogram show a right-sided extradural lesion at L3–4. The ventrodorsal view shows a slight deviation of the right contrast column medially but this lesion is more evident on the oblique projections.

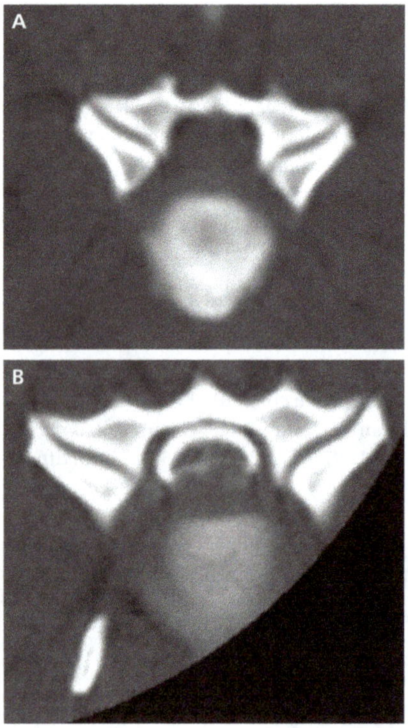

Figure 7.13 Noncontrast CT (A) and CT-myelography (B) demonstrate a ventral extradural spinal cord compression. The noncontrast CT shows slight loss of the epidural fat but compared with the CT-myelogram it underestimates the severity of the compressive lesion.

the suspicion of intervertebral disc herniation may be high, this diagnosis is not known prior to proceeding to imaging. When all types of lesions are combined the sensitivity of unenhanced CT decreases to 66% [26]. This is because the sensitivity of CT for the detection of lesions other than mineralized intervertebral disc extrusions is significantly decreased (40%) [29]. It has also been shown that interobserver agreement for CT is poor and agreement is only good for large-volume mineralized intervertebral disc herniations [26,29]. Dogs with chronic intervertebral disc herniation are more likely to be detected on unenhanced CT because the disc material is more likely to be mineralized (chronic disc material, 745 ± 288 HU; acute disc material, 219 ± 95 HU) [31,51]. A more recent case series of 11 Dachshunds showed that in four cases lesions were missed on precontrast CT and one case had a lesion noted on precontrast CT but not on CT myelography, while some cases were diagnosed with CT myelography but not on myelography [32]. Israel et al. [31] showed that myelography was more sensitive in dogs weighing less than 5 kg. Therefore, if no mineralized disc material is evident on noncontrast CT, then CT myelography should be performed as it is often required to obtain the correct diagnosis [29].

Rather than intrathecal contrast, CT with intravenous contrast has been evaluated for the diagnosis of intervertebral disc herniation with variable results [29,53]. In one study, contrast-enhanced CT provided no additional information compared with unenhanced CT [29]. This is likely because the venous sinuses in the thoracolumbar region are not as evident as they are in the cervical region. The other study did not evaluate contrast-enhanced CT relative to unenhanced but did conclude that contrast-enhanced CT and CT myelography were equally sensitive in the diagnosis of intervertebral disc herniation [53].

MRI is equivalent or superior to myelography and CT for localizing spinal cord compression due to intervertebral disc herniation [42,54,55]. MRI also facilitates assessment of the spinal cord parenchyma for edema and myelomalacia which can be prognostic indicators. Spinal cord edema is characterized by T2 hyperintensity and swelling of the spinal cord. Hemorrhagic myelomalacia can also be seen as a decreased signal on gradient echo (T2*) images [56]. Although spinal cord lesions can provide insight into prognosis, the degree of spinal cord compression is not correlated with neurological status at presentation or the outcome [57]. Heavily T2-weighted images demonstrate the subarachnoid space similarly to myelography and can be useful in determining the site and severity of acute spinal cord compression as length of spinal cord compression has been associated with lower odds of returning to ambulation [58,59]. Contrast enhancement can occur in intervertebral disc herniation due to focal meningitis and formation of granulation tissue but is not related to clinical signs or pathological features [60,61].

Lumbosacral Disease

Many of the signs of lumbosacral disease are the same as seen with intervertebral disc disease. Myelography is limited in evaluating lumbosacral disease due to the variability in termination of the dural sac (between L6 and S1). Approximately 20% of dogs have a dural sac that ends cranial to the sacrum [62]. Additionally, myelography does not allow evaluation of lateral lesions such as stenosis of the intervertebral foramen [63]. As a result CT and MRI are superior tests for the evaluation of the lumbosacral region.

Signs of nerve root compression related to lumbosacral degeneration include loss of epidural fat, bulging of the intervertebral disc, narrowing of the intervertebral foramen, soft tissue opacity in the intervertebral foramen, subluxation and osteoarthrosis of the articular processes [64]. In most cases epidural fibrosis, hypertrophy of the ligamentum flavum, or herniated disc material is the cause of the compression. These lesions may demonstrate contrast enhancement in the lateral recesses and dorsal and ventral vertebral canal that can be detected on CT and MRI [65–67]. Accurate assessment of lateral recess involvement is important as it will influence the surgical plan [65].

Cervical Stenotic Myelopathy

Cervical stenotic myelopathy occurs due to protrusion of the intervertebral disc and/or enlargement of the articular processes. Dorsolateral compression of the spinal cord from enlargement of the articular processes results in a triangular shape to the spinal cord. On conventional myelography this is difficult to detect with routine orthogonal projections [27]. Cross-sectional images easily demonstrate the triangular shape of the vertebral canal caused by enlargement of the articular processes. This also allows for the differentiation between spinal cord compression and spinal cord atrophy [27]. CT has also been shown to detect abnormalities of the articular processes with greater frequency than radiography or MRI [68]. MRI is more accurate than myelography in diagnosing cervical stenotic myelopathy, with greater interobserver agreement [69]. Overall, all modalities have good agreement and should be considered complementary [68].

Flexion and extension views can be readily obtained with all imaging modalities, but as they can result in neurological deterioration they are infrequently used. If these views are to be performed, obtaining them under fluoroscopy can be beneficial by providing a real-time assessment of the degree of compression so that the procedure can be stopped if the lesion is severe. Traction views can be obtained with any imaging modality but one study indicated that myelography characterized more lesions as dynamic than MRI [69]. Since a gold standard for characterizing a lesion as dynamic is not available, it is not clear whether this represents true-positive or false-positive results (i.e., which modality is correct).

Over-interpretation of cervical lesions on MRI has been reported by several authors, with degenerative changes being evident in clinically normal animals [68–70]. Although there is generally good agreement on the primary site of compression, there is poor interobserver agreement in evaluation of the articular processes and foramenal stenosis [71]. However, the direct multiplanar imaging of MRI and ability to assess the spinal cord is advantageous. Chronic compressive lesions can lead to spinal cord atrophy, gliosis, and syringomyelia. Signal changes on MRI have been correlated with histological changes in people [72]. A T2 hyperintensity with normal signal on T1 images is due to mild loss of nerve cells, gliosis, edema, demyelination, and Wallerian degeneration. Lesions that are hyperintense on T2-weighted images and hypointense on T2-weighted images are associated with severe changes such as necrosis and myelomalacia. In human patients with cervical spondylotic myelopathy, an increased T2 signal intensity only is thought to represent a potentially reversible change while a lesion that has increased T2 signal intensity and decreased T1 signal intensity is likely irreversible and a poor prognostic indicator [73]. In one study, 55% of dogs had signal intensity changes in the spinal cord but these changes were assessed in relation to clinical signs or prognosis [68,69].

Other Extradural Lesions

The sensitivity of CT to bony lysis in vertebral tumors is dramatically higher than that of radiographs [30]. CT can detect a density change of 0.5% while radiographs require a change of at least 10% to be evident [74]. Intravenous contrast administration is required to determine the extent of the soft tissue mass in order to plan therapy appropriately. Concurrent myelography may be required to better characterize the spinal cord lesion (extradural vs. intradural–extramedullary vs. intramedullary) [30].

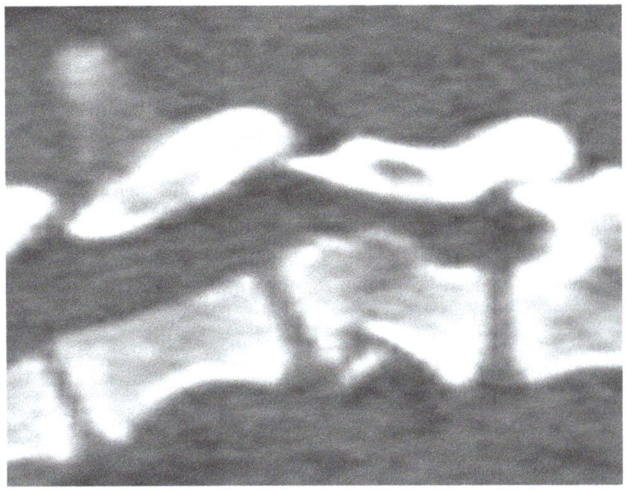

Figure 7.14 Sagittal reformatted images of an L2 vertebral body fracture shows comminution of the vertebral body and moderate displacement of the fracture with narrowing of the vertebral canal.

CT may be superior to MRI for the evaluation of spinal trauma. The fine anatomical detail provided by the ability to acquire 1-mm or submillimeter slices and to subsequently perform multiplanar and three-dimensional reconstructions aid in the diagnosis and surgical planning for vertebral fractures [42] (Figure 7.14). An added advantage of CT is that due to the speed of acquisition, it can be performed in sedated patients. Since acute hemorrhage is hyperdense on CT, it allows for concurrent evaluation of extradural compression by hemorrhage.

Intramedullary Spinal Cord Lesions

Although all imaging modalities can detect spinal cord enlargement due to intramedullary spinal cord disease, the superior contrast resolution of MRI provides additional characterization of the lesion (Figure 7.15). As most intramedullary lesions have a similar appearance on MRI (hyperintense to spinal cord on T2-weighted images, isointense to spinal cord on T1-weighted images, and variable degrees of contrast enhancement), there is considerable overlap in the differential diagnosis. Ischemia, acute noncompressive intervertebral

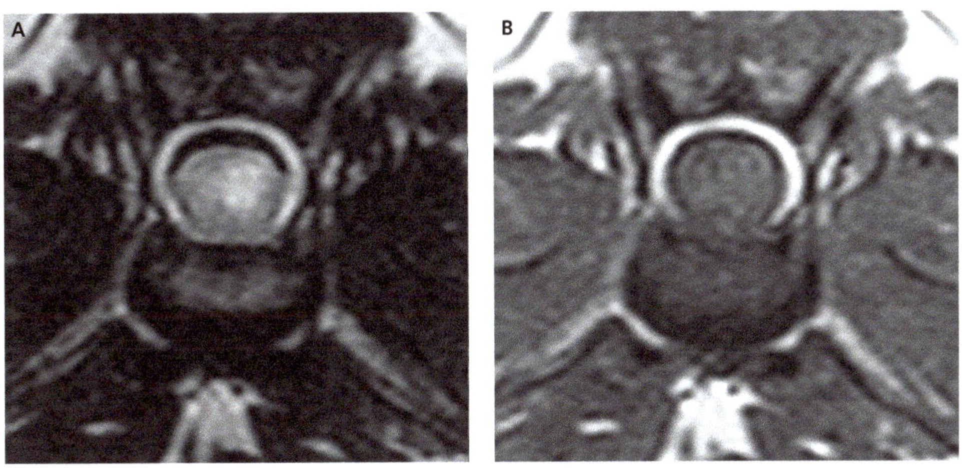

Figure 7.15 Transverse T2-weighted (A) and T1-weighted (B) MRI of the lumbar vertebral column. A focal intramedullary lesion that is hyperintense to the spinal cord on the T2-weighted image and isointense to the spinal cord on the T1-weighted image is present in the mid to left spinal cord. This lesion did not contrast enhance.

disc herniations, and intramedullary neoplasms tend to be focal lesions while inflammatory disease is often multifocal and may be associated with meningeal enhancement. Lack of signal from the CSF on this sequence has also been associated with meningitis [40]. Ischemia frequently affects one half of the spinal cord.

Myelomalacia can occur with severe exogenous trauma or intervertebral disc herniation. Spinal cord swelling and opacification of the spinal cord during myelography can be seen in dogs with myelomalacia [75]. Spinal cord opacification can be subtle, and therefore CT post myelography may be a more sensitive indicator of myelomalacia than myelography alone. Characteristics of myelomalacia on MRI are those of severe edema (T2 hyperintensity) or hemorrhage [56].

Conclusions

Although it is generally accepted that MRI is superior to myelography and CT for neuroimaging, it is important to recognize that for many spinal problems all these tests have similar sensitivities and specificities. Additionally, for certain problems such as spinal trauma the superior spatial resolution of CT can be advantageous. Therefore, when MRI is not readily available or cost-effective these other modalities remain appropriate options for imaging spinal disease in the dog and cat.

Numerous studies have compared myelography, unenhanced CT, contrast-enhanced CT, CT myelography, and MRI for the evaluation of intervertebral disc disease [25,26,29–31,51]. All studies are limited by the fact that the gold standard used is surgery. It is not practical or ethical to explore all potential sites of intervertebral disc extrusion in clinical patients and it is possible, although unlikely, that sites of intervertebral disc extrusion are not detected with any modality and that false-negative results occur. As a result surgery as a gold standard results in bias [26,44].

In spite of these limitations it is generally accepted that MRI is the best imaging modality for the assessment of spinal cord disease and when available and cost is not a concern should be the recommended test. However, CT, CT myelography, and myelography all have an acceptable sensitivity and specificity in the detection of intervertebral disc herniation and can be used when MRI is not available or affordable. Additionally, the information from all modalities can be complementary and a multimodality approach may be required for some diseases. Although MRI can provide information regarding prognosis, it has also been shown that the choice of imaging test does not correlate with patient outcome [45,59,76].

Video clips to accompany this book can be found on the companion website at:
www.wiley.com/go/shores/neurosurgery

References

1 Gibbons S, Macias C, De Stefani A, Pinchbeck G, McKee W. The value of oblique versus ventrodorsal myelographic views for lesion lateralisation in canine thoracolumbar disc disease. *J Small Anim Pract* 2006;47:658–662.

2 Tanaka H, Nakayama M, Takase K. Usefulness of myelography with multiple views in diagnosis of circumferential location of disc material in dogs with thoracolumber intervertebral disc herniation. *J Vet Med Sci* 2004;66:827–833.

3 Widmer WR, Thrall D. Canine and feline intervertebral disc disease, myelography, and spinal cord diseases. In: Thrall D (ed.) *Textbook of Veteirnary Diagnostic Radiology*, 5th edn. St Louis, MO: Saunders Elsevier, 2007.

4 Wheeler S, Davies J. Iohexol myelography in the dog and cat: a series of one hundred cases, and a comparison with metrizamide and iopamidol. *J Small Anim Pract* 1985;26:247–256.

5 Widmer WR. Iohexol and iopamidol: new contrast media for veterinary myelography. *J Am Vet Med Assoc* 1989;194:1714–1716.

6 Widmer WR, Blevins W. Veterinary myelography: a review of contrast media, adverse effects, and technique. J Am Anim Hosp Assoc 1991;27:163–177.

7 Fatone G, Lamagna F, Pasolini MP, Potena A, Brunetti A. Myelography in the dog with non-ionic contrast media at different iodine concentrations. *J Small Anim Pract* 1997;38:292–294.

8 DeLahunta A, Glass E. *Veterinary Neuroanatomy and Clinical Neurology*, 3rd edn. St Louis, MO: Saunders/Elsevier; 2008.

9 Lamb CR. Common difficulties with myelographic diagnosis of acute intervertebral disc disease in the dog. *J Small Anim Pract* 1994;35:549–558.

10 Barone G, Ziemer LS, Shofer FS, Steinberg SA. Risk factors associated with development of seizures after use of iohexol for myelography in dogs: 182 cases (1998). *J Am Vet Med Assoc* 2002;220:1499–1502.

11 da Costa RC, Parent JM, Dobson H. Incidence of and risk factors for seizures after myelography performed with iohexol in dogs: 503 cases (2002–2004). *J Am Vet Med Assoc* 2011;238:1296–1300.

12 McKee WM, Penderis J, Dennis R. Radiology corner: obstruction of contrast medium flow during cervical myelography. *Vet Radiol Ultrasound* 2000;41:342–343.

13 Kirberger RM, Roos CJ, Lubbe AM. The radiological diagnosis of thracolumbar disc disease in the Dachshund. *Vet Radiol Ultrasound* 1992;33:255–261.

14 McCartney WT. Lumbar myelography in 79 dogs, using different puncture sites. *Vet Rec* 1997;141:417–419.

15 Tilmant L, Ackerman N, Spencer CP. Mechanical aspects of subarachnoid space puncture in the dog. *Vet Radiol* 1984;50:227–232.

16 Kishimoto M, Yamada K, Ueno H, Kobayashi Y, Wisner ER. Spinal cord effects from lumbar myelographic injection technique in the dog. *J Vet Med Sci* 2004;66:67–69.

17 Kirberger RM, Wrigley RH. Myelography in the dog: review of patients with contrast medium in the central canal. *Vet Radiol Ultrasound* 1993;34:253–258.

18 Lexmaulova L, Zatloukal J, Proks P, Dvorak M, Srnec R, Rauser P et al. Incidence of seizures associated with iopamidol or iomeprol myelography in dogs with intervertebral disk disease: 161 cases (2000–2002). *J Vet Emerg Crit Care* 2009;19:611–616.

19 Carroll GL, Keene BW, Forrest LJ. Asystole associated with iohexol myelography in a dog. *Vet Radiol Ultrasound* 1997;38:284–287.

20 Lamb CR. The dorsoventral cervical myelogram. *Vet Radiol Ultrasound* 1995;36:201–202.

21 Matteucci ML, Ramirez O III, Thrall DE. Radiographic diagnosis: effect of right vs. left lateral recumbency on myelographic appearance of a lateralized extradural mass. *Vet Radiol Ultrasound* 1999;40:351–352.

22 Nykamp S, Scrivani P. Feline myelography. *Vet Radiol Ultrasound* 2001;42:532–533.

23 Seiler G, Kinns J, Dennison S, Saunders J, Schwarz T. Vertebral column and spinal cord. In: Schwarz T, Saunders J (eds) *Veterinary Computed Tomography*. Chichester, West Sussex: Wiley-Blackwell, 2011: 209–228.

24 Kinns J, Malinowski R, McEvoy F, Schwarz T, Zwingenberger A. Special software applications. In: Schwarz T, Saunders J (eds) *Veterinary Computed Tomography*. Chichester, West Sussex: Wiley-Blackwell, 2011: 67–74.

25 Hecht S, Thomas WB, Marioni-Henry K, Echandi RL, Matthews AR, Adams WH. Myelography vs. computed tomography in the evaluation of acute thoracolumbar intervertebral disk extrusion in chondrodystrophic dogs. *Vet Radiol Ultrasound* 2009;50:353–359.

26 Newcomb B, Arble J, Rochat M, Pechman R, Payton M. Comparison of computed tomography and myelography to a reference standard of computed tomographic myelography for evaluation of dogs with intervertebral disc disease. *Vet Surg* 2012;41:207–214.

27 Sharp NJH, Cofone M, Robertson ID, DeCarlo A, Smith GK, Thrall DE. Computed tomography in the evaluation of caual cervical spondylomyopathy of the Doberman Pinscher. *Vet Radiol Ultrasound* 1995;36:100–108.

28 Hara Y, Tagawa M, Ejima H, Orima H, Fujita M. Usefulness of computed tomography after myelography for surgery on dogs with cervical intervertebral disc protrusion. *J Vet Med Sci* 1994;56:791–794.

29 Dennison SE, Drees R, Rylander H, Yandell BS, Milovancev M, Pettigrew R, et al. Evaluation of different computed tomography techniques and myelography for the diagnosis of acute canine myelopathy. *Vet Radiol Ultrasound* 2010;51:254–258.

30 Drost WT, Love NE, Berry CR. Comparison of radiography, myelography and computed tomography for the evaluation of canine vertebral and spinal cord tumors in sixteen dogs. *Vet Radiol Ultrasound* 1996;37:28–33.

31 Israel SK, Levine JM, Kerwin SC, Levine GJ, Fosgate GT. The relative sensitivity of computed tomography and myelography for identification of thoracolumbar intervertebral disk herniations in dogs. *Vet Radiol Ultrasound* 2009;50:247–252.

32 Shimizu J, Yamada K, Mochida K, Kako T, Muroya N, Teratani Y et al. Comparison of the diagnosis of intervertebral disc herniation in dogs by CT before and after contrast enhancement of the subarachnoid space. *Vet Rec* 2009;165:200–202.

33 Bettmann MA. Angiographic contrast agents: conventional and new media compared. *AJR Am J Roentgenol* 1982;139:787–794.

34 Vance A, Nelson M, Hofmeister EH. Adverse reactions following administration of an ionic iodinated contrast media in anesthetized dogs. *J Am Anim Hosp Assoc* 2012;48:172–175.

35 Dennis R, Herrtage ME. Low osmolar contrast media: a review. *Vet Radiol* 1989;30:2–12.

36 Wallack S. *The Handbook of Veterinary Contrast Radiography*. Solana Beach, CA: San Diego Veterinary Imaging, Inc., 2003.

37 Holland M. Contrast agents. *Vet Clin North Am Small Anim Pract* 1993;23:269–279.

38 Dennis R. Optimal magnetic resonance imaging of the spine. *Vet Radiol Ultrasound* 2011;52(1 Suppl 1):S72–S80.

39 D'Anjou MA, Carmel EN, Tidwell AS. Value of fat suppression in gadolinium-enhanced magnetic resonance neuroimaging. *Vet Radiol Ultrasound* 2011; 52(1 Suppl 1):S85–S90.

40 Pease A, Sullivan S, Olby N, Galano H, Cerda-Gonzalez S, Robertson ID et al. Value of a single-shot turbo spin-echo pulse sequence for assessing the architecture of the subarachnoid space and the constitutive nature of cerebrospinal fluid. *Vet Radiol Ultrasound* 2006;47:254–259.

41 Tidwell AS, Specht A, Blaeser L, Kent M. Magnetic resonance imaging features of extradural hematomas assoicated with intervertebral disc herniation in a dog. *Vet Radiol Ultrasound* 2002;43:319–324.

42 Robertson I, Thrall DE. Imaging dogs with suspected disc herniation: pros and cons of myelography, computed tomography, and magnetic resonance. *Vet Radiol Ultrasound* 2011;52(1 Suppl 1):S81–S84.

43 Olby N, Dyce J, Houlton J. Correlation of plain radiographic and lumbar myelographic findings in thoracolumbar disc disease. *J Small Anim Pract* 1994;35:345–350.

44 Schulz KS, Walker M, Moon M, Waldron D, Slater M, McDonald DE. Correlation of clinical, radiographic, and surgical localization of intervertebral disc extrusion in small-breed dogs: a prospective study of 50 cases. *Vet Surg* 1998;27:105–111.

45 Parry AT, Harris A, Upjohn MM, Chandler K, Lamb CR. Does choice of imaging modality affect outcome in dogs with thoracolumbar spinal conditions? *J Small Anim Pract* 2010;51:312–317.

46 Taeymans O, Saunders JH, vanBree H. Radiology corner: canine myelography. *Vet Radiol Ultrasound* 2002;43:550–551.

47 Bos AS, Brisson BA, Holmberg DL, Nykamp SG. Use of the ventrodorsal myelographic view to predict lateralization of extruded disk material in small-breed dogs with thoracolumbar intervertebral disk extrusion: 104 cases (2004–2005). *J Am Vet Med Assoc* 2007;230:1860–1865.

48 Scrivani PV, Barthez PY, Leveille R. The fallibility of the myelographic "double line" sign. *Vet Radiol Ultrasound* 1996;37:264–265.

49 Stickle R, Lowrie C, Oakley R. Radiology corner: another example of the myelographic "double line" sign. *Vet Radiol Ultrasound* 1998;39:543.

50 Duval J, Dewey C, Roberts R, Aron D. Spinal cord swelling as a myelographic indicator of prognosis: a retrospective study in dogs with intervertebral disc disease and loss of deep pain perception. *Vet Surg* 1996;25:6–12.

51 Olby NJ, Munana KR, Sharp NJH, Thrall DE. The computed tomographic appearance of acute thoracolumbar intervertebral disc herniations in dogs. *Vet Radiol Ultrasound* 2000;41:396–402.

52 Newcomb B, Arble J, Rochat M, Pechman R, Payton M. Comparison of computed tomography and myelography to a reference standard of computed tomographic myelography for evaluation of dogs with intervertebral disc disease. *Vet Surg* 2011;41:207–214.

53 Schroeder R, Pelsue DH, Park RD, Gasso D, Bruecker KA. Contrast-enhanced CT for localizing compressive thoracolumbar intervertebral disc extrusion. *J Am Anim Hosp Assoc* 2011;47:203–209.

54 Bos AS, Brisson BA, Nykamp SG, Poma R, Foster RA. Accuracy, intermethod agreement, and inter-reviewer agreement for use of magnetic resonance imaging and myelography in small-breed dogs with naturally occurring first-time intervertebral disk extrusion. *J Am Vet Med Assoc* 2012;240: 969–977.

55 Cooper JJ, Young BD, Griffin JF, Fosgate GT, Levine LM. Comparison between noncontrast computed tomography and magnetic resonance imaging for detection and characterization of thoracolumbar myelopathy caoused by intervertebrak disk herniation in dogs. *Vet Radiol Ultrasound* 2014;55:182–189.

56 Platt SR, McConnell JF, Bestbier M. Magnetic resonance imaging characteristics of ascending hemorrhagic myelomalacia in a dog. *Vet Radiol Ultrasound* 2006;47: 78–82.

57 Penning V, Platt SR, Dennis R, Cappello R, Adams V. Association of spinal cord compression seen on magnetic resonance imaging with clinical outcome in 67 dogs with thoracolumbar intervertebral disc extrusion. *J Small Anim Pract* 2006;47: 644–650.

58 Mankin JM, Hecht S, Thomas WB. Agreement between T2 and HASTE sequences in the evaluation of thoracolumbar intervertebral disc disease in dogs. *Vet Radiol Ultrasound* 2012;53:162–166.

59 Levine JM, Fosgate GT, Chen AV, Rushing R, Nghiem PP, Platt SR et al. Magnetic resonance imaging in dogs with neurologic impairment due to acute thoracic and lumbar intervertebral disk herniation. *J Vet Intern Med* 2009;23:1220–1226.

60 Kippenes H, Silver GM, Gavin P, Bagley RS, Tucker R. Magnetic resonance imaging of extradural spinal cord masses: distinguishing contrast-enhancing disc disease from neoplasia [Astract]. *Vet Radiol Ultrasound* 2000;41:572.

61 Freeman AC, Platt SR, Kent M, Howerth E, Holmes SP. Magnetic resonance imaging enhancement of intervertebral disc disease in 30 dogs following chemical fat saturation. *J Small Anim Pract* 2012;53:120–125.

62 Lang J. Flexion-extension myelography of the canine cauda equina. *Vet Radiol* 1988;29:242–257.

63 Ramirez O III, Thrall DE. A review of imaging techniques for canine cauda equina syndrome. *Vet Radiol Ultrasound* 1998;39:283–296.

64 Jones JC, Sorjonen DC, Simpson ST, Coates JR, Lenz S, Hathcock J et al. Comparison between computed tomographic and surgical findings in nine large-breed dogs with lumbosacral stenosis. *Vet Radiol Ultrasound* 1996;37:247–256.

65 Jones JC, Shires PK, Inzana KD, Sponenberg DP, Massicotte C, Renberg W et al. Evaluation of canine lumbosacral stenosis using intravenous contrast-enhanced computed tomography. *Vet Radiol Ultrasound* 1999;40:108–114.

66 Adams WH, Daniel GB, Pardo AD, Selcer RR. Magnetic resonance imaging of the caudal lumbar and lumbosacral spine in 13 dogs (1990–1993). *Vet Radiol Ultrasound* 1995;36:3–13.

67 deHaan JJ, Shelton SB, Ackerman N. Magnetic resonance imaging in the diagnosis of degenerative lumbosacral stenosis in four dogs. *Vet Surg* 1993;22:1–4.

68 De Decker S, Gielen IMVL, Duchateau L, Corzo-Menéndez N, van Bree HJJ, Kromhout K et al. Intraobserver, interobserver, and intermethod agreement for results of myelography, computed tomography-myelography, and low-field magnetic resonance imaging in dogs with disk-associated wobbler syndrome. *J Am Vet Med Assoc* 2011;238:1601–1608.

69 da Costa RC, Parent J, Dobson H, Holmberg D, Partlow G. Comparison of magnetic resonance imaging and myelography in 18 Doberman pinscher dogs with cervical spondylomyelopathy. *Vet Radiol Ultrasound* 2006;47:523–531.

70 Martin-Vaquero P, da Costa RC. Magnetic resonance imaging features of Great Danes with and without clincial signs of cervical spondylomyelopathy. *J Am Vet Med Assoc* 2014;245:393–400.

71 Martin-Vaquero P, da Costa RC, Drost WT. Comparison of noncontrast computed tomography and high-field magnetic resonance imaging in the evaluation of Great Danes with cervical spondylomyelopathy. *Vet Radiol Ultrasound* 2014;55:496–505.

72 Ohshio I, Hatayama A, Kaneda K, Takahara M, Nagashima K. Correlation between histopathologic features and magnetic resonance images of spinal cord lesions. *Spine* 1993;18:1140–1149.

73 Suri A, Chabbra RPS, Mehta VS, Gaikwad S, Pandey RM. Effect of intramedullary signal changes on the surgical outcome of patients with cervical spondylotic myelopathy. *Spine J* 2003;3:33–45.

74 Sande RD. Radiography, myelography, computed tomography, and magnetic resonance imaging of the spine. *Vet Clin North Am Small Anim Pract* 1992;22:811–831.

75 Lu D, Lamb CR, Targett MP. Results of myelography in seven dogs with myelomalacia. *Vet Radiol Ultrasound* 2002;43:326–330.

76 Ito D, Matsunaga S, Jeffery ND, Sasaki N, Nishimura R, Mochizuki M et al. Prognostic value of magnetic resonance imaging in dogs with paraplegia caused by thoracolumbar intervertebral disk extrusion: 77 cases (2000–2003). *J Am Vet Med Assoc* 2005;227:1454–1460.

8 Lumbar Cerebrospinal Fluid Taps

Luis Gaitero

Introduction

Lumbar puncture (tap) is an essential component in the investigation of neurological disease. The technique is originally credited to Quincke's description from 1891 [1]. The main indications for lumbar puncture [2] are:

1. obtain a sample of CSF for diagnostic purposes;
2. inject radiopaque contrast materials (myelography);
3. administer therapeutic drugs (antibiotics, chemotherapeutics);
4. measure CSF pressure;
5. reduce CSF volume for therapeutic purposes (as in benign intracranial hypertension).

CSF collection and myelography are the most common indications in veterinary medicine.

CSF analysis is valuable in the investigation of many neurological disorders and samples can be collected from the cerebellomedullary (atlanto-occipital) or the lumbar cisterns. Although the CSF flows rostrocaudally and caudorostrally, it does so in a predominantly rostrocaudal direction. To enhance the chances of detecting abnormalities, collecting from a site caudal to the lesion is desirable. Consequently, lumbar CSF collection would be highly indicated in thoracic and lumbar lesions; indeed, a lumbar CSF sample could be recommended over a cerebellomedullary one in any spinal lesion caudal to C1. The lumbar tap is technically more difficult and demanding than the cerebellomedullary one, provides smaller CSF volumes, and is associated with a higher likelihood of iatrogenic blood contamination. As a result, obtaining a sample from both sites to enhance the chances of detecting abnormal CSF findings is acceptable, performing the cerebellomedullary first to decrease the risk of CSF blood contamination [3].

Similarly, myelograms can be performed through a cerebellomedullary or a lumbar puncture. Although a lumbar puncture procedure is more challenging, lumbar myelography has multiple advantages over cerebellomedullary, mainly a lower risk of iatrogenic trauma and better image quality and lesion delineation, particularly in thoracic and lumbar compressive lesions as the contrast can be forced forward under pressure around the compression site. The contrast injection is more prone to deposit epidurally during a lumbar myelographic procedure.

Anatomical Considerations

The three layers of meninges covering the central nervous system (CNS) are the dura mater, arachnoid, and pia mater. The CSF is contained in the subarachnoid space. Lumbar puncture is performed at the interarcuate space between L5 and L6 or on space cranially (L4–L5) to minimize the risk of direct damage to the spinal cord by the needle while still gaining access to the subarachnoid space. At these locations, the spinal cord has tapered into the conus medullaris and is surrounded by the cauda equina, both of which are less likely than the cord itself to be damaged by needle insertion. The lumbar cistern, the fluid-filled subarachnoid space extending beyond the last segment of the spinal cord, rarely extends to the lumbosacral junction in dogs, whereas in cats collection may be attempted at L6–L7 or even the lumbosacral space. However, considering the variation in the location of the spinal cord segments relative to vertebrae between dogs of different sizes (with the relationship of spinal cord segment to vertebra being more cranial in large dogs than in small breeds), L4–L5 puncture could be more successful than L5–L6 in large dogs [4–6].

Access to a caudal lumbar intervertebral space requires insertion of a spinal needle through skin, subcutaneous fascia, ligaments, and epaxial muscles. The dorsal paraspinal musculature can be divided into three longitudinal muscle masses formed by numerous overlapping fascicles: from lateral to medial, the iliocostalis system, the longissimus system, and the transversospinalis system [4]. The transversospinalis system is the most medial and deepest epaxial muscle mass and consists of a number of different systems of fascicles, which join one vertebra. In the caudal lumbar region, the musculus multifidus pars lumborum and musculus interspinales are the deepest muscles of this epaxial medial mass. The multifidus lumborum is a strong homogeneous muscle composed of numerous individual portions that overlap in segments, extending from

Current Techniques in Canine and Feline Neurosurgery, First Edition. Edited by Andy Shores and Brigitte A. Brisson.
© 2017 John Wiley & Sons, Inc. Published 2017 by John Wiley & Sons, Inc.
Companion website: www.wiley.com/go/shores/neurosurgery

the mamillary processes of caudally lying lumbar vertebrae to laterally on the ends of the spinous processes of a vertebra lying two segments cranially, immediately beneath the supraspinous ligament. The lumbar portion of the interspinales muscle is covered by the multifidus, running between contiguous edges of spinous processes.

With regard to ligaments of the caudal lumbar spine, three are described: from dorsal to ventral, the supraspinous, the interspinous, and the ligamentum flavum (interarcuate or yellow) [4]. In the dog and cat, as compared to humans, the supraspinous in the lumbar spine is imperceptible and the interspinous ligaments are poorly developed except dorsally, perhaps because of the major degree of flexion of the lumbar spine exhibited by dogs and cats [7]. The weak interspinous ligaments, interspersed with muscle bundles of the musculus interspinalis, connect adjacent vertebral spines. Ventrally to the interspinous ligament lies a much more consistent ligamentum flavum or interarcuate (yellow) ligament, consisting of connective tissue between the arches of each adjacent vertebra. Because of its consistency, a "popping" can sometimes be noticed when the spinal needle perforates this ligament. Ventral to the flavum ligament lies the epidural space in the vertebral canal, which separates the ligaments and the vertebral arches from the dura covering the spinal cord. The caudal lumbar dural sac and subarachnoid space (lumbar cistern), where CSF collection and intrathecal injection of substances is performed, extend approximately 2 cm beyond the end of the spinal cord, approximately at the level of the L6–L7 intervertebral disc in large and medium-sized dogs and at the lumbosacral junction in small-breed dogs and cats [4]. A pair of valveless internal vertebral venous plexuses are located on the floor of the vertebral canal, decreasing in size caudal to the level of the fourth or fifth lumbar vertebra.

Procedure

Technically, lumbar taps are more difficult to perform than cerebellomedullary cistern puncture, and are more likely to result in iatrogenic blood contamination. A successful lumbar puncture technique requires practice. Using a lumbar spine skeleton model for constant referral to anatomical structures is helpful. Fluoroscopy guidance simplifies accurate needle placement but is not essential. As previously mentioned, lumbar puncture is performed at L5–L6 or L4–L5 in dogs, while a more caudal L6–L7 or lumbosacral space can be attempted in cats. Lumbar puncture in small animals requires general anesthesia in order to prevent movement while proceeding.

Preparation and Equipment

A sufficiently large area of surrounding skin should be shaved (from around L4 to L7 with the midline centered on the spinous processes) and cleaned with an aseptic solution (Figure 8.1). The operator performs a surgical scrub and dons sterile gloves. Equipment required for a lumbar tap includes:

- hair clippers;
- sterile surgical gloves;
- spinal needle 20–22 gauge, 1.5–3.5 inch (3.8–8.9 cm), depending on the size of the patient;
- sterile glass tubes free of anticoagulant for CSF collection.

Use of a stylet in the needle is considered essential, not only to decrease the risk of promoting an infection in the vertebral canal, but to avoid introduction of epidermal fragments into the subarachnoid space, potentially resulting in implantation of desquamated keratinized cells and iatrogenic intraspinal epidermoid tumors [8]. In humans, 40% of intraspinal epidermoid tumors are considered a late complication of lumbar puncture and associated with using nonstylet needles [9].

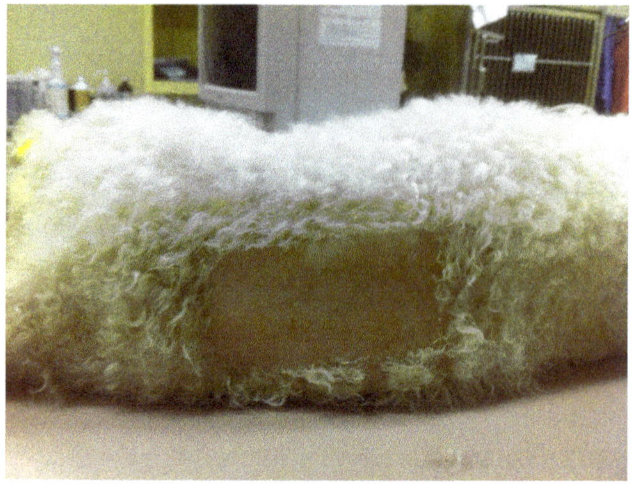

Figure 8.1 Aseptically prepared skin area for a lumbar tap.

In humans, the incidence of headache after lumbar puncture is related to the diameter of the needle: smaller needle sizes (smaller hole in the dura) are associated with reduced frequency of headache [10]. Use of atraumatic (pencil-point) spinal needles instead of the conventional "cutting" needle also reduces this risk [11]. Obviously, this complication is difficult to prove in veterinary patients. On the other hand, the narrower (22G) longer needles (2.5–3.0 inch) are more flexible and more difficult to place. In most large dogs, it is necessary to use 20G needles to reduce needle bending. Most smaller dogs require only a 22G 1.5-inch needle.

Position

Correct patient positioning is key to a successful tap. The author prefers to position the patient in right lateral recumbency with the clipped lumbar area away from the operator, and maintaining the pelvic limbs in neutral position with a pad between the limbs to keep them as parallel as possible (Figure 8.2). If the operator is left-handed, left lateral recumbency is preferred. The operator is then facing the ventral abdomen of the patient and needs to bend over the animal to insert the needle (Figure 8.3). It is extremely important to keep the lumbar spine of the patient as straight and parallel to the table as possible. This keeps the midline of the caudal lumbar spine more parallel to the insertion of the needle; otherwise the needle could be inserted in an excessively lateralized angle away from the desired interarcuate foramen. Proper positioning can be further accomplished by placing small pads or towels under the lumbar spine and under the ventral abdomen, and confirmed through lateral survey radiographs or fluoroscopy, aiming for overlapping of bilateral spinal anatomical components (ribs, lumbar transverse processes, wings of the ilium).

The patient can be positioned in sternal recumbency instead of lateral. The sternal position prevents the spine being excessively rotated, tilted or laterally flexed, as it can be in the case of lateral recumbency. However, the lateral recumbency position is more comfortable for the operator and the whole procedure, particularly if sequential images are obtained over time during a myelographic study to assess the progression of the contrast. Some clinicians

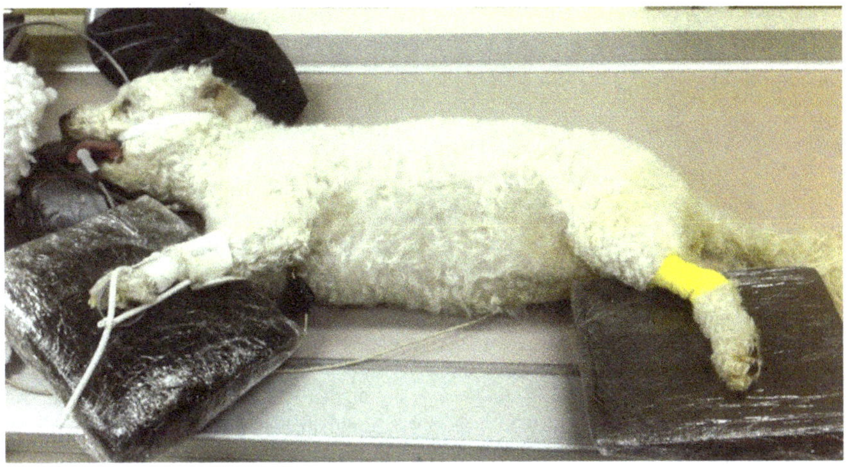

Figure 8.2 Correct positioning of the patient in right lateral recumbency for a lumbar tap.

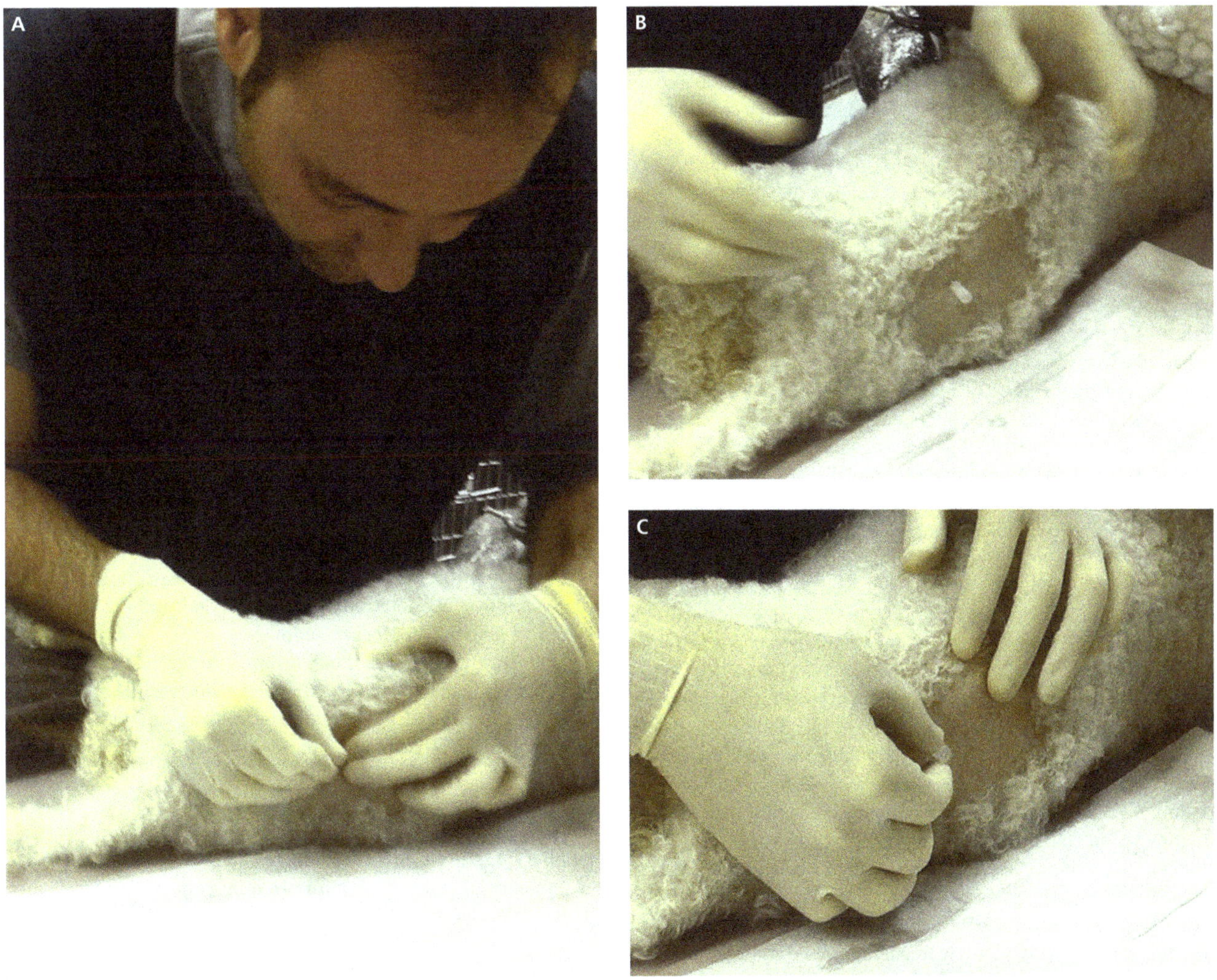

Figure 8.3 Lumbar puncture at L5–L6. (A) Operator bending over the patient facing abdomen, identifying L6 spinous process with left hand, and inserting spinal needle in its caudal aspect. (B) Once spinal needle is suspected to be in contact with the floor of the vertebral canal, remove stylet and check for CSF flow. (C) If CSF is not present, readjust needle rotating and withdrawing it until CSF flows.

recommend performing the lumbar puncture in lateral recumbency in a kyphotic position with the pelvic limbs advanced and flexed in an attempt to maximize the aperture of the interarcuate space. One study demonstrated that positioning a dog in sternal recumbency with the spine flexed produced a significantly larger L5–L6 interarcuate space aperture compared with lateral recumbency with the spine flexed, while both positions were superior to the lateral neutral [12].

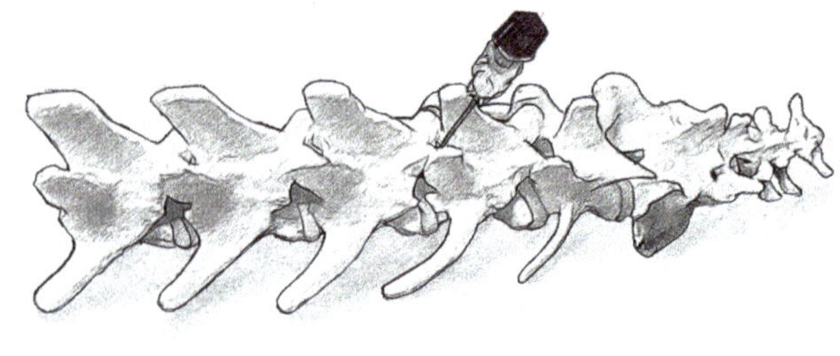

Figure 8.4 Lumbar puncture at L5–L6. Spinal needle inserted in the caudal aspect of L6 spinous process, mildly lateral, pointing cranioventrally at 45° angle aiming for the midline, and advanced into the vertebral canal through the L5–L6 interarcuate space. *Source*: Courtesy of Dr. Andrea Sanchez.

Technique

The lumbar puncture is performed through a midline approach. Bending over the patient, the appropriate L5–L6 intervertebral space is identified by palpating the cranial border of the wings of the ilium (iliac crests) using the nondominant hand, and putting the fingers of that hand on each to maintain the relationship while proceeding (Figure 8.3). The spinous process located in the midline and level with the iliac crests is L7, while immediately cranial to the iliac crests is L6. Assessing the caudal lumbar spine with survey radiographs or fluoroscopy also assists in locating the various spinous processes, especially in obese animals. While palpating the spinous process of L6 with the nondominant hand, the dominant hand is used to insert the spinal needle just mildly lateral to the caudal aspect of the L6 spinous process. The spinal needle is inserted pointing cranially at about 45° (range 30–60°) perpendicularly to the long axis of the spine[1], and advanced cranioventrally toward the midline of the spine in order to reach the L5–L6 interarcuate space (Figure 8.4). The most medial epaxial muscles (multifidus pars lumborum and interspinales) and the interspinous ligament are penetrated, and if bone is contacted the needle should be slowly moved a few millimeters cranially or caudally over the roof of the vertebra until a soft consistency is felt, corresponding to the ligamentum flavum. Resistance suddenly decreases after penetrating this ligament and accessing the vertebral canal; frequently, tail or pelvic limb twitching can be observed as the needle irritates the cauda equina nerve roots. The reported "popping" as the needle penetrates the flavum ligament is uncommonly felt. Even though the spinal needle penetrates the spinal cord during a lumbar CSF tap, this does not appear to cause any clinical problems. The needle is inserted until it contacts the bone of the ventral aspect of the spinal canal to reach the ventral subarachnoid space; then, the stylet is removed to assess presence or absence of CSF fluid and collect it (Figure 8.3). If CSF is not flowing, the needle is slowly readjusted, rotating it and changing the orientation of the bevel. If CSF flow is still not observed, the needle is slowly withdrawn and rotated without abandoning the vertebral canal until CSF is visible.

If L5–L6 puncture is not successful, a second needle can be inserted at L4–L5. It is relatively frequent in acute compressive myelopathies, such as intervertebral disc extrusion, that even if the needle is adequately positioned in the L5–L6 subarachnoid space, no CSF flows due to blockage at a more cranial level. If the main goal is to perform a lumbar myelogram but a CSF sample for analysis is not essential for diagnostic work-up, a small amount of contrast media (0.2–0.3 mL) can be injected as a trial after confirming radiographically the correct positioning of the spinal needle. Adequate injection into the subarachnoid space can be confirmed radiographically by the presence of myelogram and differentiated from epidurographic, subdural, or nonvertebral canal injections as solid contrast lines delineating dorsally and ventrally the lumbar cistern and even the nerve roots inside the cistern (Figure 8.5). If no myelogram is obtained after that, repositioning a second needle to L4–L5 should be tried without removing the L5–L6 needle to avoid leakage of contrast into the epidural canal through the previous L5–L6 dural hole (Figure 8.5). When injecting contrast, the bevel of the spinal needle should be oriented in the direction of desired flow of contrast.

Approximately, 1 mL of CSF per 5 kg body weight can be safely removed at one time for analysis, although only 1–1.5 mL is usually collected [5]. The rate of CSF flow is usually slower than from the cerebellomedullary cistern, and the fluid quantity retrieved is less. Compression of the jugular veins by an assistant will greatly increase the flow of CSF. The fluid should be collected in a sterile glass tube, preferably without EDTA, since it can cause falsely elevated protein concentrations and falsely low cell concentrations in small samples, and it is bactericidal, interfering with CSF culture if needed. During collection, CSF should not be aspirated by using negative pressure applied with a syringe attached directly to the needle hub. Aspiration can cause a rapid decrease in CSF pressure, which may trigger hemorrhage or herniation.

As previously discussed, lumbar myelography is safer and typically results in better-quality images as the contrast material flows forward under pressure to outline lesions, particularly in the thoracic and lumbar spine. Compared with cerebellomedullary injections, the lumbar needle often penetrates the spinal cord and is more likely to deposit some contrast epidurally. The calculated dose of contrast (0.3–0.5 mL/kg body weight) is slowly injected. It is very important to only used aqueous-based nonionic contrast material that is approved for intrathecal use (i.e., Isovue-M®). The author prefers to always administer a test injection (0.2–0.3 mL) to ensure the contrast is in the subarachnoid space before administering the remainder of the calculated contrast dose.

When the procedure is completed, the lumbar puncture needle can be removed without reinserting the stylet[2], and the area can be compressed to prevent local bleeding.

An ultrasound-guided lumbar puncture technique has been reported in the dog to facilitate the introduction of the needle while avoiding exposure of the operator to ionizing radiation if fluoroscopic guidance is used [13].

Contraindications and Complications

Lumbar puncture is usually a simple and safe technique, but there are some risks that can be minimized by employing proper anesthetic and collection techniques, and by excluding patients that have an increased risk of complications.

Contraindications for Lumbar CSF Tap

1. *Elevated intracranial pressure*: potentially leads to fatal brain herniation, typically cerebellar through the foramen magnum, rapidly precipitated by the removal of CSF and resulting in apnea

[1] *Editors' note*: Another placement technique involves insertion of the needle perpendicular to the axis of the spinal cord at a point just barely medial to the spinous process of the L6 vertebra in an L5–L6 puncture. The needle is advanced very slightly medially and ventrally through the interarcuate space. Using this technique, a smaller cross-sectional area of the spinal cord is traversed by the needle.

[2] *Editors' note*: In cases of lumbar puncture and myelography, the stylet is generally replaced before needle removal to prevent any contrast material from being deposited into the spinal cord parenchyma.

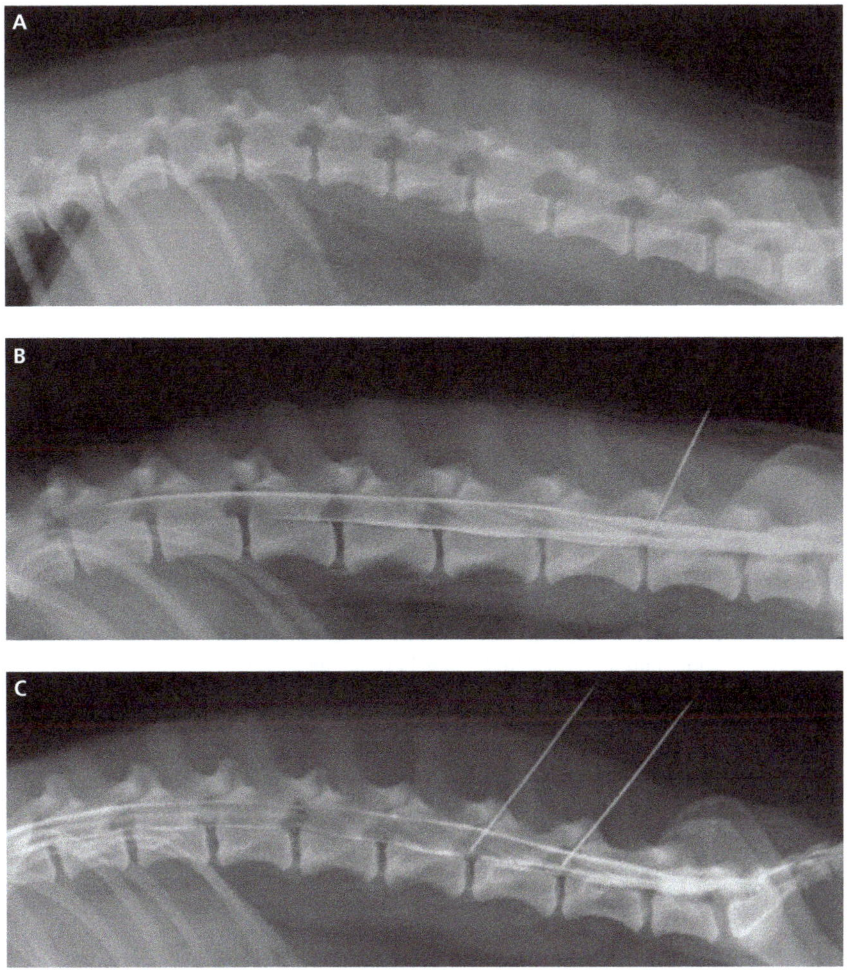

Figure 8.5 (A) Lateral radiograph of caudal spine. Substantial overlapping of bilateral anatomical components (ribs, lumbar transverse processes, wings of ilium) confirms proper patient positioning. (B) Lateral radiograph showing adequate spinal needle placement at L5–L6 and myelographic study. (C) Lateral radiograph showing proper needle placement at L4–L5 and myelography and previously inserted L5–L6 spinal needle still in place.

and death. Increased intracranial pressure can be suspected when the patient shows progressive obtundation, papilledema, bilateral miosis, and/or decerebrate rigidity. When these clinical signs are observed, the puncture should not be performed until advanced imaging (CT or MRI) of the brain excludes the presence of large space-occupying lesions or findings associated with suspected increased intracranial pressure (cerebellar herniation, mass effect, severe brain edema, severe hydrocephalus). There is no advantage of lumbar versus cerebellomedullary CSF collection in terms of brain herniation risk. In humans, lumbar puncture has been reported to cause herniation or impaction of the cord in patients with spinal mass lesions [14].

2 *Elevated risk of anesthetic complications*: CSF collection in small animals requires general anesthesia in order to prevent movement. Although generally not recommended, lumbar puncture may be attempted with heavy sedation and local anesthesia if the patient presents an unacceptable anesthetic risk.
3 *Hemorrhagic diathesis*: in patients with thrombocytopenia or coagulopathies, or taking oral anticoagulants, there is a risk of iatrogenic CNS hemorrhage.
4 *Suspected active intracranial hemorrhage.*
5 *Skin or soft tissue infection around the lumbar puncture site*, because of the possibility of introducing infection into the intrathecal compartment.
6 *Central canal dilation with myelography*: if the end of the needle is placed in the central canal or if the contrast material is injected rapidly with high pressure, the media may enter the central canal and cause it to dilate. The consequences can include paresis and extreme pain.

A good evaluation of the potential risks and benefits from obtaining a CSF sample for analysis by the clinician is vital. In the case of hemorrhagic diathesis or infected lumbar skin, if CSF analysis proves to be essential for diagnostic and therapeutic purposes, the procedure can be attempted with efforts made to reverse the coagulopathy (if at all possible) and limit the chances of spreading the skin infection.

Potential Complications of Lumbar CSF Tap

1 *Brain herniation*: sudden release of CSF pressure distally can result in herniation.
2 *Spinal cord trauma*: preexisting trauma to the area being tapped or ongoing thrombocytopenia or other clotting disorder could result in intraspinal hemorrhage.
3 *Iatrogenic hemorrhage*: due to inadvertent trauma to the venous sinuses, or dural or arachnoid vessels. Generally, this is of little consequence, although blood contamination can prevent adequate CSF sample interpretation. However, occasionally extensive spinal epidural, subdural, subarachnoid, intraspinal or even intracranial bleeding may be induced [15,16].
4 *Failure to obtain CSF ("dry tap")*: can result from the presence of spinal disease narrowing the interarcuate space (as in degenerative joint disease). In these cases another attempt should be made in the interspace cranially or caudally. If the needle is adequately

positioned in the subarachnoid space but no fluid can be obtained, this suggests that the space is blocked at a higher level (as in acute intervertebral disc extrusions) or that the lumbar cistern is infiltrated by a spinal lesion or adhesive arachnoiditis.

5 *Meningitis, discospondylitis, epidural abscess*: caused by poor sterile technique.
6 *Others* (not reported in small animals):
   - Iatrogenic intraspinal epidermoid cyst [8,9].
   - Headache: common in humans, occurring in approximately 10–15% of patients after lumbar puncture [14]. Difficult to demonstrate in animals. The risk is reduced by using the smallest caliber possible of nontraumatic spinal needle [10,11].

Indications for Lumbar CSF Analysis

CSF evaluation is a crucial component of the neurological diagnostic plan, particularly when an inflammatory CNS condition is suspected. CSF is routinely assessed for physical properties (color, clarity), total and differential nucleated cell count and cytology, and total protein concentration; normal general reference ranges are provided in Table 8.1. An extensive revision on CSF sample analysis, interpretation, and abnormal findings is beyond the scope of this chapter and the reader is referred to more specific sources in the veterinary literature [17,18].

CSF analysis (Table 8.1) is especially useful in diagnosing CNS inflammatory diseases (meningitis, encephalitis, myelitis), as it often reveals an increased inflammatory cell count and protein concentration (Figures 8.6, 8.7 and 8.8). However, although CSF analysis provides valuable data since abnormalities in CSF cytology and protein are relatively sensitive indicators of CNS disease, these are mostly nonspecific and the clinician should be careful not over-interpreting the findings. CSF analysis helps to narrow the differential diagnosis and rule out some conditions but must be interpreted cautiously in the context of the specific case signalment, history, clinical signs, and neuroimaging. The main indications for collection of a lumbar CSF sample for analytical purposes are as follows.

1 *Thoracolumbar myelopathies*: particularly to identify and characterize inflammatory/infectious conditions (myelitis, meningitis, meningomyelitis).
2 *CSF collection prior to myelography*: contrast agents are low-grade leptomeningeal irritants and change the characteristics of the CSF producing mild inflammation [19]; thus a fluid sample must be collected before injection of contrast if CSF evaluation is required later. A study in normal dogs showed that CSF nucleated cell count returned to normal range within

Table 8.1 Normal lumbar CSF values in dogs.

Physical characteristics (clarity, color, viscosity): clear, colorless, same viscosity as water
Total cell count
Red blood cells: 0/μL
White cells: 0–3/μL
Lymphocytes: 60–70% (small, well differentiated)
Monocytes: 30–40%
Differential cell count and cytology
Occasional neutrophils, eosinophils (<2%)
Choroid plexus and ependymal cells, squamous cells, chondrocytes, hematopoietic cells: rare
Total protein: <45 mg/dL

Source: Data from Vernau et al. [17] and Wamsley and Alleman [18].

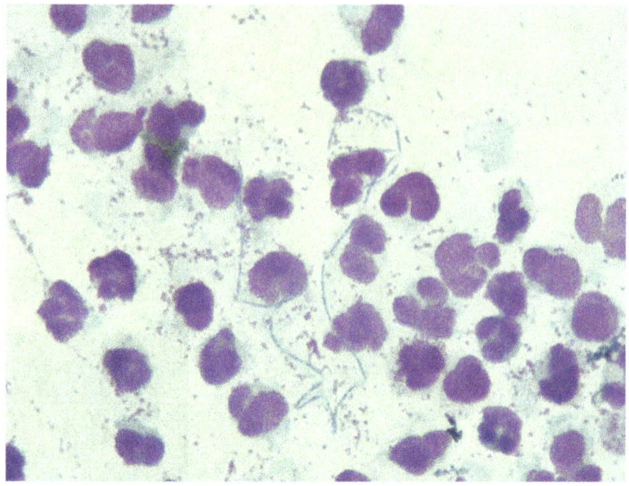

Figure 8.6 Cerebrospinal fluid (dog): neutrophilic pleocytosis showing numerous degenerated neutrophils and microorganisms consistent with a diagnosis of bacterial meningitis.

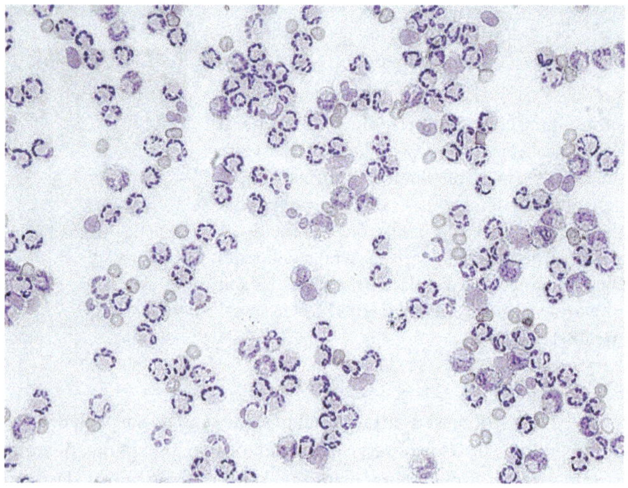

Figure 8.7 Cerebrospinal fluid (dog): neutrophilic pleocytosis with predominance of mature nondegenerated neutrophils consistent with a diagnosis of steroid-responsive meningitis arteritis.

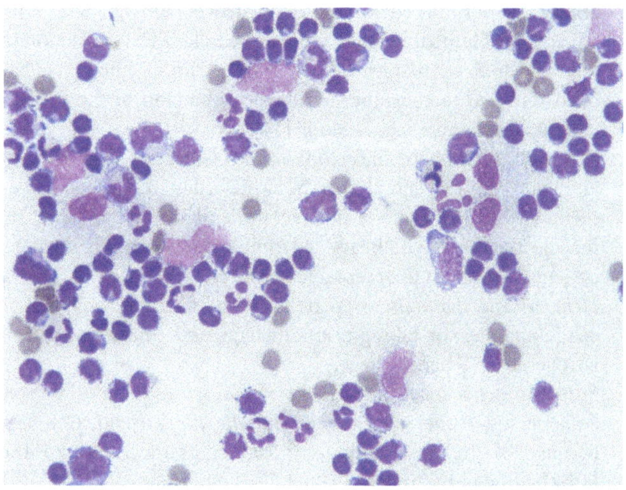

Figure 8.8 Cerebrospinal fluid (dog): mixed cell pleocytosis with a predominant population of mononuclear monocytes and lymphocytes consistent with granulomatous meningoencephalomyelitis.

82 hours of myelography, and CSF protein elevation resolved after 8 days [20]. However, a lumbar sample cannot always be obtained, as occasionally happens after an acute intervertebral disc extrusion. In this scenario, the clinician frequently faces the dilemma of delaying the myelographic procedure, and potential emergency decompressive surgery, until a cerebellomedullary sample is obtained, or to continue the myelographic study without collecting CSF. Obviously, clinician experience and knowledge of the most likely differential diagnosis and adequate consideration of potential advantages and disadvantages are essential.

3 *Radiculopathies*: meninges enclose the nerve roots distally until they become peripheral nerves. Therefore, diseases affecting the spinal nerve roots may alter the CSF, especially polyradiculoneuritis.

4 *Cerebellomedullary puncture* is contraindicated due to anatomical or mechanical restrictions, mainly atlantoaxial subluxation.

> Video clips to accompany this book can be found on the companion website at:
> www.wiley.com/go/shores/neurosurgery

References

1 Quincke H. Die lumbalpunktion des hydrocephalus. *Klin Wochenschr* 1891;28:929–933, 965–968.

2 Sharief M. Lumbar puncture and CSF examination. *Medicine* 2004;12:44–46.

3 Thomson CE. Analysis of cerebrospinal fluid from the cerebellomedullary and lumbar cisterns of dogs with focal neurologic disease: 145 cases (1985–1988). *J Am Vet Med Assoc* 1990;196:1841–1844.

4 Evans HE. *Miller's Anatomy of the Dog*. Philadelphia, PA: WB Saunders, 1993.

5 Dewey CW, Ducoté JM. Neurodiagnostics. In: Dewey CW (ed.) *A Practical Guide to Canine and Feline Neurology*, 2nd edn. Ames, IA: Wiley-Blackwell, 1983: 85–113.

6 De Lahunta A, Glass E. Cerebrospinal fluid and hydrocephalus. In: De Lahunta A, Glass E (eds) *Veterinary Neuroanatomy and Clinical Neurology*, 3rd edn. St Louis, MO: Saunders Elsevier, 2009: 54–86.

7 Heylings DJA. Supraspinous and interspinous ligaments in dog, cat and baboon. *J Anat* 1980;130:223–228.

8 Batnitzsky S, Keucher TR, Mealey J Jr, Campbell RL. Iatrogenic intraspinal epidermoid tumors. *JAMA* 1988;238:148–150.

9 Per H, Kumandaş S, Gümüş H, Yikilmaz A, Kurtsoy A. Iatrogenic epidermoid tumor: late complication of lumbar puncture. *J Child Neurol* 2008;22: 332–336.

10 Armon C, Evans RW. Addendum to assessment: prevention of post-lumbar puncture headaches: report of the Therapeutics and Technology Assessment Subcommittee of the American Academy of Neurology. *Neurology* 2005;65:510–512.

11 Hammond ER, Wang Z, Bhulani N, McArthur JC, Levy M. Needle type and the risk of post-lumbar puncture headache in the outpatient neurology clinic. *J Neurol Sci* 2011;306:24–28.

12 Puggioni A, Arnett R, Clegg T, Glyde M, Tobin E, McAllister H. Influence of patient positioning on the L5-L6 mid-laminar distance. *Vet Radiol Ultrasound* 2006;48:449–452.

13 Etienne A, Peeters D, Busoni V. Ultrasonographic percutaneous anatomy of the caudal lumbar region and ultrasound-guided lumbar puncture in the dog. *Vet Radiol Ultrasound* 201;51:528–532.

14 Sternbach G. Lumbar puncture. *J Emerg Med* 1985;2:199–203.

15 Platt SR, Dennis R, Murphy K, De Stefani A. Hematomyelia secondary to lumbar cerebrospinal fluid acquisition in a dog. *Vet Radiol Ultrasound* 2005;46: 468–481.

16 Packer RA, Bergman RL, Coates JR et al. Intracranial subarachnoid hemorrhage following lumbar myelography in two dogs. *Vet Radiol Ultrasound* 2008;48:323–328.

17 Vernau W, Vernau KA, Bailey CS. Cerebrospinal fluid. In: Kaneko JJ, Harvey JW, Bruss ML (eds) *Clinical Biochemistry of Domestic Animals*, 6th edn. Burlington, MA: Academic Press, 2008: 769–819.

18 Wamsley H, Alleman AR. Clinical pathology. In: Platt SR, Olby NJ (eds) *BSAVA Manual of Canine and Feline Neurology*, 3rd edn. Gloucester, UK: British Small Animal Veterinary Association, 2004: 35–52.

19 Widmer WR. Cerebrospinal fluid changes after iopamidol and metrizamide myelography in clinically normal dogs. *Am J Vet Res* 1992;53:396–401.

20 Cook LB, Bergman RL, Johnson MC, Coates JR, Henry GA. Effects of iohexol myelography on cerebrospinal fluid analysis in normal dogs. *J Vet Intern Med* 2003;18:400–401.

9 Muscle and Nerve Biopsy

Michaela Beasley

Introduction

Biopsies of muscles and nerves are indicated for a variety of neuromuscular diseases, mononeuropathies and polyneuropathies, and infectious, inflammatory and metabolic myopathies. Biopsies should follow neurological examination, minimum database, and electrodiagnostic testing. This information allows the examiner to select the appropriate biopsy sites: thoracic limb, pelvic limb or both, proximal or distal sites, or severely affected versus less severely affected structures. When practical, biopsies are collected contralateral to the side where a majority of the electrodiagnostics were performed. This avoids needle insertion artifacts. In acute disease a severely affected muscle should be chosen. However, in chronic disease the most affected muscles may only show fibrotic infiltration and not the underlying disease process; therefore, less severely affected muscle are chosen [1–4]. Even the best sample can become useless without appropriate handling and shipping to a qualified pathologist, trained specifically in neuropathology [2–4]. Readers are strongly encouraged to contact their submission laboratory for specific instructions on shipment and their comfort level in reviewing your samples. At a minimum, formalin-fixed muscle and nerve biopsies and fresh refrigerated muscle biopsies are submitted using overnight shipping in an insulated container. Samples are taken on a day when their arrival at the laboratory will not fall on a weekend or long holiday.

Techniques

Techniques for obtaining muscle and nerve biopsies are described in this chapter and include descriptions of performing an open biopsy for the cranial tibial, biceps femoris, gastrocnemius, and triceps brachii muscles. Fascicular nerve biopsy techniques are described for the ulnar, common peroneal, and tibial nerves, all containing mixed sensory and motor components. This technique, which samples 30–50% of the nerve diameter, preserves the neurological function of the nerve while being a representative sample of the entire nerve diameter. Nonetheless, owners are warned that, rarely, conscious proprioceptive deficits can be seen for a few days following the procedure [5].

Pelvic Limb

In the pelvic limb, the common peroneal nerve and biceps femoris and gastrocnemius muscles are biopsied through a single curved incision centered behind the stifle. Alternatively, the tibial nerve and cranial tibial muscle can be biopsied through two separate but smaller linear incisions. For both options, the leg is clipped and the skin surgically prepared with chlorhexidine or betadine. The author prefers to remove the hair and prepare the leg on both the lateral and medial surface in a hanging leg type preparation. A sterile towel or drape is placed under the leg to give a sterile ventral field, followed by a second towel placed over the foot to allow manipulation of the leg if necessary. A fenestrated paper drape can then be placed over the leg or a third surgical towel/drape placed over the remaining hair dorsal to the prepared area (Figure 9.1).

The cranial tibial muscle and tibial nerve offer a distal muscle and nerve for biopsy. These can be biopsied through one incision in some small dogs and cats, but often require two separate incisions. The leg is clipped and prepared as described above. A linear proximal to distal incision is made overlying the cranial tibial muscle located on the craniolateral aspect of the tibia just distal to the stifle. The fascia of the cranial tibial muscle is incised in line with the skin incision and a $1 \times 1 \times 2$ cm block of muscle removed using a #11 scalpel blade. This block of tissue is separated into two 1 cm^2 blocks. One piece should be put in 10% buffered formalin and the other wrapped in gauze moistened with physiological saline. After the procedure, the muscle is placed in a 10-mL red-top tube or similar container for shipping. If excessive bleeding from the muscle biopsy site is encountered, absorbable hemostatic gelatin sponge is placed in the defect and the muscle fascia closed over it (Figure 9.2). The subcutaneous tissue and skin are closed in routine fashion.

The tibial nerve is located in a nerve/artery/vein (neurovascular) bundle between the gastrocnemius tendon and distal tibia. A proximal to distal linear incision is made distal to the lateral saphenous vein extending to the tibiotarsal junction. Here it is important for

Current Techniques in Canine and Feline Neurosurgery, First Edition. Edited by Andy Shores and Brigitte A. Brisson.
© 2017 John Wiley & Sons, Inc. Published 2017 by John Wiley & Sons, Inc.
Companion website: www.wiley.com/go/shores/neurosurgery

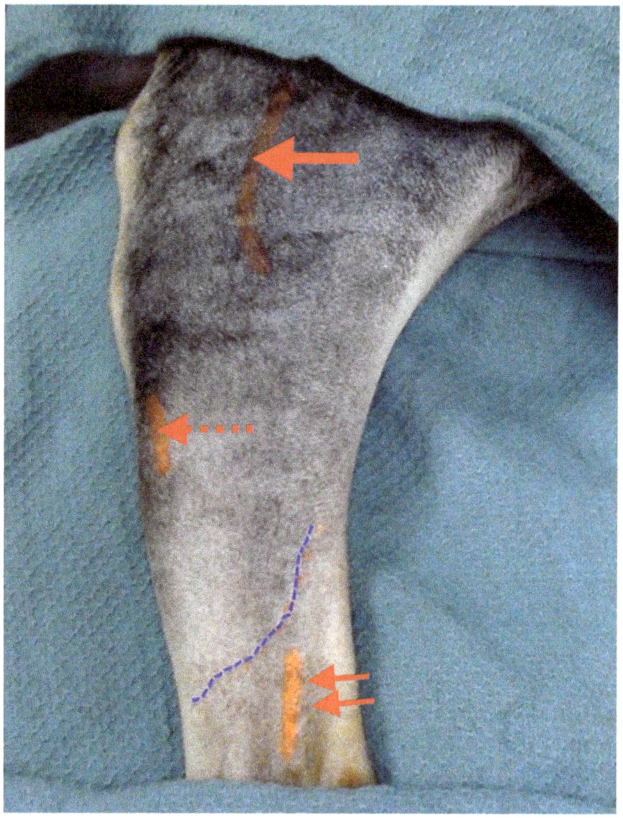

Figure 9.1 Pelvic limb (lateral distal femur and tibia) shown draped for muscle and nerve biopsies. The dotted line indicates the lateral saphenous vein, to be avoided during biopsy of the tibial nerve. The solid arrow indicates the incision for biopsy of the biceps femoris and gastrocnemius muscles as well as common peroneal nerve. The dashed arrow indicates incision for biopsy of cranial tibial muscle and double arrow indicates incision for biopsy of tibial nerve.

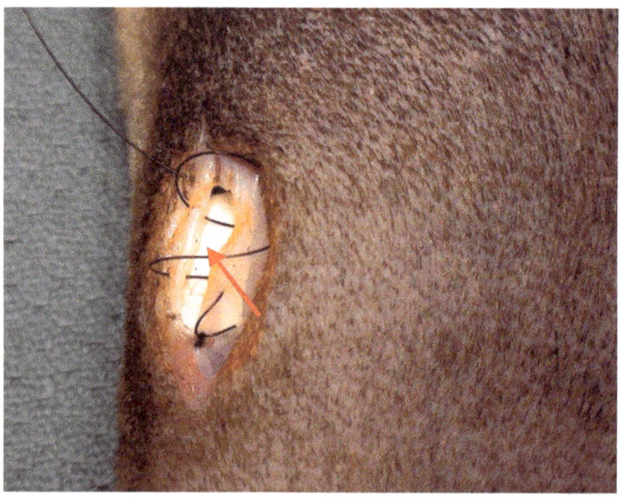

Figure 9.2 A biopsy of the cranial tibial muscle has been taken, an absorbable hemostatic sponge (arrow) has been placed in the defect, and the fascia closed using a simple continuous suture pattern.

identification to "strum" the nerve between the tip of the index finger and nail of the thumb through the sterile gloves. Having initially clipped and prepared in a hanging-leg fashion makes it easier to use this strumming technique while maintaining a sterile field. One should feel the multitude of perineurium bundles passing between the tip of the index finger and nail of the thumb. It is critical to separate the associated artery and vein from the nerve. This not only decreases morbidity by leaving the vasculature intact, but also ensures a diagnostic sample is taken and not a sample from only some of the surrounding connective tissue. To start, a hemostat is used to separate the nerve, artery, and vein bundle from surrounding tissue in a 360° dissection. Next, hemostats are used to separate the nerve from the rest of the bundle. This can be performed by pushing on the edge of the nerve with the closed tips of hemostats and with downward pressure opening the hemostats to strip away fascia and connective tissue (Figure 9.3). Once the bundle is identified and completely isolated, a fascicular biopsy is made [5].

The tibial nerve is split in a proximal to distal direction for the length of the biopsy with a #11 or #15 scalpel blade. It may be beneficial to have a second scalpel handle or other structure under the nerve to provide a cutting surface (Figure 9.4). The nerve is split so that one-third of its width is taken for the biopsy [5]. Thumb forceps are used to grasp the nerve biopsy at its most proximal dissection (Figure 9.5). This is the only time the nerve will be grasped in order to minimize trauma to the biopsy specimen. An alternative to manipulating the nerve with forceps is to suture one-third of the width of the nerve at the most proximal aspect of dissection leaving a suture tag to hold. Then the proximal end of the biopsy is always severed first in a transverse manner followed by the distal aspect (Figure 9.6). This is to minimize patient discomfort as, even in a surgical plane of anesthesia, sectioning of an intact nerve will arouse the patient because of intense pain. The sample is then either pinned or tied to a previously prepared piece of tongue depressor or tied to the wooden end of a cotton-tipped applicator. This ensures the nerve will not contract during shipment. The entire sample is placed in 10% formalin.

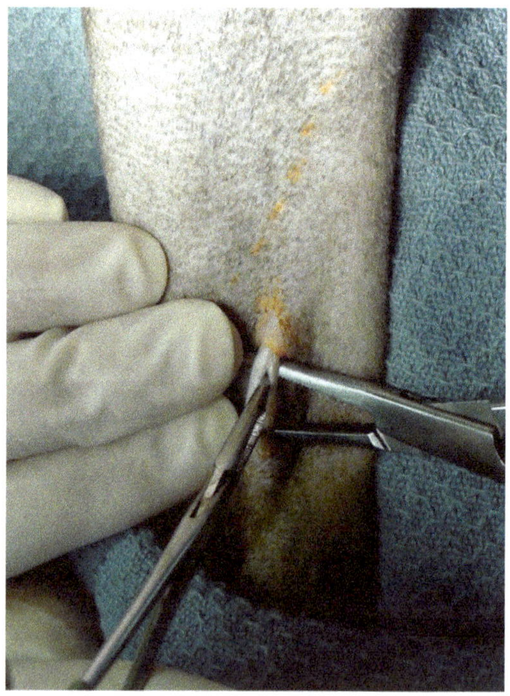

Figure 9.3 A pair of hemostats has been placed under the tibial nerve bundle after 360° dissection and a second pair is being used to dissect away surrounding vasculature and connective tissue.

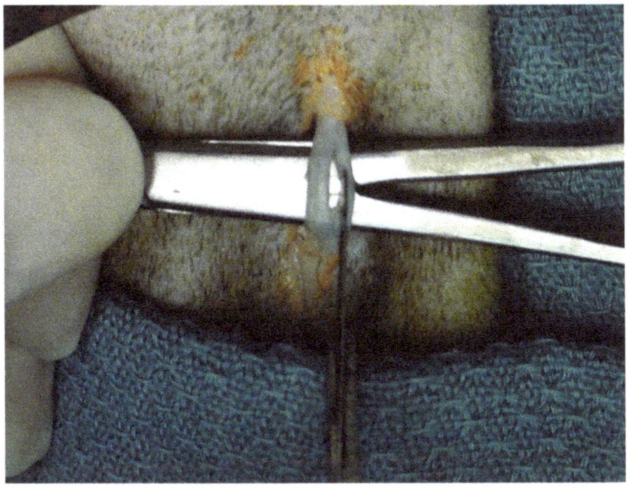

Figure 9.4 With a solid surface under the tibial nerve, a scalpel blade is used to split the nerve into one-third and two-third sections in a proximal to distal direction.

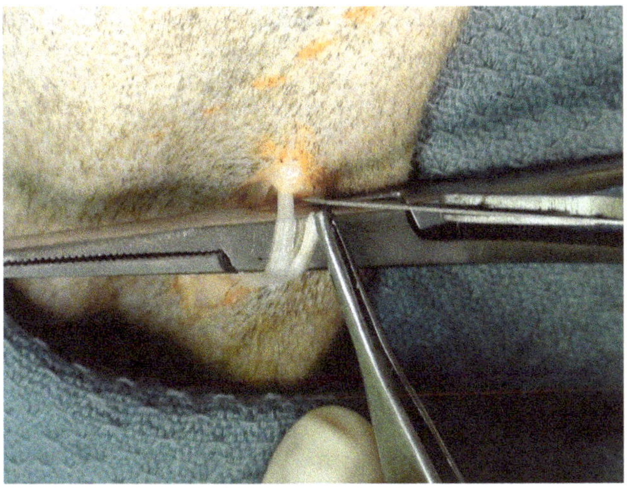

Figure 9.5 The nerve has been split with a scalpel blade and the proximal end is held and transected with a scalpel blade.

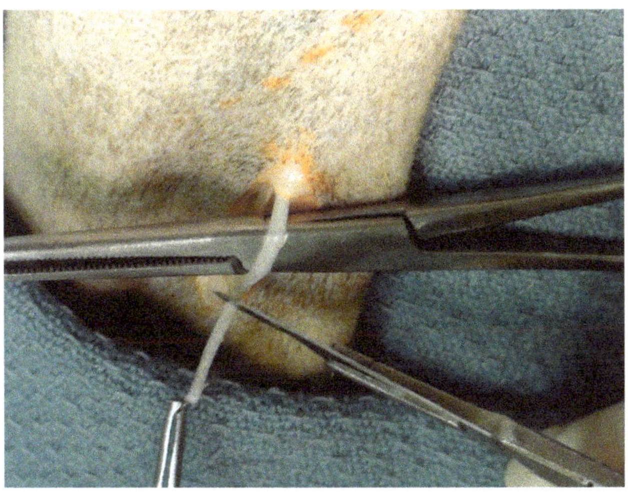

Figure 9.6 Once the proximal aspect has been severed, the biopsy sample can be cut at the distal end and prepared as described in the text.

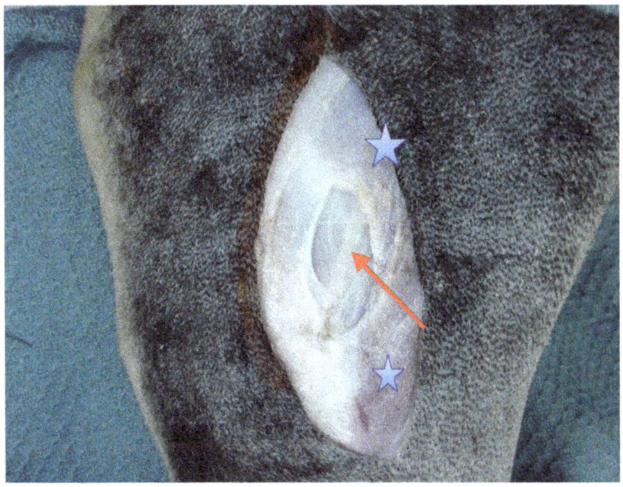

Figure 9.7 An incision has been made in the skin and fascia revealing the underlying common peroneal nerve (arrow). The sites for biopsy of the proximal biceps femoris and distal gastrocnemius are marked with stars.

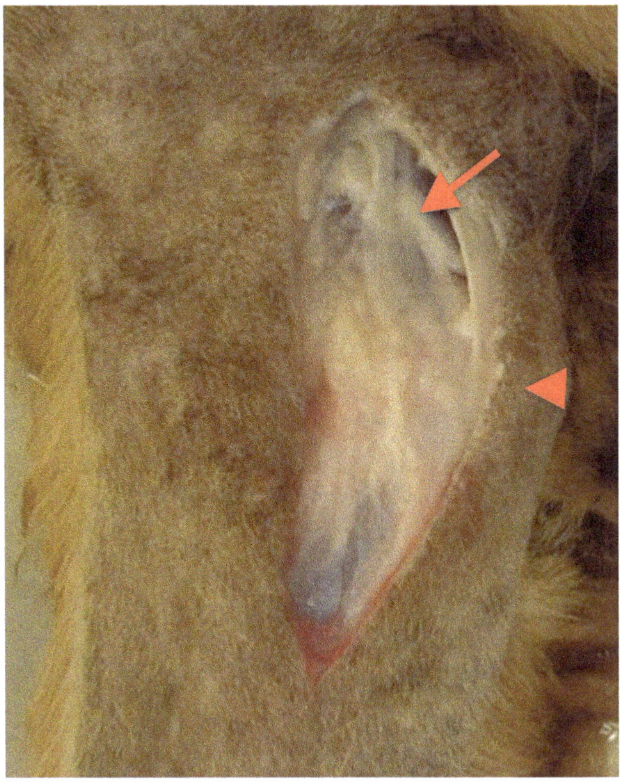

Figure 9.8 The medial aspect of the forelimb over the elbow has been clipped. An assistant is holding the opposite leg out of the field. A linear incision centered caudally has been made in a proximal to distal direction. The olecranon is marked with an arrowhead and the ulnar nerve bundle with an arrow.

The preparation of the tongue depressor is done to ensure it will fit into the planned sample container. In this case a 10-mL red-top tube is usually chosen. The subcutaneous tissue and skin are closed in routine fashion.

Sampling of the common peroneal nerve and biceps femoris and gastrocnemius muscles requires a proximal to distal curvilinear

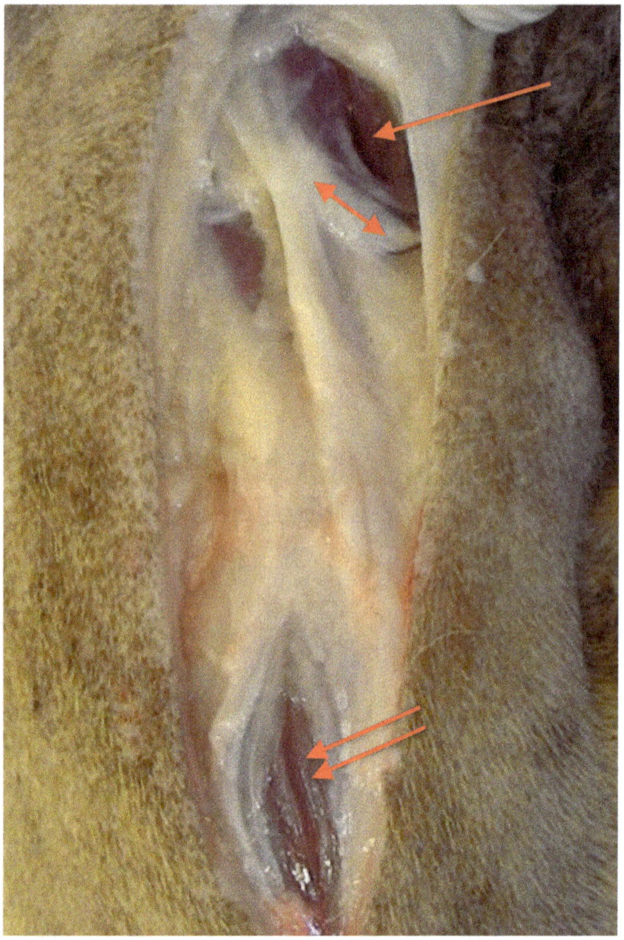

Figure 9.9 Fascia cleared for biopsy of the biceps muscle (single arrow) and superficial digital flexor muscle (double arrow) as well as ulnar nerve (double arrowhead).

incision to be made centered caudal to the stifle. After incising through the skin and subcutaneous tissues, the biceps femoris muscle is visualized and a 1 × 1 × 2 cm block of tissue is excised using a #11 scalpel blade and processed as described earlier. Next, the biceps fascia is incised behind the stifle taking care to only incise this fascia and no underlying tissue. Reflection of the fascia caudally reveals the underlying common peroneal nerve (Figure 9.7). The fascicular biopsy is performed as described above. The incision in the biceps fascia is closed followed by biopsy of the lateral head of the gastrocnemius muscle. The procedure concludes with subcutaneous tissue and skin closure.

Thoracic Limb

In the thoracic limb, the ulnar nerve and medial head of the triceps brachii and superficial digital flexor muscles are biopsied through a single incision (Figures 9.8 and 9.9). The ulnar nerve is also contained in a neurovascular bundle, so care is taken as with the tibial nerve. The medial aspect of the thoracic limb is clipped and prepared. An assistant may be needed to hold the upper thoracic limb out of the field. A linear proximal to distal incision centered over the medial aspect of the elbow is made. After dissection through the subcutaneous tissue, the ulnar nerve is seen coursing in a cranial to caudal direction just distal to the medial condyle of the humerus and olecranon. The medial head of the triceps is biopsied proximal to the ulnar nerve and the superficial digital flexor muscle biopsied distal to the nerve. These samples are prepared as above and the fascia, subcutaneous tissue, and skin closed.

Video clips to accompany this book can be found on the companion website at:
www.wiley.com/go/shores/neurosurgery

References

1 Braund KG. Nerve and muscle biopsy techniques. *Prog Vet Neurol* 1991;2:35–56.
2 Dickinson PJ, LeCouteur RA. Muscle and nerve biopsy. *Vet Clin North Am Small Animal Pract* 2002;32:63–102.
3 Lecouteur RA, Williams DC. Neurodiagnostics. In: Tobias KM, Johnston SA (eds) *Veterinary Surgery: Small Animal*. St Louis, MO: Elsevier Saunders, 2012: 351–356.
4 Lorenz MD, Coates JR, Kent M. Confirming a diagnosis. In: *Handbook of Veterinary Neurology*, 5th edn. St Louis, MO: Elsevier Saunders, 2011: 89.
5 Braund KG, Walker TL, Vandevelde M. Fascicular nerve biopsy in the dog. *Am J Vet Res* 1979;40:1025–1030.

SECTION II

Intracranial Procedures

10 Transfrontal Craniotomy

Ane Uriarte and Rodolfo Cappello

Introduction

The rostral cerebrum comprises the brain tissue rostral to the cruciate sulcus and pyriform lobe. The blood supply is maintained by the rostral and middle cerebral arteries (Figure 10.1) [1]. In dogs, the blood reaching the rostral half of the brain is from the internal carotid. In cats, the entire adult brain is supplied by maxillary blood [2]. The frontal bone, frontal sinus, and cribriform plate protect the frontal lobe of the cerebrum (Figures 10.2 and 10.3). The size and shape of the frontal sinus varies with the breed and skull type. In general, brachycephalic breeds have a smaller or absent frontal sinus compared with mesocephalic dogs, while dolichocephalic breeds have a larger and longer frontal sinus (Figure 10.4).

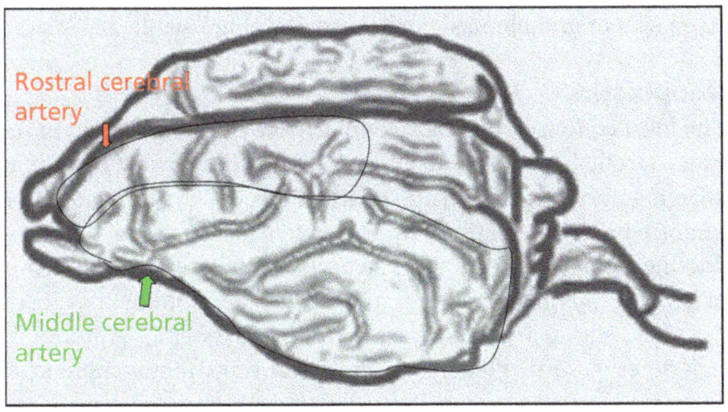

Figure 10.1 Blood supply of the frontal lobe.

The history of the study of frontal lobe function is one of the most complicated and contradictory chapters in the investigation of brain physiology [3]. Multiple studies were performed in the past on lobotomized dogs [4,5]. Pavlov regarded the frontal lobes in dogs as an essential and the most complex component of the motor cortex, participating in the selection of necessary "goal-directed movements." It seems the frontal lobes determine the adaptive capacities of dogs with regard to their repeated patterns and their capacity for rapid and appropriate change of task [6]. More recent studies performed in a canine model of aging (the frontal lobe seems sensitive to normal aging) have shown that reduced frontal lobe volume correlates with impaired performance on measures of executive function, including inhibitory control and complex working memory [7].

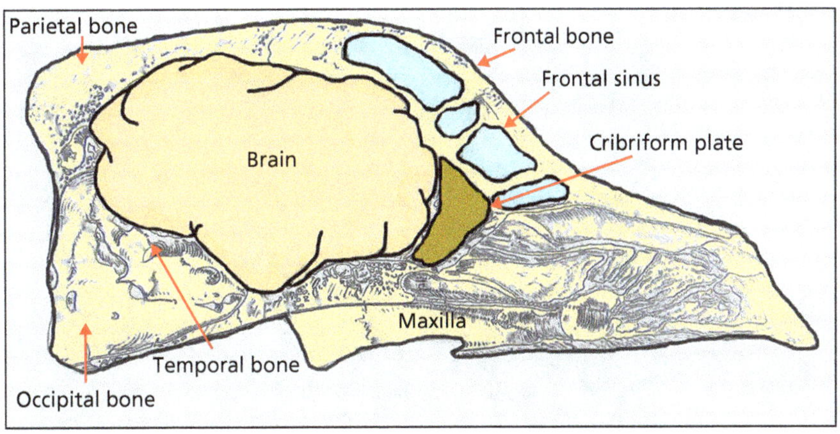

Figure 10.2 Schematic drawing of the major structures surrounding the frontal lobe.

Current Techniques in Canine and Feline Neurosurgery, First Edition. Edited by Andy Shores and Brigitte A. Brisson.
© 2017 John Wiley & Sons, Inc. Published 2017 by John Wiley & Sons, Inc.
Companion website: www.wiley.com/go/shores/neurosurgery

Despite the multiple tasks of the frontal lobe, "silent" areas have been identified experimentally in the frontal lobes of animals. "Silent" areas of the cerebral cortex can be stimulated mechanically, chemically, or electrically without producing an obvious motor or sensory response. Lesions produced experimentally in frontal lobe areas are reported to cause no signs, seizures, or behavior changes such as uncontrolled rage or apathy [8]. Generalized seizures commonly precede abnormalities in the neurological examination when the lesion is localized on the frontal lobe. Slow-growing or small tumors have traditionally been regarded as the cause of this observation, although prefrontal location has been proposed to result in seizures without neurological deficits in dogs [9]. Consequently, the absence of neurological deficits on initial examination appears to be an unlikely predictor of space-occupying masses in the rostral cerebrum. Therefore, it is not uncommon for the neurosurgeon to encounter large tumors in this area. Transfrontal craniotomies in dogs have been related to severe postsurgical complications such as general seizures and postoperative surgical infection in the first described frontal craniotomies [10–12].

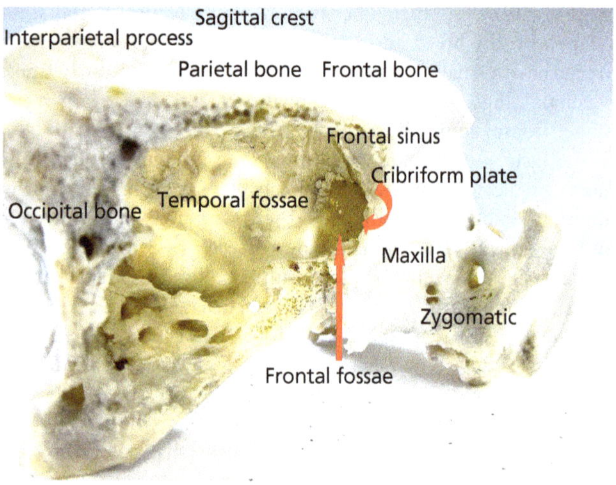

Figure 10.3 View from a partially opened skull showing the principal bony structures.

Transfrontal craniotomy is limited by the anatomy of the area, extent of the tumor, and exposure provided by the surgical approach: a good exposure provided by an adequate surgical approach is important for the success of the technique and avoids postsurgical complications. Transfrontal craniotomy in veterinary medicine was described in dogs in 1972 by Parker and Cunningham [11], by DeWet et al. in 1982 [12], and by Kostolich and Dulisch in 1987 [10]. These approaches combined a rostrotentorial approach with a transfrontal approach and proximal transfrontal sinus approach with destruction of the cribriform plate. Clear visualization with adequate exposure was limited by these surgical approaches. Moreover, severe postoperative complications were recorded [10]. In 2000, Glass et al. [13] proposed a modified bilateral transfrontal sinus approach in five dogs, and in 2011 Uriarte et al. [14] described a bilateral and unilateral transfrontal sinus approach in seven dogs with frontal meningiomas. Both papers demonstrated a satisfactory exposure of the frontal lobe without major postsurgical complications.

Indications

Transfrontal craniotomies/craniectomies are indicated for exposure of the dorsal frontal cortices (approximately the cruciate sulci), olfactory bulbs, and ethmoidal areas. The types of lesions with indications for surgery include neoplastic, vascular (primary or secondary hemorrhages), head trauma (depression fracture), infectious (abscesses or granulomas), and congenital abnormalities.

Neoplastic

The most common surgically approachable pathology found in the canine frontal lobe is a neoplastic lesion. In a review of tumors affecting the rostral cerebrum, meningioma was the most common tumor type (30%), followed by astrocytoma (16%), nasal neuroendocrine carcinoma (14%), and neuroblastoma (12%) [8]. Excision of frontal meningiomas by transfrontal craniotomy has been described successfully in a case series by Glass et al. [13] and by Uriarte et al. [14]. Bilateral or unilateral transfrontal approaches allow easy access to tumors located on the olfactory lobe and dorsal frontal lobe (Figures 10.5 and 10.6).

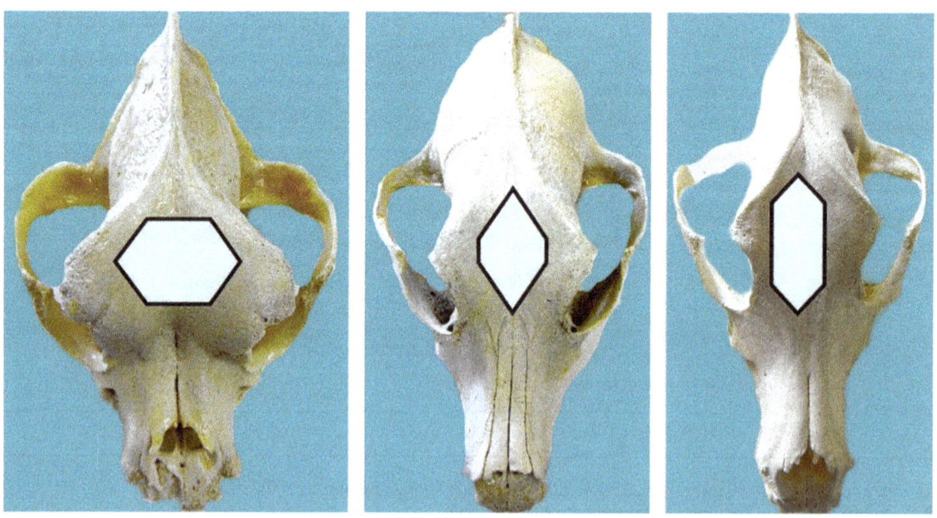

Figure 10.4 Three skulls from brachycephalic, mesocephalic, and dolichocephalic dogs with their related frontal sinuses.

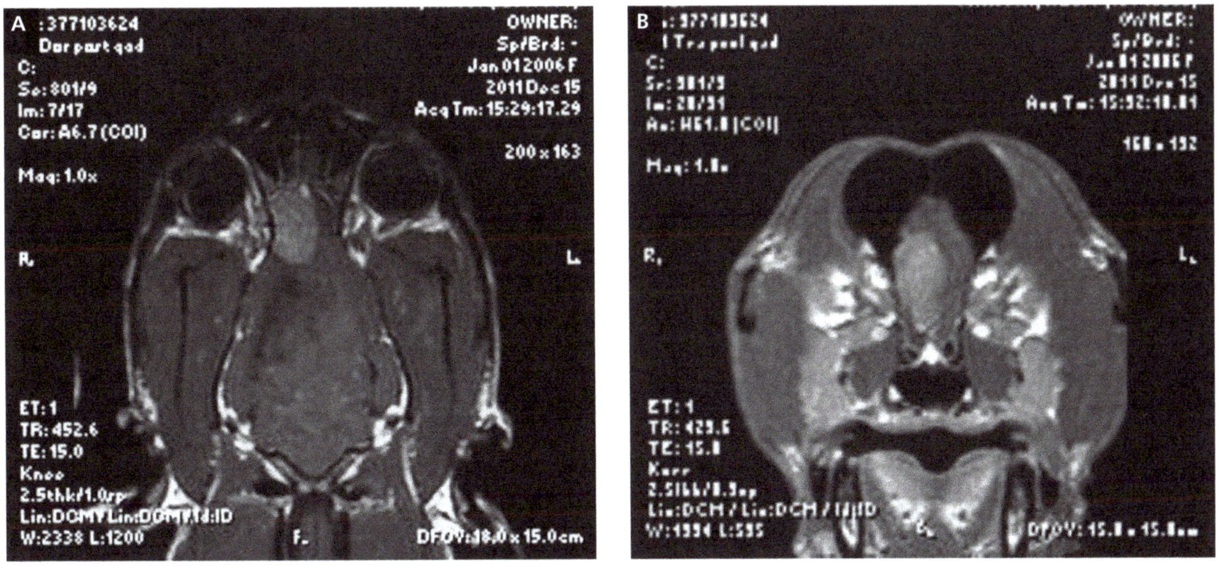

Figure 10.5 A 9-year-old female Hungarian Vizla dog. The dog was referred after a generalized seizure was recorded 24 hours previously. The histopathology results after surgical removal were consistent with a meningioma, atypical type. (A) Dorsal T1-weighted postgadolinium MRI of the brain. There is evidence of a mass affecting the right olfactory and frontal lobe causing a marked midline shift to the left. This mass shows heterogeneous contrast enhancement. (B) Transverse T1-weighted postgadolinium MRI of the brain at the level of the frontal lobe. There is heterogeneous contrast enhancement of the mass located on the right frontal lobe. There is a mass effect.

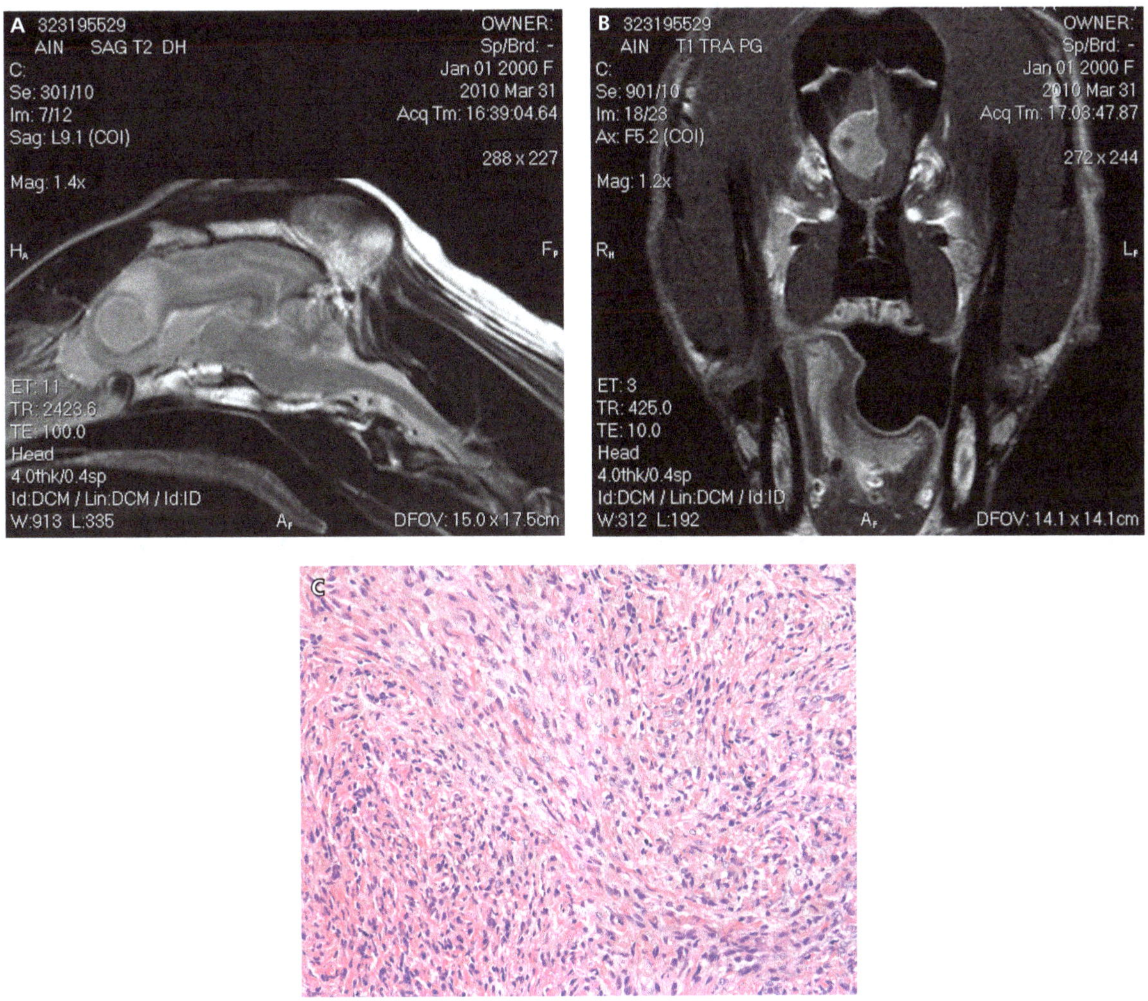

Figure 10.6 A 12-year-old female German Shepherd dog presented for intermittent behavioral changes and a generalized seizure 2 months before referral. The histopathology results (C) after surgical removal were consistent with a meningioma, fibroblastic microcystic subtype. (A) Sagittal T2-weighted MRI of the brain. There is evidence of a hyperintense well-defined mass affecting the frontal lobe. There is perilesional edema. (B) Transverse T1-weighted postgadolinium MRI of the brain at the level of the frontal lobe. There is evidence of a mass effect affecting the right frontal lobe causing a midline shift to the left. This mass shows heterogeneous contrast enhancement. There is a dural tail sign associated with the longitudinal fissure. (C) Spindle cells with elongated nuclei haphazardly arranged in small bundles. H&E staining, ×20. *Source*: (C) Courtesy of Dr. Jim Cooley.

Vascular

Hemorrhage on the frontal lobe which necessitates surgical decompression is uncommon. However, if the neurological symptoms are severe, persist, or deteriorate, transfrontal craniotomy to allow decompression might be required [15]. The frontal lobe is supplied by the rostral and middle cerebral arteries (see Figure 10.1). Rupture of a blood vessel wall (artery or vein) causing hemorrhage can be classified as primary or secondary depending on the underlying cause of bleeding. Primary hemorrhage originates from the spontaneous rupture of small damaged vessels, while secondary hemorrhage has been reported in dogs in association with various causes, such as rupture of congenital vascular abnormalities, hemorrhage into brain tumors, inflammatory disease, brain infarction, or impaired coagulation [16]. Extradural, subdural, epidural, subarachnoid, and intraparenchymal hemorrhage has been reported in dogs and cats following head injury [15,17,18].

Trauma

The frontal lobe is protected by the skull and the frontal sinus (see Figures 10.2 and 10.3). However, penetrating trauma can reach the frontal lobe [15,19] through the frontal sinus and cribriform plate (Figure 10.7). If the neurological signs are severe and deteriorate secondary to a skull depression, hemorrhage, or a hypertensive pneumocephalus, transfrontal craniotomy might be indicated [15,20].

Infectious

Frontal lobe abscess or empyema, are often secondary to head trauma or migrating foreign bodies (Figure 10.8). A transfrontal approach might be needed to decompress, debride and culture suppurative material [20]. Access to a more ventral empyema might not be achieved with this technique (Figure 10.8). Nevertheless, sample collection for culture or biopsy (ultrasound guided if needed) is possible through the transfrontal approach.

Frontal lobe extension from aspergillosis is uncommon in veterinary medicine. However, in humans, neurosurgical intervention (frontotemporal craniotomy) in combination with antifungal therapy remains the treatment of choice to improve survival in CNS aspergillosis [21].

Malformation

Congenital malformations affecting the frontal lobe cortex include: anencephaly, meningocele, exencephaly, lipomeningocele, and holoprosencephaly–arrhinencephaly. Meningoencephalocele is a protrusion of cerebral tissue and meninges through a congenital defect in the cranial bones (cranioschisis or cranium bifidum) whereas herniation of only meninges is a meningocele [22]. Meningoencephalocele is the most common of these two malformations, but microscopic examination is commonly required to appreciate the difference. Generalized seizures not responding to medical treatment is the main neurological sign when the meningocele only affects the frontal lobe [23,24]. Transfrontal craniotomy with excision of a meningoencephalocele and closure of the dural defect was an effective treatment for an intranasal meningoencephalocele in a dog, and was described by Martlé et al. [24].

Surgical Technique (Video 10.1)

Several techniques have been described [10,11,13,14]. The techniques vary by the region (olfactory vs. frontal lobes) and the type of intervention necessary. The approach to the frontal lobe and olfactory bulb is generally approached via the diamond-shaped or trapezoidal-shaped bone flap over the rostral extent of the frontal bone sinus [13,14]. Bilateral and unilateral approaches have been described. However, the unilateral approach has limited visibility and restricted access to the frontal and olfactory lobes.

The dog is positioned in sternal recumbency; the head can be raised by air cushions or sand bags and the table inclined so the head

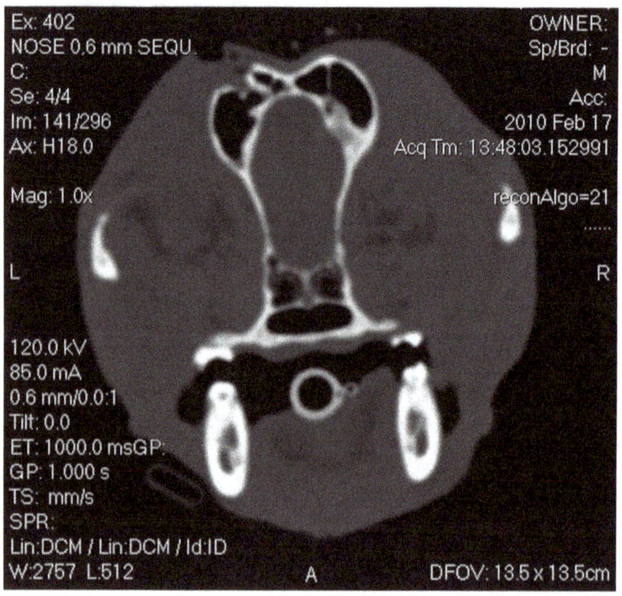

Figure 10.7 CT scan of a 9-year-old Border Terrier that was hit on the head with a pickaxe. The fracture is affecting the left frontal bone. The calvarium, periorbital space, and cribriform plate are intact. The dog was neurologically normal.

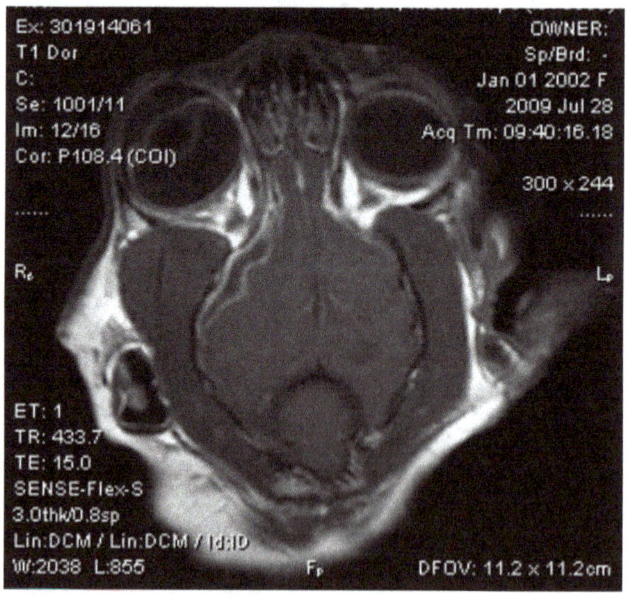

Figure 10.8 A 5-year-old female Domestic Shorthair cat that was referred for depression, coughing, and retching of several weeks' duration. The referring veterinarian had extracted two fragments of grass awn from the oropharynx. Dorsal T1-weighted postgadolinium MRI of the brain shows a right frontal–temporal lobe lesion that exhibited a subdural space ring enhancement after gadolinium administration. A similar lesion can be seen in the right caudal nasal passage involving the right cribriform plate. The final diagnosis was cerebral empyema.

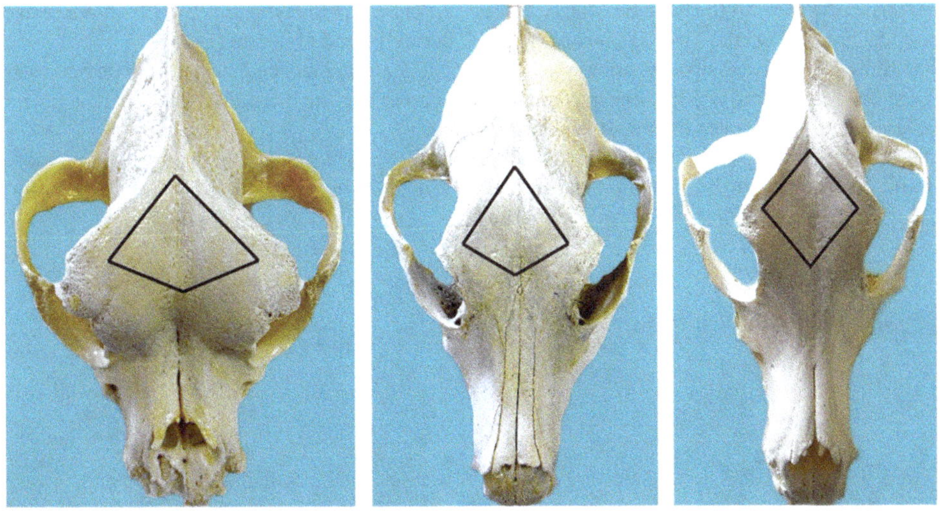

Figure 10.9 Schematic representation of the diamond-shaped osteotomy in different skulls. The limits of the craniotomy extend rostro-medially from the junction of the nasal bones to the medial portion of the zygomatic process of the orbit and caudally from the zygomatic process of the orbit to the junction of the frontal–parietal sutures.

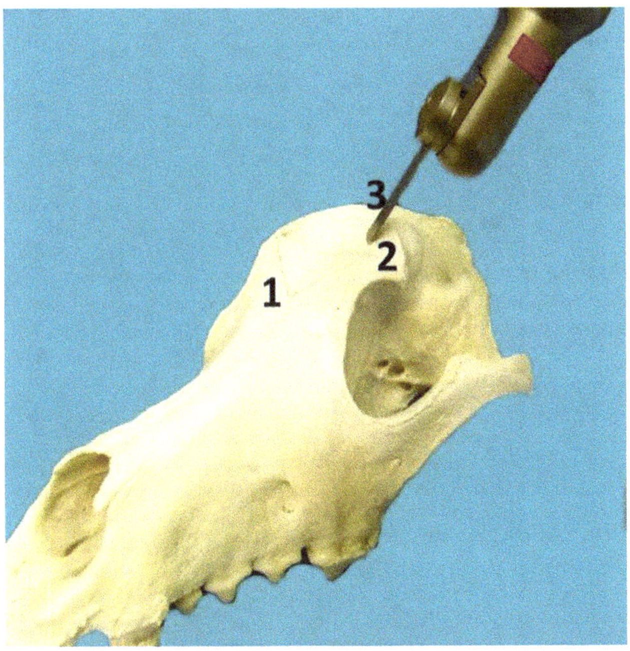

Figure 10.10 Starting the craniotomy. The diamond shaped-osteotomy is performed using an oscillating saw. Note the inclination of the blade by approximately 30° to facilitate the repositioning of the bone flap. The limits of the craniotomy extend rostro-medially from the junction of the nasal bones (1) to the medial portion of the zygomatic process of the orbit (2) and caudally from the zygomatic process of the orbit to the junction of the frontal–parietal sutures (3).

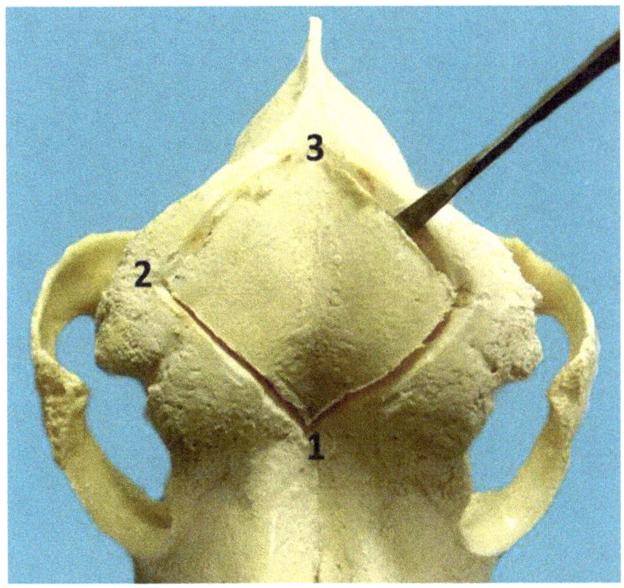

Figure 10.11 Once the frontal bone is cut, small periosteal elevators are inserted into the bone incision and care is taken to check that there are no residual bone connections which can make detachment of the bone flap difficult and increase the possibility of fracturing or damaging the flap. 1, Junction of nasal bones; 2, zygomatic process of the orbit; 3, frontal–parietal sutures.

is slightly above the rest of the body and at 90° with the neck. During positioning care should be taken to avoid pressure on the jugular veins. The body can be strapped at the level of the shoulders and pelvis to immobilize the dog and allow movement of the table in all directions during the surgical procedure, if these are necessary, to facilitate the visualization of the frontal and olfactory lobes.

The head is surgically prepared, clipping from the occipital protuberance to the orbital protuberance and nasal bones. A midline incision is performed from the caudal edge of the nasal bone to the caudal margin of the frontal sinus passing the bregma point. The incision varies slightly depending on the conformation of the head (Figure 10.9). The underling subcutaneous tissues including the periosteum are reflected laterally with periosteal elevators.

A diamond-shaped or trapezoidal-shaped craniotomy is performed using an oscillating saw. It is recommended that the blade is inclined by 30° to facilitate the reposition of the bone flap (Figure 10.10). The limits of the craniotomy extend rostro-medially from the junction of the nasal bones to the medial portion of the zygomatic process of the orbit and caudally from the zygomatic process of the orbit to the junction of the frontal–parietal sutures (Figures 10.11, 10.12 and 10.13). Once the frontal bone is cut, a small periosteal elevator is inserted into the bone incision. Care is taken to check for residual bone connections that can make detachment of the bone flap difficult and increase the possibility of fracturing or damaging the flap (Figure 10.11). Prior to detachment of the flap it is advisable to predrill the holes (Figure 10.13) for the sutures or wire fixation of the flap at the end of the surgery. The flap is elevated dorsally and detached from the septum of the frontal sinus. The bone is wrapped in moistened gauze sponges and saved for closure. This type of approach allows replacement of the bone flap at the end of the surgery.

The sinuses can be irrigated with povidone-iodine solution prior to accessing the brain. However, there is no general consensus on

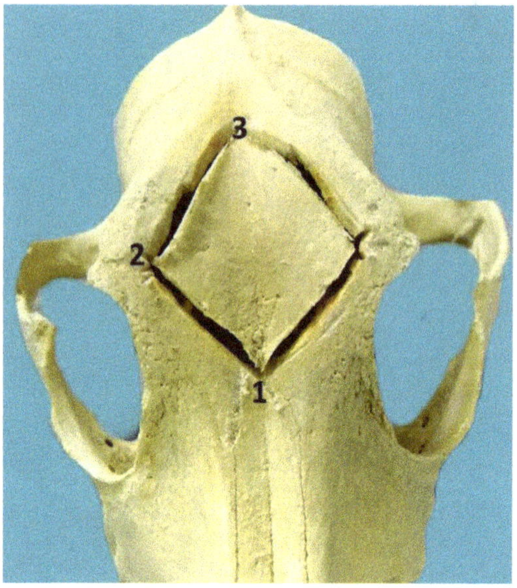

Figure 10.12 Mesocephalic cranium. 1, Junction of nasal bones; 2, zygomatic process of the orbit; 3, frontal–parietal sutures.

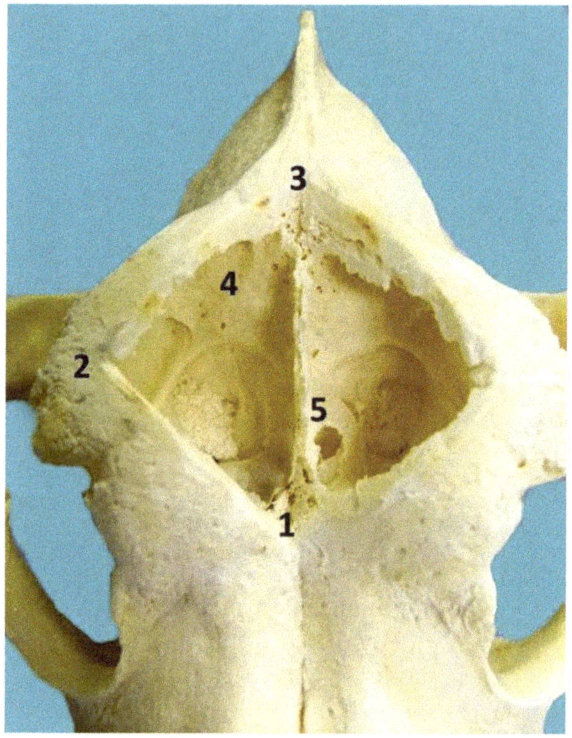

Figure 10.14 Brachycephalic cranium. 1, Junction of nasal bones; 2, zygomatic process of the orbit; 3, frontal–parietal sutures; 4, internal table of frontal bone; 5, cribriform plate.

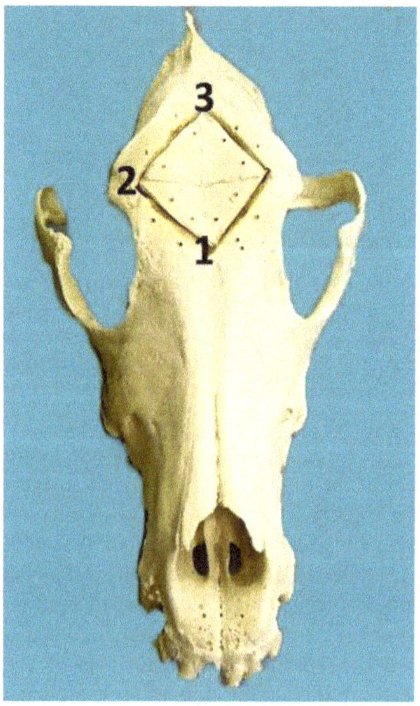

Figure 10.13 Dolichocephalic cranium. The osteotomy is completed. Before elevating the bone flap, holes for placing the suture at the end of the surgery are predrilled. 1, Junction of nasal bones; 2, zygomatic process of the orbit; 3, frontal–parietal sutures.

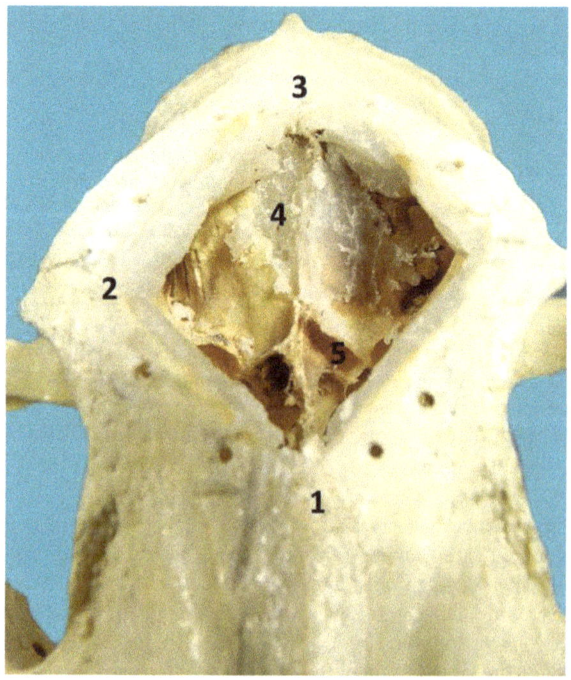

Figure 10.15 Mesocephalic cranium. 1, Junction of nasal bones; 2, zygomatic process of the orbit; 3, frontal–parietal sutures; 4, internal table of frontal bone; 5, cribriform plate.

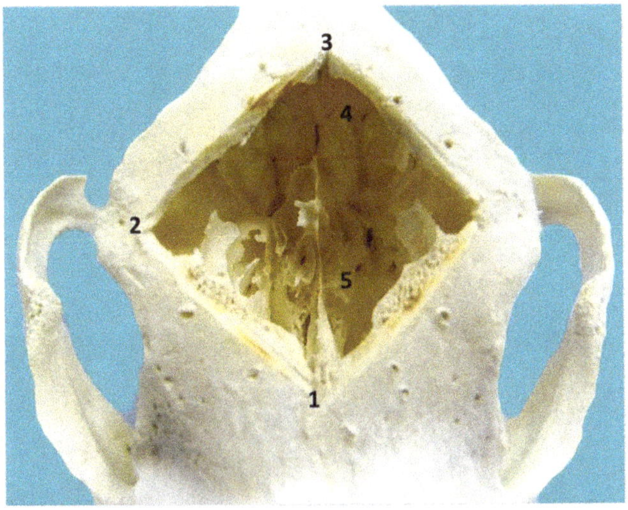

Figure 10.16 Dolichocephalic cranium. 1, Junction of nasal bones; 2, zygomatic process of the orbit; 3, frontal–parietal sutures; 4, internal table of frontal bone; 5, cribriform plate.

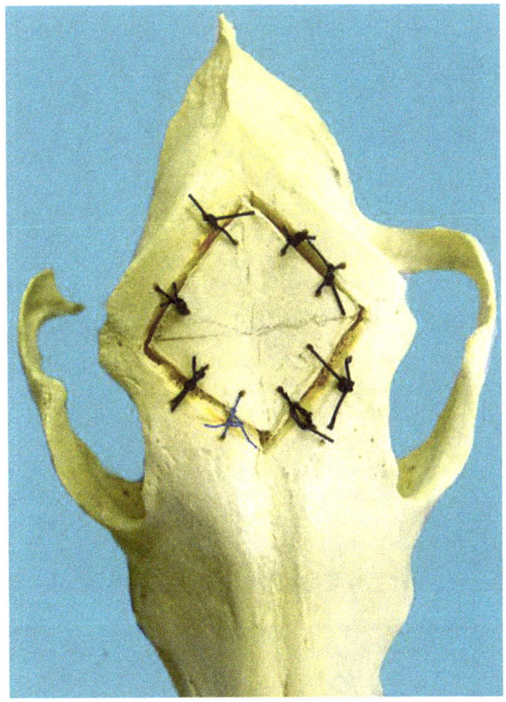

Figure 10.17 Repositioning of bone flap, with sutures placed in the predrilled holes to secure the flap.

the necessity of this procedure. Similarly, there are anecdotal reports of isolating the frontal sinus by packing them with bone wax or gelatin sponge. After the cavity of the frontal sinus is reached the thin bone of the septum of the frontal sinus and the ectoturbinate is gently removed with rongeurs (Figures 10.14, 10.15 and 10.16). Depending on the access desired small Lempert or Kerrison rongeurs can be used. The internal table of the frontal bone overlying the frontal and olfactory lobes can be removed with rongeurs or high-speed drill making sure not to damage the meningeal vessels. The bone in this region is much thinner than any other part of the skull. The dorsal sagittal sinus originates from the osseous nasal septum and the olfactory lobes and transverses caudally in the attached edge of the falx cerebri. It lies ventrally to the sagittal suture and interparietal bone process of the occipital bone. The sagittal sinus collects blood from the dipoic veins (cerebral veins). In this region it is not easily identified, although the rostral origin is visible at the level of the projection of the mid portion of the zygomatic arch [25]. Although rostral damage to the dorsal sagittal sinus in this area is unlikely to cause problems, it is best avoided. Arteries of this region originate mainly from the rostral cerebral arteries; these are end terminal arteries and damage does not cause severe brain necrosis.

Once the dura mater is exposed, this is incised with a #11 scalpel blade. The dura can be lifted with a nerve hook or blunt dental scraper and the incision continued as desired. The dura is often involved in the disease process and large portions will be removed. Removal of the tumor can be performed via delicate blunt dissection or with the use of an ultrasonic aspirator [15]. Meningiomas can be highly vascularized and great care should be taken with visualization of the blood vessel associated with the tumor and appropriately cauterized with bipolar cautery. The authors have found it useful to cauterize vessels while abundantly irrigating with saline and aspiration. This allows visualization of the blood vessel and makes the bipolar cauterization more effective. In tumors of the olfactory lobe is often difficult to spare the normal tissue and complete resection of the olfactory bulb can be made without serious consequences. Different techniques have been suggested for closure of the dura; however, most of the time this is impossible. Several authors recommend watertight dural closure using fascial or synthetic grafts. However, nonclosure of the dura is possible as long as precautions are taken to avoid postsurgical infections and pneumocephalus. Postoperative antibiotics are often recommended and bacteriological swab culture is suggested to facilitate the choice of antibiotic therapy.

The bone flap is returned to its original position and fixed with polypropylene sutures or wires. Because wires create MRI and CT artifacts, they should be avoided if further investigations are necessary (Figure 10.17). Once the bone is placed, the fascia and skin are closed routinely. In cases of craniectomy, the bone defect can be closed by simple fascial closure or using polymethylmethacrylate (PMMA) at the end of surgery. PMMA has been found to increase infection in some human studies, but there are no studies in veterinary neurosurgery and most of the reports are anecdotal. However, a good seal and aesthetic results are obtained with this approach. The advantage of this closure is the opportunity to modify the approach by using a high-speed drill and performing a craniectomy by extending the bone defect caudally and cranially as necessary, allowing adaptation to the conformation of the head and increasing visualization of the frontal and olfactory lobes. This technique can also be used in cats.

Complications

General complications of transfrontal craniotomies are those described previously for intracranial surgery: infections at the surgical site, increased intracranial pressure, seizures, and pneumonia [10,11,26]. However, hypertensive pneumocephalus and fistula with cerebrospinal fluid (CSF) leakage should be specifically discussed when using this surgical approach.

Pneumocephalus (asymptomatic intracranial air) after craniectomy is a common occurrence in humans. However, the transformation

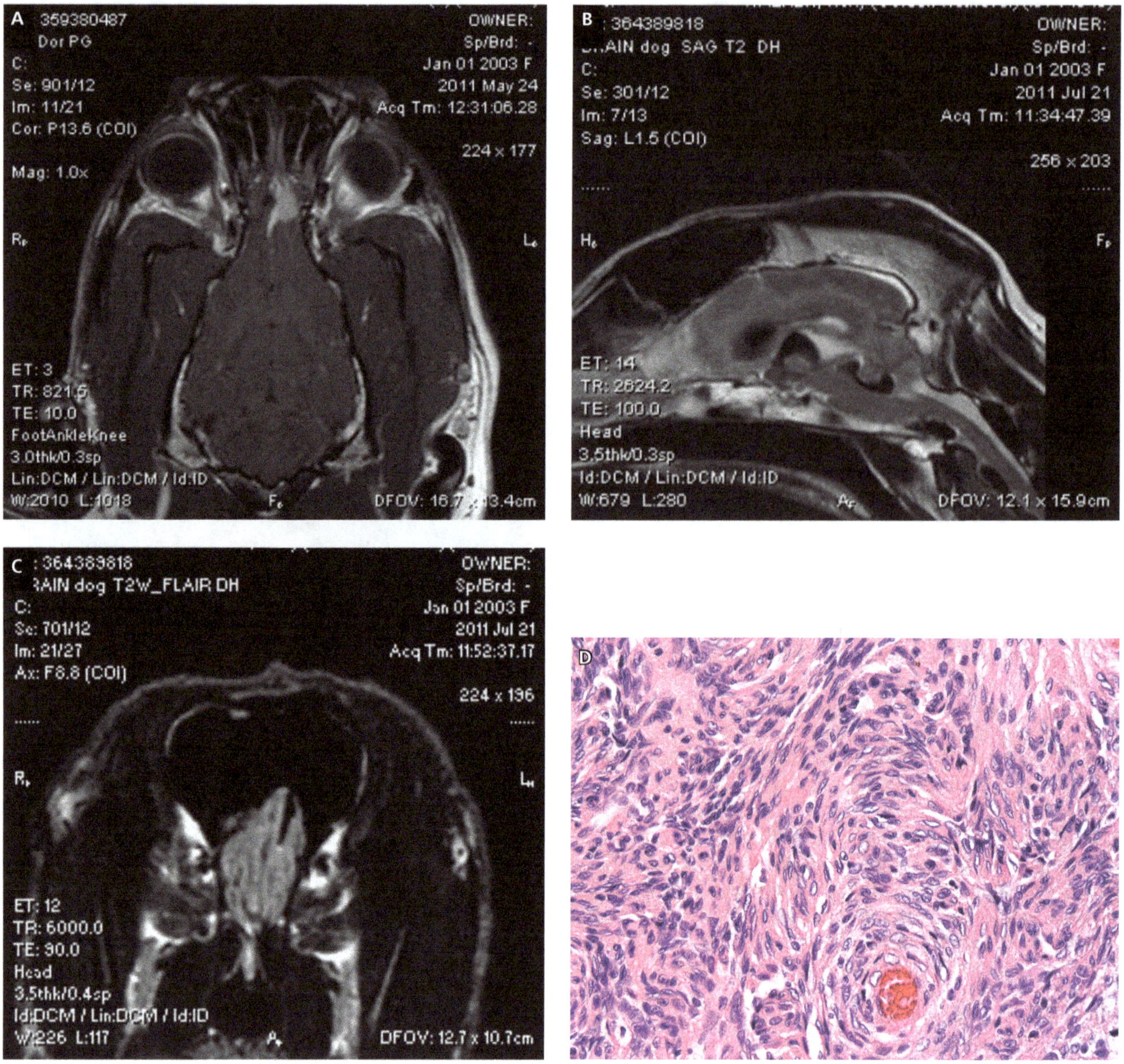

Figure 10.18 An 8-year-old male Golden Retriever presented with a history of generalized seizures for 2 months. The images in (B) and (C) were obtained 20 days after the surgery, when he was presented for neck pain and depression. (A) Dorsal T1-weighted postgadolinium MRI of the brain before surgery. There is evidence of a mass affecting the left olfactory and frontal lobe. This mass shows homogeneous contrast enhancement and a dural tail sign associated with the longitudinal fissure. (B) Sagittal T2-weighted MRI of the brain. There is signal void in the lateral, third and fourth ventricles. There is also signal void in the subarachnoid space of the cervical spine. These images are consistent with pneumocephalus and pneumorrhachis. (C) Transverse T2-weighted FLAIR image of the brain at the level of the frontal lobe. There is signal void in the dorsal aspect of the left frontal lobe. This might represent the fistula. (D) Sheets of cells with indistinct cell borders, elongate to ovoid nuclei, and mostly one prominent nucleolus, consistent with a transitional meningioma. H&E staining, ×40. *Source*: (D) Courtesy of Dr. Jim Cooley.

of pneumocephalus into tension pneumocephalus (symptomatic intracranial air) is a rare phenomenon and has been rarely described in veterinary medicine [20,27–30]. Damage of the cribriform plate seems the most common reason [27–29]. Transfrontal craniotomies can result in a large postoperative dural defect. Moreover, disruption of the cribriform plate and ethmoturbinates results in increased exposure of the surgical site. This might explain the high risk of tension pneumocephalus in humans following transfrontal craniotomies. Repair of the dural defect is not considered essential with the transfrontal approach. However, reviewing the literature, we can appreciate that in the cases of hypertensive pneumocephalus and CSF leakage described, no attempt to close the dural defect was made.

Clinical signs of hypertensive pneumocephalus are nonspecific and consistent with a diffuse anatomical localization. Depression, pain, seizures, and abnormal behavior are classically described [27–29]. This clinical presentation is similar to meningoencephalitis, which is also a possible postsurgical complication. The diagnosis can only be made after diagnostic imaging evaluation and CSF analysis. In the particular case of ventricular pneumocephalus, evaluation of skull radiographs may show radiolucent areas corresponding to the lateral ventricles. CT can clearly demonstrate intracranial air bubbles or a porencephalic cyst near the site of a fistula [31]. CT cisternography helps directly visualize contrast passing through defects in the skull [32]. MRI can offer another alternative to these imaging techniques. Air within the ventricles is visible as a signal void on both T1-weighted and T2-weighted images (Figure 10.18) [27].

Management of asymptomatic pneumocephalus when associated with trauma or surgery might be rest and close monitoring. However, if clinical signs progress, a medical or surgical procedure should be initiated. Supplemental oxygen to increase the rate of absorption of intracranial air is a common human neurosurgical practice. Surgical therapy for hypertensive pneumocephalus consists of relieving the tension within the cavity and closure of the dural tear. It had been reported that dead spaces and fistulae can be treated by closing them with a free graft of temporalis fascia, with fat [10], or hemostatic sponges [28]. This should limit desiccation of the brain parenchyma in contact with air in the frontal sinuses and prevent further entry of air into the ventricles or leakage of CSF.

Closure of a craniotomy flap involves placing 22- to 24-gauge stainless steel orthopedic wire or size 0 to 2-0 nonabsorbable monofilament suture materials through predrilled holes at strategic locations around the bone fragment [11,13]. Alternatively, the use of interlaced suture to lace or suspend the bone flap has also been described. Although inexpensive in their implementation, these techniques can be associated with disadvantages like bone fragment sequestration and material breakdown. Use of a rivet-like titanium clamp closure system to replace an external frontal bone flap after transfrontal craniotomy has been described. This technique enhances stability, reduces surgical time, and the clamps are MRI compatible but the system is expensive and requires specific instrumentation [33].

There are some situations where the craniotomy flap cannot be replaced, such as when there is bone pathology (hyperostosis) or the bone has been damaged during the drilling. In the case series of Uriarte et al. [14], a PMMA prosthesis was placed to cover the bony defect created by the transfrontal approach, as the bone flap could not be restituted. In our hospital, we have used this technique for replacement of craniotomy defects without any complications to date.

> Video clips to accompany this book can be found on the companion website at:
> www.wiley.com/go/shores/neurosurgery

References

1 Meyer H. The brain. In: Evans HO, Christensen GC (eds) *Miller's Anatomy of the Dog*, 2nd edn. Philadelphia, PA: WB Saunders, 1979: 686, 844.

2 King AS. *Physiological and Clinical Anatomy of the Domestic Mammals. Vol. 1. Central Nervous System*. Oxford: Blackwell Science, 1999: 4.

3 Batuey AS. Integrative role of the frontal lobes in dogs. *Neurosci Behav Physiol* 1969;3:99–106.

4 Lichtenstein PE. Studies of anxiety: II. The effects of lobotomy on a feeding inhibition in dogs. *J Comp Physiol Psychol* 1950;6:419–427.

5 Pavlov IP. *Conditioned Reflexes: An Investigation of the Physiological Activity of the Cerebral Cortex*. Translated and Edited by G. V. Anrep. London: Oxford University Press, 1927.

6 Kozloz AP, Vartanyan GA. Activity of frontal cortex neurons of the dog with change in motoric conditioned reflex programs. *Neurosci Behav Physiol* 1996;26:273–276.

7 Tapp PD, Siwak CT, Gao FQ et al. Frontal lobe volume, function, and beta-amyloid pathology in a canine model of aging. *J Neurosci* 2004;24:8205–8213.

8 Foster ES, Carrillo JM, Patnaik AK. Clinical signs of tumors affecting the rostral cerebrum in 43 dogs. *J Vet Intern Med* 1988;2:71–74.

9 Patnaik AK, Lieberman PH, Erlandson RA, Shaker E, Hurvitz AI. Paranasal meningioma in the dog: a clinicopathologic study of ten cases. *Vet Pathol* 1986;23: 362–368.

10 Kostolich M, Dulisch ML. Surgical approach to the canine olfactory bulb for meningioma removal. *Vet Surg* 1987;16:273–277.

11 Parker AJ, Cunningham JG. Transfrontal craniotomy in the dog. *Vet Rec* 1972;90:622–624.

12 DeWet PD, Ali II, Peterson DN. Surgical approach to the rostral cranial fossa by radical transfrontal craniotomy in the dog. *J S Afr Vet Assoc* 1982;53:40–41.

13 Glass EN, Kapatkin AS, Vite CH, Steinberg SA. A modified bilateral transfrontal sinus approach to the canine frontal lobe and olfactory bulb: surgical technique and five cases. *J Am Anim Hosp Assoc* 2000;36:43–50.

14 Uriarte A, Moissonnier P, Thibaud JL et al. Surgical treatment and radiation therapy of frontal lobe meningiomas in 7 dogs. *Can Vet J* 2011;7:748–752.

15 Cabassu JB, Cabassu JP, Brochier L, Catheland S, Ivanoff S. Surgical treatment of a traumatic intracranial epidural haematoma in a dog. *Vet Comp Orthop Traumatol* 2008;21:457–461.

16 Garosi LS, Platt SR, McConnell JF, Wray JD, Smith KC. Intracranial haemorrhage associated with *Angiostrongylus vasorum* infection in three dogs. *J Small Anim Pract* 2005;46:93–99.

17 Summers BA, Cummings JF, de Lahunta A. Injuries to the central nervous system. In: *Veterinary Neuropathology*. St Louis, MO: Mosby Year Book, 1995: 189–207.

18 Dewey C, Downs M, Aron D et al. Acute traumatic intracranial hemorrhage in dogs and cats: a retrospective evaluation of 23 cases. *Vet Comp Orthop Traumatol* 1993;6:153–159.

19 Tan Y, Zhou S, Liu Y, Li Z. A gross and microscopic study of cerebral injuries accompanying maxillofacial high-velocity projectile wounding in dogs. *J Oral Maxillofac Surg* 1998;56:345–348.

20 Haley AC, Abramson C. Traumatic pneumocephalus in a dog. *J Am Vet Med Assoc* 2009;234:1295–1298.

21 Kasper EM, Bartek J Jr, Johnson S, Kasper BS, Pavlakis M, Wong M. Post-transplant aspergillosis and the role of combined neurosurgical and antifungal therapies under belatacept immunosuppression. *Surg Neurol Int* 2011;2:75.

22 de Lahunta A, Glass E. Development of the nervous system: malformation. In: *Veterinary Neuroanatomy and Clinical Neurology*, 3rd edn. St Louis, MO: Saunders Elsevier, 2009: 40.

23 Jeffery N. Ethmoidal encephalocoele associated with seizures in a puppy. *J Small Anim Pract* 2005;46:89–92.

24 Martlé VA, Caemaert J, Tshamala M et al. Surgical treatment of a canine intranasal meningoencephalocele. *Vet Surg* 2009;38:515–519.

25 Carreira LM, Ferreira A, Burilo FL. The dorsal sagittal venous sinus anatomical variations in brachycephalic, dolichocephalic, and mesocephalic dogs and their significance for brain surgery. *Anat Rec* 2011;294:1920–1929.

26 Fransson BA, Bagley RS, Gay JM et al. Pneumonia after intracranial surgery in dogs. *Vet Surg* 2001;30:432–439.

27 Garosi LS, Penderis J, Brearley MJ, Brearley JC, Dennis R, Kirkpatrick PJ. Intraventricular tension pneumocephalus as a complication of transfrontal craniectomy: a case report. *Vet Surg* 2002;31:226–231.

28 Cavanaugh RP, Aiken SW, Schatzberg SJ. Intraventricular tension pneumocephalus and cervical subarachnoid pneumorrhachis in a bull mastiff dog after craniotomy. *J Small Anim Pract* 2008;49:244–248.

29 Fletcher, DJ, Snyder JM, Messinger SJ, Chiu AG, Vite CH. Ventricular pneumocephalus septic meningoencephalitis secondary to dorsal rhinotomy and nasal polypectomy in a dog. *J Am Vet Med Assoc* 2006;229:240–245.

30 Thieman K, Echandi RL, Arendse A, Henry G. Imaging diagnosis: trauma-induced tension pneumocephalus. *Vet Radiol Ultrasound* 2008;49:362–364.

31 Aoyama I, Kondo A, Nin K, Shimotake K. Pneumocephalus associated with benign brain tumor: report of two cases. *Surg Neurol* 1991;36:32–36.

32 Ahmadi J, Weiss MH, Segall HD, Schultz DH, Zee C-S, Giannotta SL. Evaluation of cerebrospinal fluid rhinorrhea by metrizamide computed tomographic cisternography. *Neurosurgery* 1985;16:54–60.

33 Gordon PN, Kornegay JN, Lattimer JC, Cook CR, Tucker-Warhover T. Use of a rivet-like titanium clamp closure system to replace an external frontal bone flap after transfrontal craniotomy in a dog. *J Am Vet Med Assoc* 2005;226:752–755, 731–732.

11 Lateral (Rostrotentorial) Craniotomy/Craniectomy

Andy Shores

Introduction

This approach was developed and published by Dr. J.E. Oliver in the mid 1960s [1]. The basics have changed little in the ensuing half-century. Dr. Oliver described this approach for exposing the "frontal, parietal, temporal, and occipital lobes" [2]. Indications for this approach include intracranial tumors (Figure 11.1), aberrant blood vessels (congenital, acquired) [3], traumatic brain injury (Figure 11.2), brain abscesses, and cerebral biopsy [4].

Regions of the brain in dogs and cats are not as clearly definable as in humans; however, for orientation purposes, the regions to consider are the olfactory, frontal, parietal, temporal, and occipital. Variations of the lateral craniectomy are used to approach all of these regions except for the olfactory lobe. The olfactory lobe and some lesions of the frontal lobe are best approached using transfrontal craniotomy.

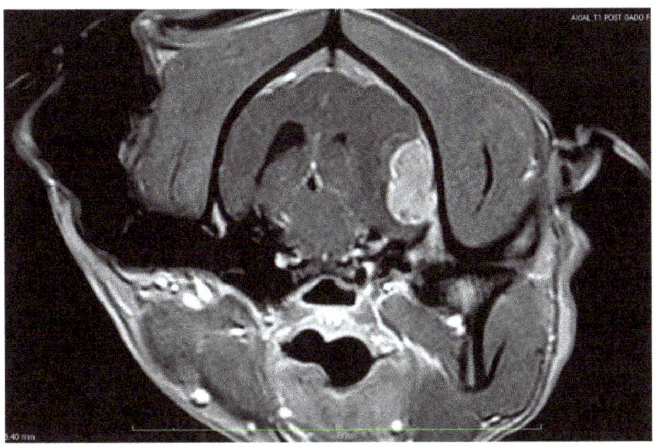

Figure 11.1 Transverse T1-weighted postcontrast MRI of a canine meningioma. This mass would be approached using a lateral rostrotentorial craniectomy.

Craniectomies are far more commonly performed than craniotomies in veterinary neurosurgery. Because the large temporalis muscle covers the skull defect, cosmetic defects are uncommon, and the muscle mass affords more than adequate protection of the exposed cortex after closure. The author always uses a dural substitute (biological or synthetic) and usually places a synthetic polypropylene mesh over the skull defect. These measures help prevent adhesions between muscle and cortical tissue.

Patient Preparation and Positioning

Standards for preoperative patient preparation apply, concluding in clipping the head on both sides, laterally to below the zygomatic arches, rostrally to just dorsal to the orbit, caudally to the level of C1, with a sterile skin preparation after the patient is positioned on the operating table (Figure 11.3). Because the ears are draped out of the operating field in most procedures, it is unnecessary to clip the outer ear pinna.

The patient is positioned on a padded operating table in sternal recumbency. Beaded Styrofoam vacuum bags, sand bags, or a head stand are used to position the head with the mandible parallel to the table without pressure on the jugular veins. It is very important to have the head positioned correctly and firmly fixed in position to prevent movement during the procedure. If the planned lateral craniectomy is considerably more ventral than midline, having the head rotated slightly away from the surgeon can aid in gaining adequate exposure. The surgeon should be in the operating room at the time of positioning to ensure it is correctly done for the planned procedure. After the final sterile preparation, the patient is quarter draped and the surgery can begin.

Surgical Technique

A curvilinear (horseshoe-shaped) incision is made beginning just caudal and medial to the lateral canthus of the eye, to the dorsal midline, and then curving caudally and ventrally to behind the ear

Current Techniques in Canine and Feline Neurosurgery, First Edition. Edited by Andy Shores and Brigitte A. Brisson.
© 2017 John Wiley & Sons, Inc. Published 2017 by John Wiley & Sons, Inc.
Companion website: www.wiley.com/go/shores/neurosurgery

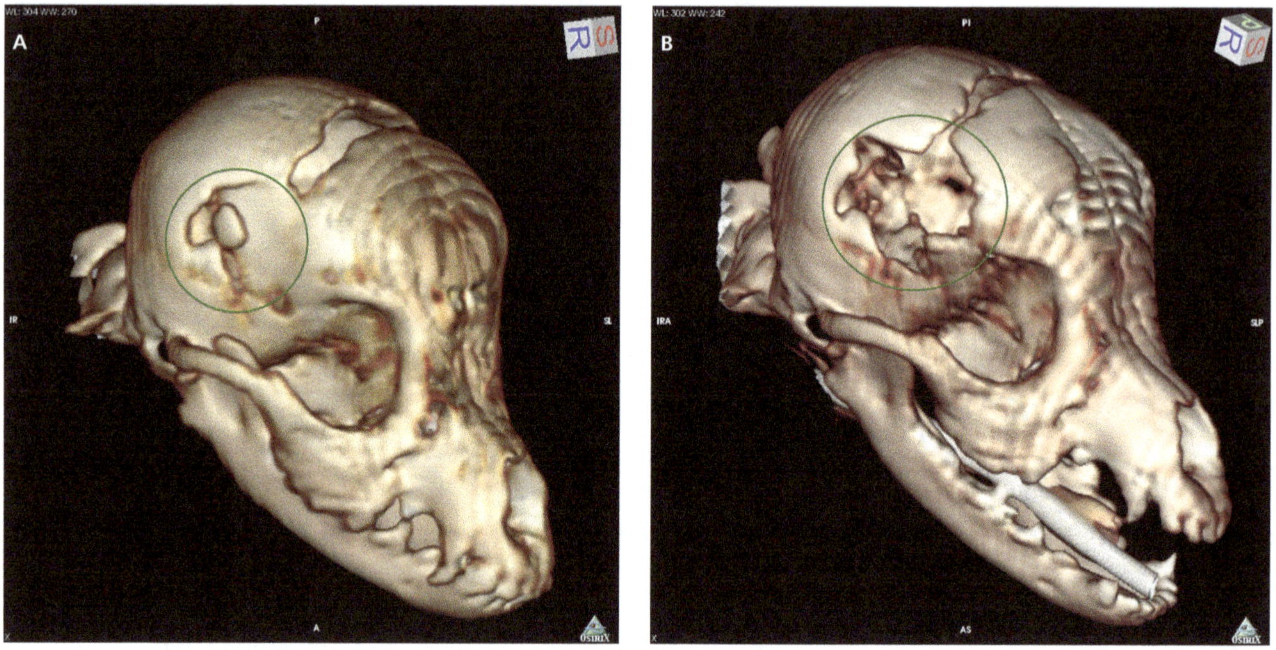

Figure 11.2 A massive depressed skull fracture of the right frontal and parietal bones in a 3-month-old Yorkshire Terrier caused by a bite wound to the head. (A) Preoperative and (B) postoperative three-dimensional reconstruction of the CT scan. The areas within the circle represent the location of the depressed segment.

(Figure 11.4A). The subcutaneous tissue is undermined and reflected ventrally; however, subcutaneous dissection at the cranial aspect of the incision is limited so the branch of the auriculopalpebral nerve is avoided, so this tissue is not cut but can be reflected ventrally with the temporalis muscle.

The temporalis muscle is incised in a similar horseshoe fashion using an electroscalpel. The incision can extend rostrally to the border of the skin incision, to a point 2–4 mm lateral to its attachment to the skull, and caudally behind the ear as needed for exposure. A periosteal elevator is used to undermine the temporalis muscle. The author prefers a rounded, wide-blade, wooden-handled periosteal elevator in large dogs and a Freer elevator-dissector in small dogs and cats. As the muscle is elevated, it is reflected ventrally (Figure 11.4B); the inner surface of the muscle is kept moistened throughout the procedure with frequent bathing in warm saline.

Reflection of the muscle exposes portions of the frontal, parietal, temporal, and sphenoid bones (Figure 11.5). Location of the craniectomy is determined by the location of the lesion and the reason for the surgery. Less invasive procedures (placement of ventriculoperitoneal shunt, marsupialization of the ventricle, evacuation of blood clots, skull fracture elevations) may require only one or two burr-holes. Removal of intracranial tumors, of course, does require a considerably larger opening. The borders of the craniectomy are determined in preoperative planning. Usually, four burr-holes are made, one at each corner of the boundaries, using a perforator or a high-speed nitrogen-powered drill with a rounded bit (Figure 11.6). The burr-holes should penetrate the inner cortical bone but optimally not damage the dura. Each burr-hole is inspected with a small probe to ensure the inner cortical layer is perforated.

The four completed burr-holes are connected to complete the bone flap using a small burr with the high-speed nitrogen-powered drill or a craniotome, preferably with a pediatric dura guard. The dorsal, rostral, and caudal connections are made. If the drill is used, the span of bone between the ventral burr-holes is connected, but only grooved and not through the full thickness of the bone. After ensuring the rostral, dorsal, and caudal connections are complete, a periosteal elevator is carefully inserted under the flap and above the dura to pry the flap, breaking through the groove placed in the ventral aspect of the flap (Figure 11.7A). If the craniotome with a dura guard is used, this ventral aspect is cut in similar fashion to the rest of the flap.

As the bone flap becomes loose, the surgeon tries to elevate any dural attachments as the bone is slowly removed. If this is not done, the underlying dura can tear and sometimes result in considerable hemorrhage from the middle meningeal artery and its branches. Bipolar cautery is used to control this and any hemorrhage from the bone is controlled with a coating of bone wax.

If necessary, the craniectomy can be extended using Lempert or Kerrison rongeurs to accommodate exposure of the lesion.

The exposed dura is inspected and the surgeon prepares to open it and create a flap (Figure 11.7B). A number 12 blade is used to make the initial opening, then the edge of the dura is grasped with jeweler's forceps and scissors (tenotomy, Potts) are used to complete the flap (Figure 11.8). The dural incisions are made along the dorsal, rostral, and caudal edges of the opening after ligating or cauterizing the middle meningeal artery as ventrally as possible. Two long 5-0 synthetic absorbable stay sutures are placed on the rostral and caudal corners of the dura and clamped with small hemostats before reflecting it ventrally over the exposed reflected muscle tissue.

All exposed tissues, and most especially the cortical surface, are kept moist throughout the procedure with warm sterile saline solution. If the surgeon chooses to replace the bone flap at the end of the procedure, it is kept in a moistened wrap of sterile gauze sponges.

Extraaxial lesions, such as meningiomas, may be visible from the surface; however, this is often not the case. Based on the preoperative planning and the advanced imaging, the approximate locale of the lesion (tumor) is determined. A far better method of visualizing intraaxial and extraaxial masses is with the use of intraoperative ultrasound. This is a very useful tool and the process/technique has

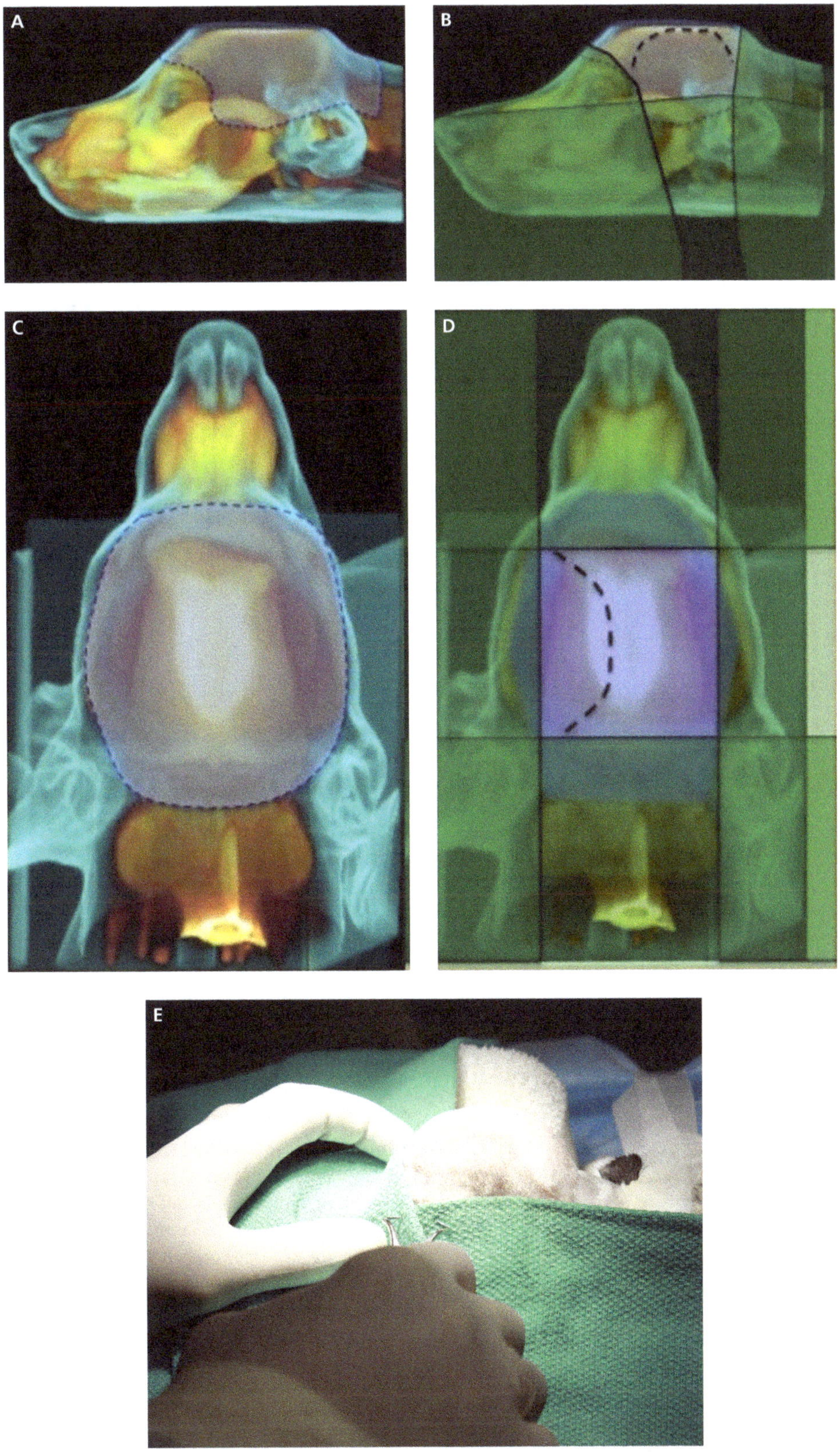

Figure 11.3 Positioning, preparation, and draping areas for the lateral rostrotentorial approach. Areas within the dotted lines in the lateral (A) and dorsal (B) illustrations of the skull represent the region clipped and prepared for surgery. Lateral (C) and dorsal (D) illustrations of the draping for the lateral rostrotentorial approach. The dashed line represents the incision line. Lateral view (E) of a live animal positioned and being draped for the lateral rostrotentorial approach. *Source*: illustrations A–D: Andy Shores.

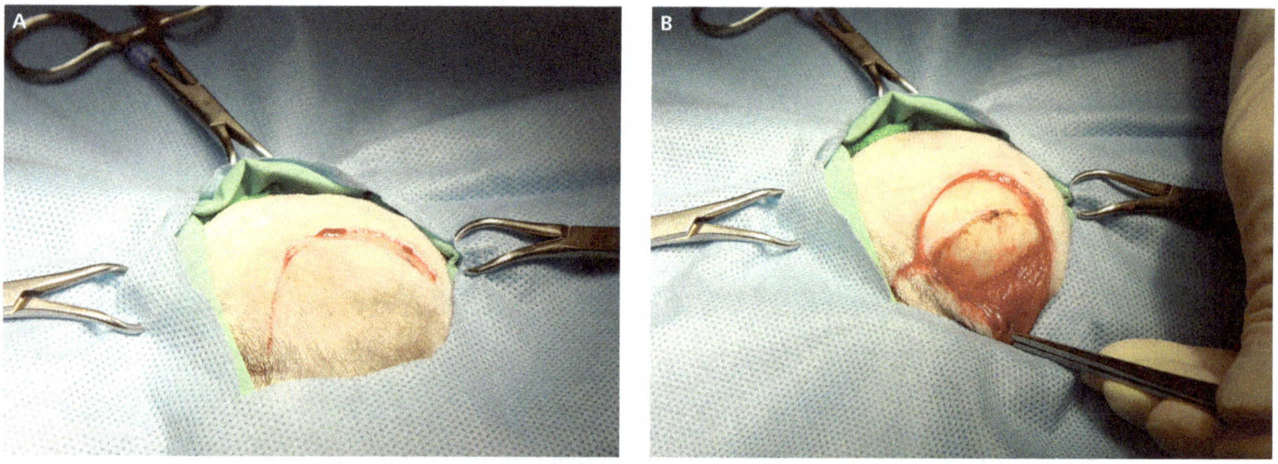

Figure 11.4 (A) Curvilinear (horseshoe) incision is made beginning just caudal and medial to the lateral canthus of the eye, to the dorsal midline and then curving caudally and ventrally to behind the ear. (B) Reflected temporalis muscle.

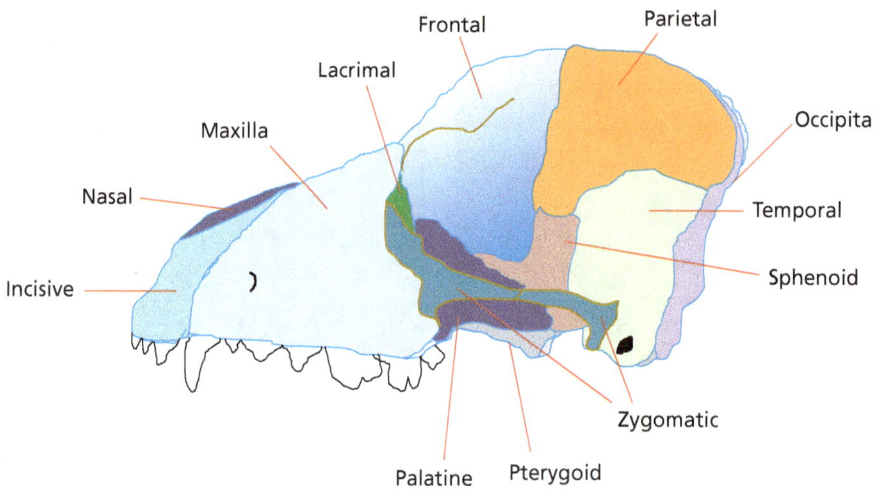

Figure 11.5 Bones of the canine skull. *Source*: illustration by Andy Shores.

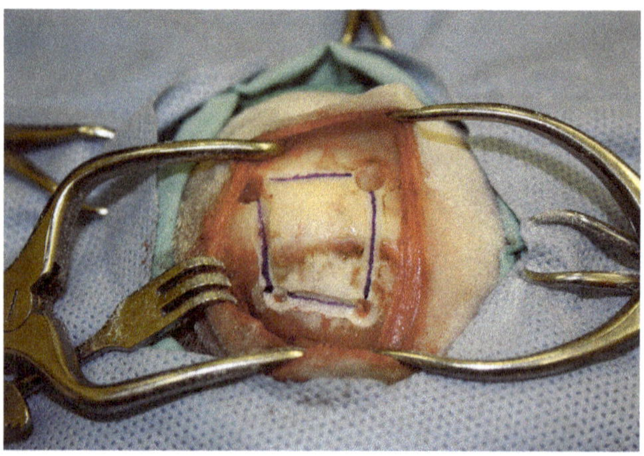

Figure 11.6 Four burr-holes are made in the skull. Marked lines are the borders for the bone flap to complete the craniectomy.

been described [5]. Figure 11.9 shows the operating room set-up for ultrasonography and an ultrasound image of an intraaxial tumor. In addition, a recent publication describes the use of a stereotactic apparatus for use in small animals [6].

Often, the exposed cortex must be incised to access the mass. The approach is always through the gyri and not the sulci to avoid additional hemorrhage. The texture and coloration of the mass is different from normal tissue, but the differences may be slight to moderate. Borders of the mass and normal cortical tissue are easily distinguished using ultrasound.

The author utilizes the ultrasonic aspirator unit for removal of the mass (Figure 11.10). Bipolar cautery and suction can also be used. The surgeon must be aware of keeping the surrounding tissues moist and use extreme care to avoid excessive hemorrhage. In the author's experience, cortical swelling during the procedure is often associated with excessive or undetected hemorrhage.

Following removal or debulking of the mass, the field is copiously lavaged with normal saline solution and the site is inspected

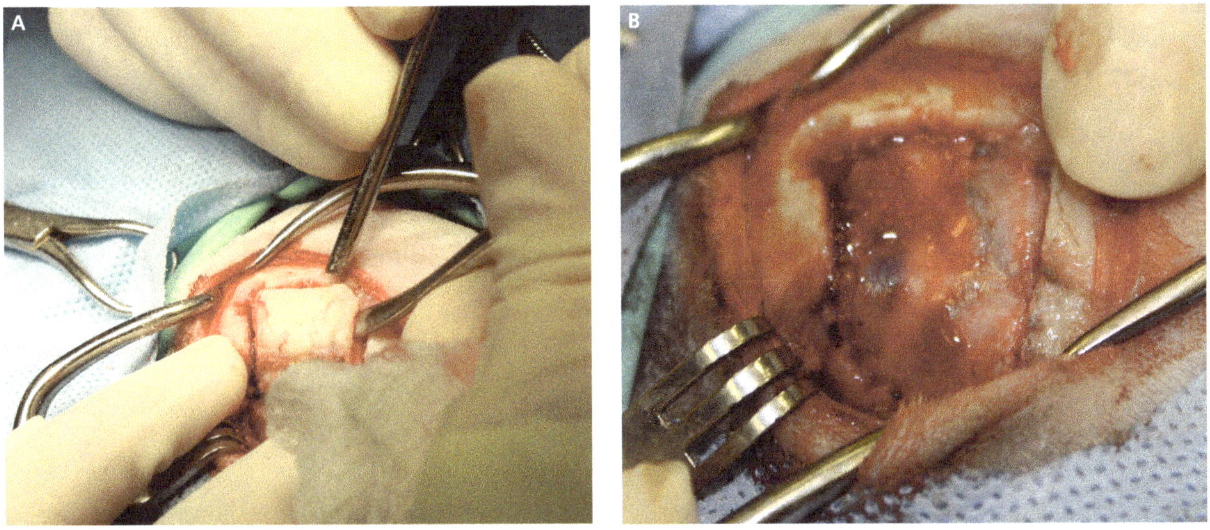

Figure 11.7 The completed craniectomy. (A) Elevation of bone flap using periosteal elevator. (B) The bone flap has been removed, exposing the underlying dura.

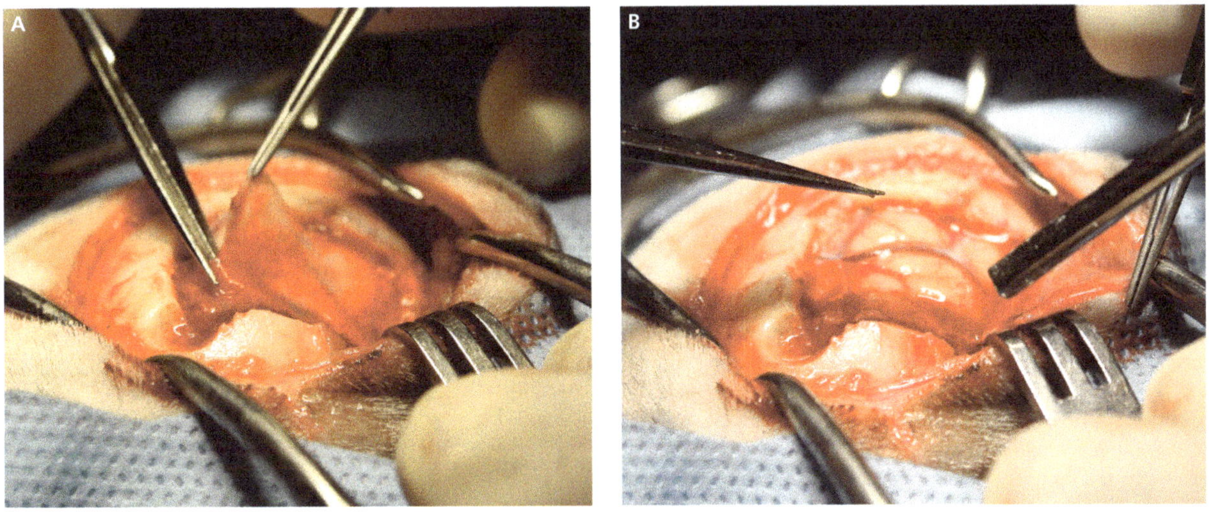

Figure 11.8 (A) Incising the dura and arachnoid. (B) The completed dural flap, exposing the cortical tissue.

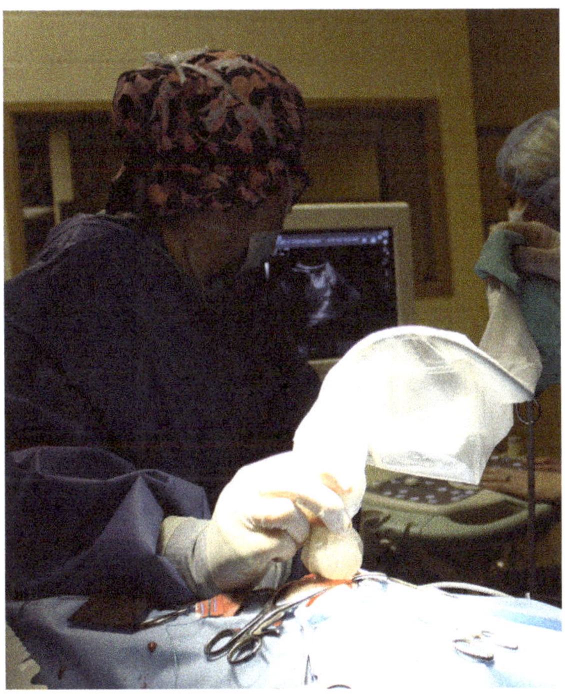

Figure 11.9 Operating room set-up for ultrasonography. The ultrasound is shrouded in a sterile sleeve and placed softly on the cortical tissue using a saline interface. The surgeon is able to see the screen in real time to visualize the mass and surrounding vasculature.

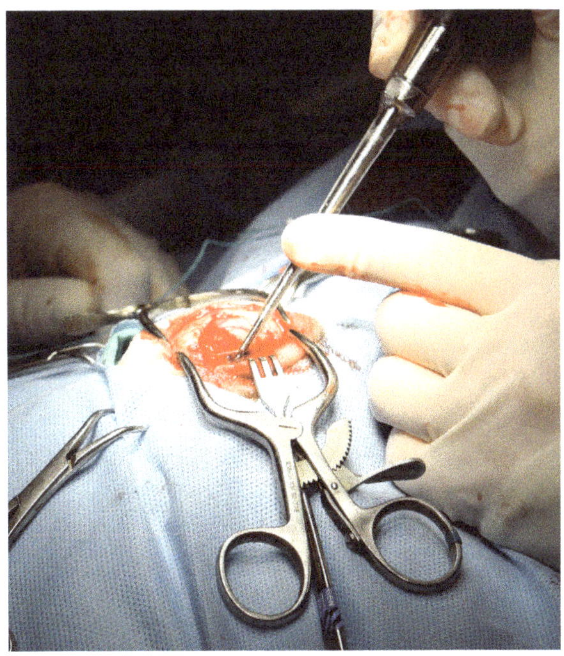

Figure 11.10 Ultrasonic aspirator hand-piece employed by the surgeon to begin removal of the mass after visualizing it on the ultrasound screen.

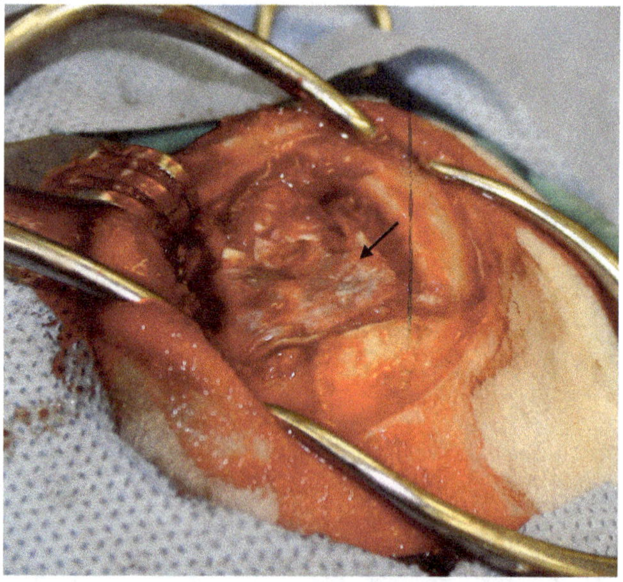

Figure 11.11 A dural substitute material (arrow) has been placed over the cortical tissue. This material can be used with the remaining dura or by itself as a scaffolding for regrowth of the dura.

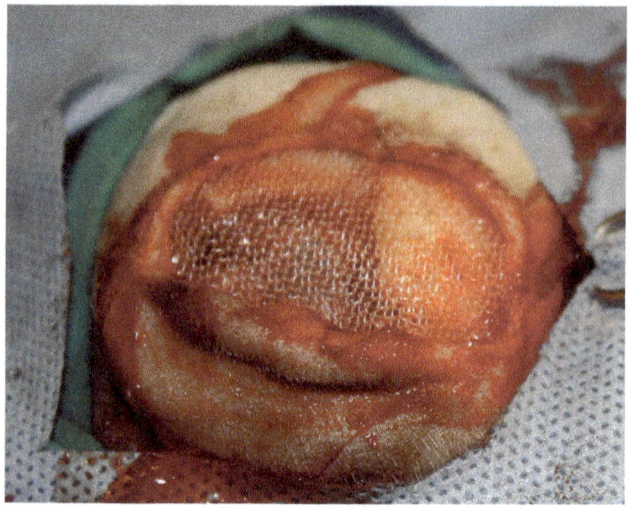

Figure 11.12 A polypropylene mesh is placed over the craniectomy site. This material is biologically inert and can be attached to the borders of the craniectomy using small drill holes and 2-0 absorbable or nonabsorbable monofilament sutures or can be sutured to the thin fascia underlying the temporalis muscle.

for any continued hemorrhage. Closure begins with a dural covering. Most often the dura is torn, can contain neoplastic cells, or is otherwise inadequate for complete coverage of the exposed cortical tissue. A dural substitute can be fashioned from the temporalis muscle fascia or a commercially available product (DuraGen®, Integra Corporation; ACell Vet®, ACell, Inc.; Biodesign® Dural Graft; COOK® Biotech) is used (Figure 11.11). If the dura or dural substitute is sutured, 5-0 or 6-0 absorbable monofilament suture is used in a simple interrupted pattern.

Generally, the bone flap is not replaced since there is adequate muscle covering; however, if replaced, 2-0 absorbable or nonabsorbable sutures are placed in holes drilled into the bone flap and the connecting area of the skull. An alternative used by the author is a polypropylene mesh to cover the defect (Figure 11.12). The mesh can be sutured to the bone as described for flap replacement or to the fascia underneath the temporalis muscle.

The incised temporalis muscle fascia is sutured to remaining temporalis fascia attached to the skull. The overlying interscutularias muscle, other subcutaneous tissue, and the skin are closed to complete the procedure.

Video clips to accompany this book can be found on the companion website at:
www.wiley.com/go/shores/neurosurgery

References

1 Oliver JE Jr. *Canine cranial surgery*. Thesis, Auburn University, 1966.

2 Oliver JE Jr. Cranial surgery. In: Oliver JE, Hoerlein BF, Mayhew IG (eds) *Veterinary Neurology*. Philadelphia, PA: WB Saunders, 1987: 470–492.

3 Shores A, Cooper TG, Gartrell CL et al. Cerebrovascular disease in small animals: clinical characteristics. In: *Proceedings of the 9th Annual Veterinary Medical Forum, New Orleans, May 1991*. Lakewood, CO: American College of Veterinary Internal Medicine, 1991: 777–780.

4 Bagley RS. Brain. In: Slatter D (ed.) *Textbook of Veterinary Surgery*, 3rd edn. Philadelphia, PA: WB Saunders, 2003: 1163–1173.

5 Shores A, Holland M, Hudson J. Intraoperative ultrasound for intracranial surgery. In: McFarlane D, Sellon R (eds) *Proceedings of the American College of Veterinary Internal Medicine Forum 2012*. Lakewood, CO: American College of Veterinary Internal Medicine, 2012. Available at http://www.vin.com/acvim/2012/Default.htm

6 Chen AV, Wininger FA, Frey S et al. Description and validation of a magnetic resonance imaging-guided stereotactic brain biopsy device in the dog. *Vet Radiol Ultrasound* 2012;53:150–156.

12 Suboccipital Craniectomy/Foramen Magnum Decompression

Erin Y. Akin and Andy Shores

Indications

This procedure was first described by Oliver [1], and while the indications for foramen magnum decompression (FMD) have changed, the basic procedure has stayed much the same [2–5]. The procedure is used to expose the caudal cerebellum, dorsal aspect of the caudal medulla, and the most cranial aspect of the cervical spinal cord [2,4]. Indications for suboccipital decompression and FMD include the following.

1. Neoplasms involving structures of the caudal fossa:
   a. cerebellum, dorsal aspect of caudal brainstem;
   b. cranial cervical spinal cord (Figures 12.1, 12.2 and 12.3).
2. Quadrigeminal diverticula (Figure 12.4).
3. Chiari-like malformation (Figure 12.5).
4. Cerebellar biopsy.

Surgical Anatomy

An illustration of the caudal aspect of the canine skull is shown in Figure 12.6. The cervicoauricular–occipital complex comprises the superficial muscles encountered on the dorsal midline. Cranial to the C3 vertebra the deeper dorsal cervical muscles include the cleidocervicalis, sterno-occipitalis, sternomastoideus, rhomboideus, splenius, semispinalis capitis biventer, and complexus. All these make some attachment to the occipital bone and are reflected during the dissection process [2,6].

In addition to the numerous arteries and veins associated with the muscle attachments, the muscular and occipital branches of the great auricular artery represent the vessels most commonly encountered. At least one of these branches also anastomoses with the ascending branch of the omocervical artery [6].

The nuchal ligament attaches to the spinous process of the axis. The cranial aspect of the axis is the origin of the dorsal atlantoaxial ligament that attaches to the dorsal arch of the atlas. Surgical anatomy for the cat is very similar; however, the nuchal ligament does not exist in this species.

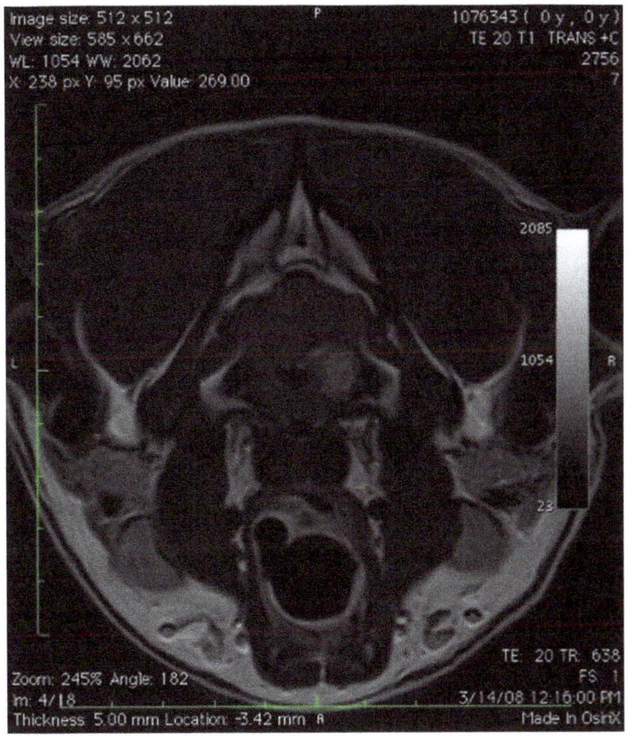

Figure 12.1 Transverse T1-weighted postcontrast MRI of choroid plexus tumor.

Patient Positioning

The patient is placed in sternal recumbency on the operating table, with the head ventroflexed perpendicular to the axis of the spine (Figure 12.7). The positioning is similar to that used for a patient undergoing a cisternal spinal tap in dorsal recumbency, with the

Current Techniques in Canine and Feline Neurosurgery, First Edition. Edited by Andy Shores and Brigitte A. Brisson.
© 2017 John Wiley & Sons, Inc. Published 2017 by John Wiley & Sons, Inc.
Companion website: www.wiley.com/go/shores/neurosurgery

neck slightly arched to afford better access to the occipital bone and foramen magnum. The patient is secured in this position with tape, sandbags, or a head restraint device, avoiding any direct pressure on the jugular veins. The site is clipped and aseptically prepared over the dorsal aspect of the head and cervical area. The prepared area should extend rostrally to caudally from the bregma to the level of the fourth cervical vertebra and the width should be just lateral to the width of the wings of the atlas on each side. An area over the dorsal aspect of the ilial wing is also clipped and prepared for harvesting a fat graft to be used over the FMD [2,4]. Tilting the patient's head 30° away from the side of the lesion increases exposure of structures lateral to the midline [7,8].

Surgical Technique (Video 12.1)

A fat graft is harvested. This procedure is performed first and gloves and instruments are discarded prior to beginning the craniectomy approach. The fat is wrapped in a warm saline-soaked gauze sponge and preserved until later in the procedure [9]. A dorsal midline incision is made, extending from 1–2 cm rostral to the external occipital protuberance to the caudal aspect of the spinous process of C2. The subcutaneous tissues and fat are incised along the midline and retracted, exposing the underlying superficial cervical musculature. The superficial cervical musculature is incised using an electroscalpel along the median raphe. This exposes the deeper cervical muscles and the dissection continues

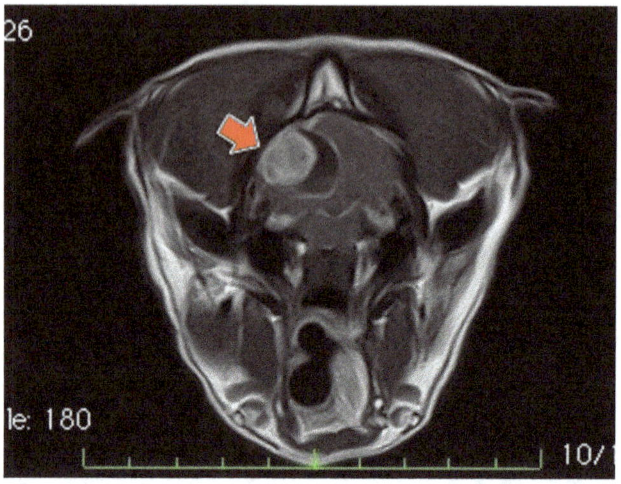

Figure 12.2 Transverse T2-weighted MRI of a cystic cerebellar mass (arrow).

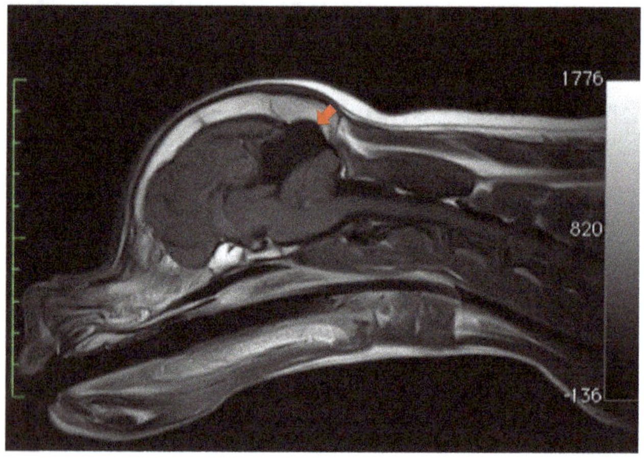

Figure 12.4 Sagittal T1-weighted MRI of a subarachnoid diverticulum (arrow) showing severe compression of the cerebellum.

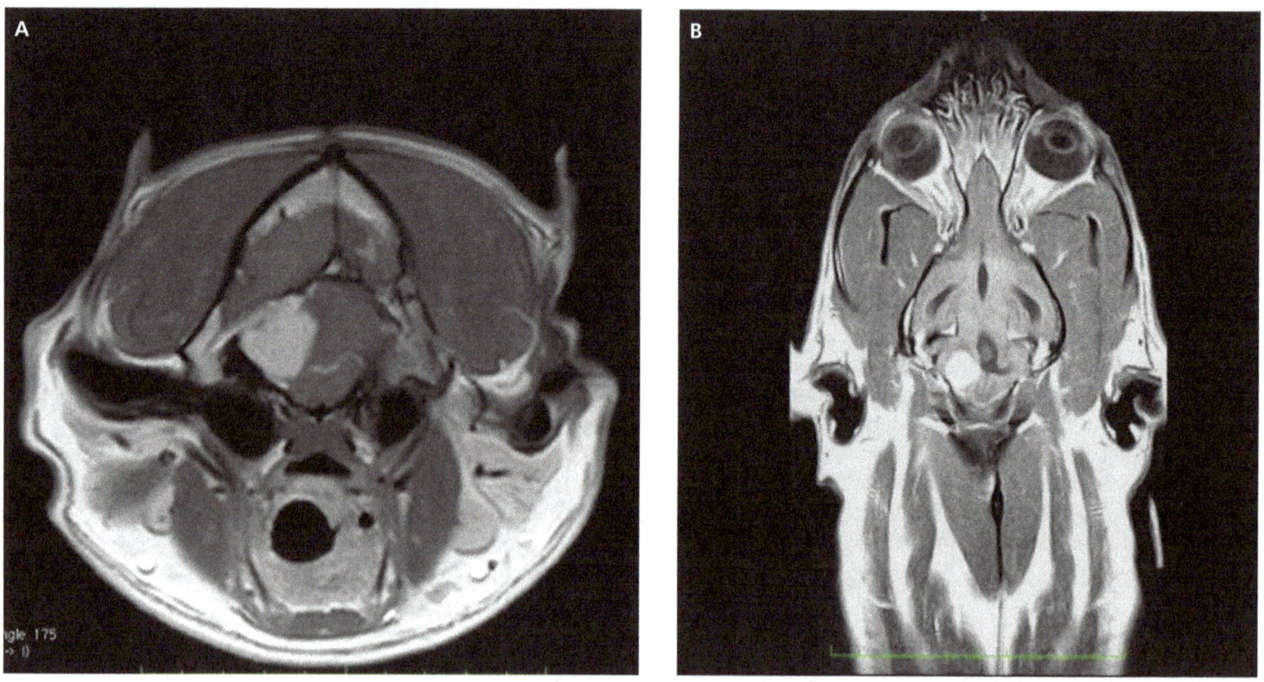

Figure 12.3 (A) Transverse and (B) dorsal T1-weighted postcontrast MRI of meningioma located in the cerebello-pontomedullary angle. This mass was biopsied and partially removed prior to patient undergoing radiation therapy.

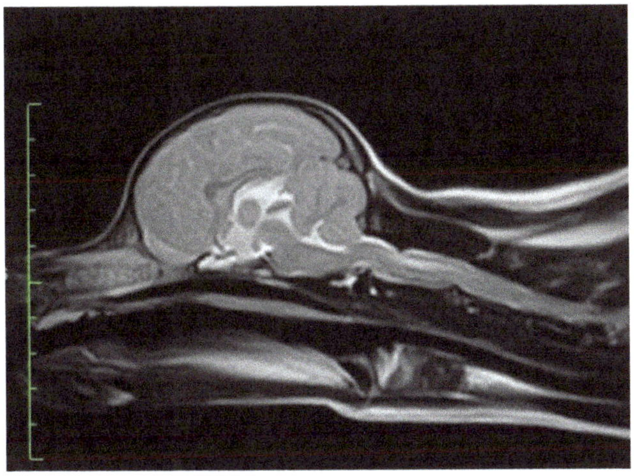

Figure 12.5 Sagittal T2-weighted MRI of canine patient with Chiari-like malformation changes (cerebellar herniation and syringomyelia).

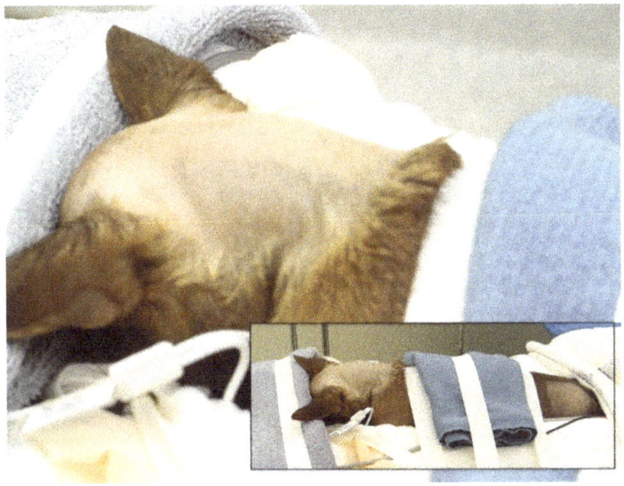

Figure 12.7 Patient positioning for suboccipital craniectomy/foramen magnum decompression. Note the additional area surgically prepared (*inset*) over the dorsal aspect of the wing of the ilium for harvesting a fat graft.

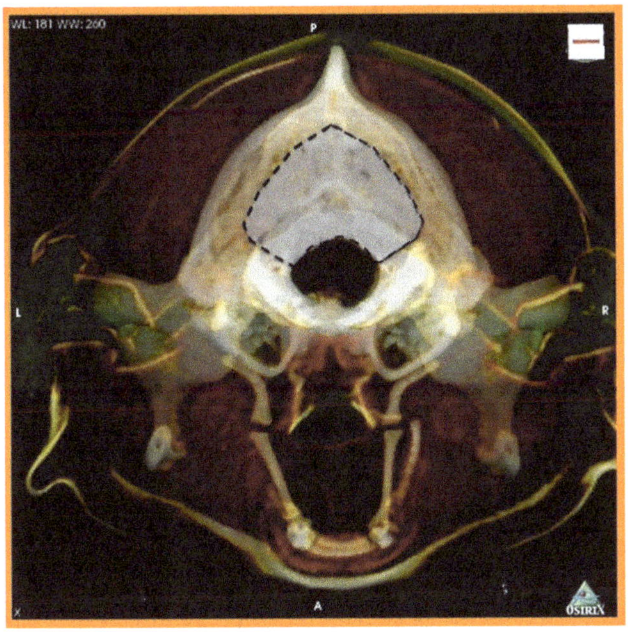

Figure 12.6 Illustration showing caudal aspect of the canine skull. The area encompassed by the dotted lines represents the area removed for most suboccipital craniectomy/foramen magnum decompression procedures.

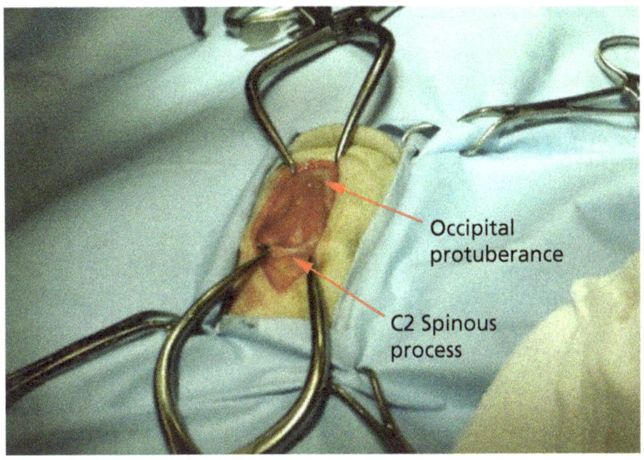

Figure 12.8 Intraoperative photo showing dissection through the superficial cervical musculature with an incision extending caudally from rostral to the occipital protuberance to the caudal aspect of the C2 spinous process.

along the midline through the biventer cervicis muscles and rectus capitis dorsalis (Figure **12.8**) [2–5]. The cranial attachment of the nuchal ligament can be palpated as it attaches to C2 and the occipital protuberance is exposed. A Freer periosteal elevator is used to elevate the musculature from the occipital bone, the dorsal arch of C1, and the spinous process of C2. Frequently, the various muscle arterial and venous branches are encountered and can produce considerable hemorrhage. At some juncture, branches of the great auricular artery are breached on both sides and require bipolar cautery to control [4,5].

The surgeon must carefully evaluate the structure of each patient's occipital bone before beginning periosteal elevation of the muscles. Some patients, especially the smaller breeds, will have extensive occipital dysplasia and the muscles lie just dorsal to a thin periosteal membrane or simply directly overlie the dural membrane (Figure 12.9). Vigorous dissection in these instances can cause severe damage to the cerebellum.

Gelpi or other self-retaining retractors are placed at the cranial and caudal aspects of the exposure. Hemostasis is achieved with monopolar or bipolar electrocautery. The exposed tissues are periodically lavaged with warmed sterile saline solution.

At this juncture, the surgeon inspects the area to ensure adequate exposure for the procedure. For intracranial tumor removal, the dissection can be carried laterally and dorsally to the nuchal line and occipital protuberance, respectively. The occipital condyles are the ventrolateral extent of the dissection and the foramen magnum is the ventrocaudal extent. Often, slightly less lateral exposure is used for FMD procedures in the surgical treatment of Chiari-like syndrome. The dorsal atlanto-axial membrane spans the gap between the caudal ventral extent of the occipital bone and the dorsal arch of C1. This membrane is fibrous and usually thickened in patients with Chiari-like

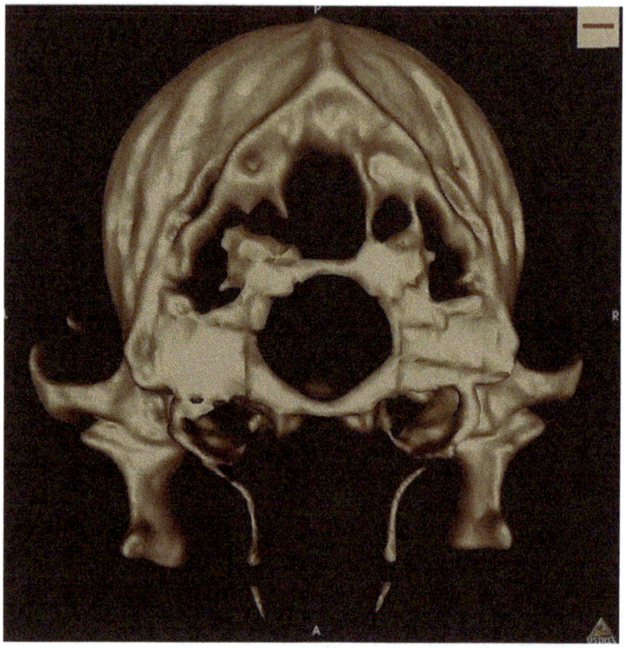

Figure 12.9 Three-dimensional CT reconstruction of severe occipital dysplasia in a Chihuahua with Chiari-like malformation. The surgeon must exercise extreme care in dissecting the musculature from the occipital area to avoid damaging the neural structures in this region when this defect is present.

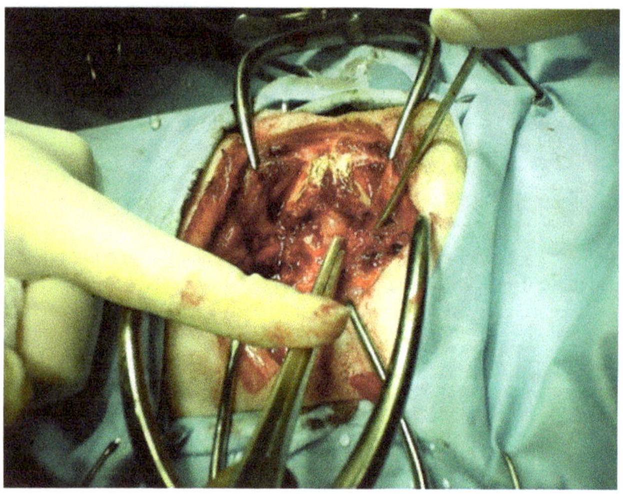

Figure 12.10 Kerrison rongeurs being used to perform the craniectomy.

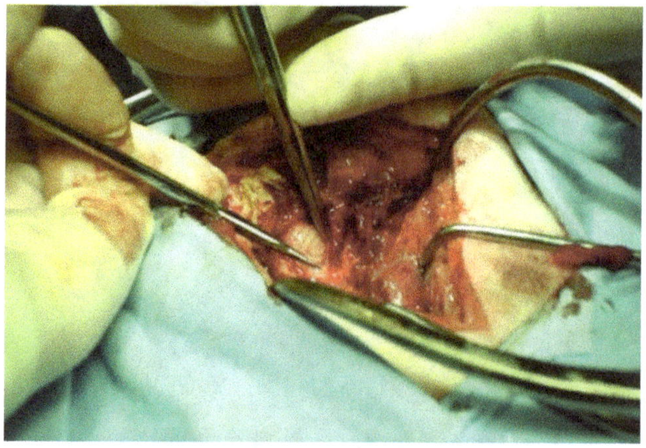

Figure 12.11 Tenotomy scissors are used to extend the incision through the meninges after the initial opening is created using a #12 scalpel blade.

malformation. Incising this structure and the underlying meningeal layers exposes the neuropil and results in a copious flow of cerebrospinal fluid.

After completing the exposure, the craniectomy is performed. The occipital bone has irregular undulations and therefore varying thickness of the bone. In patients with severe occipital dysplasia or a very thin occipital bone, only the use of Kerrison and Lempert rongeurs is necessary to perform the craniectomy and dorsal laminectomy of C1 (Figure 12.10). Thicker bone requires the use of a high-powered nitrogen drill to begin the process [4]. One or more burr-holes are made lateral to the midline. The opening is expanded using the aforementioned rongeurs. The boundaries of the bony defect can extend from just ventral to the nuchal line laterally, just below the occipital protuberance dorsally, and ventrally to the foramen magnum. These limits avoid the dorsal sagittal sinus, confluens sinum, and the transverse sinus. Ventrolaterally, the occipital condyles are the border. This much exposure may not be necessary and the surgeon should plan the dissection and craniectomy accordingly. For instance, if the procedure is addressing drainage of a quadrigeminal cyst (usually dorsal to the cerebellum), this much ventral exposure is unnecessary.

If the surgeon ventures too far in the ventrolateral bony dissection, the condylar vein that drains the sigmoid sinus is encountered. Bleeding here can be substantial and must be controlled by packing with an absorbable gelatin sponge or neurosurgical patties.

With the initial exposure completed, any continued hemorrhage from surrounding structures is controlled with bipolar cautery and the tissues are lavaged with sterile saline before continuing. The exposed meninges are incised longitudinally with a #12 scalpel blade. After the initial opening, the incision is continued rostrally and caudally with Potts or tenotomy scissors (Figure 12.11). This includes incising through the dorsal atlantoaxial membrane that may be vascular. When the desired length of the meningeal incision is achieved, the incision is extended at each end from medial to lateral on both sides, making the completed incision (viewed laterally) in the shape of the letter H. This allows reflection of the meninges laterally for improved exposure. Stay sutures (6-0) can be placed in the meninges to maintain retraction (Figure 12.12).

The remainder of the procedure is dictated by the original indication for the surgery. Any handling of the nervous system tissue must be done with extreme care and generally involves the use of lint-free cellulose spears. The obex and caudal aspect of the fourth ventricle are exposed with gentle dorsal traction of the vermis and carefully incising the thin transparent tissue covering the obex. Adhesions are often present with chronic Chiari-like malformation; such adhesions are cleared using the cellulose spears.

Quadrigeminal diverticula, if not immediately apparent over the dorsal aspect of the cerebellum, can be visualized by gently retracting the cerebellum ventrally, sometimes with slight medial retraction. Well-encapsulated tumors arising from the region of the lateral cerebellomedullary junction are visualized with medial retraction of one cerebellar hemisphere. These masses can be biopsied and on occasion completely excised; however, exposure is generally limited and may require combination with a rostrotentorial craniectomy and occlusion of the transverse sinus [4]. The use of an ultrasonic surgical aspirator improves the opportunity for tumor removal and biopsy.

The most frequently encountered indication for a suboccipital craniectomy is surgical treatment of Chiari-like malformation. In this procedure, the meninges are incised in the manner described earlier and are then marsupialized by suturing laterally to the adjacent muscle fascia using 5-0 or 6-0 absorbable synthetic monofilament suture. Usually two simple interrupted sutures on each side are sufficient. Frequently in this condition, the cerebellum is found extending under the dorsal arch of C1. Approximately one-third to half of the dorsal arch is removed with Kerrison rongeurs to facilitate adequate decompression. Copious amounts of CSF will flood the surgical site and require suctioning. Next, a duroplasty is performed using sheet of a commercially available porcine submucosal product or a synthetic dural replacement to serve as scaffolding for regrowth of the dura.

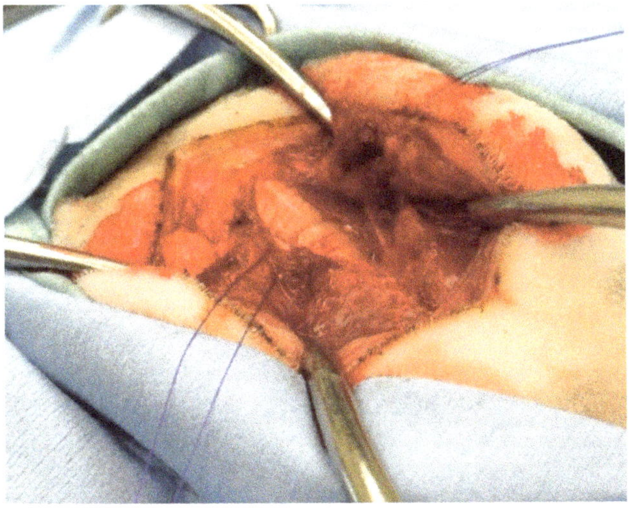

Figure 12.12 6-0 stay sutures placed through the lateral aspect of the incised meninges to maintain traction and improve exposure.

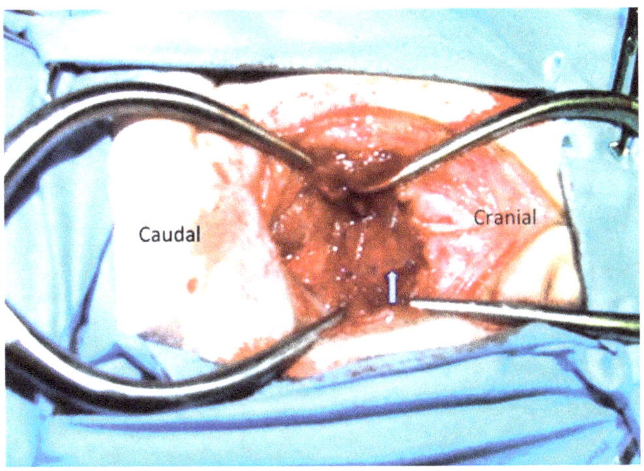

Figure 12.13 Intraoperative photograph showing nearly completed duroplasty using a sheet of commercially available porcine submucosal product (arrow). This product is placed over the exposed cerebellum and cervical spinal cord in surgery for Chiari-like malformation. This material is cut to the desired size and sutured to the edges of the cut meninges in a tent-like fashion using simple interrupted sutures of 5-0 or 6-0 absorbable synthetic monofilament suture. The duroplasty is intended to serve as scaffolding for regrowth of the dura and also serves to protect the underlying neural tissue from adhesions.

The material is cut to the desired size and sutured in a tent-like fashion using simple interrupted sutures of a 5-0 or 6-0 absorbable synthetic monofilament suture (Figure 12.13) [9]. In most patients, four simple interrupted sutures are placed on each side to connect the duroplasty material to the marsupialized dura, and then one suture rostrally and caudally if necessary. A watertight seal does not appear necessary as is often stated in the human neurosurgical literature.

After achieving complete hemostasis, a previously obtained fat graft from the gluteal region is rinsed with saline and placed over the duroplasty (Figure 12.14), followed by a sheet of absorbable gelatin foam. The fat graft is usually 5–7 mm thick and of sufficient size for an anticipated 30% reduction in size during the revascularization phase [10].

The incision is closed beginning with apposing the dorsal cervical musculature on the midline in a simple continuous pattern with monofilament absorbable suture. If necessary, muscle attachments can be sutured rostrally to remaining muscle attachments to the occipital bone or to the temporalis fascia. The subcutaneous tissues

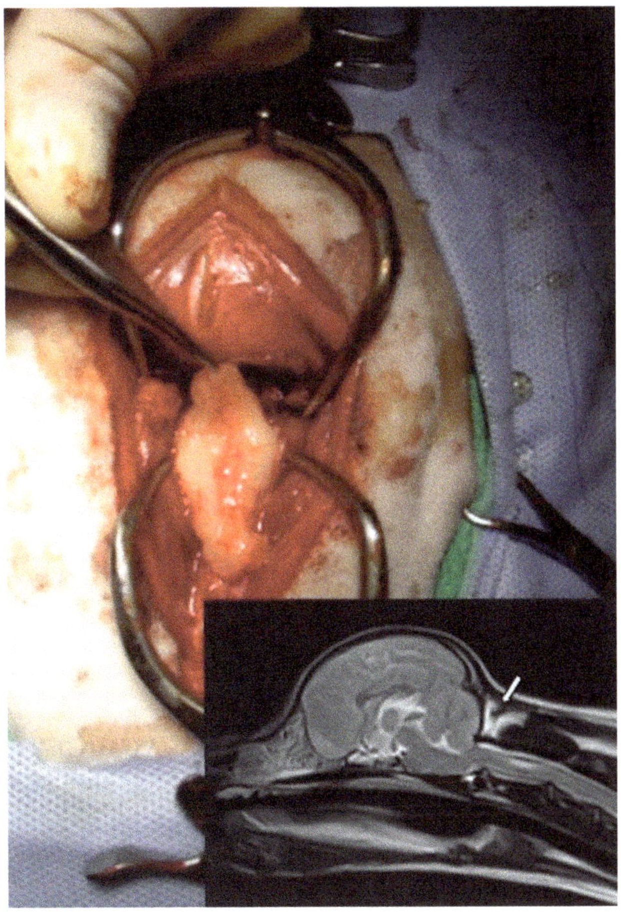

Figure 12.14 A fat graft is positioned over the craniectomy site. This is often covered with an absorbable gelatin sponge and the musculature is sutured over the graft. (*Inset*) Sagittal T2-weighted MRI shows the fat graft in place 2 years after surgery (arrow).

and skin are closed in routine fashion. The incision site is covered with a sterile waterproof bandage.

The results of the authors' experience indicates that this procedure is clinically effective and the use of titanium mesh, additional hardware, and polymethylmethacrylate offers no advantage in canine Chiari-like malformation patients.

Video clips to accompany this book can be found on the companion website at:
www.wiley.com/go/shores/neurosurgery

References

1 Oliver JE. Surgical approaches to the canine brain. *J Am Vet Med Assoc* 1968;29:353–378.

2 Vermeersch K, Ham LV, Caemaert J et al. Suboccipital craniectomy, dorsal laminectomy of C1, durotomy and dural graft placement as a treatment for syringohydromyelia with cerebellar tonsil herniation in Cavalier King Charles Spaniels. *Vet Surg* 2004;33:355–360.

3 Dewey C, Marino D, Bailey KS et al. Foramen magnum decompression with cranioplasty for treatment of caudal occipital malformation syndrome in dogs. *Vet Surg* 2007;36:406–414.

4 Bagley RS. Surgical approaches to the central nervous system: brain. In: Slatter DH (ed.) *Textbook of Small Animal Surgery*, 3rd edn. Philadelphia, PA: WB Saunders, 2003: 1167–1169.

5 Shores A. Neurosurgical techniques. In: Braund KG (ed.) *Clinical Syndromes in Veterinary Neurology*, 2nd edn. St Louis, MO: Mosby Year Book, 1994: 429–430.

6 Evans, HE. The muscular system. In: *Miller's Anatomy of the Dog*, 3rd edn. Philadelphia, PA: WB Saunders, 1993.

7 Shores A. Intracranial surgery. In: Slatter DH (ed.) *Textbook of Small Animal Surgery*, 2nd edn. Philadelphia, PA: WB Saunders, 1993: 1122–1135.

8 Shores A. Successes and failures in the surgical management of caudal occipital malformation syndrome in dogs. In: McFarlane D (ed.) *Proceedings of the American College of Veterinary Internal Medicine Forum 2010*. Lakewood, CO: American College of Veterinary Internal Medicine, 2010.

9 Akin EY, Ortinau NH, Shores A et al. Foramen magnum decompression with free autogenous adipose tissue graft for treatment of caudal occipital malformation syndrome in dogs. Poster presentation at ACVS Symposium, October 2009, Washington, DC.

10 Trevor, PB, Martin RA, Saunders GK, Trotter EJ. Healing characteristics of free and pedicle fat grafts after dorsal laminectomy and durotomy in dogs. *Vet Surg* 1991;5:282–290.

13 Surgical Treatment of Skull Tumors

Michelle Oblak and Andy Shores

Indications

Skull tumors are an uncommon primary bone tumor in the dog. Affected dogs have two classic presentations: the young dog with a protracted history of a slowly growing mass, or the geriatric dog with a newly discovered mass [1–3]. Rarely, these masses can invade into the surrounding soft tissues and brain parenchyma, but more commonly these are tumors of bone that act as space-occupying lesions [1,3–5]. In most cases, patients are asymptomatic [3–6]. Clinical signs may be seen if the tumor is in an area near the temporomandibular joint or orbit, or if it invades the sinus. Rarely, parenchymal compression can result in circling, ataxia, seizures, or other neurological abnormalities associated with the region of the brain affected. Most dogs present because of a progressive mass effect on the head but it is important to be aware that there may still be significant brain compression, despite a lack of clinical signs [4–6].

Any type of primary bone tumor can also develop in the skull but the most common differential diagnoses for primary skull tumors include multilobular osteochondrosarcoma, osteoma, and osteosarcoma [1–8]. Less commonly primary chondrosarcoma, squamous cell carcinoma, and fibrosarcoma can also occur in this location [6,8].

When a patient presents for a suspected skull tumor, the diagnostic work-up is similar to that of any other tumor. Staging may include a full physical examination and health screening (complete blood count, biochemistry profile and urinalysis, three-view thoracic radiographs, abdominal ultrasound) in addition to further diagnostic evaluation. When the mass is malignant, fine-needle aspiration and cytology may yield a diagnostic result [9]. If incisional biopsy of the mass is to be undertaken, it should be performed after advanced imaging is obtained and with the surgical approach in mind, as the biopsy tract will need to be removed during definitive surgery [10,11]. Definitive diagnosis and prognostication from biopsies can be challenging due to the small sample sizes [12,13]. Often a Jamshidi bone marrow biopsy needle or Michele Trephine bone biopsy instrument is required to obtain an adequate sample of the tumor. In these cases, depth should be measured in advance from radiographs or computed tomography (CT) images and it is important to exercise caution when placing force on the biopsy needle as the center of the mass can be softer, resulting in disruption of the medial tumor capsule or iatrogenic brain trauma.

Preoperative Imaging

Skull radiographs can be helpful for evaluating the size of the mass and extent of cranial vault involvement. CT and magnetic resonance imaging (MRI) may be used independently or in combination depending on the clinical signs and expected soft tissue changes [4,5,14]. Often the choice of advanced imaging modality will be determined based on personal preference as well as availability. While CT can provide good anatomical localization and overview for surgical planning, MRI is more sensitive for any potential parenchymal changes and can also help to better delineate important vascular structures [14].

During evaluation of advanced imaging results, close attention should be paid to the proximity of the dorsal sagittal and transverse venous sinuses, evidence of contrast enhancement within the temporalis muscle, and involvement of the frontal sinus or cribriform plate. In addition, imaging will allow for a determination of the extent of the resultant skull defect and consideration of reconstruction options.

One significant advantage of incorporating CT into the planning process is the ability to reconstruct images. Multiple planes and three-dimensional reconstruction can help with preoperative visualization and planning, as well as for client education (Figure 13.1, Video 13.1). In complex cases where further insight and planning is required, three-dimensional printing of the skull and associated mass can further assist with surgical preparation and planning (Figure 13.2).

Surgical Anatomy

The main bone regions of the cranium include the frontal, parietal, temporal, and occipital bones [15]. The cribriform plate separates the cranial cavity from the nasal sinuses. The majority

Current Techniques in Canine and Feline Neurosurgery, First Edition. Edited by Andy Shores and Brigitte A. Brisson.
© 2017 John Wiley & Sons, Inc. Published 2017 by John Wiley & Sons, Inc.
Companion website: www.wiley.com/go/shores/neurosurgery

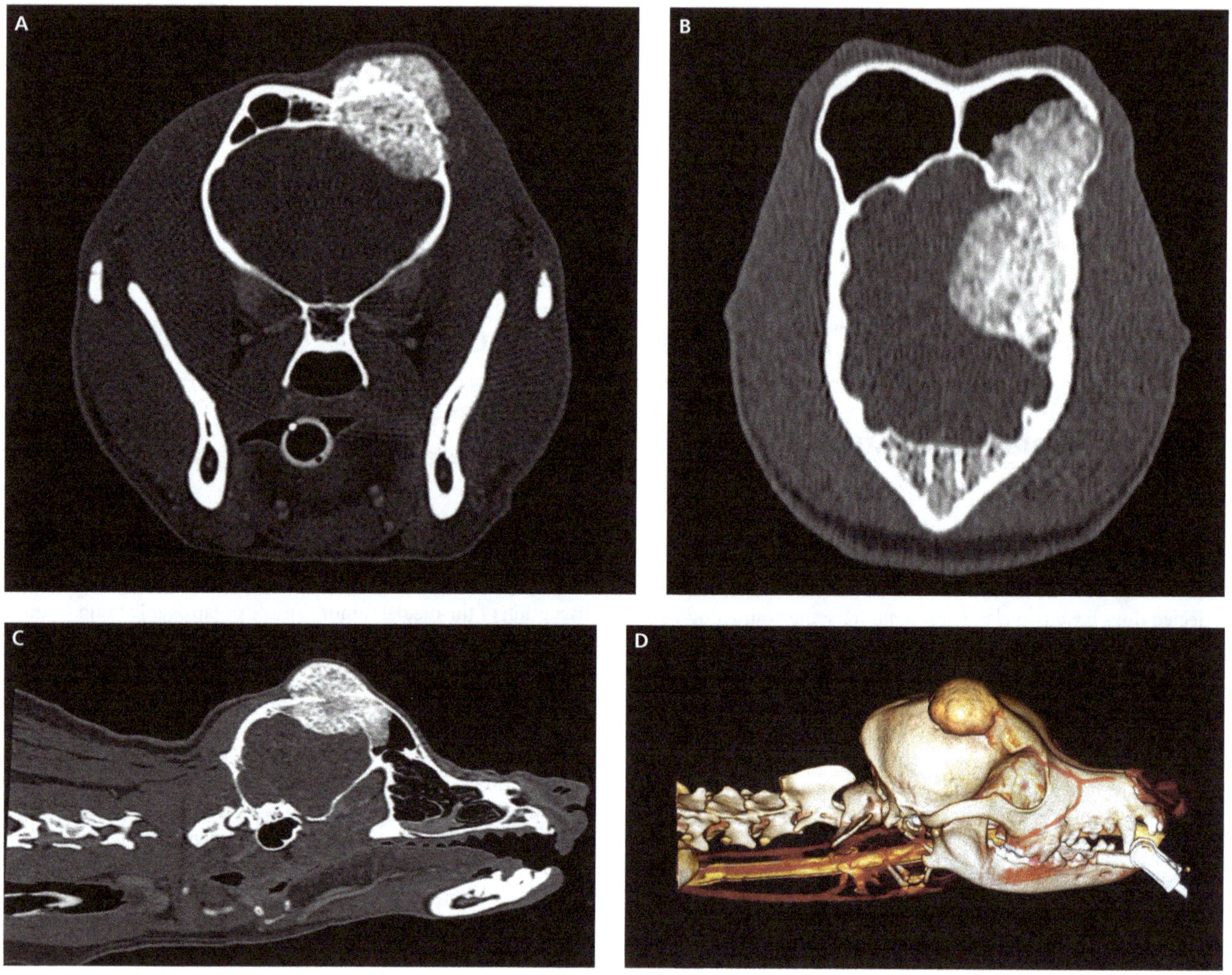

Figure 13.1 (A) Transverse, (B) dorsal and (C) sagittal reconstructed CT images of a skull osteosarcoma. (D) A virtual three-dimensional reconstruction has also been created for planning.

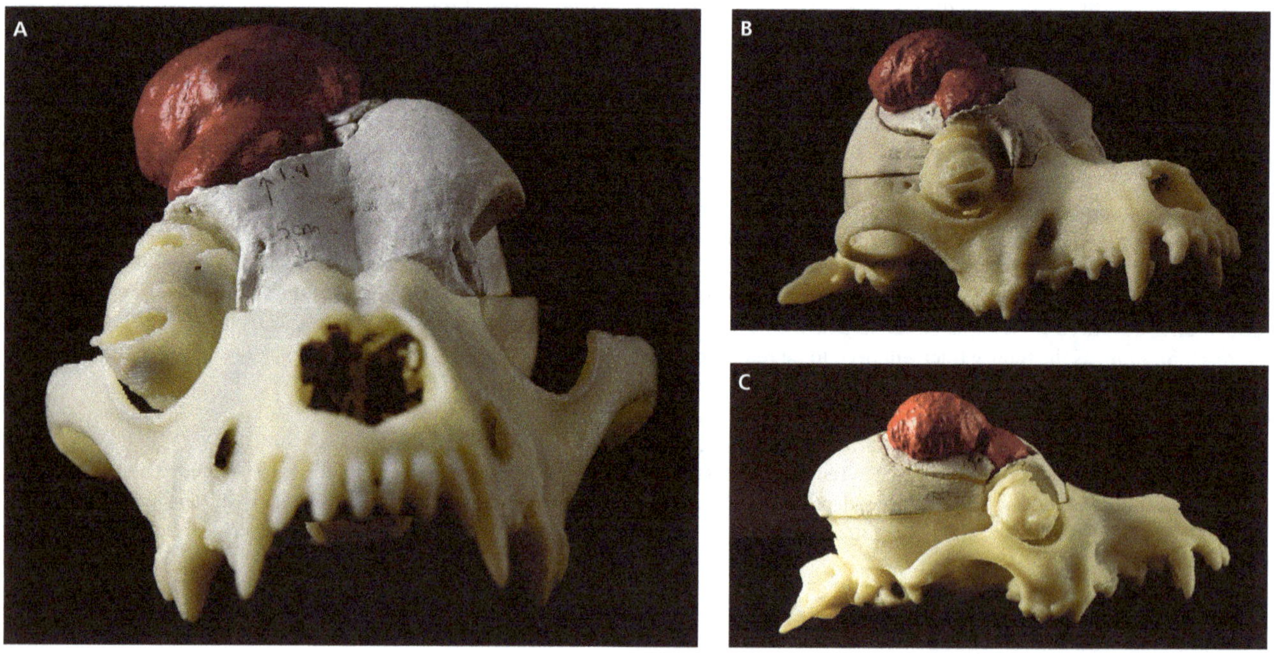

Figure 13.2 A three-dimensional printed skull can help with visualization and preoperative surgical planning, allowing for margin measurement and reconstruction planning.

of the muscles of the skull attach to the mandible and maxilla for mastication [16]. The main muscular group encountered during craniectomy is the temporalis muscle. The margins of the temporalis muscle include the orbital ligament and frontal crest cranially, the zygomatic arch laterally, the external sagittal crest medially, and the dorsal nuchal line caudally [17] (Figure 13.3). The most significant vessels that may be encountered during routine craniectomy include the dorsal sagittal and transverse sinuses, which lie within the dura [18] (Figure 13.4). The dorsal sagittal sinus extends along the midline rostrally, from the cribriform plate to the occipital bone, and enters the skull at the level of the tentorium [18].

Patient Positioning

Craniectomy for skull tumors requires extensive preoperative planning and a wide clip and surgical preparation. In cases of primary bone tumors, the skin should be freely moveable over the mass and therefore does not require extensive resection (except for the biopsy tract). The patient will be placed in sternal recumbency or slightly oblique to allow for easy access to the entire head (Figure 13.5). A vacuum bag or patient positioning device can help to ensure the animal remains in the same position throughout surgery. Patients should receive antimicrobial prophylaxis 30 min prior to the start of surgery and every 90 min thereafter.

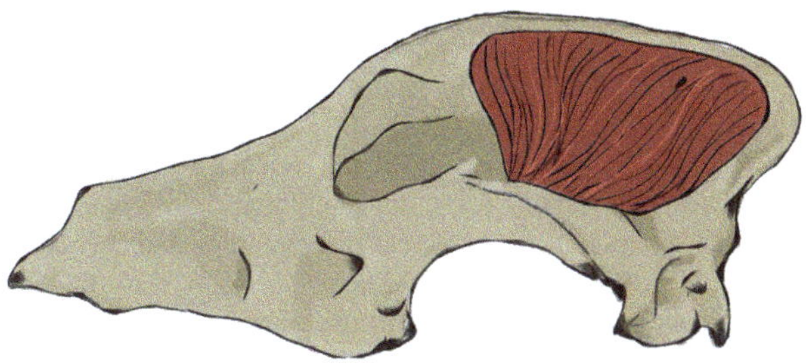

Figure 13.3 Illustration of the temporalis muscle, which is encountered during dorsal or rostral craniectomy and can be used for reconstruction of the defect. *Source*: Courtesy of Emily Wong.

Surgical Technique

The surgical approach to the mass will vary depending on its location but whenever possible should be curvilinear to allow access to the entire region of the skull and temporalis fascia. When a skin incision is created, the biopsy tract should be removed in cases of malignancy, with a 1-cm margin, and this entire tract of tissue should remain with the mass (Figure 13.6). Following skin incision, depending on the location, the temporalis fascia and muscle may be identified overlying the mass. For bony tumors that are not growing into this fascia it should be preserved for closure. Depending on the location of the mass, the temporalis fascia may be incised on the medial or lateral border. The temporalis muscle is then preserved, or removed as a margin associated with the mass, to expose the skull using a combination of sharp dissection, electrocoagulation, and periosteal elevation.

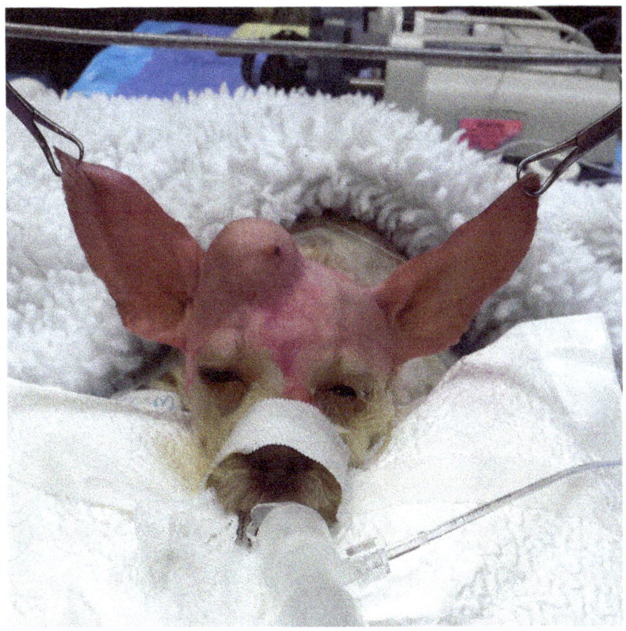

Figure 13.5 The patient is positioned in sternal recumbency with the assistance of a vacuum bag. The entire head is clipped and prepared for surgery.

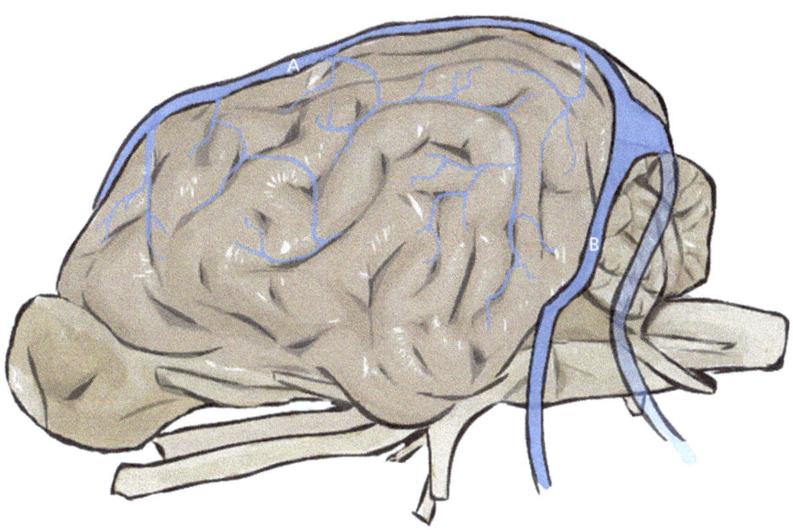

Figure 13.4 Illustration of the sinuses that may be encountered during craniectomy. Care must be taken to avoid damage to the dorsal sagittal sinus (A) and paired transverse sinuses (B), which are located within the dura and can be disrupted during bone removal. *Source*: Courtesy of Emily Wong.

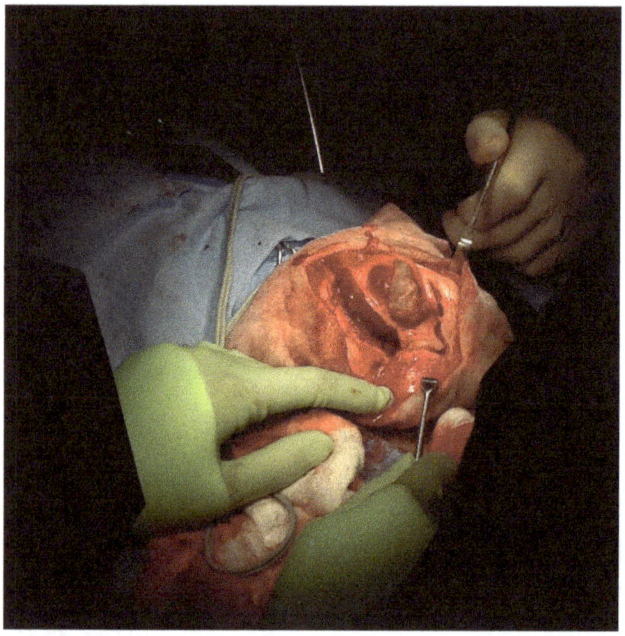

Figure 13.6 Incision through the skin and temporalis fascia and muscle. The biopsy tract is being removed with the mass. In this case, the mass had invaded the temporalis fascia so it could not be preserved.

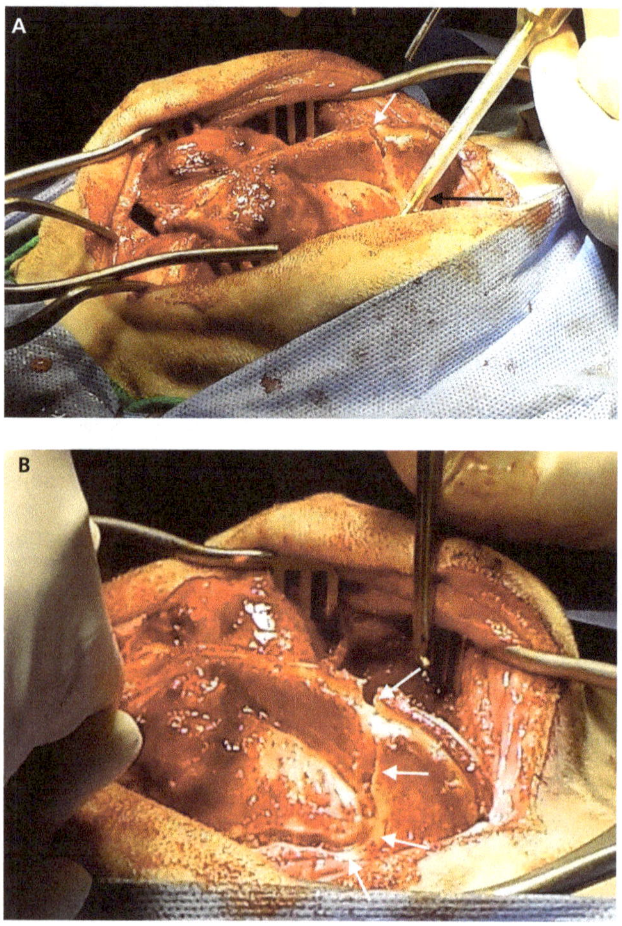

Figure 13.7 (A) Resection of the skull mass with the bone-cutting CUSA NXT 35 kHz Neuro Tip (black arrow). White arrow points to cut through the mid-sagittal crest of the skull. (B) White arrows outline the cutting line caudal to the mass. Using this method, no bone dust is produced.

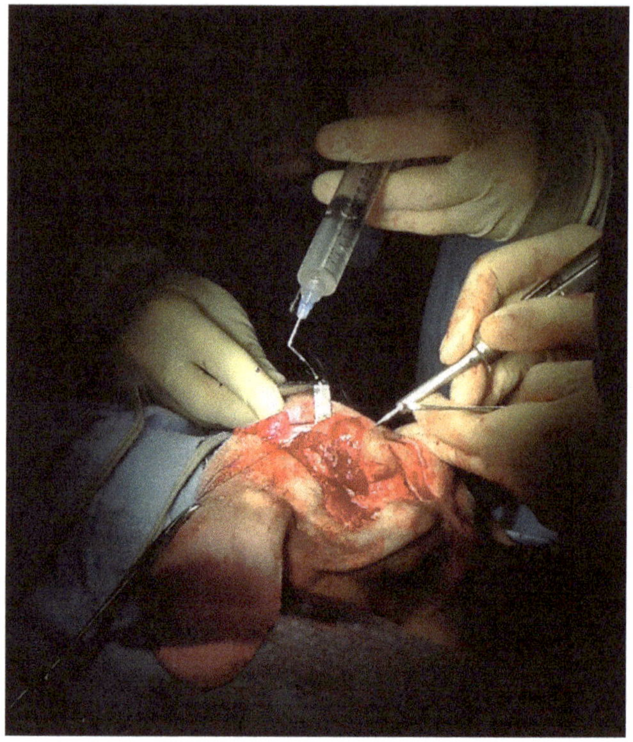

Figure 13.8 A pneumatic drill is used to make a circumferential incision in the skull. Continuous irrigation during drilling will help dissipate the heat from the bone and surrounding tissues.

Since local recurrence is a significant concern with both malignant and benign tumors, a 1–2 cm safety margin of bone beyond the mass is planned to reduce local recurrence [2,3,19]. This margin should be identified and marked based on planning from advanced imaging. It is important that imaging is consulted for this approach as the mass may have a more substantial internal component than what is externally visible. If skull excision is based on the visible mass, there is an increased risk of disruption of the mass during drilling with subsequent incomplete margins.

A pneumatic drill and burr is then used to make a circumferential incision into the skull. Alternatively, the CUSA NXT 35 kHz Neuro Tip (Integra LifeSciences Corporation, Plainsboro, NJ) can been used to cut through the skull, thereby avoiding the bone dust that could seed the area with tumor cells (Figure 13.7). Bone thickness should be determined on the preoperative CT and can vary significantly. Saline irrigation over the burr and bone is used to minimize heat conduction and necrosis (Figure 13.8). When using a drill and burr, the incision is continued until the inner periosteum can be palpated as soft circumferentially and a curette or rongeur can be used to complete the incision. Following circumferential incision, the bone segment should be moveable and should be removed carefully as it can be closely associated with or adherent to the dura or sinuses. A damp cotton-tipped applicator, curette, or Freer periosteal elevator can be useful to gently separate the bone segment from the dura (Video 13.2). Any minor bleeding encountered can be addressed with a hemostatic sponge, bipolar electrocoagulation with lavage or gentle pressure. The resected segment should then be evaluated to ensure that an adequate margin has been achieved in all directions and further bone removed as necessary with rongeurs. Gentle irrigation of the site is performed

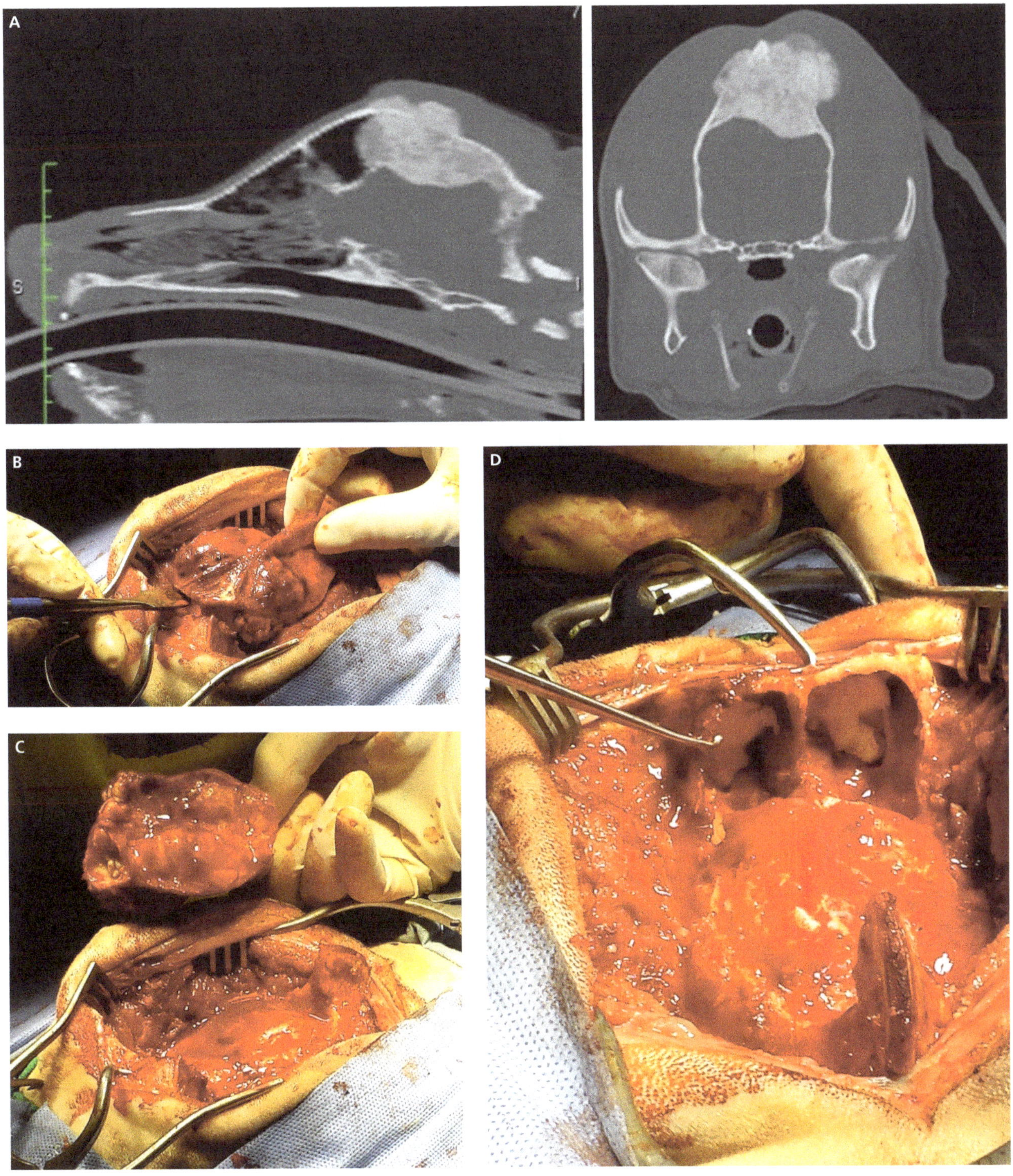

Figure 13.9 (A) Sagittal and transverse images of the skull mass preoperatively. (B) Skull mass after resection with CUSA. (C) Removal of the skull mass. (D) Skull defect after mass removal. (Note that the frontal sinuses have been flushed with Betadyne solution prior to the resection and the entrance into the nasal cavity has been packed with gelatin sponges and bone wax.)

prior to reconstruction. If desired, Vetrix® BioSIS ECM (Vetrix Inc., Cumming, GA) can be placed over the exposed brain to decrease the risk of adhesions. Closure will vary depending on the size and location of the resultant defect. In many cases the preserved temporalis fascia can be used to cover the defect with closure of the subcutaneous and skin in routine fashion.

Some of the extremely large skull masses require extensive resection and reconstruction, which can be performed with creation of a polymethylmethacrylate (PMMA) prosthesis or titanium mesh [20,21]. Advantages of this reconstruction method include improved cosmesis and increased protection of the exposed brain from accidental trauma. The main disadvantages include cost,

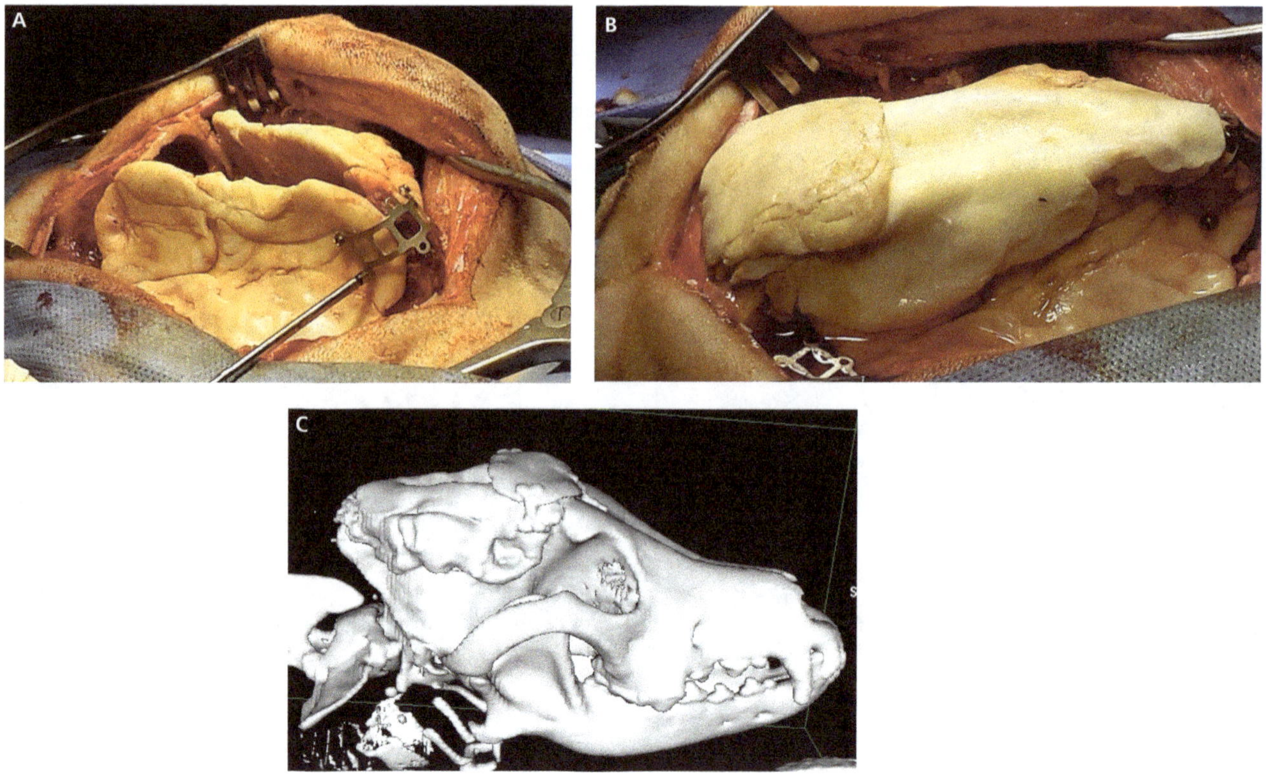

Figure 13.10 (A) First stage of skull reconstruction using PMMA. (B) Completed reconstruction. (C) Postoperative three-dimensional CT reconstruction of PMMA prosthesis.

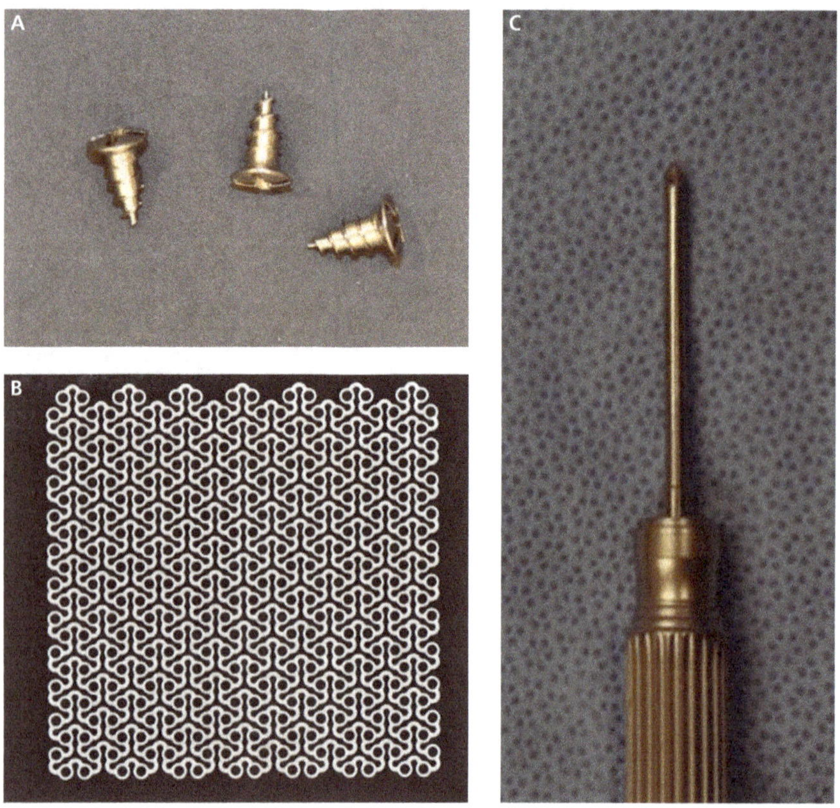

Figure 13.11 (A) Self-drilling/self-tapping screws. (B) Contourable titanium mesh. (C) Screwdriver. *Source*: Courtesy of Noel Moens.

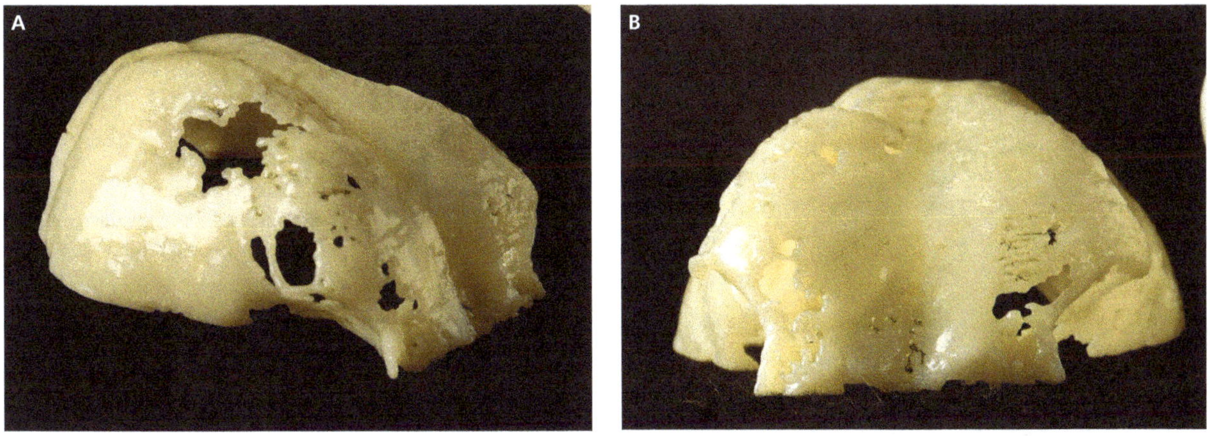

Figure 13.12 (A, B) A custom-printed sterilizable three-dimensional printed skull cap can be used intraoperatively to help contour the titanium plate in a manner that closely resembles the normal skull.

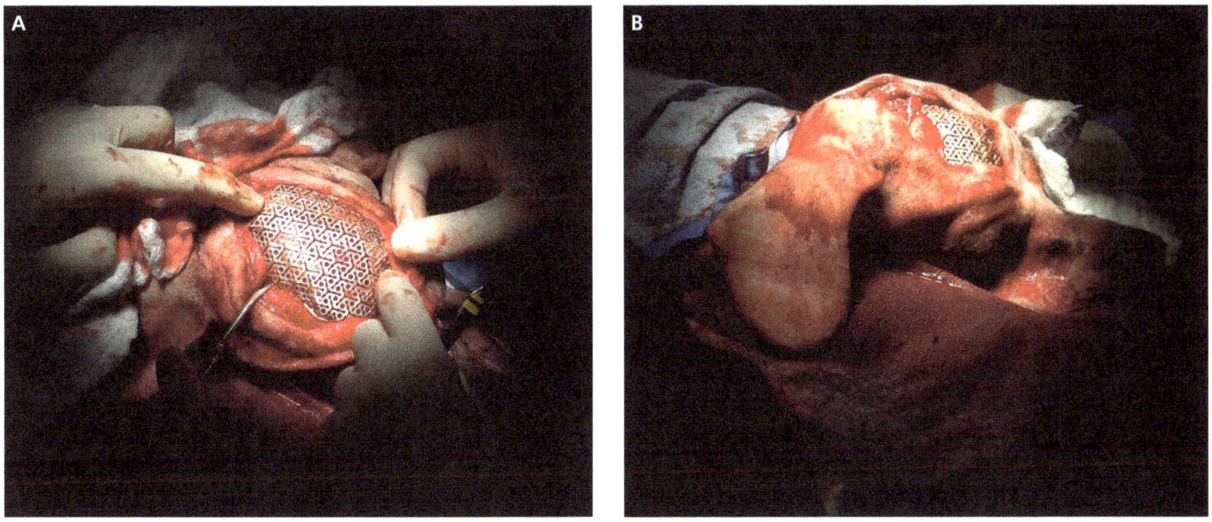

Figure 13.13 (A) Placement of an intraoperatively contoured titanium mesh that has been fixed in place with small bone screws. (B) Appearance of the mesh following closure of any remaining temporalis muscle prior to subcutaneous and skin closure.

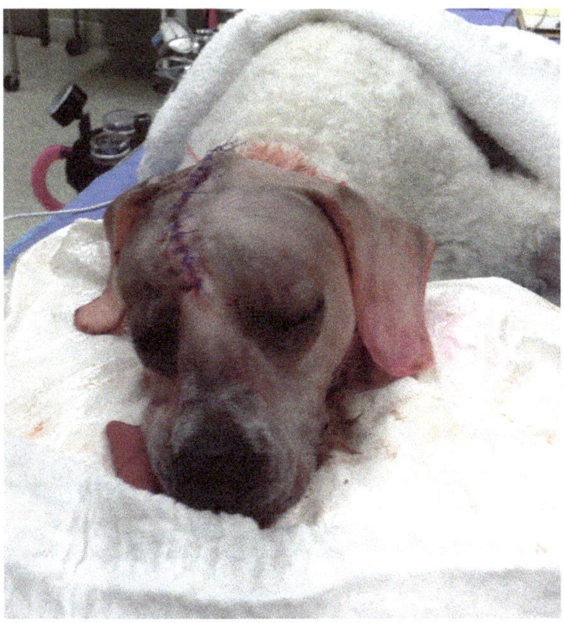

Figure 13.14 Postoperative appearance of the patient in Figure 13.13 following reconstruction and closure.

increased procedure time, and a potential increased risk of infection leading to empyema or need to remove the implant.

PMMA has been successfully used to reconstruct large defects in the canine calvarium [20]. A preformed molded PMMA prosthetic implant can be used or the PMMA prosthesis can be sculpted at the time of surgery (Figures 13.9 and 13.10).

Surgical titanium mesh is available in a variety of styles and sizes. The standard mesh is 0.6 mm thick and is easily contoured by hand. Equipment required includes the mesh, associated self-drilling/self-tapping screws, specialized screwdriver, and fine wire cutters (Figure 13.11). Reconstruction mesh benders and cutters can be purchased but are not a requirement to use this implant. Following removal of the affected bone segment, contouring of the mesh is performed to reconstruct the region of bone that has been removed. The mesh is first cut to size and then gently manipulated to reconstruct the defect. If desired, a three-dimensional printed sterilizable model of the normal contour of the skull can be used for planning and contouring during reconstruction (Figure 13.12).

The mesh is then fixed to the skull with self-drilling/self-tapping screws that have been premeasured based on preoperative imaging (Figure 13.13). Predrilling is recommended if the bone is greater than 5 mm thick, which is uncommon in veterinary

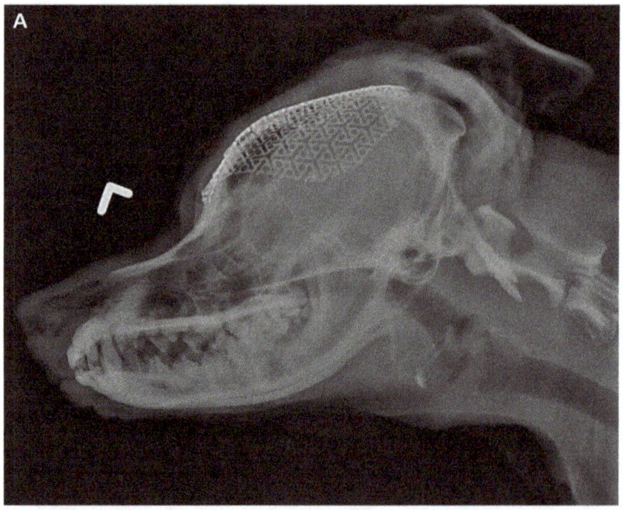

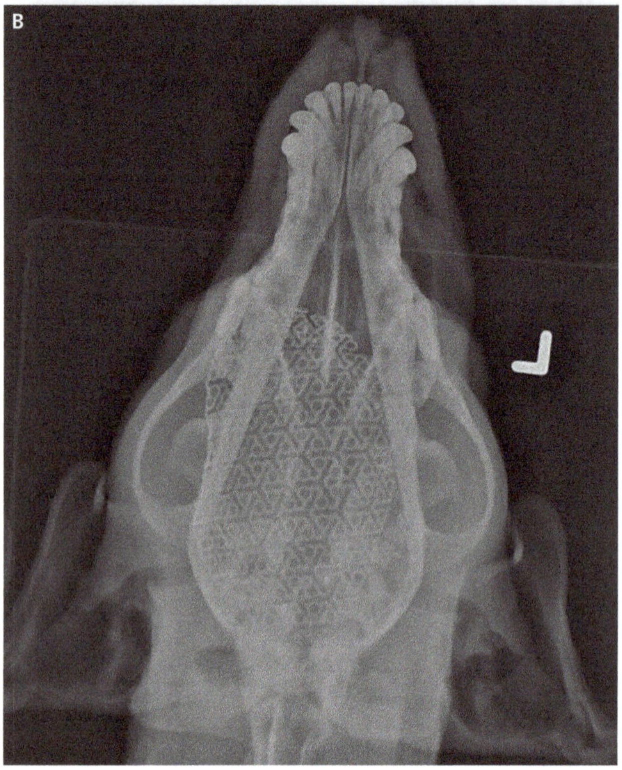

Figure 13.15 Postoperative skull radiographs of the patient in Figure 13.13 showing the position of the implant and providing a comparison for future evaluation.

patients. The screw heads are specific to the mesh selected. Depending on the size of the defect, six to eight screws are typically used to ensure adequate fixation. Following fixation of the mesh, any remaining temporalis muscle or fascia is secured to cover the implant as much as possible and the subcutaneous tissue and skin are closed in routine fashion (Figure 13.14). Postoperative skull radiographs and/or CT are performed as a reference point for future monitoring (Figure 13.15).

Postoperative Considerations

Patients are recovered in an intensive care unit. A single dose of mannitol is administered prior to anesthetic recovery and can be repeated if necessary based on neurological signs. Patients are monitored closely for evidence of increased intracranial pressure. Pain is controlled with an opioid constant-rate infusion. Typical patients are discharged 48–72 hours postoperatively if their recovery is uncomplicated. Antibiotic prophylaxis is continued while the patient is in hospital and for 7 days following discharge.

Video clips to accompany this book can be found on the companion website at:
www.wiley.com/go/shores/neurosurgery

References

1 Goldschmidt MH, Thrall DE. Benign bone tumors in the dog. In: Newton CD, Nunamaker DM (eds) *Textbook of Small Animal Orthopaedics*. Philadelphia, PA: JB Lippincott, 1985: 899–907.
2 Selmic LE, Lafferty MH, Kamstock DA et al. Outcome and prognostic factors for osteosarcoma of the maxilla, mandible, or calvarium in dogs: 183 cases (1986–2012). *J Am Vet Med Assoc* 2014;245:930–938.
3 Dernell WS, Straw RC, Cooper MF, Powers BE, Larue S, Withrow SJ. Multilobular osteochondrosarcoma in 39 dogs: 1979–1993. *J Am Anim Hosp Assoc* 1998;34:11–18.
4 Lipsitz D, Levitski RE, Berry WL. Magnetic resonance imaging features of multilobular osteochondrosarcoma in 3 dogs. *Vet Radiol Ultrasound* 2001;42:14–19.
5 Hathcock JT, Newton JC. Computed tomographic characteristics of multilobular tumor of bone involving the cranium in 7 dogs and zygomatic arch in 2 dogs. *Vet Radiol Ultrasound* 2000;41:214–217.
6 Kim H, Nakaichi M, Itamoto K, Taura Y. Primary chondrosarcoma in the skull of a dog. *J Vet Sci* 2007;8:99–101.
7 Johnson KA, Cooley AJ, Darien DL. Zygomatic osteoma with atypical heterogeneity in a dog. *J Comp Pathol* 1996;114:199–203.
8 Kealy JK, McAllister H, Graham JP. The skull and vertebral column. In: *Diagnostic Radiology and Ultrasonography of the Dog and Cat*. St Louis, MO: Saunders Elsevier, 2010: 447–543.
9 Jorda M, Rey L, Hanly A, Ganjei-Azar P. Fine-needle aspiration cytology of bone. *Cancer Cytopathol* 2000;90:47–54.
10 Sabel MS, Diehl KM, Chang AE. Principles of surgical therapy in oncology. In: Chang AE, Hayes DF, Pass HI et al. (eds) *Oncology: An Evidence-Based Approach*. Berlin: Springer Science & Business Media, 2006: 58–72.
11 Mohana R, Faisham W, Zulmi W, Nawfar AS, Effat O, Salzihan MS. The incidence of malignant infiltration in the biopsy tract of osteosarcoma. *Malays Orthop J* 2007;1:7–10.
12 Wadhwa N. Osteosarcoma: diagnostic dilemmas in histopathology and prognostic factors. *Indian J Orthop* 2014;48:247–254.
13 Rozeman LB, Cleton-Jansen AM, Hogendoorn PCW. Pathology of primary malignant bone and cartilage tumours. *Int Orthop* 2006;30:437–444.
14 Kraus DH, Lanzieri CE, Wanamaker JR, Little JR, Lavertu P. Complementary use of computed tomography and magnetic resonance imaging in assessing skull base lesions. *Laryngoscope* 1992;102:623–629.
15 Evans HE, de Lahunta A. Anatomy of the skeleton. In: *Miller's Anatomy of the Dog*, 4th edn. St Louis, MO: Elsevier Saunders, 2013: 80–158.
16 Ström D, Holm S, Clemensson E, Haraldson T, Carlsson GE. Gross anatomy of the craniomandibular joint and masticatory muscles of the dog. *Arch Oral Biol* 1988;33:597–604.
17 Tomlinson J, Presnell KR. Use of the temporalis muscle flap in the dog. *Vet Surg* 1981;10:77–79.
18 de Lahunta A, Glass E, Kent M. Neuroanatomy gross description and atlas of transverse sections and magnetic resonance images. In: *Veterinary Neuroanatomy and Clinical Neurology*, 4th edn. St Louis, MO: Elsevier Saunders, 2015: 6–45.
19 Boston SE. Craniectomy and orbitectomy in dogs and cats. *Can Vet J* 2010;51:537–540.
20 Bryant KJ, Steinberg H, McAnulty JF. Cranioplasty by means of molded polymethylmethacrylate prosthetic reconstruction after radical excision of neoplasms of the skull in 2 dogs. *J Am Vet Med Assoc* 2003;233:67–72.
21 Bordelon JT, Rochat MC. Use of a titanium mesh for cranioplasty following radical rostrotentorial craniectomy to remove an ossifying fibroma in a dog. *J Am Vet Med Assoc* 2007;231:1692–1695.

14 Shunt Placement and Marsupialization in Treatment of Hydrocephalus and Quadrigeminal Diverticula

William Thomas and Jill Narak

Hydrocephalus

Hydrocephalus is active distension of the ventricular system of the brain caused by obstruction of flow of cerebrospinal fluid (CSF) from its point of production to its point of absorption. Obstruction can be caused by developmental abnormalities or acquired lesions such as neoplasia or inflammatory lesions. A number of conditions such as infarction and necrosis can result in decreased volume of brain parenchyma in which the loss of brain tissue leaves a vacant space filled passively with CSF. Although this was previously called hydrocephalus ex vacuo, such conditions do not cause active distension of the ventricles and are therefore not classified as hydrocephalus and do not require specific treatment [1].

Definitive treatment of hydrocephalus is directed at the underlying cause if possible. Medical therapy is used to delay surgery, to manage acute deterioration, and when surgery is not an option or not indicated. Acetazolamide, furosemide, or omeprazole are used to decrease CSF formation. Glucocorticoids, such as prednisone, are also commonly used. Although these drugs can provide temporary relief, medical therapy does not provide long-term benefit and definitive treatment is a surgical procedure to divert CSF, most commonly implantation of a ventriculoperitoneal shunt.

Clinical Features

Based on the age of onset, hydrocephalus can be broadly classified as pediatric or acquired. Pediatric hydrocephalus is caused by developmental abnormalities and clinical signs are usually apparent by several months of age. Toy and brachycephalic dogs are at increased risk but the condition occurs sporadically in other breeds of dogs and cats. In most cases an obvious site of obstruction is not apparent, but may be due to obstruction at the level of the subarachnoid space or arachnoid villi, which is difficult to detect. Another possibility is intraventricular obstruction during a critical stage of development in which the obstructive lesion later resolves, leaving only the ventricular enlargement. Pediatric hydrocephalus may also be associated with other malformations such as meningomyelocele, Chiari-like malformation, Dandy–Walker syndrome, and arachnoid diverticula. Signs of pediatric hydrocephalus include an enlarged dome-shaped head with persistent fontanelles and open cranial sutures. There may be ventral or ventrolateral strabismus, due to either malformation of the orbit or brainstem dysfunction. Neurological deficits include abnormal behavior, cognitive dysfunction (such as inability to become house-trained), disturbed consciousness, ataxia, circling, blindness, seizures, and vestibular dysfunction. Affected patients are often fragile and can worsen later in life coincident with other diseases or minor head trauma.

Acquired hydrocephalus can develop at any age due to diseases such as tumors and inflammatory disease. Neurological deficits are similar to those in young patients, but if hydrocephalus develops after the cranial sutures have closed, malformation of the skull does not develop.

Diagnostic Evaluation

The diagnosis of hydrocephalus is based on clinical and imaging features. Magnetic resonance imaging (MRI) is the best modality to assess ventricular size and other lesions. Obstructing masses such as tumors, granulomas, and diverticula may be identified, especially on postcontrast images. MRI is more sensitive than computed tomography (CT) in demonstrating small focal lesions, especially those in the caudal fossa. CT is usually sufficient for follow-up of previously diagnosed patients and those with an existing shunt. Ultrasound is practical for assessing ventricular size in patients with a persistent fontanelle. Enlarged ventricles are easily seen with any of these techniques, although there is poor correlation between clinical signs and ventricular size.

Current Techniques in Canine and Feline Neurosurgery, First Edition. Edited by Andy Shores and Brigitte A. Brisson.
© 2017 John Wiley & Sons, Inc. Published 2017 by John Wiley & Sons, Inc.
Companion website: www.wiley.com/go/shores/neurosurgery

Evidence of increased intraventricular pressure includes periventricular edema, enlargement of the temporal horns, and effacement of sulci. These findings suggest acute, active hydrocephalus and are an indication for treatment, as compared with chronic, relatively compensated hydrocephalus with normal intraventricular pressure, in which case surgery may not be beneficial. Periventricular edema starts at the dorsolateral angles of the lateral ventricles and spreads into the adjacent white matter. This is evident on CT as blurring or loss of the normally sharp ventricular margins. Periventricular edema is best appreciated on T2-weighted MRI as increased intensity compared with normal white matter. Heavily T2-weighted fluid-attenuated inversion recovery (FLAIR) sequences are useful in detecting subtle periventricular lesions. In doubtful cases, careful observation with serial imaging is indicated [2] (Figure 14.1).

Analysis of CSF is helpful in cases of suspected meningoencephalitis. Imaging is performed first to identify any shifting of brain tissue, such as caudal cerebellar herniation, or other abnormalities that may increase the risk of CSF collection from the cerebellomedullary cistern. In some cases it may be safer to collect CSF from an enlarged lateral ventricle through a persistent fontanelle. Removal of CSF is sometimes used as a temporary measure to decrease intraventricular pressure and to help predict which patients will benefit from surgical shunting. In patients with a fontanelle, an enlarged lateral ventricle can be punctured with a 25G needle inserted at the lateral aspect of the fontanelle, avoiding the sagittal sinus on the midline. Ultrasound is helpful in determining the depth of the center of the ventricle. Approximately 2 mL of CSF can be safely removed in most patients.

Indications for Surgery

A young patient with clinical signs, ventriculomegaly, and evidence of increased intraventricular pressure is a clear indication for a CSF diversionary procedure. Progressive ventriculomegaly over time is also an indication to treat unless it is secondary to cortical atrophy. Older patients with stable clinical signs and stable ventriculomegaly are generally not considered for treatment [2].

Equipment

Ventriculoperitoneal shunts comprise three basic elements: a ventricular catheter, valve, and peritoneal catheter. There are many variations of these components available on the market. Pediatric or low-profile versions designed for small infants work well in small dogs and cats. Some systems also include a CSF reservoir that can be pumped to check patency and an access port that can be aspirated percutaneously to collect CSF. Antibiotic-impregnated shunts are available that have been shown to decrease the rate of shunt infection in human patients [3] (Figure 14.2).

Ventricular Catheter

The ventricular catheter can be straight or right-angled and usually has multiple holes in the last 10 mm. Some systems consist of a separate ventricular catheter and distal tube connected at the time of surgery while others use a single-piece design. When the ventricular catheter is inserted, if bleeding occurs it is best to allow drainage of fluid until it clears before attaching to the valve; otherwise the blood can occlude the valve. For this reason, separate ventricular catheters are preferred [4].

Valves

The most common valve is a differential pressure valve, which opens when the pressure difference across the valve exceeds a predetermined threshold. Most manufacturers provide fixed pressure valves in ranges of three or four categories, for example very low (<1 cmH_2O), low (1–4 cmH_2O), medium (4–8 cmH_2O), and high (>8 cmH_2O). Externally adjustable ("programmable") valves are also available that allow the clinician to percutaneously adjust the opening pressure as the patient's clinical course changes. Flow rate through the valve depends on the differential pressure and the resistance in the shunt system. Two different valves may have the same opening pressure and completely different resistance and therefore behave differently.

Diaphragm valves are the most commonly produced and involve deflection of a silicone membrane in response to pressure. Some shunts employ a slit valve, usually at the distal end. These valves

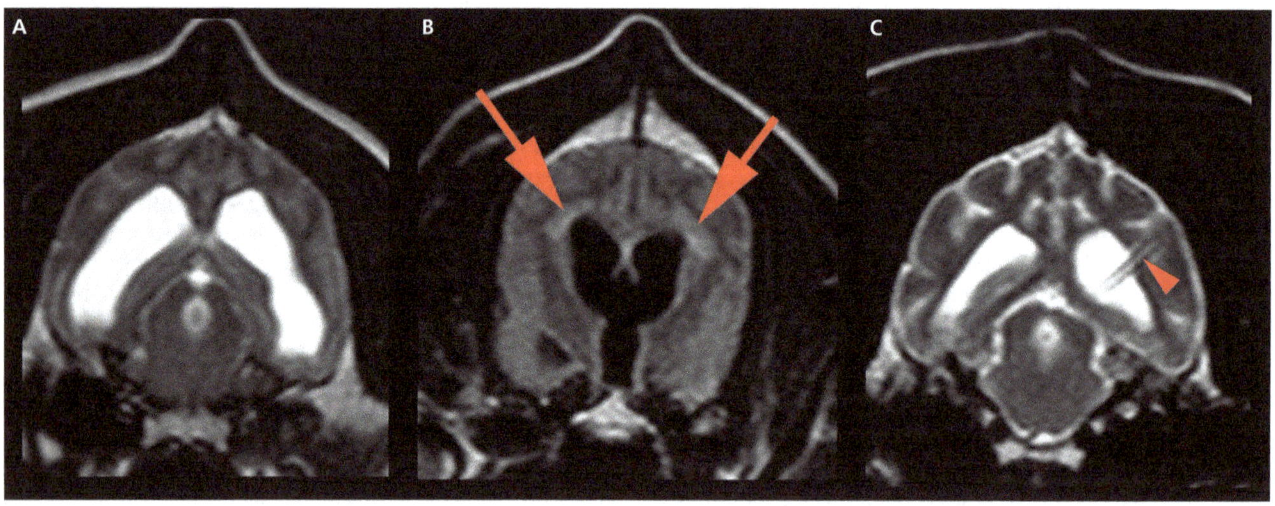

Figure 14.1 MRI of hydrocephalus. (A) T2-weighted transverse image at the level of the midbrain. There is enlargement of the lateral ventricles and effacement of the cerebral sulci. (B) FLAIR transverse image at the level of the third ventricle. There is hyperintensity adjacent to the dorsolateral aspects of the lateral ventricles (arrows). (C) T2-weighted image at the level of the midbrain 2 months after placement of a ventriculoperitoneal shunt. The lateral ventricles are smaller and the cerebral sulci are more prominent compared with preoperative imaging. The ventricular catheter is evident in the lateral ventricle (arrowhead).

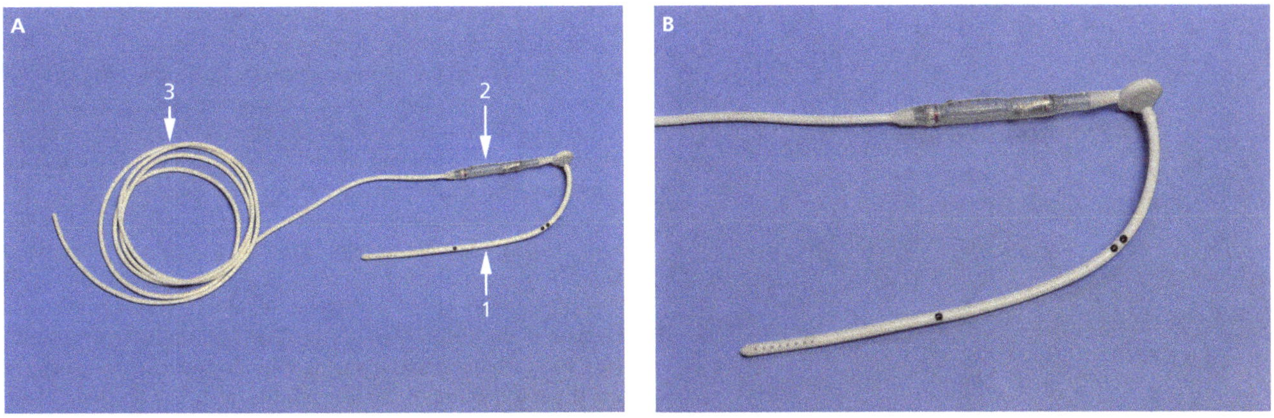

Figure 14.2 (A) Ventriculoperitoneal shunt showing the ventricular catheter (1), valve (2), and peritoneal catheter (3). (B) Close-up of the ventricular catheter and valve.

consist of one or more slits in the tubing that open and close based on the thickness and stiffness of the material. In human patients distal slits are associated with a greater incidence of shunt obstruction due to omentum or proteinaceous debris [5].

When the patient assumes an upright posture the effect of gravity on the long column of fluid has a significant effect on the pressure differential across the valve. Because the head is not open to atmospheric pressure, fluid will flow until the intraventricular pressure drops to negative to balance this pressure difference. This gravitational effect is called siphoning and can cause over-shunting. Siphon control devices and antisiphon devices detect negative pressure and increase resistance, theoretically preventing over-shunting. Gravity-actuated valves attempt to reduce siphoning by increasing opening pressure with the assistance of gravity when the patient sits or stands. Although siphoning has been shown to occur in laboratory dogs when they are in an upright posture, it is unclear how significant siphoning is in veterinary patients [6].

No data are available to determine which particular shunt should be recommended. In human patients, randomized trials comparing a standard differential valve to both siphon-limiting valves and flow-limiting valves have failed to show any difference in terms of overall shunt failure [7]. Another randomized trial compared an externally adjustable valve with fixed pressure valves and outcomes were nearly identical [8]. Similarly, there are no data to indicate the ideal opening pressure for veterinary patients. In human pediatric patients, medium- or high-pressure valves are more likely to fail than low-pressure valves, usually due to obstruction of the ventricular catheter associated with smaller ventricles [9]. For most cases, the surgeon should become familiar with a specific system and use that product consistently.

Preoperative Preparation

Shunt surgery has a high failure rate and requires meticulous attention to detail. Many complications are avoidable, such as intraparenchymal placement of the ventricular catheter, extraperitoneal placement of the distal catheter, and disconnection or migration of a shunt. A number of human studies have shown that prophylactic perioperative antibiotics are effective at reducing infection [10]. One protocol is cefazolin 20 mg/kg intravenously just before surgery, repeated every 90 min during surgery and then every 6 hours until 24 hours after surgery. The urinary bladder is emptied to avoid damage when placing the distal catheter.

The patient is positioned so there is a flat plane between the cranial and abdominal incision sites. This is aided by placing a rolled towel under the neck. Using preoperative brain imaging as a guide, the site of insertion of the ventricular catheter is chosen so that the catheter tip will be placed in the center of the occipital horn or frontal horn, caudal or rostral to the choroid plexus. The distance from the surface of the skull to the center of the ventricle is measured to determine the depth of insertion. The cranial incision is located 1–3 cm lateral to the nuchal crest. The abdominal incision is located 2–3 cm caudal to the last rib, about halfway between the lumbar spine and the ventral aspect of the abdomen. The patient is measured to determine the proper shunt length, planning on placing approximately one-third to half the shunt length into the abdomen. The distal catheter contributes a significant amount of the total resistance of the shunt system so care must be taken when shortening a distal catheter because this will affect the pressure–flow characteristics. Shunts with a distal slit valve cannot be cut to shorten them. The site of the burr-hole and abdominal incisions are selected and marked before draping.

The skin is clipped and surgically prepared for surgery from the skull along the entire subcutaneous pathway to the site of abdominal incision. Disposable adhesive drapes are used to cover the patient and operating table except for a small band of skin from the burr-hole site to the abdomen. A transparent adhesive sheet is applied to cover the remaining area of exposed skin (Figures 14.3 and 14.4).

Surgical Technique

For the cranial incision, the skin, subcutaneous tissue, and superficial muscles are incised. If necessary, the temporalis fascia is incised and the temporalis muscle elevated from the calvarium. A burr-hole slightly larger than the ventricular catheter and any anchoring clip is created using an air drill. Bone wax is applied for hemostasis. If the catheter is to be sutured to the skull, a second smaller burr-hole is created adjacent to the insertion site and nonabsorbable monofilament suture is preplaced by passing from the small hole to the large hole. The dura is coagulated with bipolar cautery and incised just large enough to accommodate the ventricular catheter without resistance and avoid CSF leakage around the catheter. The pia mater is carefully cauterized and nicked with a fine-tipped bipolar forceps (Figure 14.5).

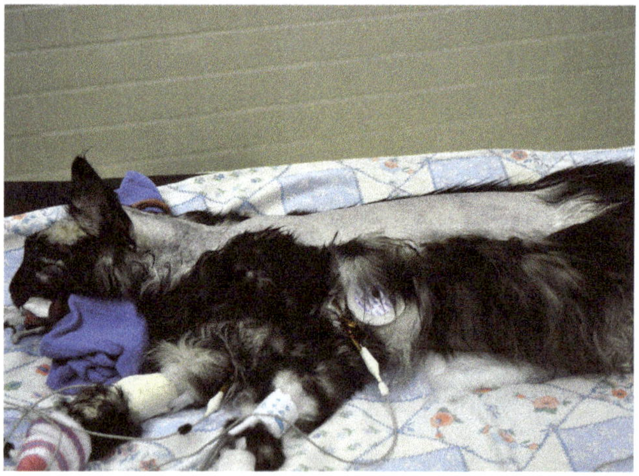

Figure 14.3 Patient positioning. The skin is clipped from the skull along the entire subcutaneous pathway to the site of abdominal incision. The patient is positioned so there is a flat plane between the cranial and abdominal incision sites with a rolled towel under the neck.

The skin and subcutaneous tissue are incised at the site of the abdominal incision. Any bleeding is controlled with bipolar cautery. To verify that the peritoneum cavity and not just the subcutaneous tissue or abdominal wall has been penetrated, a blunt forceps is passed well into the abdominal cavity. A pursestring suture is placed around the abdominal wall incision using a monofilament nonabsorbable suture material.

A subcutaneous tunnel is created connecting the two incisions using Doyen intestinal forceps. Alternatively, a shunt passer (e.g., Shunt Passer; Codman & Shurtleff, Raynham, MA) is helpful in creating this tunnel and pulling the shunt tubing from the cranial incision to the abdominal incision. The shunt passer consists of a long malleable tube containing a leader that attaches to the end of the shunt to pull the shunt through the tube. The tip of the shunt passer is inserted through the cranial incision and tunneled caudally through the subcutaneous tissues to the abdominal incision. Care must be taken during subcutaneous tunneling to avoid entering

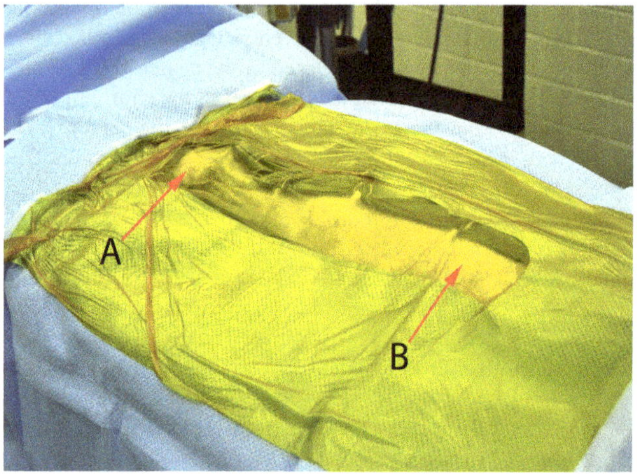

Figure 14.4 Draping of the patient. The cranial incision site (A), the path of the shunt, and the abdominal incision site (B) are draped and covered with a transparent adhesive sheet.

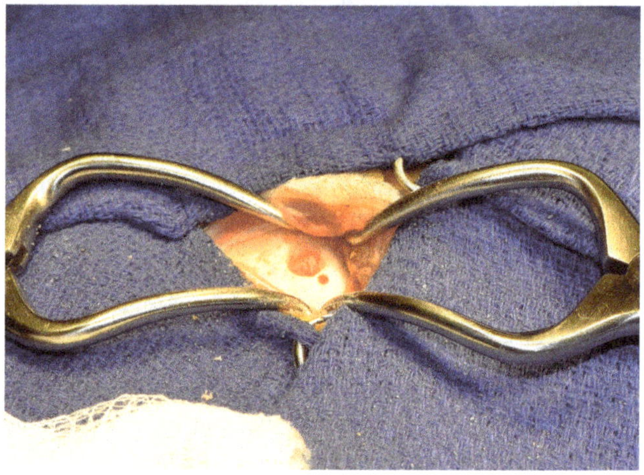

Figure 14.5 Cranial burr-holes. The temporalis fascia is incised and a portion of the temporalis muscle is reflected from the skull and retracted. A burr-hole slightly larger than the ventricular catheter and any anchoring clip is created using an air drill. A second, smaller burr-hole is created to accommodate suture to secure the ventricular catheter to the skull.

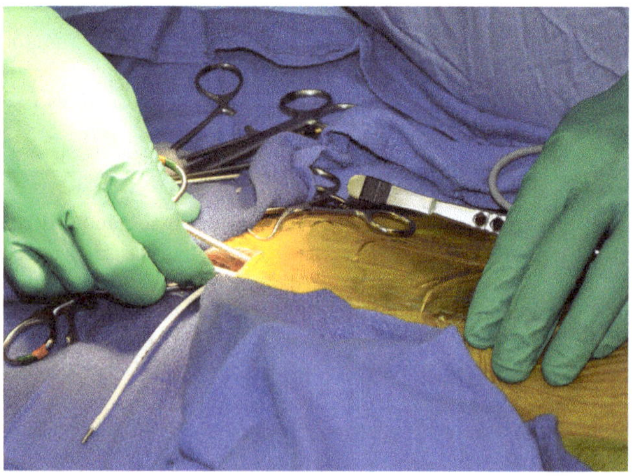

Figure 14.6 Creating a subcutaneous tunnel. Large forceps are passed subcutaneously along the pathway of the shunt from the cranial incision to the abdominal incision.

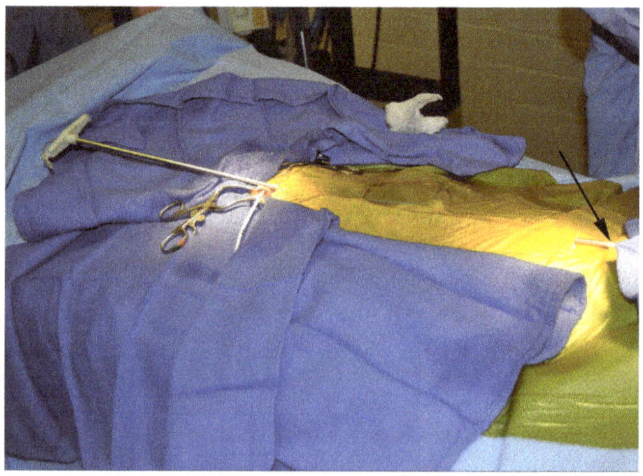

Figure 14.7 Use of a shunt passer. A malleable shunt passer is used to create the subcutaneous tunnel from the cranial incision site to the abdominal incision site. The tip of the shunt passer is visible exiting the abdominal incision site (arrow).

the chest or lacerating the skin. Bending the tunneling tube into a gentle curve helps follow the contour of the body; the tip is directed medially as it is passed over the thorax to the neck and then rotated 180° to pass over the skull. If excessive force is necessary, a separate incision in the neck is advisable [2]. The leader is attached to the distal end of the shunt and the shunt is pulled through the tube to the abdominal incision. Avoid contact between the shunt and the patient's skin as well as the surgeon's gloves by using blunt-tipped or sleeved forceps and clean surgical patties. The ventricular end of the catheter is held while the tube of the shunt passer is withdrawn through the abdominal incision. The valve is attached and irrigated with saline. It is not necessary to test the opening pressure of the valve because merely handling the valve will affect these measurements [2]. The distal end is placed into the sterile tray from the shunt package while the ventricular catheter is placed (Figures 14.6 and 14.7).

The trajectory of the ventricular catheter is determined according to external landmarks and measurements obtained from preoperative imaging. The surgeon will often feel a "pop" or loss of resistance as the catheter penetrates the ependyma and CSF flows from the catheter. If the location is uncertain, gently irrigating the catheter with saline will usually reveal pulsatile flow of CSF. Using a syringe to vigorously aspirate will only draw brain tissue into the catheter if it is placed in the parenchyma. A small amount of blood that clears is not uncommon. With more prolonged bleeding, the ventricular catheter is gently irrigated with warm saline until the CSF clears before connecting the shunt so that blood does not obstruct the valve (Figure 14.8).

The shunt is connected and secured by tying a nonabsorbable monofilament suture around the catheter over the connector. The suture is sufficiently tight to avoid subsequent disconnection but not too tight to lacerate the tubing. The peritoneal catheter is secured to the skull by tying the preplaced suture around the catheter. Alternatively, the shunt is tied to a small titanium screw placed in the skull near the burr-hole (Figures 14.9 and 14.10).

Once in place, the system is checked to ensure that it is flowing, either spontaneously or with gentle pumping of the reservoir. The distal catheter is then inserted into the abdomen and secured to the abdominal muscles with the pursestring suture in a finger-trap pattern (Figure 14.10). The scalp and abdominal subcutaneous tissue are closed with absorbable suture. The skin incisions are closed routinely.

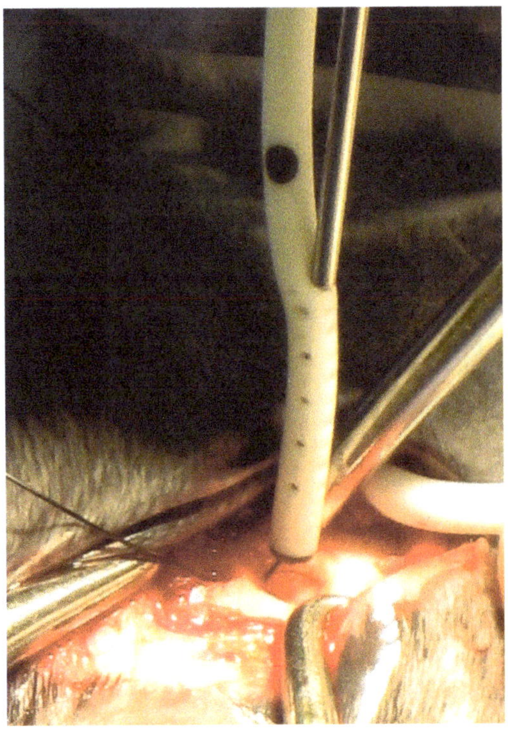

Figure 14.8 Inserting the ventricular catheter. A metal stylet is placed in the lumen of the ventricular catheter to assist inserting the catheter into the ventricle.

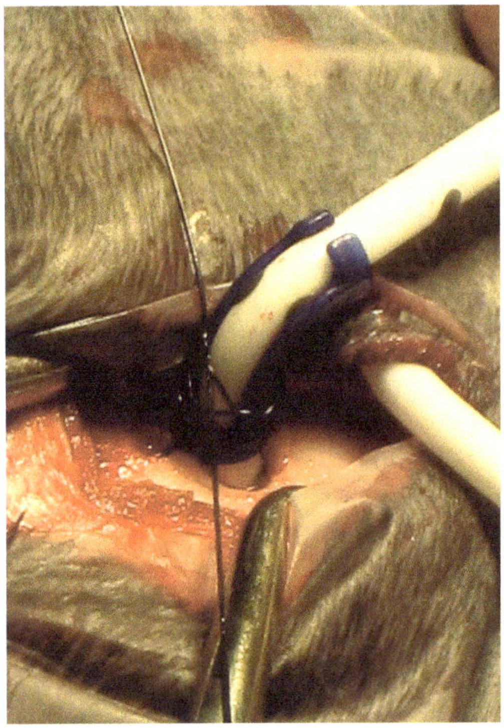

Figure 14.9 Anchoring the ventricular catheter and clip to the skull using the preplaced suture. To prevent dislodgement of the catheter, it is important to tie the suture around the catheter itself, not just to the clip.

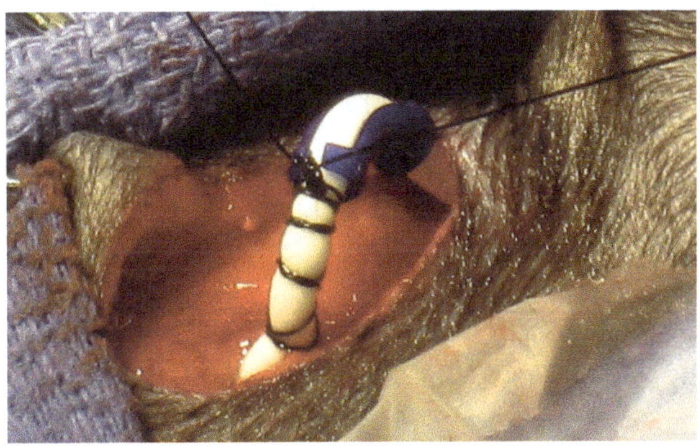

Figure 14.10 Anchoring the peritoneal catheter to the abdominal muscles.

Postoperative Management

Pain control is provided by injectable analgesics that are transitioned to oral medication. Preoperative antibiotics are occasionally continued for several days but prolonged antibiotic therapy is not indicated for uncomplicated cases. Any preoperative antiseizure medications are continued as needed. Two-view radiographs of the entire shunt from skull to abdomen are obtained to serve as a baseline for any future complications (Figure 14.11).

Preoperative neurological deficits usually resolve quickly. Patients are reassessed within the first 2 or 3 months with ultrasound, CT or MRI to measure ventricular size and serve as a baseline for subsequent follow-up.

Complications

Obstruction

Obstruction to flow can arise at any point along the shunt system but most commonly occurs at the ventricular catheter. Over-drainage probably increases the risk of obstruction because as the ventricle collapses the catheter can adhere to the ventricular wall or become embedded in the choroid plexus [11]. Obstruction of the valve is less common and usually occurs soon after shunt insertion, presumably from blood or cellular debris. Kinking of the shunt system can also cause obstruction. Obstruction causes recurrence of the original neurological signs [12,13].

Disconnection and Migration

Shunt components can become disconnected, the ventricular catheter can slide out of the ventricle, or the distal catheter can move out of the peritoneal cavity [13,14]. These complications usually occur soon after placement and are detectable on survey radiographs.

Over-drainage

Over-drainage can result in collapse of the ventricle and cerebral cortex and accumulation of extraaxial blood or fluid. This is most common in patients with very large ventricles. Subdural fluid accumulation is often asymptomatic, but a large or rapidly expanding hematoma can result in progressive neurological deficits [14].

In human patients, over-drainage can lead to very small ventricles and episodes of increased intracranial pressure and headache, called slit ventricle syndrome or noncompliant ventricle syndrome. Very small ventricles allow the brain to almost completely fill the intracranial space, which decreases the ability to compensate for transient increases in intracranial volume. Episodes of pain can occur after shunting in dogs and may be similar to slit ventricle syndrome in human patients [12].

Infection

In human patients, 8–10% of shunts become infected within 6 months [15]. A similar rate of infection has been reported in veterinary patients [13,14]. Shunt infections present as shunt obstruction, meningitis, or nonspecific signs such as fever and lethargy. Diagnosis is based on cytology and culture of CSF collected from the shunt system. Infection may resolve with 4 weeks of antibiotic therapy chosen based on culture and sensitivity [13]. Resolution of infection is documented with follow-up cytology and culture of CSF. Persistent infection requires exchange of the shunt.

Shunt Revision

Indications for shunt revision include shunt obstruction, disconnection, migration or kinking, and infection. Surgery for shunt revision is similar to initial shunt placement with a few important exceptions. If the site of obstruction is unknown, the ventricular catheter is explored first. For two-component systems, the ventricular catheter is disconnected to determine if CSF is flowing freely from the ventricular catheter. If the ventricular catheter is occluded, it is gently removed and quickly replaced with a new catheter before the ventricle collapses. Gently rotating the catheter may free an adherent catheter. If not, the metal stylet is inserted through the catheter to the tip and cautery applied to the stylet while rotating the catheter. Extremely adherent catheters are best left in place to avoid substantial hemorrhage and a second ventricular catheter placed [2]. If the valve or peritoneal catheter is occluded, it can be replaced and attached to the existing ventricular catheter.

Prognosis

Approximately 85% of dogs treated with shunting have long-term improvement; 15% of patients require shunt revision, usually due to shunt obstruction, fracture or migration [12,13].

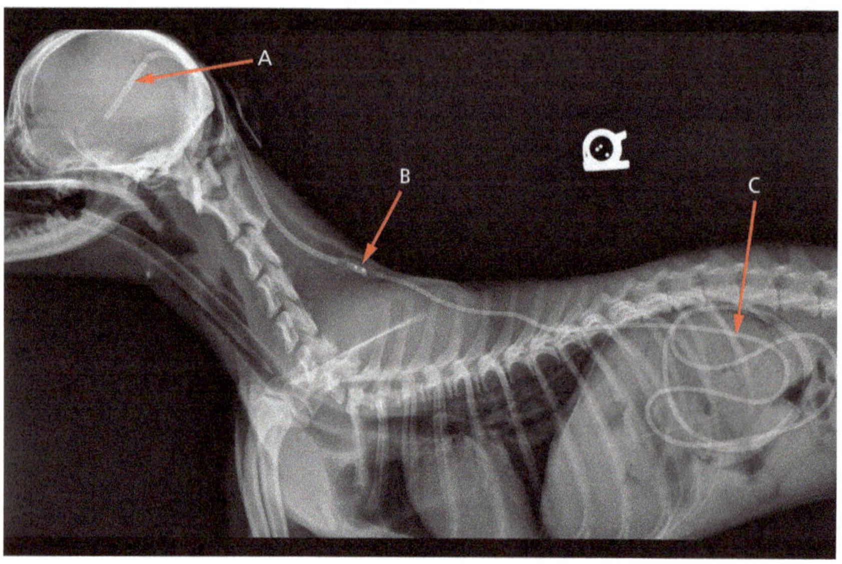

Figure 14.11 Postoperative lateral radiograph to document placement of a ventriculoperitoneal shunt. The ventricular catheter (A), valve and access port (B), and peritoneal catheter (C) are visible.

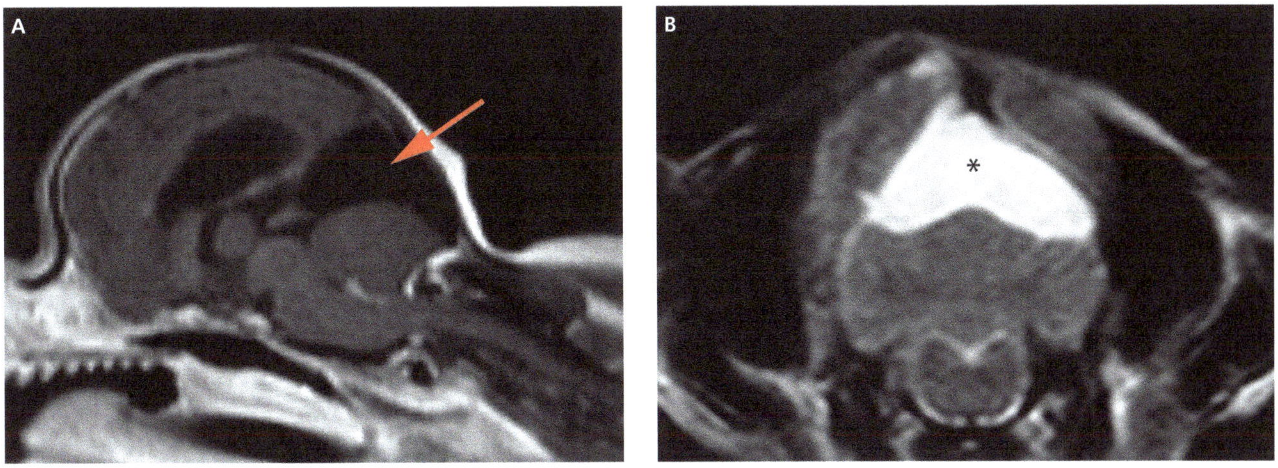

Figure 14.12 MRI of a quadrigeminal cistern. (A) Sagittal T1-weighted image after contrast administration. The diverticulum (arrow) is located dorsal to and compressing the cerebellum. The diverticulum is isointense to CSF and does not enhance. (B) Transverse T2-weighted image at the level of the diverticulum. The diverticulum (asterisk) is isointense with respect to CSF with sharp margins between the diverticulum and the surrounding brain parenchyma.

Quadrigeminal Diverticula

Arachnoid diverticula, also called intraarachnoid diverticula, are lined with arachnoidal membrane and usually contain fluid that is virtually identical to normal CSF. They may or may not communicate with the subarachnoid space. The pathogenesis is not well understood but is thought to be due to a defect early in fetal development, possibly from aberrant CSF flow that splits the developing arachnoid [16]. Most arachnoid diverticula do not expand over time but some do, possibly because some diverticula may communicate with the subarachnoid space via a one-way valve mechanism that allows CSF to enter the space during systole [16]. In dogs and cats, the most common location is the quadrigeminal cistern, dorsal to the midbrain, rostral to the cerebellum, and caudal to the occipital lobes. These are often incidental lesions and are referred to as quadrigeminal diverticula or supracollicular collections of fluid. When clinical signs occur they are related to mass effect on adjacent brain tissue or obstruction of CSF pathways.

Medical therapy is the same as for hydrocephalus, although there is limited published information regarding the efficacy of medical treatment for clinically significant quadrigeminal diverticula. Definitive treatment consists of surgical fenestration or placement of a diverticuloperitoneal shunt (Figure 14.12).

Preoperative Evaluation

Quadrigeminal diverticula are most common in small and brachycephalic breeds, with Shih Tzus being the most common. Many affected dogs develop clinical signs by 1 year of age but older dogs can also be affected. Quadrigeminal diverticula have also been reported in cats [17,18]. Seizures, ataxia, vestibular dysfunction, and neck pain are the most common neurological signs.

Diagnosis is confirmed with imaging. Quadrigeminal diverticula are located between the collicular plate and the incisural notch of the tentorium. The diverticulum does not communicate with the fourth ventricle and there is no hypoplasia of the cerebellum. In some patients, ultrasound through the foramen magnum shows the diverticulum as a large fluid-filled structure immediately rostral to the cerebellum [19]. On CT, the diverticulum is isodense with respect to CSF with sharp margins between the diverticulum and the surrounding brain parenchyma [20]. MRI is the best modality to identify concurrent lesions and distinguish the CSF-like fluid of arachnoid diverticula from the proteinaceous fluid of other fluid-filled lesions [20–22]. The walls of the diverticulum do not enhance after intravenous contrast administration. Analysis of CSF is helpful in identifying or ruling out inflammatory lesions.

The most important diagnostic consideration is distinguishing clinically significant diverticula from incidental findings. Small asymptomatic diverticula are ignored. Surgery is indicated in patients with large diverticula causing mass effect and neurological deficits. One study found the degree of mass effect correlated to the presence of clinical signs. Using mid-sagittal MRI, dogs with compression of the occipital lobe greater than 14% (compared with the expected rostrocaudal length of the forebrain) always suffered neurological signs while patients with compression of both the occipital lobe and cerebellum were more likely to have clinical signs compared to dogs with compression of only one region or no compression [21]. Since many patients have an incidental finding of a quadrigeminal diverticulum, it is important to rule out other causes of neurological signs, such as encephalitis, before a quadrigeminal diverticulum is considered clinically significant.

Surgical Techniques

Surgery involves fenestration and marsupialization of the diverticulum into the subarachnoid space or diverticuloperitoneal shunting. Fenestration avoids the ubiquitous problems of shunting, such as shunt failure and infection. Conversely, shunting requires less extensive surgical exposure and avoids reexpansion of the diverticulum if the fenestration closes. Currently there are no data to indicate which technique, if either, is better for veterinary patients.

Quadrigeminal Diverticulum Fenestration

An occipital craniectomy usually provides adequate exposure for fenestration of quadrigeminal diverticula and the technique is similar to that described for Chiari decompression (see Chapter 12). The patient is placed in sternal recumbency, with the neck ventroflexed. The dorsal aspect of the head and neck is clipped and prepared from the level of the bregma to the level of the third cervical vertebra. A dorsal midline incision is made extending from approximately 1 cm rostral to the external occipital protuberance to the middle of the spinous process of C2. The muscles are sharply incised on the midline, elevated off the occiput, and retracted laterally to expose the caudal portion of the occiput and the arch of C1. Hemorrhage is controlled with bipolar electrocautery.

A high-speed air drill and Lempert and Kerrison rongeurs are used to remove a portion of the occiput. Borders of the craniectomy are the atlanto-occipital joints laterally, the foramen magnum ventrally, and a point approximately halfway between the external occipital protuberance and the dorsal aspect of the foramen magnum dorsally. The diverticulum is located dorsal and rostral to the cerebellum. Larger diverticula are evident at the dorsal portion of the craniectomy whereas smaller diverticula may require gentle retraction of the cerebellum ventrally for exposure. The dura over the diverticulum usually has a blueish tint. The dura is incised on the midline, extending from the dorsal to the ventral aspect of the craniectomy. Any dural vessels are coagulated with bipolar cautery and the dura is sharply incised. The outer wall of the diverticulum is often adherent to the dura. Most of the outer wall of the diverticulum is excised to provide a wide communication with the subarachnoid space. There is little if any benefit in attempting to strip the inner wall of the diverticulum from the adjacent neural tissue. A collagen-based dural graft implant (Duraform; Codman & Shurtleff, Raynham, MA) is trimmed to fit the craniectomy and laid in place. Closure is routine.

If the majority of the diverticulum is located rostral to the tentorium, exposure involves a rostrotentorial craniectomy or if necessary a combined rostrotentorial/suboccipital craniectomy with sacrifice of the transverse sinus. The combined approach provides greater exposure but carries a risk of hemorrhage from the transverse sinus. Rostrotentorial craniectomy is described in Chapter 11. For a combined lateral rostrotentorial/suboccipital craniectomy, a horseshoe-shaped incision is made starting on the dorsal midline at the bregma, extending caudally to the occipital protuberance, and curving ventrally to a point just caudal to the ear. The temporalis fascia is incised lateral to the sagittal crest, leaving enough fascia medially to suture for closure. The temporalis muscle is reflected off the lateral surface of the skull down to the level of the zygomatic arch and retracted rostrally. The muscles overlying the occiput are incised along the nuchal crest on the operated side and reflected caudally. A rostrotentorial craniectomy is created in the parietal and temporal bones using an air drill as described. An occipital craniotomy is performed as described for diverticulum fenestration. The drill is then used to remove the bone overlying the lateral aspect of the transverse sinus, being careful not to penetrate the sinus. After the majority of bone is removed to expose the sinus, bone wax is placed in the dorsal and ventral aspect of the boney canal to occlude the transverse sinus. The collapsed sinus and any remaining bone are removed with a Lempert and Kerrison rongeurs. This allows the rostrotentorial craniectomy to be connected with the occipital craniectomy.

Diverticuloperitoneal Shunt

Shunting can be performed with an occipital, rostrotentorial, or a combined rostrotentorial/suboccipital craniectomy, depending on the location of the majority of the diverticula. A shunt system designed to treat hydrocephalus is used. Once the bone is removed the diverticulum is located. The site of catheter insertion is located at the ventrolateral aspect of the diverticulum adjacent to the lateral edge of the craniectomy. To confirm the diverticulum location, a 25G needle can be used to puncture the dura and a small amount of fluid aspirated. Do not remove so much fluid that the diverticulum collapses. A small hole is drilled in the bone adjacent to the site of catheter insertion and nonabsorbable monofilament suture is preplaced to secure the catheter. Alternatively, the suture can be tied to a small titanium screw inserted into the skull.

The dura is coagulated with bipolar cautery and incised just large enough to accommodate the ventricular catheter without resistance and avoid CSF leakage around the catheter. The ventricular catheter is placed into the diverticulum in a transverse orientation and secured to the edge of the craniectomy with the preplaced suture tied in a finger-trap pattern around the catheter or anchored to the titanium screw. The distal portion of the shunt is tunneled subcutaneously and inserted into the abdomen as described for ventriculoperitoneal shunt placement. The cranial and abdominal incisions are closed routinely.

Postoperative Management

Adequate analgesics are provided and any antiseizure medications continued. For patients with a diverticuloperitoneal shunt, two-view radiographs of the entire shunt from skull to abdomen are obtained. Any preoperative medications such as prednisone and diuretics are tapered as the neurological deficits resolve. If neurological deficits persist or recur later, CT or MRI is performed to assess diverticulum size.

Prognosis

The prognosis with both fenestration/marsupialization and shunting is generally good [18,20,23,24]. Neurological deficits usually resolve soon after surgery, although seizures may persist. Complications associated with diverticuloperitoneal shunting are similar to those for ventriculoperitoneal shunting, including shunt obstruction, migration, disconnection, and infection. The main complications associated with diverticulum fenestration are incomplete resolution or recurrence of the diverticulum.

Editors' Note

Fenestration and Marsupialization of the Lateral Ventricles

In human pediatric neurosurgery, neuroendoscopic fenestration of the third ventricle into the basal cistern (endoscopic third ventriculostomy or ETV) has often replaced the use of ventriculoperitoneal shunts in the treatment of hydrocephalus. The technique restores physiological CSF circulation, and implantation of external shunt valve systems can be avoided [25]. A technique using the same principle in young dogs and cats has been used successfully by one of the editors (A.S.). This technique involves a small opening into the lateral ventricle through an overlying cerebral gyrus, insertion of a small uninflated Foley catheter, inflation of the catheter, removal of the inflated catheter to enhance the size of the fenestration and to pull the ventricular lining into the opening, and finally performing a duraplasty over the fenestration to allow flow of CSF into the subarachnoid space (Figure 14.13). Short-term results have been very good in a vast majority of patients [26].

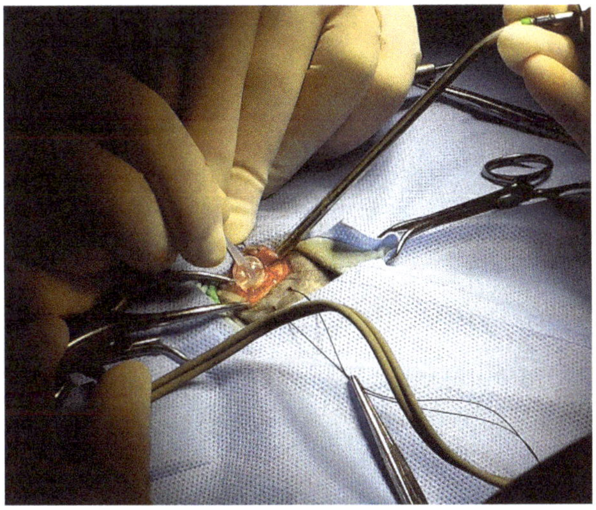

Figure 14.13 An inflated Foley catheter is removed from the lateral ventricle of a kitten with severe congenital hydrocephalus. This procedure produced a fenestration of the lateral ventricle with flow of CSF into the subarachnoid space. A duroplasty was performed over the fenestration to allow continued flow of CSF. Presented with severe central vestibular signs and seizures, the patient had no complications and quickly returned to normal neurological status. Follow-up examination 6 months after surgery revealed normal neurological status and imaging revealed a reduction in ventricular size and patency of the fenestration.

Video clips to accompany this book can be found on the companion website at: www.wiley.com/go/shores/neurosurgery

References

1 Rekate HL. A contemporary definition and classification of hydrocephalus. *Semin Pediatr Neurol* 2009;16:9–15.

2 Iantosca MR, Drake JM. Cerebrospinal fluid shunts. In: Albright AL, Pollack IF, Adelson PD (eds) *Operative Techniques in Pediatric Neurosurgery*. New York: Thieme, 2001: 3–14.

3 Klimo P Jr, Thompson CJ, Ragel BT, Boop FA. Antibiotic-impregnated shunt systems versus standard shunt systems: a meta- and cost-savings analysis. *J Neurosurg Pediatr* 2011;8:600–612.

4 Anderson RCE, Garton HJL, Kestle JRW. Treatment of hydrocephalus with shunts. In: Albright AL, Pollack IF, Adelson PD (eds) *Principles and Practice of Pediatric Neurosurgery*, 2nd edn. New York: Thieme, 2008: 109–130.

5 Cozzens JW, Chandler JP. Increased risk of distal ventriculoperitoneal shunt obstruction associated with slit valves or distal slits in the peritoneal catheter. *J Neurosurg* 1997;87:682–686.

6 Yamada S, Ducker TB, Perot PL. Dynamic changes of cerebrospinal fluid in upright and recumbent shunted experimental animals. *Childs Brain* 1975;1:187–192.

7 Kestle J, Drake J, Milner R et al. Long-term follow-up data from the Shunt Design Trial. *Pediatr Neurosurg* 2000;33:230–236.

8 Pollack IF, Albright AL, Adelson PD. A randomized, controlled study of a programmable shunt valve versus a conventional valve for patients with hydrocephalus. *Neurosurgery* 1999;45:1399–1408.

9 Robinson S, Kaufman BA, Park TS. Outcome analysis of initial neonatal shunts: does the valve make a difference? *Pediatr Neurosurg* 2002;37:287–294.

10 Ratilal B, Costa J, Sampaio C. Antibiotic prophylaxis for surgical introduction of intracranial ventricular shunts: a systematic review. *J Neurosurg Pediatr* 2008;1:48–56.

11 Sainte-Rose C, Piatt JH, Renier D et al. Mechanical complications in shunts. *Pediatr Neurosurg* 1991;17:2–9.

12 Shihab N, Davies E, Kenny PJ, Loderstedt S, Volk HA. Treatment of hydrocephalus with ventriculoperitoneal shunting in twelve dogs. *Vet Surg* 2011;40:477–484.

13 de Stefani A, de Risio L, Platt SR, Matiasek L, Lujan-Feliu-Pascual A, Garosi LS. Surgical technique, postoperative complications and outcome in 14 dogs treated for hydrocephalus by ventriculoperitoneal shunting. *Vet Surg* 2011;40:183–191.

14 Kitagawa M, Kanayama K, Sakai T. Subdural accumulation of fluid in a dog after the insertion of a ventriculoperitoneal shunt. *Vet Rec* 2005;156:206–208.

15 Campbell JW. Shunt infections. In: Albright AL, Pollack IF, Adelson PD (eds) *Principles and Practice of Pediatric Neurosurgery*, 2nd edn. New York: Thieme, 2008: 1141–1161.

16 Wilkinson CC, Winston KR. Congenital arachnoid cysts and the Dandy-Walker complex. In: Albright AL, Pollack IF, Adelson PD (eds) *Principles and Practice of Pediatric Neurosurgery*, 2nd edn. New York: Thieme, 2012: 162–186.

17 Reed S, Cho DY, Paulsen D. Quadrigeminal arachnoid cysts in a kitten and a dog. *J Vet Diagn Invest* 2009;21:707–710.

18 Lowrie M, Wessmann A, Gunn-Moore D, Penderis J. Quadrigeminal cyst management by cystoperitoneal shunt in a 4-year-old Persian cat. *J Feline Med Surg* 2009;11:711–713.

19 Saito M, Olby NJ, Spaulding K. Identification of arachnoid cysts in the quadrigeminal cistern using ultrasonography. *Vet Radiol Ultrasound* 2001;42:435–439.

20 Vernau KM, Kortz GD, Koblik PD, LeCouteur RA, Bailey CS, Pedroia V. Magnetic resonance imaging and computed tomography characteristics of intracranial intra-arachnoid cysts in 6 dogs. *Vet Radiol Ultrasound* 1997;38:171–176.

21 Matiasek LA, Platt SR, Shaw S, Dennis R. Clinical and magnetic resonance imaging characteristics of quadrigeminal cysts in dogs. *J Vet Intern Med* 2007;21:1021–1026.

22 Kitagawa M, Kanayama K, Sakai T. Quadrigeminal cisterna arachnoid cyst diagnosed by MRI in five dogs. *Aust Vet J* 2003;81:340–343.

23 Dewey CW, Krotscheck U, Bailey KS, Marino DJ. Craniotomy with cystoperitoneal shunting for treatment of intracranial arachnoid cysts in dogs. *Vet Surg* 2007;36:416–422.

24 Dewey CW, Scrivani PV, Krotscheck U, Cerda-Gonzalez S, Smith Bailey K, Marino DJ. Intracranial arachnoid cysts in dogs. *Compend Contin Educ Vet* 2009;31:160–168.

25 Guzman R, Pendharkar AV, Zerah M, Sainte-Rose C. Use of the NeuroBalloon catheter for endoscopic third ventriculostomy: technical note. *J Neurosurg Pediatr* 2013;11:302–306.

26 Shores A, Kornberg S, Beasley MB et al. Fenestration of the lateral ventricle in the management of obstructive hydrocephalus in young small animals. In: *Proceedings of the American College of Veterinary Internal Medicine Forum 2015*. Lakewood, CO: American College of Veterinary Internal Medicine, 2015. Available at http://www.vin.com/acvim/2015/Default.htm

SECTION III

Spinal Procedures

15 Atlantoaxial Subluxation

Fred Wininger

Introduction

Atlantoaxial subluxation (AAS) is a relatively common spinal instability disorder primarily seen in young toy-breed dogs [1,2], but can occur in larger breeds [3] and any patient when associated with a traumatic event. It is rarely reported in cats [2]. In the young toy breeds, the condition is generally associated with a combination of anatomical deformities coupled with an often supraphysiological movement that leads to joint laxity and subsequent compressive cervical myelopathy. Though often challenging, reduction and stabilization of these cases can be rewarding, often with complete long-term return to function.

Anatomy

Atlas and Axis

The first cervical vertebra (C1) is also known as the atlas because of its transversely elongated shape. C1 articulates with the skull cranially and the axis (C2) caudally. C1 is different from the typical cervical vertebrae in that it lacks a spinous process, has elongated transverse processes, and has concave articular processes that abut the occipital condyles of the skull. The atlantooccipital joint is also known as the "yes joint" as it allows for free dorsal/ventral movement but is limited on lateral flexibility.

C2 is notable because of its large and cranially protruding spinous process that is the site of attachment of the nuchal ligament in many species. Its transverse processes are shorter than adjacent vertebrae and its body notably longer. The ventral tubercle rises from the ventral surface of the body and is an important structure in identifying the joint during ventral approaches, as it is sharper than other midline processes of the ventral cervical spine [4].

The embryology of C1 and C2 is complex and potentially provides insight into the mechanism of AAS. The atlas arises from three bony components, two neural arches that form the vertebral arch and a body. The axis arises from seven total components [4].

C1 and C2 articulate via the caudal articular surface of C1 (fovea articularis caudalis). This is frequently known as the "no joint" as rotary movement is permitted but ligamentous structures prevent dorsal/ventral flexion. It is notable that there is no intervertebral disc between C1 and C2 and ligaments maintain the position of the vertebrae [5].

The odontoid process (dens) arises from the body of C2 and rests in the fovea of the dens (fovea dentis) on the dorsal surface of the C1 body. Interestingly, the dens is analogous to the intercentrum of C1, but during development permanently ossifies as a protuberance of C2. Occasionally, there is a malformation or dorsal notching of the dens that may lead to spinal cord compression, even while in normal reduction. Some have hypothesized that this is the result of abnormal fusion of the proatlas, a transient area of ossification at the apical tip of the dens. The proatlas fuses with the dens at 106 days after birth [4,5].

Ligaments

Dorsally, the joint is maintained via a dorsal atlantoaxial membrane connecting the spinous process of C2 with the vertebral arch of C1. The transverse atlantal ligament tethers between the ventral arches of C1 and maintains the dens in the fovea dentis in a retinaculum fashion that forms a large bursa in between. The apical ligament of the dens is actually a remnant of the primitive notochord as are the nucleus pulposi of the intervertebral discs. It is composed of the solitary apical ligament that traverses through the vertebral canal of C1 and attaches to the ventral surface of the foramen magnum and the paired lateralized alar ligaments, which attach medial to the occipital condyles [6].

Pathophysiology

AAS is likely a condition that is most frequently a developmental anomaly exacerbated by a physiological or supraphysiological/traumatic cervical movement. Contributing developmental factors include aplasia or hypoplasia of the dens, nonunion of the dens with the axis, or absence of the transverse ligament. When presenting in signalments noncharacteristic to AAS, the etiology is often purely traumatic with failure of the otherwise normal ligaments [7].

Current Techniques in Canine and Feline Neurosurgery, First Edition. Edited by Andy Shores and Brigitte A. Brisson.
© 2017 John Wiley & Sons, Inc. Published 2017 by John Wiley & Sons, Inc.
Companion website: www.wiley.com/go/shores/neurosurgery

AAS has been linked to other craniocervical junction diseases such as Chiari-like malformation (caudal occipital malformation syndrome) and atlantooccipital overlap (AOO). There is a decreased distance between the dorsal arch of the atlas and the supraoccipital bone with AOO, with the rostral aspect of the atlas either located immediately ventral to the foramen magnum or within the caudal fossa. This syndrome has been compared with basilar invagination seen in human children [8]. Though a genetic cause of AAS has been speculated, no specific mode of inheritance or candidate genes have been identified; however, the Yorkshire Terrier is most often affected [9].

Clinical Signs

AAS is most frequently seen in toy-breed dogs less than 2 years of age, although a variety of large-breed signalments have been reported. The most common clinical complaint is cervical hyperesthesia, noted in 53–77% of dogs [9,10]. Care is taken when ventroflexing the neck on examination as it may lead to displacement of the dens into the vertebral canal, and severe consequences [10]. Anatomical variation can lead to a dorsally deviated or even absent dens. An absent dens often prevents severe compressive myelopathy even in the face of significant atlantoaxial laxity. Dogs may show other clinical signs consistent with a C1–C5 myelopathy, including a proprioceptive ataxia and tetraparesis. A cranial cervical vestibular syndrome can occur, possibly associated with vestibulospinal tract injury or collateral brainstem injury [1]. In more severe cases, patients can present for brainstem disease associated with basilar artery trauma or ventilatory compromise, a potential in any high cervical injury [10].

Diagnosis

AAS should be a differential for any patient presented for a static or progressive C1–C5 myelopathy. Care is taken when preparing these patients for imaging diagnostics, especially while sedated or anesthetized as inadvertent flexion can have catastrophic consequences. The author prefers to place a soft padded bandage on the patients to maintain cervical extension during diagnostic work-up prior to surgical correction.

Traditionally, cervical radiography without myelography is the primary means of diagnosing AAS. Lateral radiographs are the preferred view with a gap of 4–5 mm between the spinous process of C2 and vertebral arch of C1 for a definitive diagnosis (Figure 15.1). Slight flexion of the cervical spine is sometimes needed to elicit the gap. This is safely performed under fluoroscopy or serial radiography. A ventrodorsal view can be helpful in identifying the dens and assessing its anatomical variations. Myelography can emphasize the degree of spinal cord compression secondary to AAS but is usually unnecessary. Myelography is difficult in these patients as positioning for a cisterna magna injection requires cervical ventroflexion and poses the risk of postprocedure seizures [12].

CT and MRI have elevated the diagnosis of AAS in that tomographic/cross-sectional imaging increases the sensitivity of AAS detection and aids in excluding concurrent cervical/skull base disease. CT is advantageous because of its speed, usually obviating the need for heavy anesthesia in these potentially higher-risk patients. CT is also preferable in creating bony three-dimensional reconstructions, which can be helpful in planning surgery and assessing the atlanto-occipital interface as well (Figure 15.2). A recent study showed a high sensitivity for detecting incomplete ossification of C1 with CT. A strong association was made between incomplete C1 ossification and AAS [13].

The superior soft tissue contrast resolution of MRI allows for visualization not only of the subluxation itself, but also the consequences on the adjacent spinal cord parenchyma, including gliosis, hematomyelia [10], degree of "kinking," and syringohydromyelia. In addition to spinal cord compression dorsal to the dens, other MRI features of AAS include an area of T2 signal dorsal to the dens and increased space in the ventral atlantoaxial joint ventral to the dens (Figures 15.3 and 15.4). Though traditionally thought of as difficult to identify by MRI, the ligaments of the atlantoaxial joint can be visualized by this modality [14]. As the brain can be simultaneously imaged, MRI allows detection of other concurrent and possibly related brain disease such as hydrocephalus, quadrigeminal cysts, AOO, and Chiari-like malformation [15].

The combination of CT and MRI is becoming more frequently advocated because of the frequency with which craniocervical junction abnormalities are being identified. The sensitivity for identifying these lesions increases with combined use of these modalities [15].

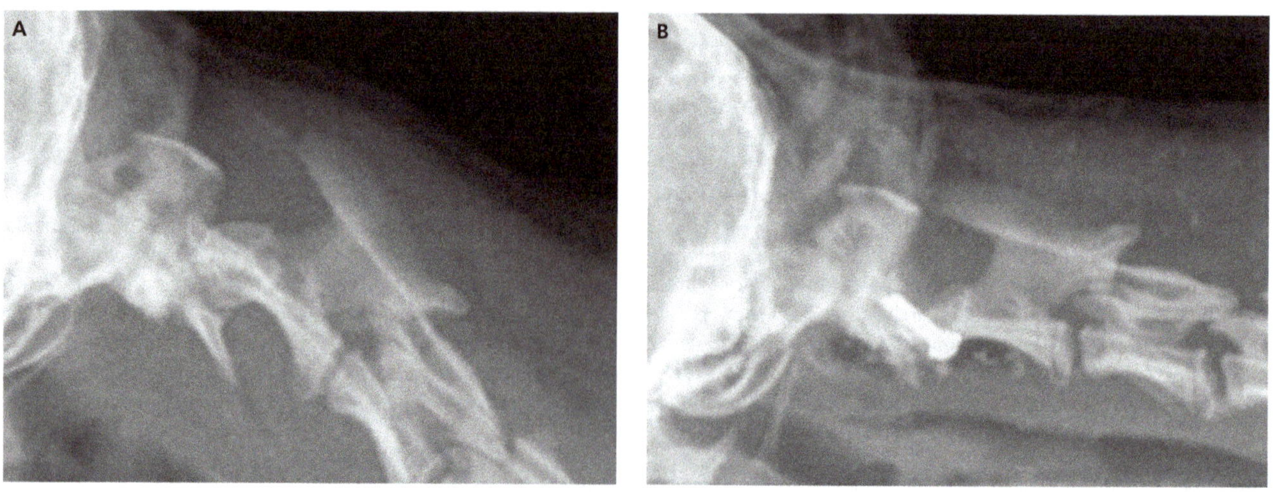

Figure 15.1 (A) Lateral cervical radiograph shows increased distance between the dorsal arch of C1 and the spinous process of C2 diagnostic for AAS. The dens is displaced dorsally into the vertebral canal. (B) Postoperative radiograph demonstrates reduction of the AAS with transarticular screw stabilization.

Medical Management

The two primary indications for medical management are patient age and financial constraints for the client. As AAS patients are most frequently toy-breed animals, those younger than 6–8 months are often not considered good candidates for surgery because of size challenges and lack of boney mineralization. Surgical correction is often delayed until there is radiographic evidence of physis closure at the vertebral endplate.

In the author's experience, the frequent replacement of the splint compounded with possible complications associated with the coaptation is often financially comparable to the surgical procedure itself. Havig et al. [16] reported on the medical management of AAS, citing a 10 of 16 case success with external coaptation when used for 1 month, particularly when the clinical signs were for less than 30 days. Ventral splinting is easier, with a contoured rigid plate made of fiberglass or orthoplast maintained in position by a modified Robert Jones type bandage (Figure 15.5).

Surgical Procedures

Surgical stabilization of AAS can be classified as dorsal and ventral approaches [1]. The ventral approaches are more commonly utilized and are reported to have a higher rate of success [9].

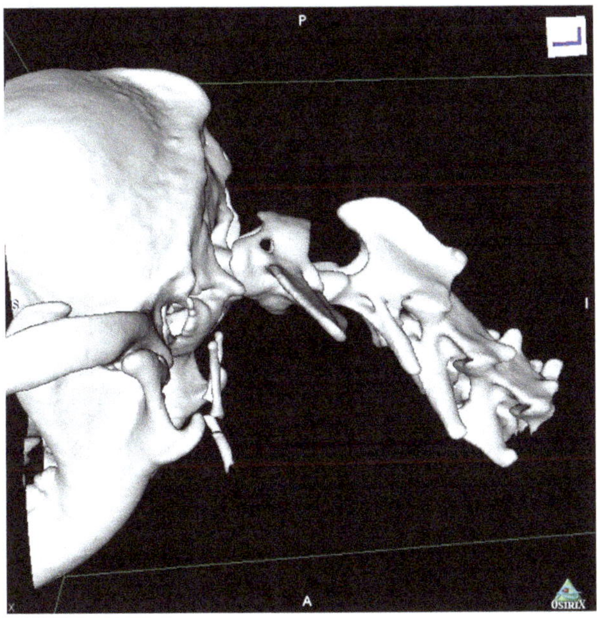

Figure 15.2 Three-dimensional CT of an atlantoaxial subluxation.

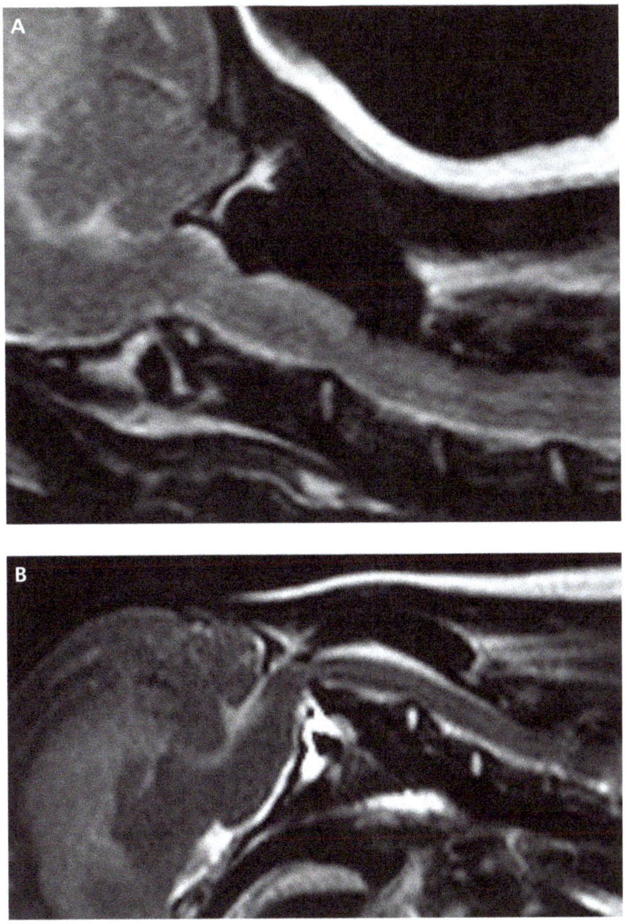

Figure 15.3 (A) Cervical neutral and (B) flexed positioning can be performed in the MRI unit. Note on the flexed view the increased space between the ventral body of C1 and the dens as well as the adjacent dorsal compressive myelopathy.

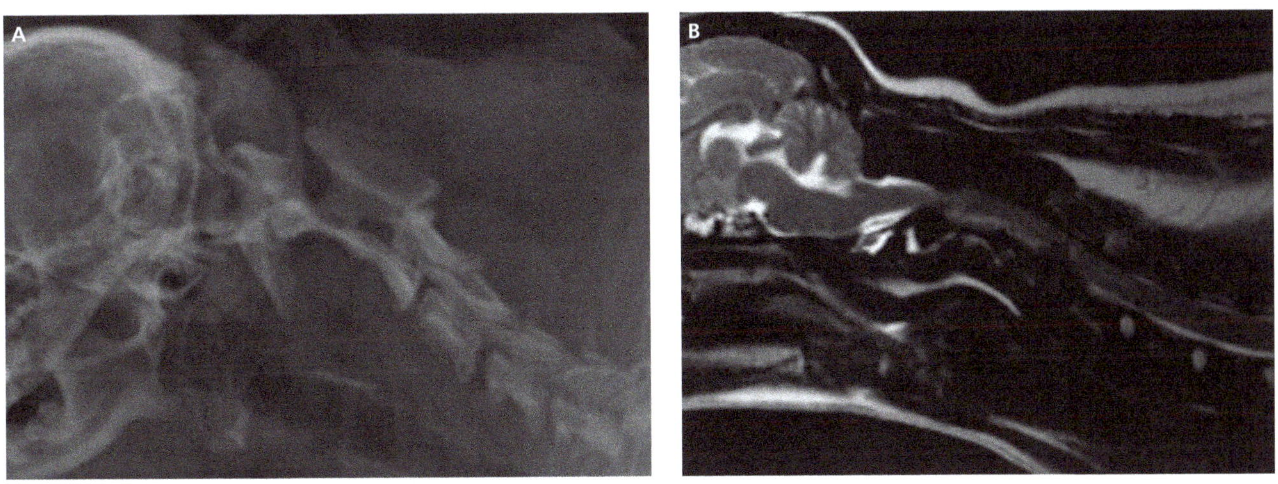

Figure 15.4 A 5-year-old female spayed Pekinese presents for a C1–C5 myelopathy. (A) Lateral radiograph demonstrates atlantoaxial subluxation and congenital fusion of the C2–C3 vertebral bodies. (B) MRI demonstrates the atlantoaxial subluxation and congenital C2–C3 fusion plus a severe compressive myelopathy secondary to intervertebral disc disease at C3–C4.

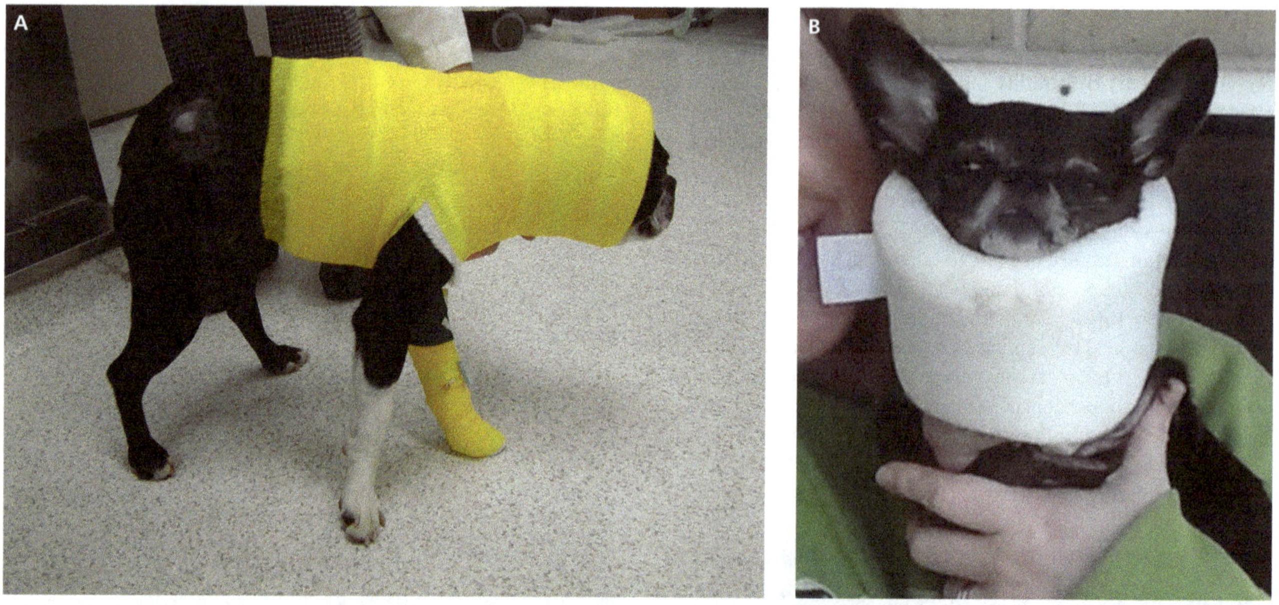

Figure 15.5 Types of external coaptation used for conservative therapy and postoperatively for approximately 6 weeks to maintain the atlantoaxial joint in an extended position to allow fusion. (A) A contoured rigid plate made of fiberglass or orthoplast maintained in position by a modified Robert Jones type bandage. (B) A soft, commercially available splint.

Dorsal Approach

The dorsal approach to the cervical spine in cases of AAS is desirable in that it has the potential for placement of a replica prosthesis for the dorsal atlantoaxial ligament. As this ligament is thought to be an important cause of failure in cases of AAS, this solution possibly provides a more physiological correction. It also provides less strain on the implants than a ventral stabilization, as this is the tension not compression surface [17]. However, the dorsal procedure is rarely performed for a number of reasons: the soft tissue approach requires a greater degree of muscle dissection, is associated with higher morbidity due to incisional complications (seroma formation, postoperative pain), and does not allow visualization of the ventral joint alignment. Most importantly, these procedures are associated with a greater degree of failure (37–49%) as they rely on long-term fibrous tissue stabilization as the prosthesis is suspected to eventually fail. This is in contrast to ventral approaches, where the goal is permanent bony arthrodesis [9]. Orthopedic wire, synthetic suture material, or nuchal ligament autogenous grafting have been used as prostheses to replicate the dorsal atlantoaxial ligament [17–19].

The challenges with these techniques include difficulty in reduction and placement of the prosthesis, which can be difficult particularly under the arch of C1, with iatrogenic spinal cord injury a frequently reported complication. Also described is failure of holding bony surfaces (both the vertebral arch of C1 and the spinous process of C2) when the implant shears (cheese wires) through the purchase [20].

More recently, a modification of the dorsal wiring technique has been reported in eight toy-breed dogs using the Kishigami device [21]. This technique does not require "feeding" the prosthesis under the C1 vertebral arch. It may also decrease the likelihood of tearing the C1 dorsal arch and allows for more physiological lateral movement. In this study, seven of eight dogs achieved good long-term reduction and stabilization (1 year). As this technique does not intend to induce arthrodesis and requires fibrous tissue to be the long-term stabilizer, its safety in larger-breed dogs is questionable. Further evaluation of this technique is needed.

A dorsal cross-pinning technique that engages the dorsal spinous process of C2 and the wings of C1 has been described [22]. This technique may be biomechanically superior to other dorsal approaches and the implants do not approach the neuraxis. Long-term studies on the efficacy of this technique have not been performed.

Ventral Approach

The ventral approach for AAS stabilization is much more commonly performed because of the ease of approach and high rate of stabilization success (Video 15.1).

The area from the caudal aspect of the mandibular rami to the caudal cervical region is aseptically prepared. A ventral midline incision is made from the caudal aspect of the mandible to 3 cm caudal to the wings of the atlas. The sternohyoid muscles are identified and separated along the midline raphe, exposing the trachea. The trachea, esophagus, and right recurrent laryngeal nerve are separated from the left carotid sheath and retracted toward the surgeon. Two landmarks for the identification of the C1–C2 junction are the caudal borders of the wings of the atlas and the sharp ventral prominence on the caudal aspect of C1. Periosteal dissection of the longus colli muscles and the rectus capitis ventralis muscles is performed along the midline with sharp dissection of their attachments to the ventral spine of C2 [23].

A modified right parasaggital approach has been described as an alternative to the midline technique [24]. This technique avoids manipulation of vital cervical structures such as the trachea, esophagus, vagosympathetic trunk, and thyroid vessels. The approach dissects though the right sternocephalicus and sternothyroideus. This approach also provides good surgical exposure, requires less dissection, provides protection of vital structures during placement of fixation devices, and may better preserve the thyroid artery.

Reduction of the AAS can be quite challenging. The dorsally recumbent surgical positioning coupled with retraction of the soft tissues laterally by Gelpi self-retaining retractors often provides partial reduction. A Hohmann retractor to lever the C2 body by the ventral arch of C1 is commonly described. The author's preferred technique is to grasp the lateral body of C2 by a large Backhaus towel clamp or AO bone grasping forceps (Figure 15.6). Ventrocaudal traction is provided until the dens can be visualized against the ventral body of C1 and the articulation is automatically correct. Alternate techniques recently described may provide a more stable reduction until implants are placed [25,26]. In this technique, a disc fenestration is made in the C2–C3 space. A Gelpi retractor is placed in the intercondyloid fissure of the occipital bone and the C2–C3 fenestration to provide over-distraction. Another technique for reduction is to use a C2 body screw as an anchor point. The body screw will later serve as part of a multi-implant construct [10].

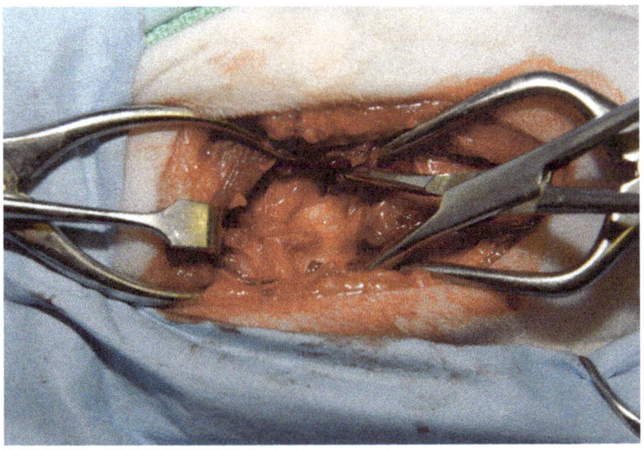

Figure 15.6 Backhaus towel clamps, fragment forceps, or AO bone grasping forceps can be used to grasp the body of C2 for reduction of the atlantoaxial joint. In this photo, a fragment forceps is attached to the body of C2 and is used to reduce the subluxation.

Means of Stabilization

Transarticular pins are the simplest method of ventral fixation described [27,28]. The pins are directed at an angle of 30° from the midline (Figure 15.7). As intraoperative assessment of this angle can be difficult, a probe can be placed in the alar notch and this point set as a target. The dorsoventral angle should engage the wings of the atlas but this can be difficult to attain because of the ventral soft tissues. A separate skin incision may be necessary for the drill to achieve the necessary angle. Newer 45-degree chucks and drills make this angle more attainable.

Pin migration and loss of reduction are cited as the most common complication. Use of positive-profile threaded pins or screws, bent exit tips, and polymethylmethacrylate (PMMA) may decrease this likelihood [29,30]. Other challenges with the technique include adequate bone purchase and potential distraction of the joint during implant placement. Placement of screws in lag fashion may therefore be preferable but add an extra step in the procedure (Figures 15.8 and 15.9) [9].

Two techniques have been described that use transarticular fixation supplemented by nonarticular screws and PMMA stabilization. Sanders et al. [31] placed transarticular screws followed by screws in the transverse processes of C1, C2, and C3 (Figure 15.10). These screws were "rebarred" with Steinman pins and cerclage wire before completing the construct with PMMA. Platt et al. [10] used a C2 body screw to facilitate joint reduction followed by transarticular Kirshner wires for temporary stabilization and incorporation of three other screws and PMMA. The techniques are likely more rigid than transarticular stabilization alone but raise questions of over-stabilization and of increasing the risk of domino lesions at adjacent intervertebral disc spaces.

A 1.5-mm five-hole butterfly locking plate has been described in three toy-breed dogs; 6-mm screws were used and laced at an angle of 10° laterally from the perpendicular in the body of the axis and variable angle in the wings of the atlas. The locking plate decreases the potential for screw pull-out and failure. Titanium implants may prove advantageous in that they allow for later MRI [32].

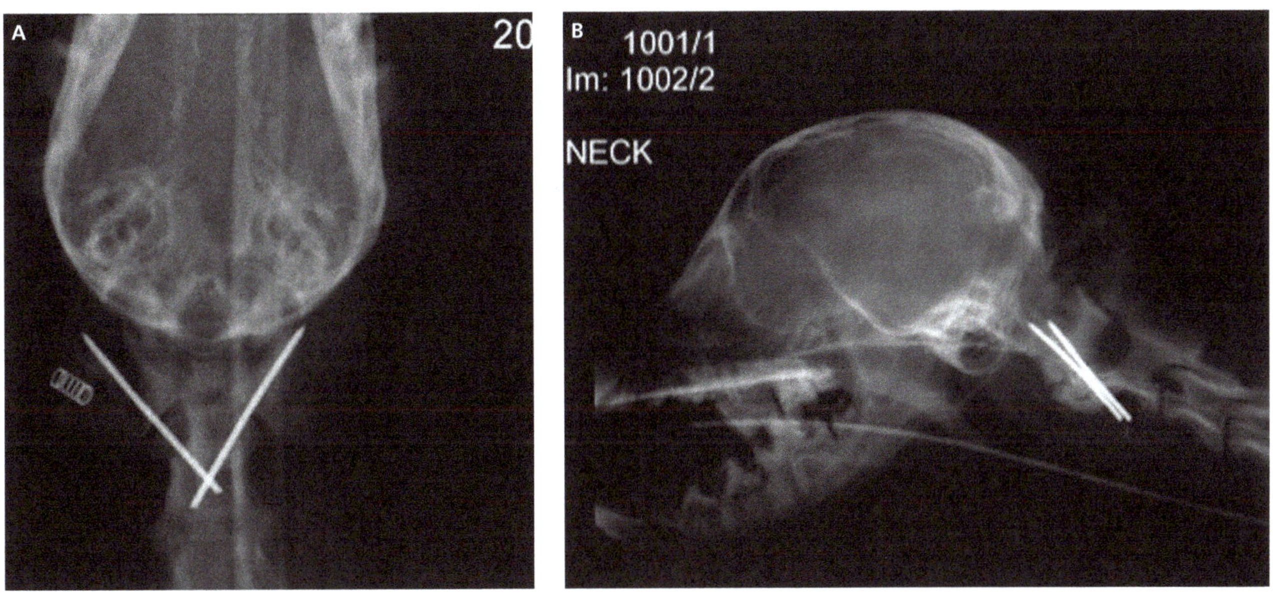

Figure 15.7 (A) Ventrodorsal and (B) lateral postoperative radiographs showing position of transarticular pins used in an atlantoaxial subluxation reduction and fixation.

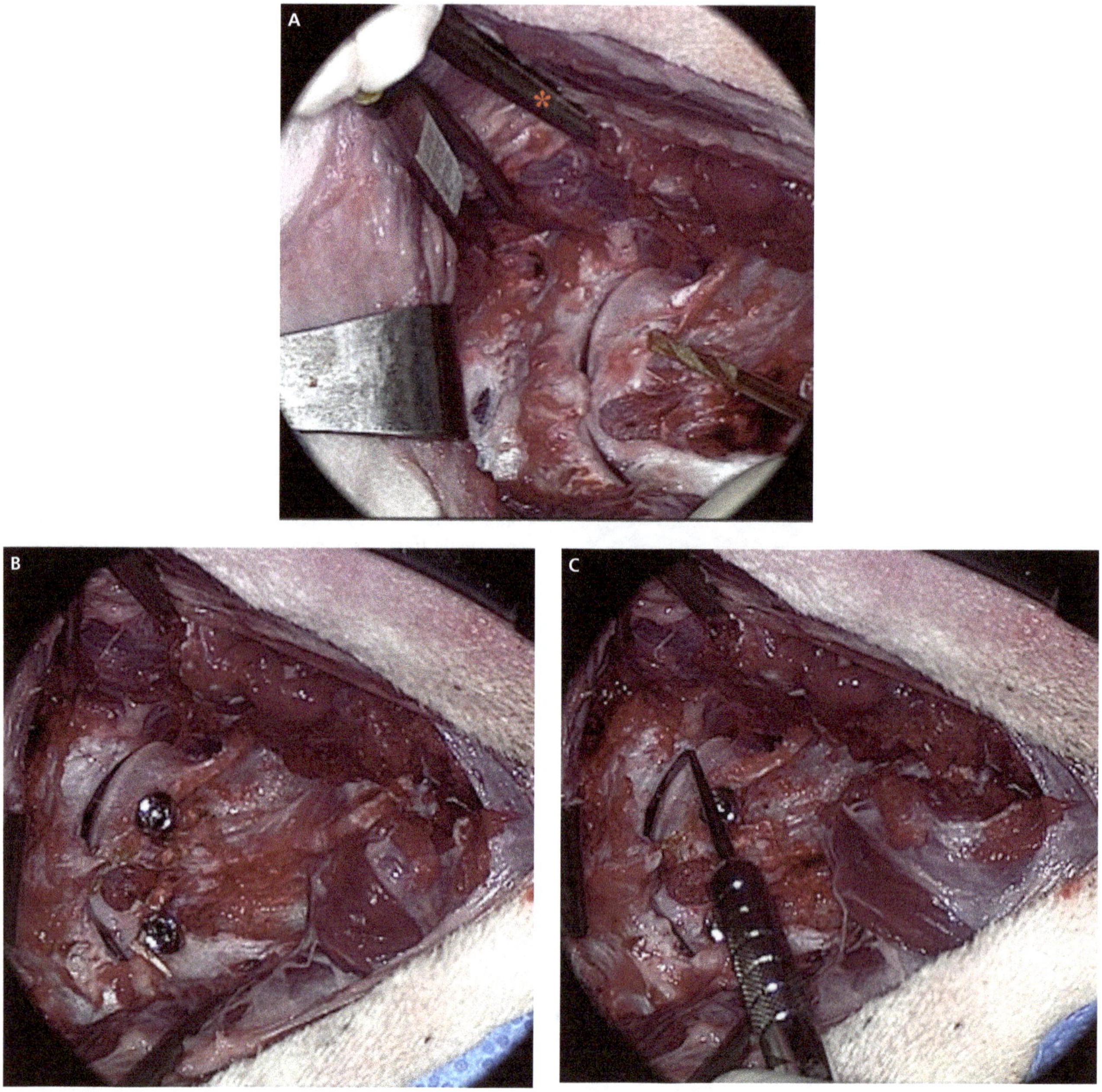

Figure 15.8 Placement of transarticular screws for ventral atlantoaxial fixation. (A) A House curette (asterisk) is placed in the alar notch for directing the angle of the screw placement from the midline. (B) Screw placements. (C) Once screws have been placed, the articular cartilage is removed and cancellous bone graft is placed in the ventral articular space.

All the ventral techniques recognize the need for long-term bony arthrodesis. A pneumatic drill or a #11 scalpel blade and small bone curette are used to remove the articular surfaces of C1 and C2. Cancellous bone autografts are used to promote osteogenesis, osteoinduction and osteoconduction [24]. Autographs or allographs can be used.

While odontectomy is described with the ventral approach, the procedure is considered difficult and necessitates more extensive C1 and C2 body osteotomies. The technique may be required in cases of severely dorsally angulated dens. However, rigid stabilization is often adequate as it prevents further mechanical trauma to the adjacent spinal cord [33].

Surgical Complications

Ventral fixation has a higher rate of success but may predispose the animal to a higher risk of surgical complications. Those reported include iatrogenic neurological trauma, focal tracheal necrosis or perforation, aspiration pneumonia, implant failure, breakage, laryngeal paralysis secondary to recurrent laryngeal neuropraxia, and Horner's syndrome secondary to trauma of the vagosympathetic trunk [34]. Dorsal complications are associated with similar cervical myelopathic effects, implant failure/malalignment, and greater pain morbidity due to muscle dissection [20]. The potential for many of these complications can be eliminated using the modified right paramedian approach described by Shores and Tepper [24].

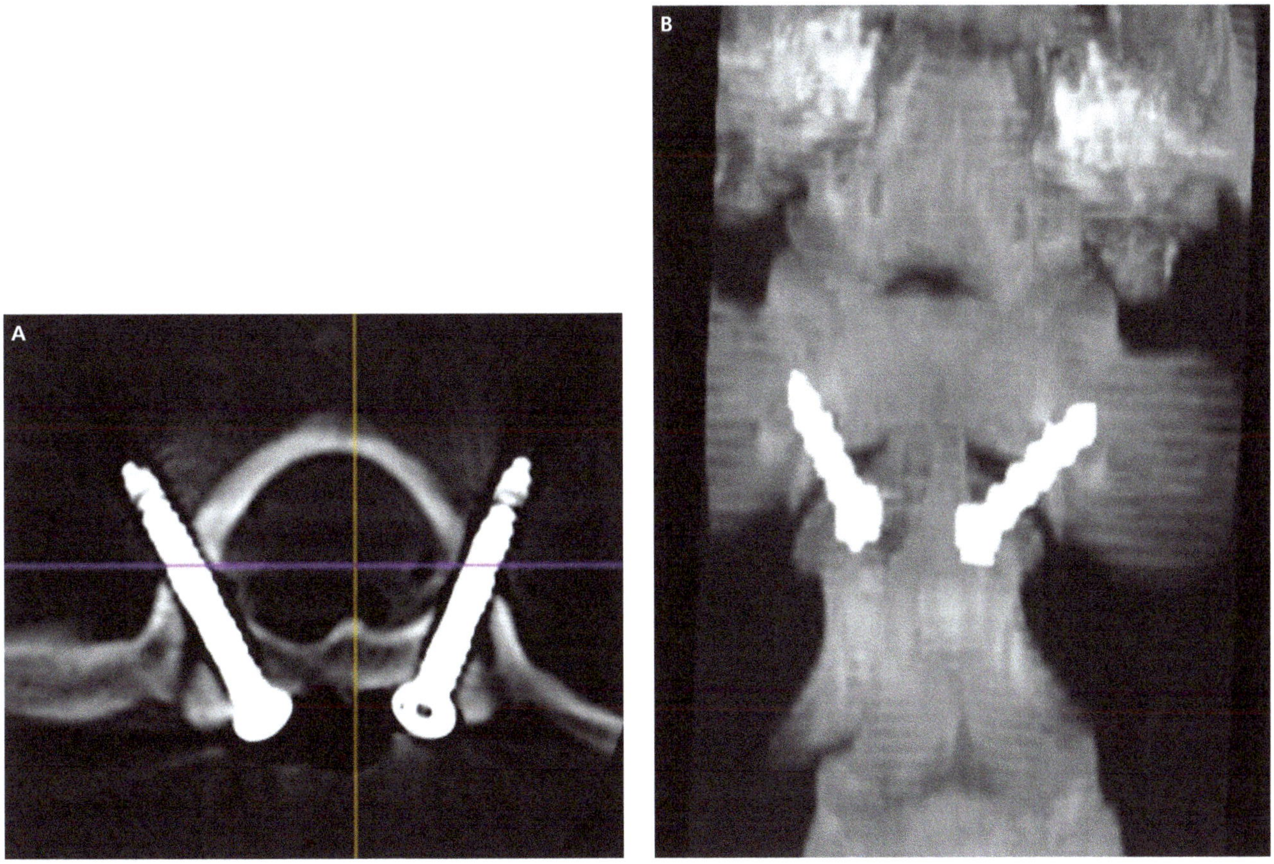

Figure 15.9 CT is an effective means of assessing implant placement because of the excellent bone definition and minor metallic artifact compared with MRI. (A) Multiplanar reconstruction (MPR) and (B) mean intensity projection (MIP) demonstrate adequate placement of transarticular screws.

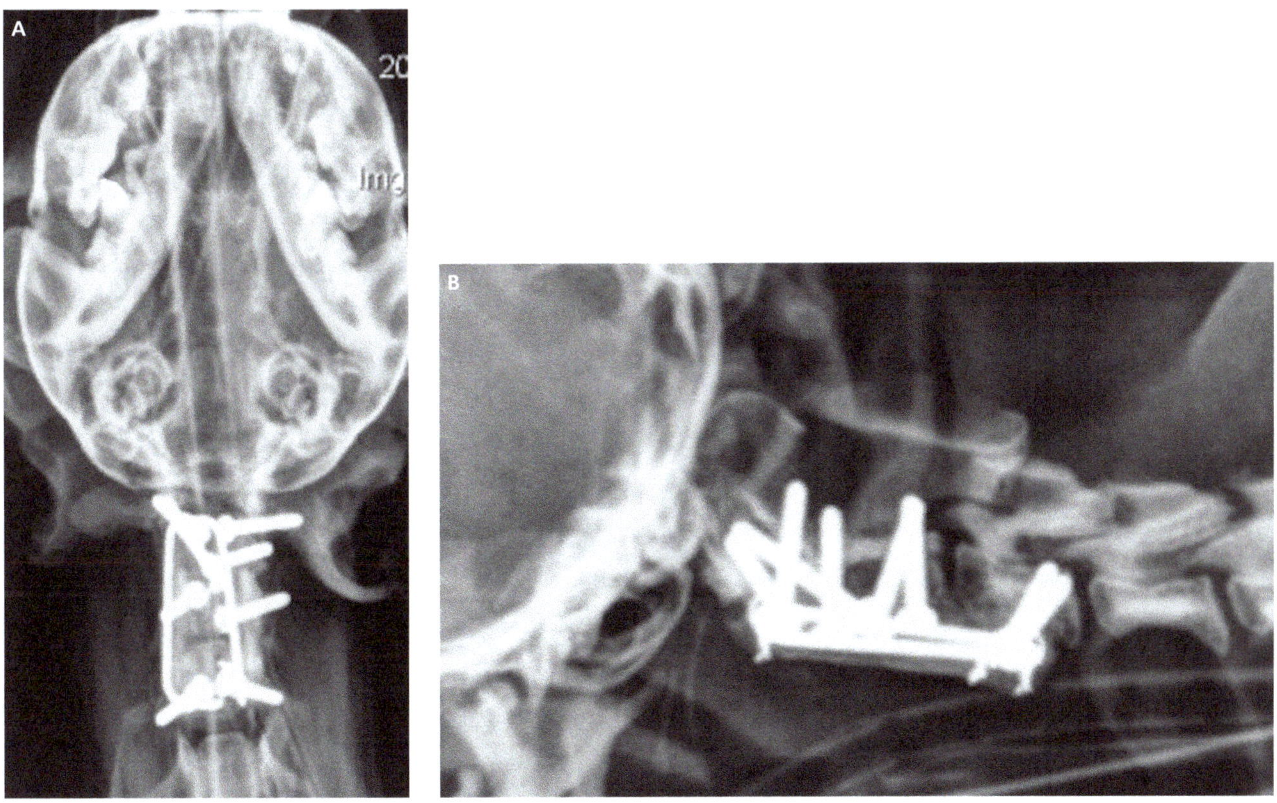

Figure 15.10 Although transarticular screws/pins are associated with a relatively low failure rate, more robust constructs have been created for stabilization. (A) Ventrodorsal and (B) lateral views of the technique described by Sanders et al. [31], supplementing transarticular screws with screws in the transverse processes of C1, C2 and C3 encased in reinforcement bars and PMMA. Cervical vertebral plates are another method used for ventral rigid stabilization.

Postoperative Management

Immediate postoperative management is directly related to possible complications associated with iatrogenic cervical myelopathic injury or the soft tissue approach itself. Capnography or blood gas monitoring is recommended up until extubation to ensure the animal can ventilate appropriately. As a neuropraxia associated with the recurrent laryngeal nerve can occur, the author prefers to hold food postoperatively for 12 hours. This is not always feasible as these small patients may not be able to maintain normoglycemia.

Because of the anatomical configuration of C1–C2 in young toy breeds, any form of fixation is initially considered marginal. Regardless of whether a dorsal or ventral approach is used, the neck is supported with a neck brace, and strict cage confinement should be enforced until radiographic evidence of union (see Figure 15.5). When applied, the goal of external coaptation is to prevent ventroflexion and is less concerned with rotation or dorso-extensive movement. As such, the brace is often contoured to allow for such movements.

Surgical Prognosis

Factors associated with a more favorable outcome following surgical stabilization include dogs less than 2 years of age at onset of clinical signs, clinical signs for less than 10 months prior to the procedure, a duration of clinical signs greater than 30 days, and an ambulatory preoperative status [10,34].

Though the procedure is often associated with high rates of success, neck pain persists in 10% of cases and clinical ataxia in 20% of cases. Should a second surgery be warranted, the literature suggests that these cases are amenable to repeat procedures with a relatively high rate of success [34].

Summary

Cases of AAS present the neurosurgeon with a unique challenge with regard to proper approach, adequate reduction, and durable stabilization in small patients with delicate anatomy. Diagnostic imaging is essential in the planning of these procedures. As these cases present sporadically in clinical practice, acquiring adequate experience to be proficient in the techniques may pose a challenge. The current body of evidence would suggest that the ventral approach with rigid stabilization by transarticular screws or multiple implants yields the most positive outcomes.

> Video clips to accompany this book can be found on the companion website at:
> www.wiley.com/go/shores/neurosurgery

References

1 Thomas WB, Sorjonen DC, Simpson ST. Surgical management of atlantoaxial subluxation in 23 dogs. *Vet Surg* 1991;20:409–412.

2 Seim III HB. Atlantoaxial instability. In: Fossum TW (ed.) *Small Animal Surgery*, 2nd edn. St Louis, MO: Mosby, 2002: 1250–1255.

3 Rochat MC, Shores A. Fixation of an atlantoaxial subluxation by use of cannulated screws. *Vet Comp Orthop Traumatol* 1999;12:43–46.

4 Watson AG, Evans HE, de Lahunta A. Ossification of the atlas–axis complex in the dog. *Anat Histol Embryol* 1986;15:122–138.

5 Watson AG, de Lahunta A, Evans HE. Prenatal development of the composite occipito-atlanto-axial synovial joint cavity in the dog. *Anat Rec* 1986;216:423–433.

6 Dyce KM, Sack WO, Wensing CJG. *Textbook of Veterinary Anatomy*, 4th edn. St Louis, MO: Saunders Elsevier, 2010: 409–410.

7 Shires PK. Atlantoaxial instability. In: Slatter D (ed.) *Textbook of Small Animal Surgery*, 3rd edn. Philadelphia, PA: WB Saunders, 2003: 1173–1180.

8 Cerda-Gonzalez S. Congenital diseases of the craniocervical junction in the dog. *Vet Clin North Am Small Anim Pract* 2009;20:121–141.

9 Denny HR, Gibbs C, Waterman A. Atlanto-axial subluxation in the dog: a review of thirty cases and an evaluation of treatment by lag screw fixation. *J Small Anim Pract* 1988;29:37–47.

10 Platt SR, Chambers JN, Cross A. A modified ventral fixation for surgical management of atlantoaxial subluxation in 19 dogs. *Vet Surg* 2004;33:349–354.

11 Kent M, Eagleson JS, Neravanda D, Schatzberg SJ, Gruenenfelder FI, Platt SR. Intraaxial spinal cord hemorrhage secondary to atlantoaxial subluxation in a dog. *J Am Anim Hosp Assoc* 2010;46:132–137.

12 Owen MC, Davis SH, Worth AJ. Imaging diagnosis: traumatic myelopathy in a dog with incomplete ossification of the dorsal lamina of the atlas. *Vet Radiol Ultrasound* 2008;49:570–572.

13 Parry AT, Upjohn MM, Schlegl K, Kneissl S, Lamb CR. Computed tomography variations in morphology of the canine atlas in dogs with and without atlantoaxial subluxation. *Vet Radiol Ultrasound* 2010;51:596–600.

14 Middleton G, Hillmann DJ, Trichel J, Bragulla HH, Gaschen L. Magnetic resonance imaging of the ligamentous structures of the occipitoatlantoaxial region in the dog. *Vet Radiol Ultrasound* 2012;53:545–551.

15 Marino DJ, Loughin CA, Dewey CW et al. Morphometric features of the craniocervical junction region in dogs with suspected Chiari-like malformation determined by combined use of magnetic resonance imaging and computed tomography. *Am J Vet Res* 2012;73:105–111.

16 Havig ME, Cornell KK, Hawthorne JC, McDonnell JJ, Selcer BA. Evaluation of nonsurgical treatment of atlantoaxial subluxation in dogs: 19 cases (1992–2001). *J Am Vet Med Assoc* 2005;227:257–262.

17 Kishigami M. Application of an atlantoaxial retractor for atlantoaxial subluxation in the cat and dog. *J Am Anim Hosp Assoc* 1984;20:413–419.

18 LeCouteur, RA, McKeown D, Johnson J, Eger CE. Stabilization of atlantoaxial subluxation in the dog, using the nuchal ligament. *J Am Vet Med Assoc* 1980;177: 1011–1017.

19 Chambers JN, Betts CW, Oliver JE. The use of nonmetallic suture material for stabilization of atlantoaxial subluxation. *J Am Anim Hosp Assoc* 1977;13:602–604.

20 van Ee RT, Pechman R, van Ee RM. Failure of the atlantoaxial tension band in two dogs. *J Am Anim Hosp Assoc* 1989;25:707–712.

21 Pujol E, Bouvy B, Omaña M, Fortuny M, Riera L, Pujol P. Use of the Kishigami atlantoaxial tension band in eight toy breed dogs with atlantoaxial subluxation. *Vet Surg* 2010;39:35–42.

22 Jeffery ND. Dorsal cross pinning of the atlantoaxial joint: new surgical technique for atlantoaxial subluxation. *J Small Anim Pract* 1996;37:26–29.

23 Piermattei DL, Johnson KA. *An Atlas of Surgical Approaches to the Bones and Joints of the Dog and Cat*, 4th edn. Philadelphia, PA: Elsevier Health, 2004: 48–51.

24 Shores A, Tepper LC, A modified ventral approach to the atlantoaxial junction in the dog. *Vet Surg* 2007;36:765–770.

25 Forterre, F, Vizcaino-Revés, N, Stahl C, Gendron K, Spreng D. An indirect reduction technique for ventral stabilization of atlantoaxial instability in miniature breed dogs. *Vet Comp Orthop Traumatol* 2012;25:332–336.

26 Pike FS, Kumar MS, Boudrieau RJ. Reduction and fixation of cranial cervical fracture/luxations using screws and polymethylmethacrylate (PMMA) cement: a distraction technique applied to the base of the skull in thirteen dogs. *Vet Surg* 2012;41:235–247.

27 Schulz KS, Waldron DR, Fahie M. Application of ventral pins and polymethylmethacrylate for the management of atlantoaxial instability: results in nine dogs. *Vet Surg* 1997;26:317–325.

28 Sorjonen DC, Shires PK. Atlantoaxial instability: a ventral surgical technique for decompression, fixation, and fusion. *Vet Surg* 1981;10:22–29.

29 Blass CE, Waldron DR, van Ee RT. Cervical stabilization in three dogs using Steinmann pins and methylmethacrylate. *J Am Anim Hosp Assoc* 1988;24:61–68.

30 Renegar WR, Stoll SG. The use of methylmethacrylate bone cement in the repair of atlantoaxial subluxation stabilization failures: case report and discussion. *J Am Anim Hosp Assoc* 1979;15:313–318.

31 Sanders SG, Bagley RS, Silver GM, Moore M, Tucker RL. Outcomes and complications associated with ventral screws, pins, and polymethylmethacrylate for atlantoaxial instability in 12 dogs. *J Am Anim Hosp Assoc* 2004;40:204–210.

32 Dickomeit M, Alves L, Pekarkova M et al. Use of a 1.5 mm butterfly locking plate for stabilization of atlantoaxial pathology in three toy breed dogs. *Vet Comp Orthop Traumatol* 2011;24:246–251.

33 Parker AJ, Park RD, Cusick PK. Abnormal odontoid proess. *Vet Rec* 1973;93: 559–561.

34 Beaver DP, Ellison GW, Lewis DD, Goring RL, Kubilis PS, Barchard C. Risk factors affecting the outcome of surgery for atlantoaxial subluxation in dogs: 46 cases (1978–1998). *J Am Vet Med Assoc* 2000;216:1104–1109.

16 Dorsal Cervical Decompression (Laminectomy/Hemilaminectomy and Laminotomy)

James M. Fingeroth

Introduction

The choice of surgical approach to the vertebral canal, dural tube, spinal cord, and nerve roots is largely predicated on the circumferential location of the targeted pathology and the nature of that pathology. The goals when making such a surgical approach are to gain access to the lesion in a manner that simultaneously maximizes the visualization and ability to treat the lesion (i.e., achieve mass removal and effectively decompress the spinal cord and nerve roots, debulk or biopsy lesions, etc.), while minimizing the need for manipulation and potential iatrogenic trauma to neurovascular structures and minimizing instability of the spinal motion segment and risk of resultant fracture or luxation.

The cervical vertebral canal is more amenable to ventral approaches than the thoracic or lumbar portions of the vertebral column in dogs and cats. And while such ventral approaches are infrequently utilized caudal to the cervical region in domestic animals, they are commonly employed in the cervical region. Therefore, the veterinary surgeon has more options in his or her approach to the cervical vertebral canal; however, there is also the burden of selecting the optimum approach, based on the principles above and published results from the literature.

Controversy exists with regard to the choice between ventral and dorsal approaches for the treatment of cervical intervertebral disc herniation and for the spectrum of diseases categorized under the heading of caudal cervical spondylomyelopathy syndrome (so-called "wobbler syndrome"). Some of this controversy and the basis for choosing a particular surgical technique are summarized in a contemporary text [1]. In this chapter I will address the main indications for a dorsally based approach, and the specifics of the involved surgical procedures.

Indications for Dorsal Decompression of the Cervical Spine

As addressed in Chapter 17, ventral approaches to the cervical vertebral canal are limited in most instances to relatively short narrow "slots" between adjacent vertebrae. The chief indication for such an approach is to effect decompression of the spinal cord and nerve roots from intervertebral disc herniations that occur centrally or just parasagittally within the vertebral canal. Ventral approaches are also used for many of the stabilizing procedures (with or without partial or complete "slots") in the treatment of spondylomyelopathy (see Chapter 17), and for placement of disc prostheses or other implants. For disc lesions more lateralized within an intervertebral foramen, or for nondisc-related lesions such as tumors, and in some cases of spondylomyelopathy, ventral approaches are usually insufficient, and dorsal (or dorsolateral) approaches are utilized [1–3]. Some advocate the use of dorsal approaches as well for ventrally or ventrolaterally herniated discs, even though this may violate one of the cardinal principles listed above, namely to minimize spinal cord manipulation and potential for iatrogenic spinal cord injury. This controversy is again addressed elsewhere [4–8]. For the treatment of other lesions, a dorsally or laterally based approach is the only effective way to adequately expose the lesion and permit the manipulations required for treatment.

Laminectomy versus Hemilaminectomy

The term "laminectomy" or "dorsal laminectomy" is frequently used to describe the complete removal of the bony lamina, whereas the term "hemilaminectomy" implies a more lateralized approach that preserves some portion of the lamina and the entire articular facet on the contralateral side and usually entails at least partial removal of the articular facet on the operative side. Often with

Current Techniques in Canine and Feline Neurosurgery, First Edition. Edited by Andy Shores and Brigitte A. Brisson.
© 2017 John Wiley & Sons, Inc. Published 2017 by John Wiley & Sons, Inc.
Companion website: www.wiley.com/go/shores/neurosurgery

dorsal laminectomies, variable amounts of the articular facets on one or both sides are removed. Extensive bilateral facetectomy is generally avoided as the degree of resultant vertebral instability produced can risk subsequent vertebral fracture/luxation.

The choice between a complete dorsal laminectomy and a more limited hemilaminectomy is based on the location of the target lesion relative to the dural tube, and the amount of space needed for both visualization and ability to introduce and utilize instruments within that space. The precision of preoperative imaging studies determines the planned approach. However, it is not uncommon for planned hemilaminectomies to be expanded into more complete dorsal laminectomies based on intraoperative findings. Figures 16.1, 16.2 and 16.3 show examples of lesions that required either a hemilaminectomy or dorsal laminetomy in the cervical region.

Dorsal Surgical Approach

Regardless of whether a complete dorsal laminectomy or hemilaminectomy is planned, the initial approach is the same. The patient is positioned in sternal recumbency. The head, neck, and vertebral column are positioned so as to minimize any rotation left or right, the introduction of any scoliosis, and to avoid increased pressure on the jugular veins (that leads to increased vertebral venous sinus pressure and greater risk for intraoperative hemorrhage). Traditionally, towels and sandbags are used for this positioning, but I prefer the use of vacuum positioners. Adhesive tape can be added cranial and caudal to the surgically prepared field to further stabilize the head and neck. It may also be advantageous to slightly elevate the head and neck. Figure 16.4 demonstrates a patient prepared and positioned for a dorsal cervical procedure. The cervical vertebral column is positioned either neutrally or somewhat flexed; extension (often misnamed "dorsiflexion") is avoided, as this would potentially narrow the interarcuate spaces. The thoracic limbs are placed cranially, or in some cases secured after crossing them ventral to the neck (the latter has been advocated for approaches to the caudal cervical and cranial thoracic vertebrae as it may help abduct the scapulae and provide more working room for dissection) [9].

Landmarks for making the skin incision are somewhat limited. Cranially, the external occipital protuberance, wings of the atlas and possibly the spinous process of the axis may be palpable, and caudally one may be able to identify the spinous process of T1 and possibly C7. Because of the extensive musculature that needs to be incised and retracted to expose the dorsal aspect of the vertebral column, a liberal midline incision is generally required to achieve adequate visualization. The cranial and caudal limits of the incision are initially guided by the longitudinal location of the lesion (i.e., cranial cervical, mid-cervical, or caudal cervical), and the incision can be lengthened as needed once deeper landmarks are identified. The epaxial musculature has a rich blood supply and even with nearly perfect midline dissection, there can be substantial hemorrhage. A combination of monopolar and bipolar electrocautery combined with tamponade usually controls most bleeding. Occasionally one can visualize and grasp a bleeding vessel with a

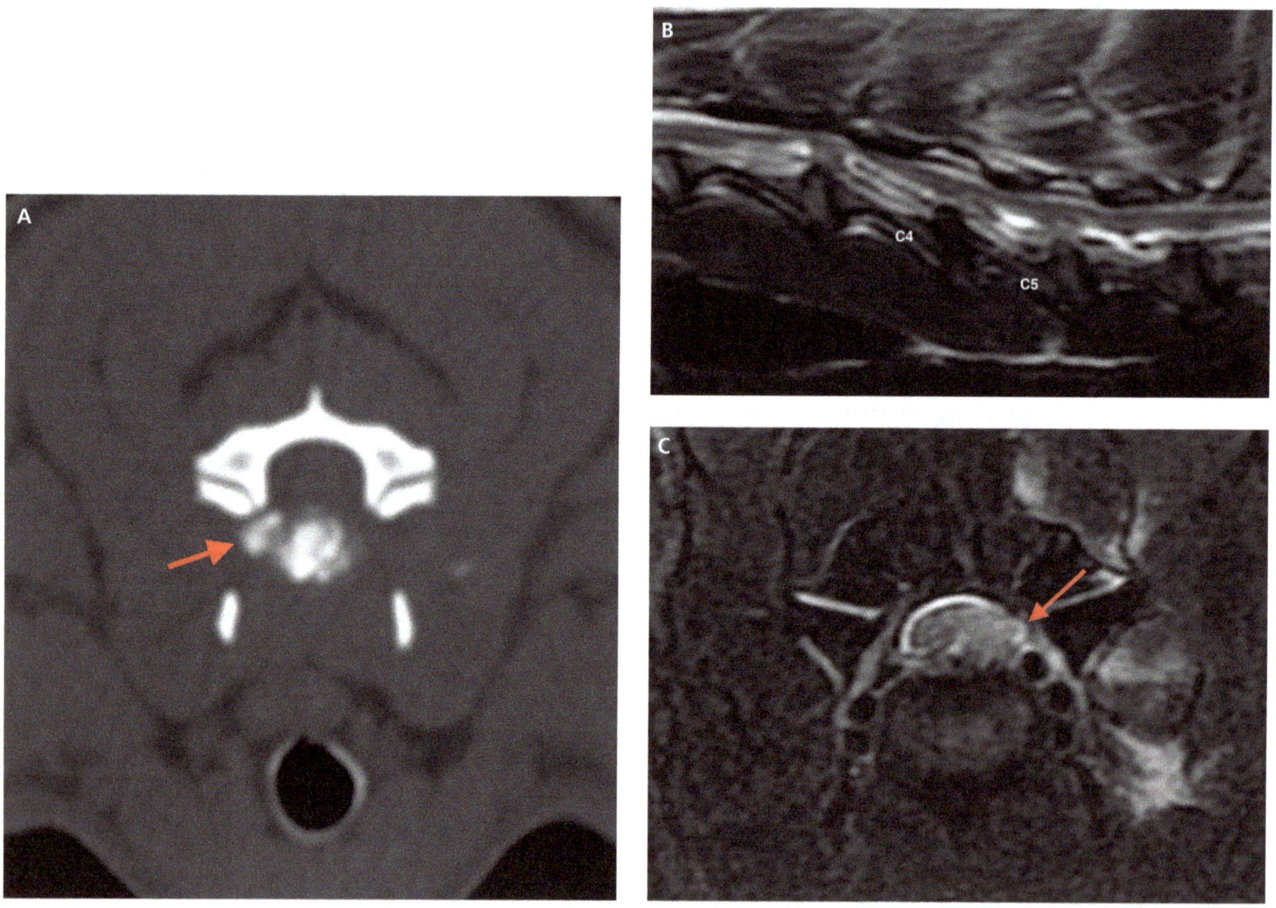

Figure 16.1 (A) Transverse CT image of a foraminal cervical disc extrusion (arrow) in a chondrodystrophic patient. (B) Sagittal T2-weighted MRI of a foraminal disc extrusion in a Great Dane at C4–C5. (C) Transverse T2-weighted MRI of same patient as in (B) showing foraminal intervertebral disc extrusion (arrow). Both patients required a cervical hemilaminectomy for adequate decompression.

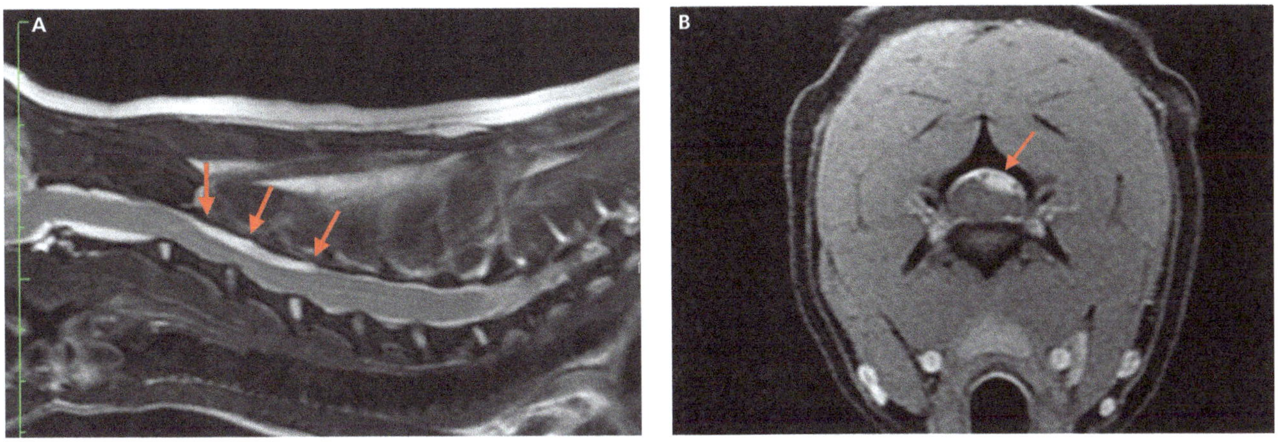

Figure 16.2 (A) Sagittal T1-weighted plus contrast and (B) transverse T2-weighted MRI of a Chihuahua with a subarachnoid mass spanning the C3 and C4 vertebrae dorsally (arrows). Exposure through a dorsal laminectomy and a durotomy revealed a stage IV *Dirofilaria immitis* larva.

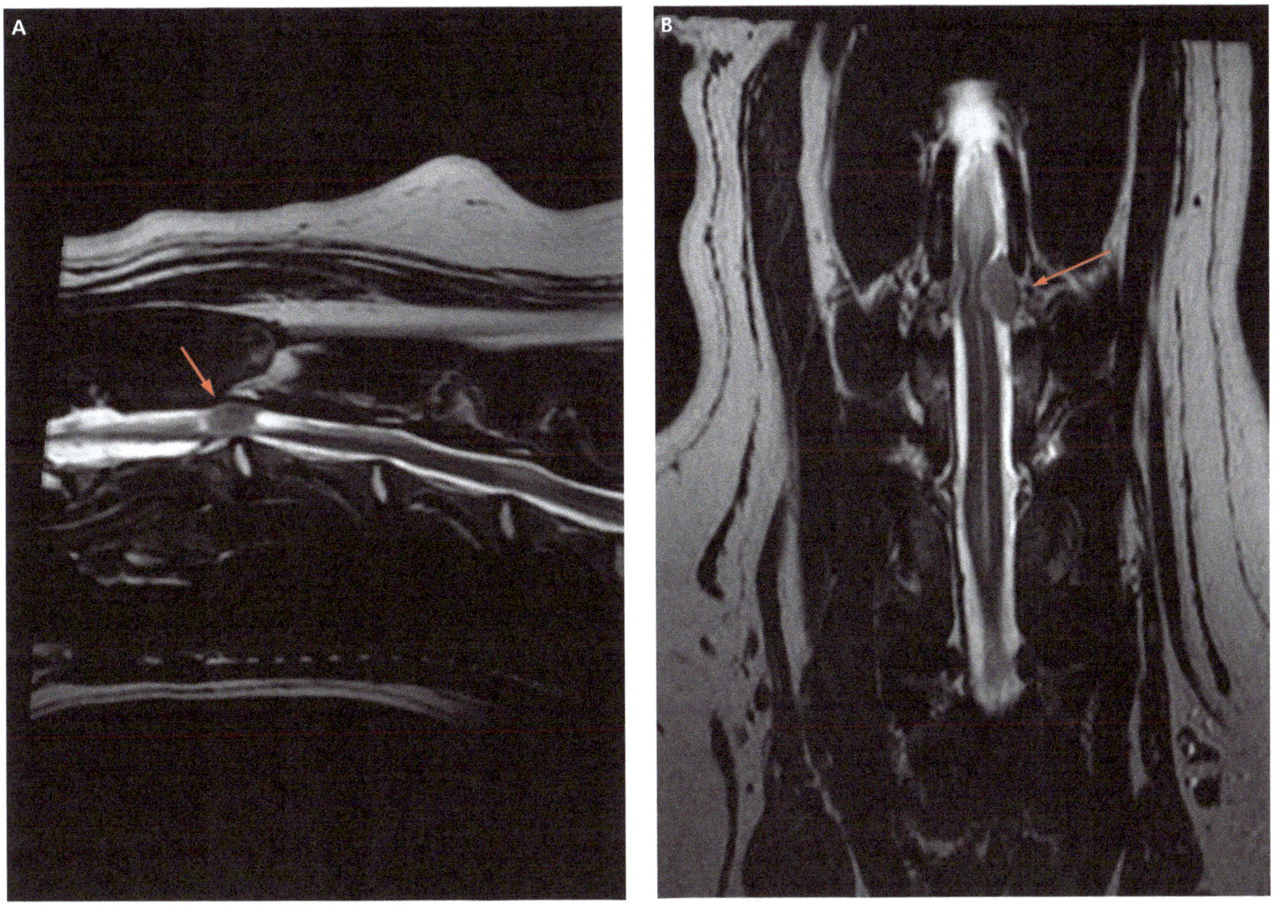

Figure 16.3 A cervical hemilaminectomy was necessary to expose and remove the intradural/extramedullary mass at C3 (arrows in A, B). (A) Sagittal and (B) dorsal T2-weighted MRI (see also Chapter 27).

hemostat to facilitate electrocoagulation. There is almost never a need for vessel ligation with suture or hemostatic clips.

The median raphes of the cleidocervicalis, trapezius and possibly rhomboideus muscles are divided and the paired biventer cervicus muscles are separated. Dorsal branches of cervical nerves may be observed and may be transected as needed without concern for functional consequences. The paired but joined nuchal ligaments are then exposed (for all intents and purposes, though, we can consider them as a single structure). Once the nuchal ligament is identified, the muscles and fascia on the side where the surgeon is positioned are incised and reflected from the ligament, with the ligament then retracted to the opposite side with self-retaining retractors. The nuchal ligaments themselves are not divided. This exposes the last group of epaxial muscles (the rectus capitis, spinalis et semispinalis cervicis, and multifidus muscles) that is carefully elevated bilaterally from the spinous processes and laminae using a periosteal elevator. Figure 16.5 illustrates the stages of dissection. Care is taken not to elevate these muscles too far laterally as there is

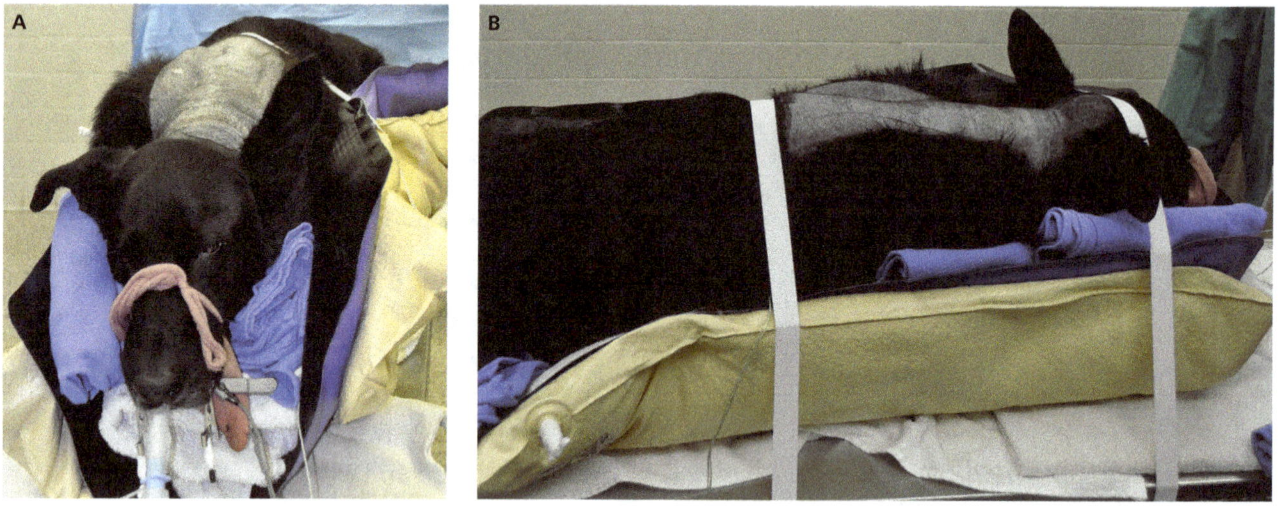

Figure 16.4 Typical patient positioning for dorsal approach to the cervical spine for laminectomy/hemilaminectomy. Effort should be made to align the head, neck, and trunk so that there is no rotation or turning of the spinal column, and that the spine is neutral or slightly flexed, and not extended. A vacuum positioner (as shown here) or sandbags and towels are used with adhesive tape to secure the head and neck so that no movement occurs intraoperatively. Compression of the jugular veins should be avoided since this could lead to dilation of the vertebral venous sinuses. The thoracic limbs are usually secured cranially as depicted here, but for approaches to the caudal cervical and cranial thoracic vertebrae it may be advantageous to cross the thoracic limbs ventral to the neck to the contralateral side in order to abduct the scapulae.

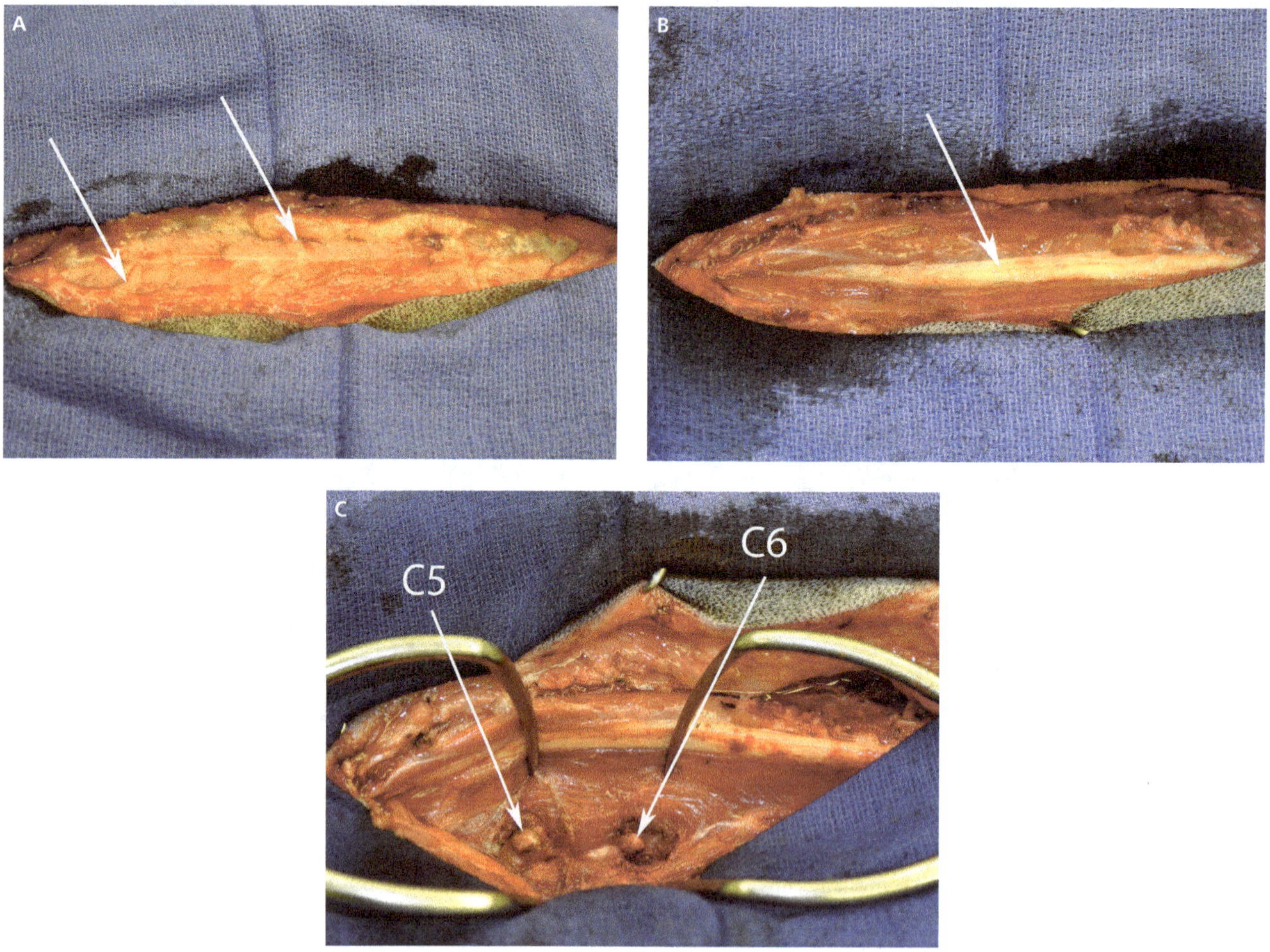

Figure 16.5 Dorsal approach to cervical spine. (A) After the skin, subcutaneous tissue, and initial fascial layers are incised on the midline, superficial nerve branches become evident (arrows). These may be sacrificed without functional consequence. (B) Separation of superficial musculature on the dorsal midline exposes the paired nuchal ligaments (arrow). These can be treated as a single ligament and retracted together to one side. (C) Self-retaining retractors have been placed to deviate the nuchal ligaments to the patient's right side (head is to the left), and the multifidus muscles have been partially elevated, exposing the spinous processes of the cervical vertebrae (arrows). *Source*: Courtesy of Dr. William B. Thomas.

a rich plexus of vascular structures surrounding the regions of the articular facets, and brisk hemorrhage could ensue. Bipolar electrocautery on appropriately sized bayonet forceps is helpful in controlling bleeding vessels and oozing that occurs throughout the dissection down to the vertebral column. Tamponade can also be achieved by placement of moistened surgical sponges or laparotomy sponges (in larger patients) between self-retaining retractors and dissected muscles.

Performance of the laminectomy procedure itself and subsequent manipulations within the vertebral canal are enhanced by the use of modest magnification (loupes) and possibly as well by supplementing overhead surgical lights with a head-mounted illumination system. Identification of the desired vertebra or vertebrae is based on palpation or visualization of the spinous process of the axis cranially, the markedly taller spinous process of T1, and then palpating or visualizing the much more truncated spinous processes of C3 through C7.

Complete Dorsal Laminectomy (C3 to Thoracic Vertebrae)

The spinous process of the vertebra to be opened is removed with double-action rongeurs. This is repeated for each contiguous vertebra where the laminectomy is to be extended. Caution is exercised during bone removal to avoid inadvertently penetrating too deeply into the vertebral canal and potentially contacting the dural tube. A high-speed drill and burrs are generally used to first outline and then deepen the proposed area of bone removal in the lamina. In general, one starts with a larger-size burr and progressively switches to burrs of smaller diameter as one advances more deeply. Smaller burrs also facilitate undercutting of the inner cortical wall and cancellous bone of the articular facets in dogs with hypertrophy and bony stenosis of the vertebral canal, as occurs in young, giant-breed dogs with the osseous-associated form of wobbler syndrome. Surgeons vary in their preference to the use of irrigation during high-speed drilling. Continuous lavage has the advantage of preventing thermal injury to the bone and adjacent tissues. However, it can become very hard to visualize the burr-bone interface when continuously under liquid. I prefer to lavage intermittently, especially if operating without assistance. In either case, it is vital to have suction at hand and a selection of various size tips (usually Frazier tips) in order to clear the surgical field of blood, bone dust, and lavage fluid. The lateral extent of the laminectomy is limited to just the medial-most aspect of each articular facet. This avoids causing excessive mechanical disruption, and also reduces the risk for encountering the vertebral artery and its branches on each side as they course through the transverse foraminae (Figure 16.6). When two or more vertebrae are to be included in the laminectomy, care is taken in the region of the interarcuate ligaments (ligamentum flavum; yellow ligament) so the burr does not sink into, or penetrate these soft tissue structures. The goal is to create a roughly rectangular defect in the outer cortical bone and cancellous bone of the lamina such that all that remains covering the vertebral canal is the thin inner cortical bone layer and the interarcuate ligament (Figure 16.7). The interarcuate ligament can then be elevated and gently incised with a #11 scalpel blade, and the same scalpel then used to dissect most of the ligamentous

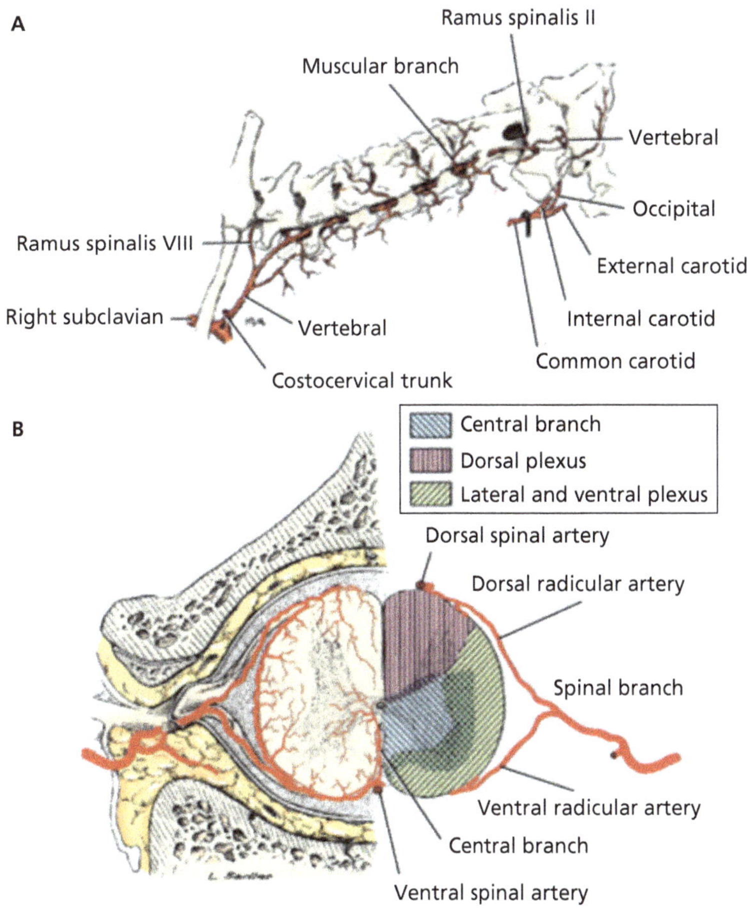

Figure 16.6 (A, B) Lateral and cross-sectional drawing of the vertebrae demonstrating the relationship of the vertebral canal and contained dural tube and the overlying lamina and articular facets. Note the location of the transverse foramina through which course the vertebral arteries. Overly aggressive facetectomy can result in brisk hemorrhage from the vertebral artery and its branches, and add considerable time to the surgical procedure in order to achieve hemostasis. *Source*: Evans HE, de Lahunta A. *Miller's Anatomy of the Dog*, 4th edn. Philadelphia: Elsevier Saunders, 2013. Reproduced with permission.

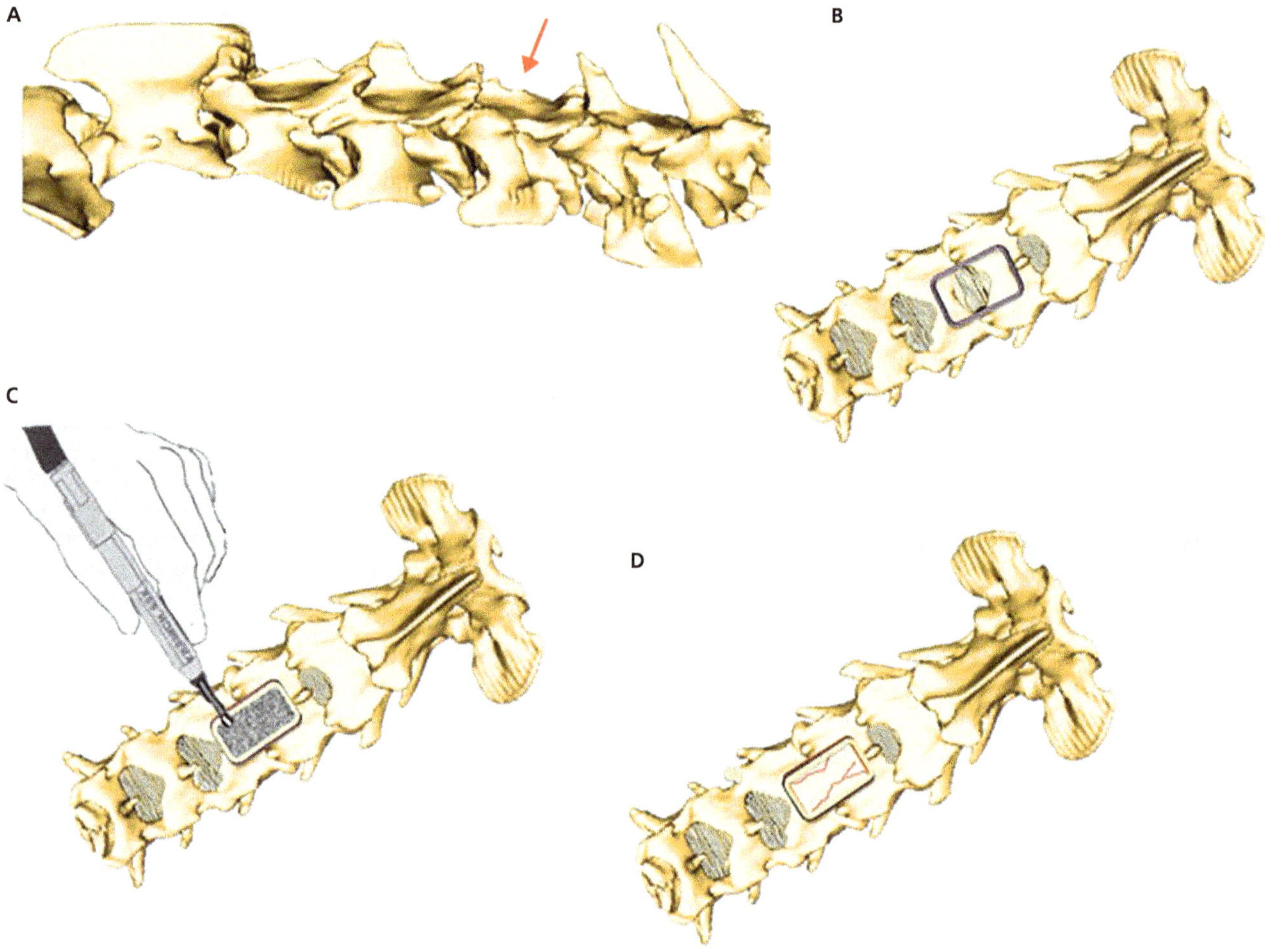

Figure 16.7 Dorsal laminectomy. After initially removing the spinous processes with rongeurs (A, arrow), a high-speed drill and burrs of gradually decreasing diameter are used to create the outline for the laminectomy (B). The outer cortical layer and underlying cancellous bone are removed to expose the thin inner cortical margin (C). The interarcuate ligament (ligamentum flavum) is seen between the adjacent vertebrae. Diploic hemorrhage from the bone can be controlled as needed with bone wax. The remainder of the laminectomy is conducted with rongeurs and curettes after removing the interarcuate ligament with a #11 scalpel blade. The completed dorsal laminectomy should be sufficiently wide, but not include the articulation (D). For hemilaminectomy the spinous processes may be preserved, and unilateral facetectomy may be more extensive than shown here. *Source*: illustration by Andy Shores.

tissue from between the adjacent vertebrae. Rongeurs are then used to complete the laminectomy. Both the high-speed drill and any rongeurs should ideally be held with two hands so as to stabilize the instruments and prevent slipping. The surgeon should have rongeurs of various designs and sizes available (see Chapter 1), but all are used in a similar manner: carefully but minimally introduced in the interarcuate space (to avoid impingement on the underlying dural tube), and small bites taken to gradually increase the size of the laminectomy opening. When the dural tube itself is not enlarged or displaced dorsally there may be a layer of epidural fat between the laminectomy and the dura mater, allowing a somewhat more aggressive use of larger rongeurs.The goal is the careful removal of bone so as to minimize or avoid any contact between the instrument and the dura. If extension of the laminectomy beyond the initial planned outline is required, this is achieved by the use of the high-speed drill and burrs or rongeurs alone, depending on the thickness of the bone in the area to be further resected. One should always try to avoid taking excessively large bites of bone with rongeurs, as closure of the instrument may cause excessive torque before the bone is cut. This torque could predispose to vertebral fracture.

Hemorrhage directly from the bone (diploic hemorrhage) is a frequent occurrence during laminectomy procedures and can obscure visualization. Bleeding vessels are typically not accessible for grasping, clamping, or electrocoagulating, and even with bipolar electrocautery one should exercise caution in proximity to the spinal cord. The most useful means of controlling such bone bleeding is through the use of sterile bone wax. Drilling or rongeuring can be continued, including through the waxed area. Dislodgement of the bone wax may occur and bleeding may recur, but can be similarly managed in a sequential fashion until the laminectomy is completed.

Once the vertebral canal has been adequately exposed the mass removal or other procedure is commenced. It should be noted that the dural tube, and spinal cord within, are largely tethered within the vertebral canal by the nerve roots and that the dural tube and spinal cord are not rigid structures. Although the dural tube may be displaced towards the lamina by a ventral or ventrolateral mass within the vertebral canal, the bulk of compression being applied to the spinal cord is at the location of the mass lesion (where it contacts and depresses into the spinal cord), and not by the secondary impingement of the dural tube against the bony lamina. Hence, laminectomy itself provides minimal to no decompressive effect for most lesions, and effective decompression of the spinal cord and/or nerve roots is usually predicated on removal of the offending mass lesion itself.

Wound closure begins with ensuring hemostasis within and around the exposed vertebral canal, and continuing to control bleeding or oozing in muscle layers as the wound is closed from deep to superficial. Hematoma and seroma formation can lead to secondary spinal cord compression [10]. There is ongoing controversy as to whether an interpositional material such as fat or cellulose sponge (e.g., Gelfoam®) should be placed over the dural tube in an effort to prevent laminectomy scar formation that might also result in secondary spinal cord compression, and specifically which material is best [11].

The muscle and fascial layers are apposed sequentially using absorbable suture material. The subcutaneous and skin closures are routine. If postsurgical MRI or CT is contemplated, sutures rather than metallic staples are used in the skin. Drains are not routinely placed but are an option if excessive dead space and/or oozing exist and concern the surgeon. Closed suction drains are much preferred over open passive drains. Neck bandaging is not routinely employed but may be chosen at the discretion of the surgeon.

Hemilaminectomy (C3–T1)

The approach and dissection to the vertebral column are identical to that described in the preceding section. Depending on the type, size, and location of the lesion as provided by preoperative imaging studies, the spinous process might be preserved or included in the bone removal. Similarly, the degree of articular facet removal is balanced between increased exposure and the desire to avoid vertebral artery trauma/hemorrhage and loss of stability.

Lateral Approach to the Cervical Vertebral Column (C3–T1)

In addition to traditional laminectomy/hemilaminectomy procedures and their shared patient positioning and muscular dissections, an alternative approach has been advocated. Unfortunately, it has also been described in the literature as a "hemilaminectomy," creating some confusion. It is more properly termed a foraminotomy and facetectomy. The approach was initially described by Lipsitz and Bailey, later modified by Rossmeisl and coworkers, and further modified by Schmied, Golini and Steffen [12–15]. It is referred to in this book as the lateral cervical approach and is discussed in greater detail in Chapter 18.

Dorsal Approach to the Occipital–Atlantoaxial Vertebral Canal (Medulla Oblongata to C2)

Lesions involving the cranial-most aspect of the vertebral canal may require some alteration to the positioning and approach utilized. Greater flexion of the head-neck junction may be indicated to increase the distance between the cranial aspect of the C2 spinous process and the dorsal arch of C1, to which it is attached by the dorsal atlantoaxial ligament. For lateralized lesions within the C1 or C2 vertebral canals a hemilaminectomy may suffice, and is preferable to a standard dorsal laminectomy that would compromise or sacrifice the spinous process of C2, the dorsal atlantoaxial ligament, or the ligamentum nuchae, any of which could predispose to loss of function, instability, and possible vertebral luxation. For large lesions at C1–C2 that would not be adequately visualized or manipulated via a limited hemilaminectomy approach, and where more dorsal exposure was desired, an alternative to laminectomy would be laminotomy of the axis [16]. In this technique, a high-speed burr and bone-cutting forceps are used to create a hinged osteotomy of the dorsal arch of C2, starting from the cranial 75% of the C2 spinous process, that can be rotated dorsally and cranially on the preserved attachment of the cranial aspect of the C2 spinous process to the dorsal arch of C1 (Figure 16.8). Combined as needed with hemilaminectomy of C1 lateral to the attachment of the dorsal atlantoaxial ligament, this approach can provide good access for removal of lesions (frequently intradural/extramedullary meningiomas that appear to have a predilection for this site), and repair of the lamina preserves the major stabilizing soft tissue structures. As needed, C1–C2 hemilaminectomy or C2 laminotomy plus C1 hemilaminectomy can be further extended through the caudal occiput for exposure of lesions extending

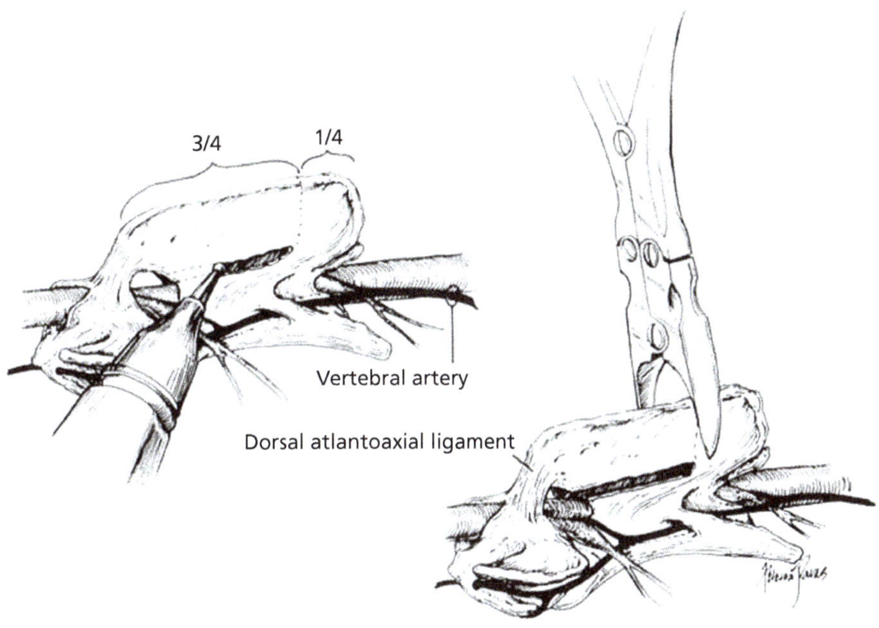

Figure 16.8 Laminotomy of C2. The dorsal atlantoaxial ligament is left intact. A high-speed pneumatic drill and small round burr are used to make lateral cuts in the vertebral arch (*left*). The vertebral artery and its radicular branches are more easily avoided with the laminotomy than with standard hemilaminectomy. A caudal transverse osteotomy is made with large bone-cutting forceps (*right*). Placement of the bone cutters is aided by scoring the bone with the burr. *Source*: Fingeroth and Smeak [16]. Reproduced with permission of John Wiley & Sons, Inc.

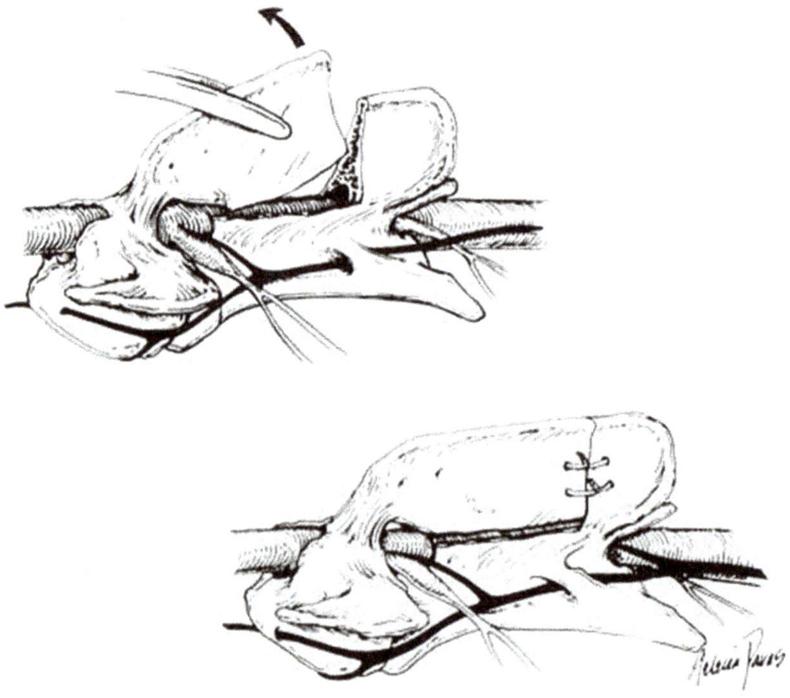

Figure 16.9 Hemostatic forceps are attached to the spinous process of C2 to elevate the laminotomy flap (*top*). Using the intact dorsal atlantoaxial ligament as a pivot point, the flap is rotated 150–180° craniad and wrapped in a moistened surgical sponge. After the neurosurgical procedure is completed, the lamina is rotated back into its normal anatomical location. Stabilization is provided by placement of two wire sutures (*bottom*). Small lateral gaps due to bone loss during the burring process are present. *Source:* Fingeroth and Smeak [16]. Reproduced with permission of John Wiley & Sons, Inc.

rostrally toward or through the foramen magnum (see Chapter 12 on suboccipital craniotomy/craniectomy techniques). If C2 laminotomy has been performed, the dorsal arch of the axis is rotated back over the exposed vertebral canal and the spinous process is stabilized with one or two cerclage wires or sutures through predrilled holes. Care should be taken with placement of any interpositional fat or cellulose sponge over the dural tube/spinal cord as this may cause secondary compression once the axis is repaired. Likewise, the creation of the laminotomy results in a thin strip of bone loss at the lateral margins, and one should take care not to force the pedicles into apposition lest the lamina end up compressing the dural tube (Figure 16.9).

> Video clips to accompany this book can be found on the companion website at:
> www.wiley.com/go/shores/neurosurgery

References

1 Felts JF, Prata RG. Cervical disk disease in the dog: intraforaminal and lateral disk extrusions. *J Am Anim Hosp Assoc* 1983;19:755–760.

2 Bagley RS, Tucker R, Harrington ML. Lateral and foraminal disk extrusion in dogs. *Compend Contin Educ Pract Vet* 1996;18:796–804.

3 De Risio L, Munana K, Murray M, Olby N, Sharp NJH, Cuddon P. Dorsal laminectomy for caudal cervical spondylomyelopathy: postoperative recovery and long-term follow-up in 20 dogs. *Vet Surg* 2002;31:418–427.

4 Fauber AE. Cervical disc disease: ventral slot versus hemilaminectomy versus dorsal laminectomy. In: Fingeroth JM, Thomas WB (eds) *Advances in Intervertebral Disc Disease in Dogs and Cats.* Ames, IA: Wiley-Blackwell, 2015: 226–231.

5 Gill PJ, Lippincott CL, Anderson SM. Dorsal laminectomy in the treatment of cervical intervertebral disk disease in small dogs: a retrospective study of 30 cases. *J Am Anim Hosp Assoc* 1996;32:77–80.

6 Funquist B. Decompressive laminectomy for cervical disk protrusion in the dog. *Acta Vet Scand* 1962;3:88–101.

7 Pettit GD, Whittaker RP. Hemilaminectomy for cervical disk protrusion in a dog. *J Am Vet Med Assoc* 1963;143:379–383.

8 Tanaka H, Nakayama M, Takase K. Usefulness of hemilaminectomy for cervical intervertebral disk disease in small dogs. *J Vet Med Sci* 2005;67:679–683.

9 Parker AJ. Surgical approach to the cervicothoracic junction. *J Am Anim Hosp Assoc* 1973;9:374.

10 Matiasek LA, Platt SR, Dennis R, Petite A. Subfascial seroma causing compressive myelopathy after cervical dorsal laminectomy. *Vet Radiol Ultrasound* 2006;47:581–584.

11 Thomas WB, Fingeroth JM. What should cover the bone defect after laminectomy/hemilaminectomy? In: Fingeroth JM, Thomas WB (eds) *Advances in Intervertebral Disc Disease in Dogs and Cats.* Ames, IA: Wiley-Blackwell, 2015: 255–258.

12 Lipsitz D, Bailey CS. Lateral approach for cervical spinal cord decompression. *Prog Vet Neurol* 1992;3:39–44.

13 Lipsitz D, Bailey CS. Clinical use of the lateral approach for cervical spinal cord and nerve root disease: eight cases. *Prog Vet Neurol* 1995;6:60–65.

14 Rossmeisl JH Jr, Lanz OI, Inzana KD, Bergman RL. A modified lateral approach to the canine cervical spine: procedural description and clinical application in 16 dogs with lateralized compressive myelopathy or radiculopathy. *Vet Surg* 2005;34:436–444.

15 Schmied O, Golini L, Steffen F. Effectiveness of cervical hemilaminectomy in canine Hansen type I and type II disk disease: a retrospective study. *J Am Anim Hosp Assoc* 2011;47:342–350.

16 Fingeroth JM, Smeak DD. Laminotomy of the axis for surgical access to the cervical spinal cord: a case report. *Vet Surg* 1989;18:123–129.

17 Ventral Cervical Decompression

Ronaldo C. da Costa

Indications

The primary indication for a ventral slot is for ventral decompression of the spinal cord caused by intervertebral disc disease (protrusion or extrusion), or disc-associated cervical spondylomyelopathy. Ventral slots can be combined with ventral fixation with pins or screws and polymethylmethacrylate (PMMA). Because of the limited visualization achieved with ventral slots, they are not an ideal technique for approaching spinal tumors.

Preparation

The dog should be positioned in dorsal recumbency. Clipping should extend from the mandible to the cranial to mid-thoracic area. Proper positioning is extremely important for successful completion of a ventral slot. If the patient is not symmetrically positioned on the table, the slot may be slightly lateralized increasing the risk of injury to the venous sinus and significant hemorrhage. It is best to finish positioning the dog after all the monitoring equipment is placed by the anesthesia personnel. A trough or a vacuum positioning pad are very helpful for keeping the spine aligned. The thoracic limbs are tied caudally and tape is used over the mandible and thoracic regions to secure the positioning of the dog on the table. It is recommended to place towels underneath the region to be approached to cause mild cervical extension and facilitate the approach. This is especially important in the caudal cervical area of deep-chested large-breed dogs (Figure 17.1). It is crucial to evaluate the positioning before draping the patient as incorrect positioning typically results from rotation of the cervical and thoracic spine.

Magnification (×2.5–3.5) and focused bright lighting greatly facilitates ventral slot procedures, especially in large dogs where the depth of the slot may hinder appropriate visualization. In deep-chested dogs, visualization of the C6–C7 disc space during drilling may also be facilitated if a right-handed surgeon is positioned on the patient's left side, rather than the typical positioning on the patient's right side.

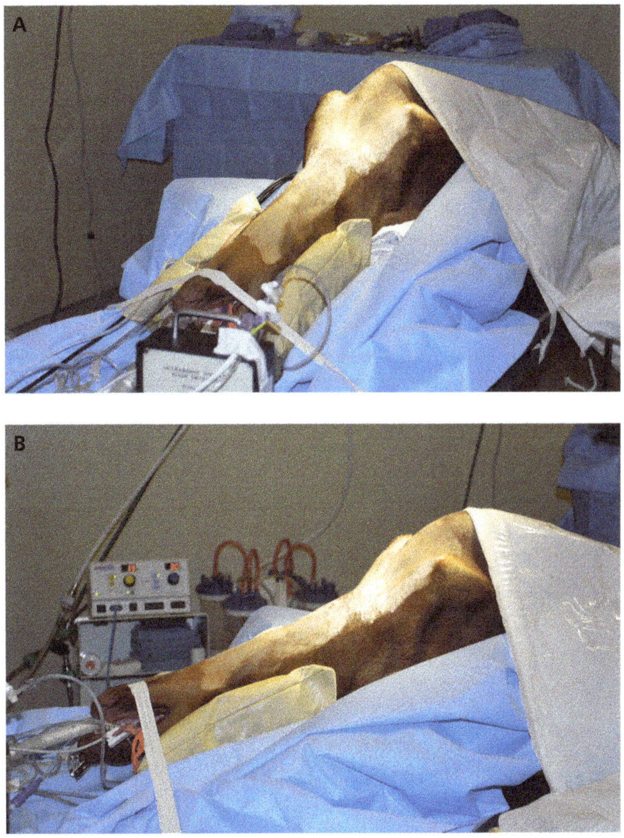

Figure 17.1 (A) Oblique view of a dog positioned in dorsal recumbency for a ventral slot. Observe the towels under the caudal cervical region and the vacuum positioning pad in the cranial cervical spine and head (yellow). (B) Lateral view. Observe the elevation of the caudal cervical spine in relation to the cranial region. This was made to facilitate approach to the caudal cervical spine (the dog was positioned for a ventral slot at C6–C7).

Current Techniques in Canine and Feline Neurosurgery, First Edition. Edited by Andy Shores and Brigitte A. Brisson.
© 2017 John Wiley & Sons, Inc. Published 2017 by John Wiley & Sons, Inc.
Companion website: www.wiley.com/go/shores/neurosurgery

Approach [1–3]

Two approaches are described for ventral slot, the median and the paramedian approaches (Figure 17.2). A ventral midline skin incision is performed from the larynx to the manubrium of the sternum. In the median approach, the paired sternocephalicus and sternohyoideus muscles are identified and both muscles are divided on the midline. The trachea is identified immediately under the sternohyoideus muscles. Digital and scissor dissection is used to expose and retract the trachea, recurrent laryngeal nerve, esophagus, and left carotid sheath towards the left, while the right carotid sheath is retracted to the right. Finger dissection is safest and most effective at this stage. Care should be exercised to avoid damage to these structures, particularly the recurrent laryngeal nerve which runs on the lateral side of the trachea. These structures can be held in retraction with blunt self-retaining retractors, such as Balfour retractors. Weitlaner retractors can also be used, but Gelpi retractors should be avoided at this stage due to the risk of damaging the neurovascular structures. Moist towels or sponges should be placed underneath the retractors to protect the tissues. In the paramedian approach, after identification of the sternocephalicus and sternohyoideus muscles, the right sternocephalicus muscle is separated from the right sternohyoideus muscle (Figure 17.2). The sternohyoideus muscles are then retracted to the left with the trachea, esophagus, and carotid sheath. This approach reduces the risk of hemorrhage from the right caudal thyroid artery and protects the trachea, right recurrent laryngeal nerve, vagosympathetic nerves, and right carotid sheath, while offering increased exposure of the caudal cervical vertebrae [4]. Retraction is maintained with blunt self-retaining retractors as described for the midline approach.

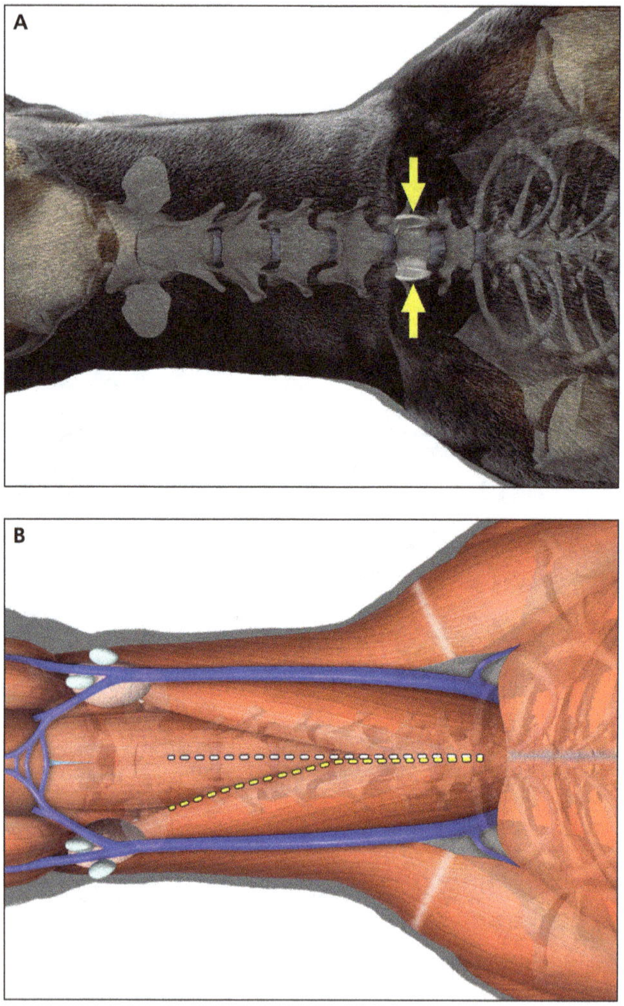

Figure 17.2 Approach to the ventral aspect of the cervical spine for a ventral slot. (A) Observe the large ventrally positioned transverse processes of the sixth cervical vertebra (arrows). Identification of C6 is important to allow identification of the correct disc space. (B) Median approach is shown by the dotted white lines over the sternohyoideus and sternocephalicus muscles. Paramedian approach is illustrated by the dotted yellow lines. After a midline skin incision and identification of the sternocephalicus and sternohyoideus muscles, the right sternocephalicus muscle is separated from the right sternohyoideus muscle in the paramedian approach. The sternohyoideus muscles are then retracted to the left with the trachea, esophagus, and carotid sheath. *Source*: Reproduced with the permission of The Ohio State University.

At this stage identification of the disc spaces for the ventral slot approach is very important. The main landmarks are the large transverse processes of the C6 vertebra and the prominent ventral process of C1 (Figure 17.2). These structures must be identified by the surgeon and assistant to avoid approaching the wrong site. The ventral tubercles of the vertebral bodies should be palpated. The ventral tubercle of C5 lies on the midline in the cranial border of the transverse processes of C6. The longus colli muscles are attached to the ventral tubercles. It is important to identify the ventral tubercles and the left and right transverse processes along the ventral aspect of the spine before incising the longus colli muscles along the intervertebral disc space to be approached. Importantly, there is no intervertebral disc between C1 and C2.

Once the intervertebral disc space has been identified and exposed, the tendinous insertions of the longus colli muscles are sharply transected. Hemostasis with bipolar cautery is important at this stage. Subperiosteal elevation of the longus colli muscle cranial and caudal to the ventral tubercle and disc space follows and retraction of the musculature is maintained using Gelpi retractors. The Lone Star® Retractor System (Cooper Surgical, Trumbull, CT) is useful in the caudal cervical region of deep-chested dogs as an alternative to long curved Gelpi retractors. Achieving adequate retraction of the musculature at C6 may be difficult due to its long ventrally positioned transverse process. Partial resection of the longus colli muscle at that location may facilitate visualization. Once the musculature is retracted and hemostasis is achieved, the ventral slot can begin.

The slot is created with a high-speed pneumatic drill. Some surgeons prefer to remove the ventral tubercle with rongeurs and to excise the annulus fibrosus with a #11 blade before drilling any bone but these steps are not necessary. When performing the slot it is important to stay on the midline and to minimize its size. Because of the angulation of the cervical intervertebral discs, the slot should begin in the cranial vertebral body. Ideally the slot should not exceed one-third of the length and width of the vertebral bodies (Figures 17.3 and 17.4) [5,6]. Drilling is performed through the outer cortex, cancellous bone, and intervertebral disc, until the inner cortex is identified. It is important to recognize the differences in color and consistency of the cancellous and cortical bone respectively. Cancellous bone is red, dark and soft, while cortical bone is white and hard. Irrigation and suction are essential for this procedure. Care should be exercised at this stage to thin the inner cortex along the cranial and caudal aspects of the slot. One should verify the thickness of the inner cortex regularly at this stage. The cortex should be thinned to a point where a soft cortical shell remains. Then, the dorsal annulus is grasped and the remaining

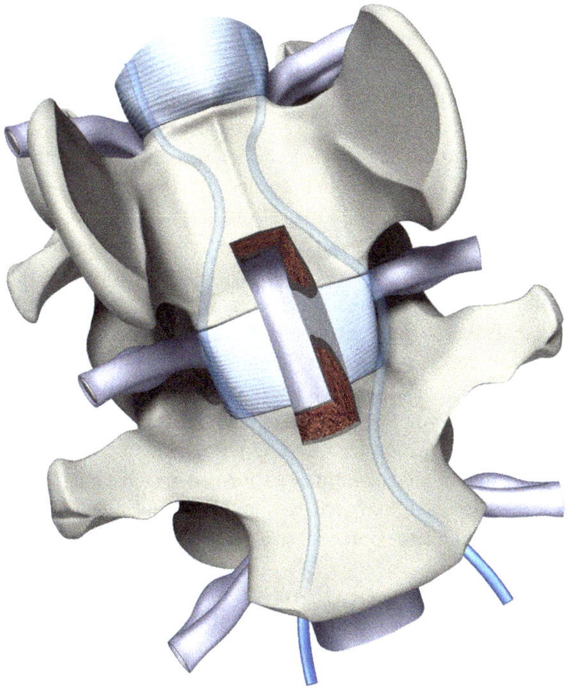

Figure 17.3 Ventral view of a ventral slot at C6–C7. The slot width and length should ideally be kept at about one-third of the vertebral bodies. The internal vertebral venous plexus is represented by the blue vessels running in the ventral aspect of the vertebral canal. *Source*: Reproduced with the permission of The Ohio State University.

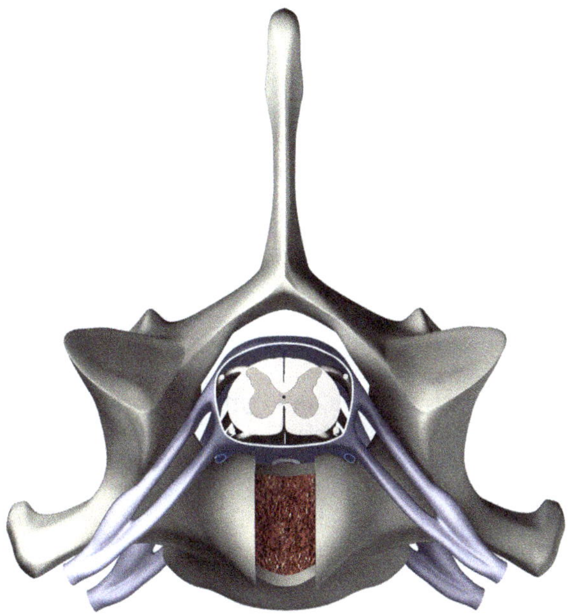

Figure 17.4 Transverse view of a ventral slot at C6–C7. The slot width should ideally be kept at about one-third of the vertebral bodies to avoid injuring the vertebral venous plexus (illustrated in blue, immediately ventral to the nerve roots). *Source*: Reproduced with the permission of The Ohio State University.

cortex and dorsal longitudinal ligament are excised with a #11 blade. Removal of the inner thin cortex can be achieved with bone curettes, Love–Kerrison rongeur, or Wayne laminectomy punch. Placing the footplate of the Love–Kerrison rongeur in the vertebral canal of small dogs can lead to spinal cord compression, thus removal of inner cortex with bone curettes is often safer in small-breed dogs. Bleeding from the cancellous bone may be controlled with bone wax. It is recommended to open the vertebral canal along the midline initially to avoid injury to the vertebral venous plexus. Caution should be exercised when widening the slot to avoid injuring the internal vertebral venous plexus, which can cause severe hemorrhage. Removal of disc material can be achieved with blunt curved nerve hooks, fine forceps, or a malleable iris spatula. All disc material should be removed, exploring laterally, cranially and caudally along the slot. After disc removal the spinal cord should be visualized and should be sitting in normal position. Lateral inspection is very important to avoid leaving disc material that compresses the nerve roots, which could lead to severe postoperative pain. Injury to the vertebral venous plexus can occur at this stage and can be controlled using gelatin sponge and by filling the surgical site with cool sterile saline for a few minutes. After a final inspection lavage is used to remove any debris and blood clots and surgical closure is performed. It is unnecessary and contraindicated to place any material in the slot site as it could interfere with bone fusion. Fusion of the slot site is expected to occur 8–12 weeks postoperatively [5,6], although not all slot sites develop fusion [7]. Apposition of the longus colli muscles is done with simple interrupted sutures. The sternohyoideus muscle is apposed using a simple continuous pattern. The subcutaneous tissues are closed in one or two layers with a simple continuous suture pattern, tacking to the fascia below to reduce dead space and the risk of seroma. The skin is closed routinely. A protective bandage can be applied over the skin incision.

Variations of Ventral Slot Procedure

Inverted Cone Technique

The technique of inverted cone is a modification of the traditional ventral slot aiming at minimizing bone removal, and therefore reducing the risk of vertebral subluxation [8]. The decompression window resembles an inverted cone in which the base of the cone lies adjacent to the ventral vertebral canal, allowing maximal surgical access cranially, caudally and laterally (Figure 17.5). The width of the ventral decompression window is limited to 20% of the cranial vertebral body. This technique allows more complete removal of the protruded disc from the vertebral canal, with less risk of hemorrhage [8]. The inverted cone slot technique also minimizes collapse of the disc space that could lead to postoperative nerve root entrapment and lameness that may be seen with the traditional slot technique [9].

Slanted Ventral Slot Technique

A slanted slot technique has been described that removes only the caudal aspect of the cranial vertebral body to access the extruded disc material [10]. It is not a transdiscal procedure like the traditional ventral slot. Using a high-speed round burr, a window is created cranial to the disc a few millimeters from the ventral tubercle. A window in the bone is made to be approximately 20% of the width and 20–25% of the length of the vertebral body toward the vertebral endplate, aiming to enter the spinal canal at the level of the dorsal portion of the annulus fibrosus. The suggested advantage of this procedure is that it provides access to the spinal canal at the site of disc herniation without removing a large portion of the annulus fibrosus, presumably preserving more stability at the surgical site than is preserved with the standard ventral slot. Because it is not a transdiscal slot, bone healing would probably occur more frequently.

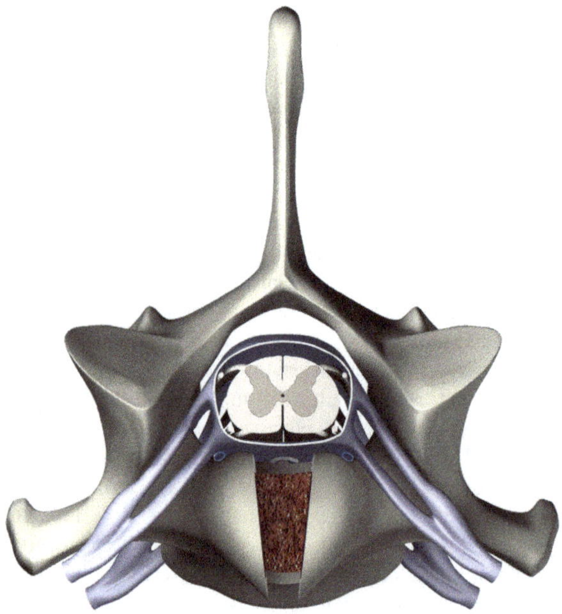

Figure 17.5 Transverse view of an inverted cone ventral slot. The decompression window resembles an inverted cone in which the base of the cone lies adjacent to the ventral vertebral canal allowing maximal surgical access cranially, caudally and laterally. This modification of the traditional ventral slot minimizes the risk of hemorrhage and subluxation. *Source*: Reproduced with the permission of The Ohio State University.

The disadvantages are the limited visualization offered by the slanted slot and the possibility of extending the slot too far cranially and damaging the vertebral venous plexus.

Video-assisted Ventral Slot

Minimally invasive spinal surgery has been used in humans for many years. This technique has been used in cervical spinal surgery in dogs by Leperlier et al. [11]. The authors used an endoscopic device designed for spinal surgery in humans without fluoroscopic guidance as described in humans. A skin incision of 2.5–5 cm was performed over the targeted disc space. Careful study of the vertebral landmarks is paramount as the approach is limited. When the technique was applied in clinical patients, a midline approach was first used to drill the ventral cortex and cancellous bone without video assistance. Video-assisted endoscopy was then used to drill the inner (dorsal) cortex and for disc removal. The slot was performed in the correct disc space in all dogs and no major complications were observed. Purported advantages of this technique are the limited invasiveness and faster recovery. The preliminary experience suggests it is a safe technique if one uses the proper instrumentation and carefully respects the local surgical anatomy.

Complications

Several complications have been reported with the ventral slot procedure. Complications range from minor hemorrhage, probably the most common complication, to death. The incidence of significant complications following ventral slot in the largest retrospective study published to date (112 dogs were studied) was 14.9%, with 6.3% of deaths associated with the procedure [12].

Hemorrhage

Significant hemorrhage can occur during the surgical approach if the patient is rotated or the midline is not identified correctly and muscle dissection is done at the level of the transverse processes, thus damaging branches of the vertebral artery. Extensive lateral retraction of the longus colli muscles can also lead to hemorrhage between the muscles and vertebral bodies from branches of the vertebral artery [2].

Hemorrhage caused by damage to the vertebral venous plexus is very common; in most cases it can be controlled and does not lead to major complications. However, death has been reported secondary to hemorrhage of the vertebral venous plexus [10,13]. In a case series of 112 dogs that underwent ventral slot, significant hemorrhage was reported in 26.7% of the cases. Hemorrhage can be worse in dogs receiving aspirin or with deficiency of von Willebrand factor. Testing for deficiency of von Willebrand factor by measuring the concentration of von Willebrand factor or by performing a buccal mucosal bleeding time should be routinely performed in Doberman Pinschers and Rottweilers. All hemorrhage should be controlled before closure, as there is a large potential space for hematoma formation.

Respiratory Complications

Two main types of respiratory complications can occur in patients undergoing surgery for cervical spinal disorders. Some patients may experience ventilatory failure associated with neurological dysfunction leading to paralysis or paresis of the respiratory musculature [14]. In contrast, some patients are able to ventilate normally, but have abnormal pulmonary gas exchange because of lung pathology such as pneumonia or atelectasis associated with recumbency and prolonged anesthesia [3,13,14].

In dogs, the neurons of the medullary respiratory center enter the spinal cord via the reticulospinal tracts and give rise to the phrenic nerve through segments 5–7 of the cervical spinal cord [14]. The reticulospinal tracts also give rise to the neurons that innervate the intercostal muscles via the segmental intercostal nerves. Most dogs with ventilatory compromise have lesions located between C2 and C4 spinal cord segments, therefore cranial to the origins of the phrenic nerve [14]. A study evaluated 263 dogs that underwent cervical spine surgery and found that 4.9% developed ventilatory failure and required positive-pressure ventilation postoperatively. Most dogs were weaned off the ventilator (mean 4.5 days) and recovered [14]. Pneumonia has also been reported as a complication of ventral slot leading to death [15].

Cardiac Dysrhythmias and Hypotension

The risk of cardiac dysrhythmias is greater with ventral slot surgery than with thoracolumbar intervertebral disc decompression surgery [16]. This is most likely associated with retraction of the carotid arteries, vagal nerve, and sympathetic trunks and anatomical disruption of the sympathetic tectotegmental tracts of the spinal cord [13,16]. Stimulation of the vagus nerve or the carotid bodies may cause bradycardia, and manipulation of the sympathetic trunks may cause premature ventricular contractions. A study evaluated 52 dogs that underwent ventral slot and found severe bradycardia and hypotension leading to death in three dogs (5.7%) [13].

Hypotension may develop secondary to cardiac dysrhythmias, prolonged anesthesia, and blood loss, factors regularly seen in dogs undergoing ventral slot surgeries. Systolic blood pressure was evaluated in 75 dogs undergoing ventral slot and 16.5% were found to develop intraoperative hypotension (<70 mmHg) [12]. It is also possible that the incidence of hypotension is even higher than described because the few studies specifically evaluating intraoperative complications were done several years ago when blood pressure monitoring was not routinely used. Aggressive monitoring of blood pressure to identify hypotension as soon as it occurs is important to minimize complications. Intraoperative hypotension may lead to postoperative neurological deterioration secondary to spinal cord hypotension during surgery.

Neurological Complications

Excessive manipulation of the spinal cord, prolonged anesthesia for a patient with a chronically compromised spinal cord, intraoperative spinal cord hypotension, and excessive cervical extension during surgery can all result in neurological deterioration after the surgical procedure. Marked neurological deterioration is uncommon but is occasionally seen. Incomplete spinal decompression was a frequent cause of neurological worsening or failure to improve after surgery leading to euthanasia in a case series of Dobermans with cervical spondylomyelopathy [15]. In this series, residual spinal cord compression was found at necropsy in six of seven dogs, even though the surgery report of these cases indicated complete spinal cord decompression [15]. Worsening of neck pain may also be seen and can be managed postoperatively with opioids, muscle relaxants, gabapentin, nonsteroidal antiinflammatory drugs (NSAIDs), or corticosteroids. If severe pain persists beyond 2 days it should be investigated. Diagnostic imaging for patients that fail to improve or those with postoperative neurological deterioration should ideally be done using CT or MRI to allow evaluation of the intervertebral foramina. Horner's syndrome is occasionally seen after a ventral slot procedure and is usually a mild temporary complication. It is caused by excessive soft tissue retraction [17].

Vertebral Instability and Subluxation

Ventral slots alter the vertebral range of motion at the surgical site which can lead to instability and subluxation. A study documented an increase of 15–20% in the range of motion in flexion and extension and lateral bending compared with the intact intervertebral region [18]. Others have found higher increases in range of motion [19]. This instability should be more significant in the first few weeks after surgery and should decrease progressively during the healing period. Instability is expected to resolve once vertebral fusion occurs 8–12 weeks postoperatively [5,6]. Vertebral body subluxation was radiographically documented in 8% (9/113) of dogs undergoing a ventral slot procedure in one study [20]. The ratio of ventral slot to vertebral body width was 0.5 or greater in seven of eight cases with confirmed subluxation. Subluxation seems to occur more commonly in small-breed dogs and in the caudal cervical region compared with the cranial cervical region [21]. Clinical signs associated with postoperative subluxation include worsening of neck pain, worsening of neurological status, and failure to neurologically improve, all occurring usually within a week of surgery. Improvement was noted in most dogs after cervical vertebral stabilization surgery.

Postoperative Care

Postoperative care of the ventral slot patient involves cage rest for most of the day with monitored leash walks using a body harness. Activity should be very limited in the first 2 weeks after surgery. Frequency and duration of walks increases progressively but free activity should only be allowed once fusion of the slot is complete or close to complete 8 weeks postoperatively. Pain control is important in the postoperative period and can be achieved with opioids such as fentanyl as a constant-rate infusion and fentanyl patches with or without NSAIDs such as meloxicam or carprofen. If muscle spasms are present, muscle relaxants such as methocarbamol or diazepam can be used. Gabapentin is also an option for patients with more severe pain. Mild cervical discomfort can be managed with tramadol. Ice packing can be performed every 4–6 hours for 24–48 hours in an attempt to reduce postsurgical swelling and seroma formation. Nonambulatory dogs should receive physical therapy, and great care should be paid to bedding and cleanliness [2].

Video clips to accompany this book can be found on the companion website at:
www.wiley.com/go/shores/neurosurgery

References

1 Coates JR, Hoffman AG, Dewey CW. Surgical approaches to the central nervous system. In: Slatter DH (ed.) *Textbook of Small Animal Surgery*, 3rd edn. Philadelphia, PA: WB Saunders, 2003:1148–1163.
2 Sharp NJH, Wheeler SJ. Cervical disc disease. In: Sharp NJH, Wheeler SJ (eds) *Small Animal Spinal Disorders: Diagnosis and Surgery*, 2nd edn. Philadelphia, PA: Elsevier Mosby, 2005:93–120.
3 Platt SR, da Costa RC. Cervical spine. In: Tobias KM, Johnston SA (eds) *Veterinary Surgery: Small Animal*. Philadelphia, PA: Elsevier, 2011:410–448.
4 Cechner PE. Ventral cervical disc fenestration in the dog: a modified technique. *J Am Anim Hosp Assoc* 1980;16:647–650.
5 Swaim SF. Ventral decompression of the cervical spinal cord in the dog. *J Am Vet Med Assoc* 1974;164:491–495.
6 Gilpin GN. Evaluation of three techniques of ventral decompression of the cervical spinal cord in the dog. *J Am Vet Med Assoc* 1976;168:325–328.
7 da Costa RC, Parent JM. One-year clinical and magnetic resonance imaging follow-up of Doberman Pinschers with cervical spondylomyelopathy treated medically or surgically. *J Am Vet Med Assoc* 2007;231:243–250.
8 Goring RL, Beale BS, Faulkner RF. The inverted cone decompression technique: a surgical treatment for cervical vertebral instability "Wobbler syndrome" in Doberman Pinschers. *J Am Anim Hosp Assoc* 1991;27:403–409.
9 Jeffery ND. The "wobbler" syndrome In: Jeffery ND (ed.) *Handbook of Small Animal Spinal Surgery*. London: WB Saunders, 1995: 169–186.
10 McCartney W. Comparison of recovery times and complication rates between a modified slanted slot and the standard ventral slot for the treatment of cervical disc disease in 20 dogs *J Small Anim Pract* 2007;48:498–501.
11 Leperlier D, Manassero M, Blot S, Thibaud JL, Viateau V. Minimally invasive video-assisted cervical ventral slot in dogs. A cadaveric study and report of 10 clinical cases *Vet Comp Orthop Traumatol* 2011;24:50–56.
12 Smith BA, Hosgood G, Kerwin SC. Ventral slot decompression for cervical intervertebral disc disease in 112 dogs. *Aust Vet Practit* 1997;27:58–64.
13 Clark DM. An analysis of intraoperative and early postoperative mortality associated with cervical spinal decompressive surgery in the dog. *J Am Anim Hosp Assoc* 1986;22:739–744.
14 Beal MW, Paglia DT, Griffin GM, Hughes D, King LG. Ventilatory failure, ventilator management, and outcome in dogs with cervical spinal disorders: 14 cases (1991–1999). *J Am Vet Med Assoc* 2001;218:1598–1602.
15 Chambers JN, Oliver JE, Bjorling DE. Update on ventral decompression for caudal cervical disk herniation in Doberman Pinschers. *J Am Anim Hosp Assoc* 1986;22:775–778.
16 Stauffer JL, Gleed RD, Short CE, Erb HN, Schukken YH. Cardiac dysrhythmias during anesthesia for cervical decompression in the dog. *Am J Vet Res* 1988;49:1143–1146.
17 Boydell P. Horner's syndrome following cervical spinal surgery in the dog. *J Small Anim Pract* 1995;36:510–512.
18 Fauber AE, Wade JA, Lipka AE, McCabe JB, Aper RL. Effect of width of disk fenestration and a ventral slot on biomechanics of the canine C5–C6 vertebral motion unit. *Am J Vet Res* 2006;67:1844–1848.
19 Koehler CL, Stover SM, LeCouteur RA, Schulz KS, Hawkins DA. Effect of a ventral slot procedure and of smooth or positive-profile threaded pins with polymethylmethacrylate fixation on intervertebral biomechanics at treated and adjacent canine cervical vertebral motion units. *Am J Vet Res* 2005;66:678–687.
20 Lemarie RJ, Kerwin SC, Partington BP, Hosgood G. Vertebral subluxation following ventral cervical decompression in the dog. *J Am Anim Hosp Assoc* 2000;36:348–358.
21 Fitch RB, Kerwin SC, Hosgood G. Caudal cervical intervertebral disk disease in the small dog: role of distraction and stabilization in ventral slot decompression. *J Am Anim Hosp Assoc* 2000;36:68–74.

18 Lateral Cervical Approach

Amy Fauber and Robert Bergman

Introduction

It is not uncommon for the neurosurgeon to encounter lateralizing disease in the cervical spine. A lateral approach to the spinal cord or nerve roots can be very useful for intervertebral disc disease, trauma, neoplasia such as nerve sheath tumors, and other spinal cord disease such as cervical spondylomyelopathy due to bulbous articular facets. Lesions of the cervical spine located in the intervertebral foramen or spinal nerve root or involving the articular facet may require a lateral approach. Specifically, portions of the subaxial cervical spine, C3–C4 to C7–T1 present a distinct challenge in obtaining adequate exposure to the region of interest.

Clinical Evaluation

Various clinical presentations of animals with a lateralized cervical lesion may be noted. "Root signature" is a commonly encountered clinical sign [1]. An animal with this sign may hold up the affected limb periodically. Forelimb lameness may also be a presenting complaint. Following a thorough orthopedic examination, a complete neurological evaluation is recommended. Careful attention should be given to signs of front and pelvic limb lameness, weakness or ataxia that is predominantly one-sided. In some dogs with a herniated disc located in the intervertebral foramen, episodic pain may be the only clinical sign noted. Patients may or may not have significant cervical pain on palpation of the spine. Flexor withdrawal should be evaluated in both front limbs. With lesions involving the caudal aspect of the cervical spine, flexor withdrawal may be weak, incomplete, or absent. Some animals exhibit marked hyperesthesia in the affected limb and for these patients generally the lesion localization will be confined to the C6–T2 spinal cord segments. It has been reported that a weak flexor withdrawal may result from a lesion cranial to C6 spinal cord segment [2]. With chronic lesions, or profound nerve root compression, there may be marked muscle atrophy of the affected limb.

Diagnosis

Electrodiagnostic evaluation, specifically electromyography (EMG), may also be used to identify denervation and lesion distribution. EMG can be used in the determination of neurogenic atrophy from disuse atrophy. This can be helpful when a lameness is difficult to diagnose. EMG does not preclude imaging [3]. Identification of the underlying cause for lateralized clinical signs is generally done by advanced imaging (MRI, CT, or CT-myelography). Survey radiography of the cervical spine for intervertebral disc disease has a low sensitivity of about 35% for accurately identifying the location of a disc herniation [4]. Myelography without CT may not identify intraforaminal discs and it is recommended that when a lateralized lesion is suspected that CT be used concurrently [5]. CT without intrathecal contrast may be useful for chondrodystrophic dogs, although a normal study does not rule out the possibility of underlying disease [6]. CT protocols of the cervical spine have been described [7]. MRI characteristics of nerve sheath tumors and intraspinal nerve sheath tumors have been described [8]. Both types of tumor tend to be most frequently found in the cervical spine [8,9]. The authors prefer MRI, as it is the most sensitive form of imaging for soft tissue and neurological disease processes [10,11].

Indications for a Lateral Cervical Approach

Lateral approaches to the cervical spine have been described previously in a limited number of reports [12–14]. Exposure to this portion of the spine can be technically difficult. This approach may be avoided in favor of a less optimal form of exposure if the clinician is not experienced with this surgical approach.

A lateral approach can be particularly helpful for multiple neurological diseases that require decompression. Hansen type I intervertebral disc material will sometimes lodge in the intervertebral foramen (Figure 18.1). Residual disc within the intervertebral foramen can serve as a source of ongoing radicular pain. A ventral slot

Current Techniques in Canine and Feline Neurosurgery, First Edition. Edited by Andy Shores and Brigitte A. Brisson.
© 2017 John Wiley & Sons, Inc. Published 2017 by John Wiley & Sons, Inc.
Companion website: www.wiley.com/go/shores/neurosurgery

does not allow for exposure of the nerve root, while a dorsal approach may not allow adequate decompression of the ventral aspect of the spinal cord. Lateral exposure allows for clear visibility of the spinal nerve in addition to allowing access to the dorsal and lateral aspects of the spinal canal.

A variation of a hemilaminectomy has been suggested for use in small dogs [15]. A case series of 41 dogs in which a hemilaminectomy was used to treat type I and type II intervertebral disc disease has been described. In this report, dogs with type I disc disease tended to have a better outcome following surgery [16].

The modified dorsal–lateral approach is commonly used by the authors for treatment of facet-related cervical spondylomyelopathy (Figure 18.2). The lateral approach is used to remove an abnormal facet and then a separate approach is used to perform a discectomy and fusion. The lateral removal of a malformed articular facet is technically easier and less likely to cause excessive spinal cord manipulation compared with a dorsal laminectomy that is used for access to abnormal facets. While the exposure of the affected facet is not particularly difficult in a large dog, the bone can be quite thick and require extensive drilling. This approach to treatment has been used to decompress the spinal cord at more than one level in dogs with multilevel cervical spondylomyelopathy by the authors.

Neoplasia that affects the spinal cord or nerve roots of the cervical spine may require lateral exposure to the cervical spine. This type of exposure allows the clinician to follow the tumor as it exits the intervertebral foramen. It also provides enough access to perform a durotomy at the location where the tumor enters the spinal cord. Tumors the authors have treated using this approach include osteosarcoma, meningioma, chondrosarcoma, and nerve sheath tumors (Figure 18.3).

Surgical Anatomy and Approaches

The anatomy in the lateral and dorsal cervical spine is complex (Figure 18.4). Most neurosurgeons are familiar with the ventral anatomy of the neck but the complex muscle attachments and vascular anatomy of the dorsal and lateral cervical spine can make a neurosurgeon less likely to attempt a lateral approach.

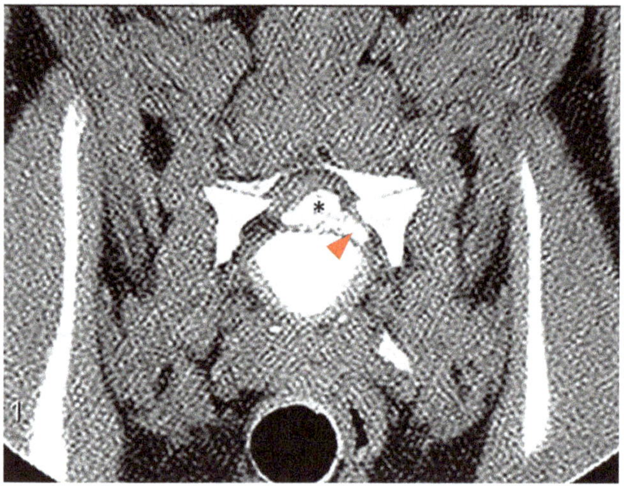

Figure 18.1 Transverse CT at the level of C5–C6. There is a large ventrolateral extradural spinal cord compression (asterisk) with extension into the intervertebral foramen (arrowhead).

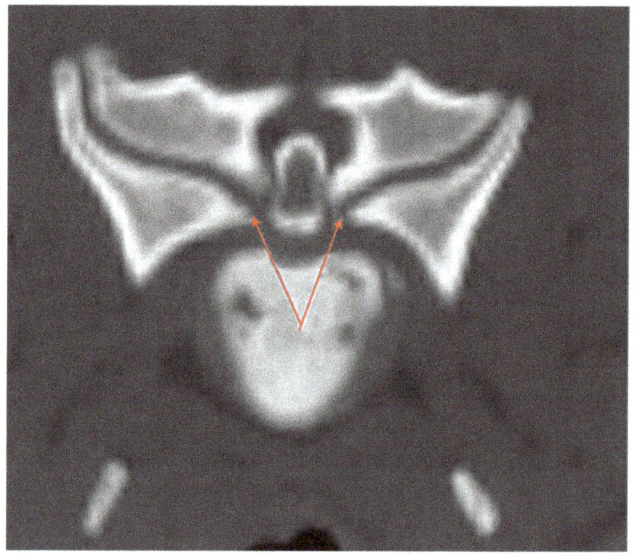

Figure 18.2 Transverse CT-myelography at C5–C6 demonstrating lateral compression of the spinal cord due to bulbous facets (arrows).

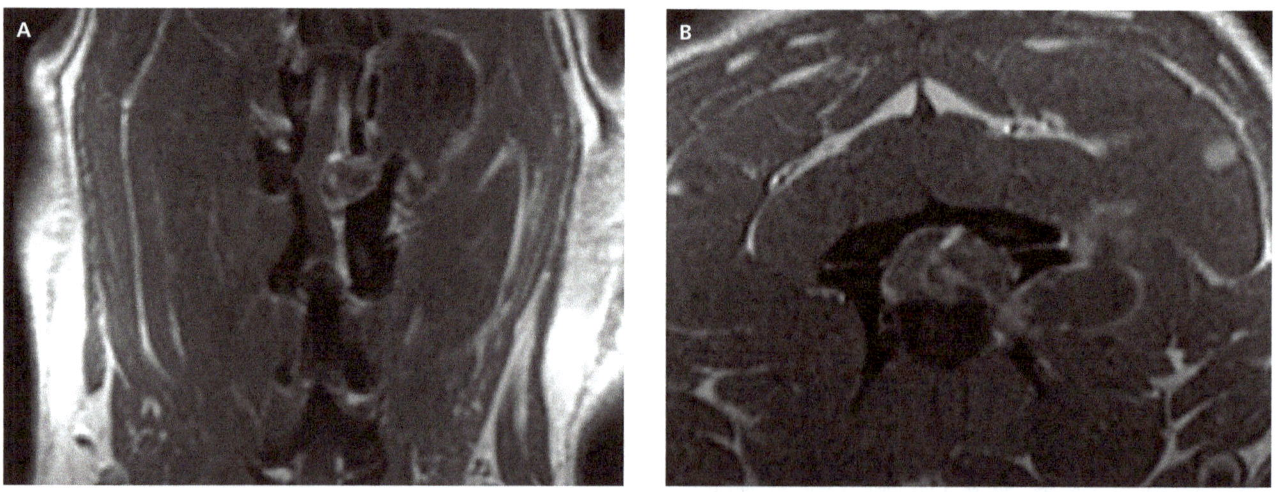

Figure 18.3 (A, B) Dorsal and transverse T1-weighted, gadolinium-contrast MRI demonstrating lateralizing compression of the spinal cord due to neoplasia.

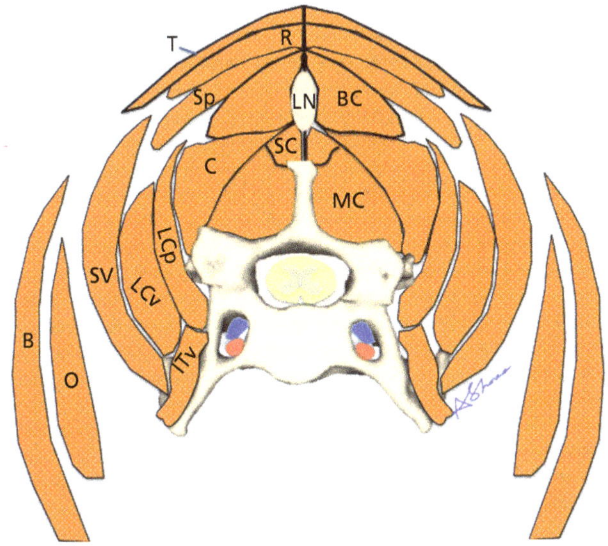

Figure 18.4 Canine fifth cervical vertebra and associated musculature: cross-sectional anatomy. T, trapezius; R, rhomboideus; Sp, splenius; BC, biventer cervicalis; LN, ligamentm nuchae; SC, spinalis cervicalis; MC, multifidus cervicis; LCp, longissimus capitis; LCv, longissimus cervicis; SV, serratus ventralis; ITv, intertransversarii; O, omotransversarius; B, brachiocephalicus.

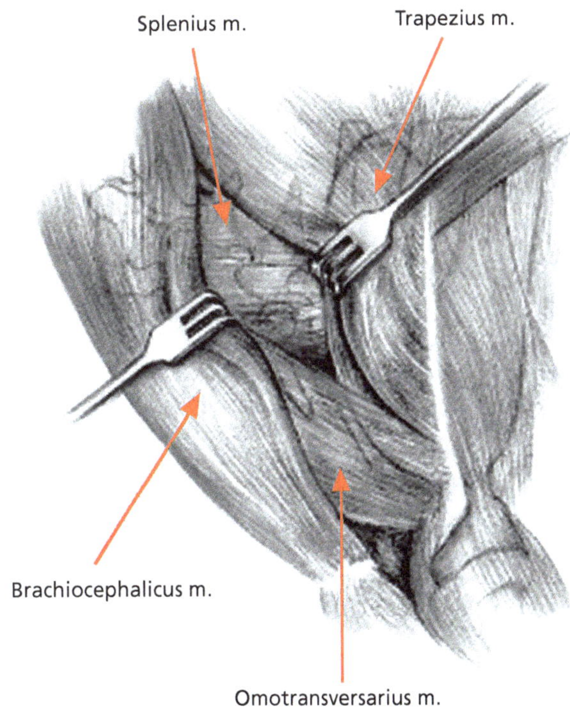

Figure 18.5 Superficial lateral approach to the caudal cervical canine spine, with the skin and platysma muscle removed. Craniolateral retraction of the brachiocephalicus and caudo-dorsolateral retraction of the trapezius muscles is facilitated by the fascial plane that naturally divides these two muscles, and exposes the underlying splenius muscle. The serratus ventralis muscle has been incorporated into the caudal retractor. *Source*: Rossmeisl et al. [14]. Reproduced with permission of John Wiley & Sons, Inc.

Postoperative morbidity and lack of exposure of the ventrolateral and ventral spinal canal with a traditional dorsal approach and limited exposure to only the ventral spinal canal from a ventral slot make a lateral approach a necessity for cases with lateralizing disease. Three techniques have been described for an approach to the lateral cervical spine.

Lateral Approach

This approach allows exposure of the lateral spinal canal [12,13]. The patient is placed in lateral recumbency with the affected side up and positioned with the forelimb pulled caudally. After the transverse processes of the affected site are identified with palpation, an incision is made in the skin and platysma from C2 to the cranial border of the scapula. The brachiocephalicus and trapezius muscles are then identified and the superficial cervical artery and vein are retracted or ligated and transected. The brachiocephalicus muscle is then incised and the splenius and serratus ventralis muscles are exposed. The omotransversarius muscle is then retracted after it is dissected from adjacent connective tissue. The serratus ventralis muscle is incised perpendicular to its muscle fibers. The insertion of the serratus ventralis to the transverse processes of the cervical vertebrae should not be disturbed. The longissimus cervicis and longissimus capitis muscle are bluntly dissected and retracted ventrally. Correct localization can be determined by palpating the prominent transverse process of C6. The C5–C6 articular facet can then be identified and the correct surgical site can be determined by counting articular facets rostrally or caudally. Once the correct articular facet is identified, dissection is continued between the longissimus capitis muscle and the complexus muscle. The tendinous attachments of the multifidus cervicis muscle are sharply transected from the articular facets. A periosteal elevator is used to elevate the longissimus capitis muscle dorsally and the intertransversarii cervicis muscle is retracted ventrally. The vertebral artery and vein are avoided as they run through the transverse foramen, and the intervertebral foramen is avoided. The facet and laminae at the affected site are then removed to allow exposure of the lateral and ventral spinal canal. Care should be taken when performing the facetectomy as the interarcuate branches of the internal vertebral venous plexus can be found in the interarcuate ligament. This vessel should be ligated and transected. A free fat graft can be placed over the laminectomy site. Reapposition of the serratus ventralis and brachiocephalicus muscle is performed with horizontal mattress sutures. The subcutaneous tissue and skin are closed according to the surgeon's preference.

Modified Lateral Approach

The patient is placed in lateral recumbency and the forelimb is pulled caudally [14]. A curvilinear incision is made over the cervical articular facets from C2 to the cranial aspect of the scapula. The platysma is incised and the brachiocephalicus and trapezius muscles are visualized. The brachiocephalicus muscle is bluntly dissected using a grid approach. The serratus ventralis muscle is also bluntly dissected from the longissimus muscles. For caudal lesions the fascial plane between the brachiocephalicus muscle and trapezius muscle is bluntly dissected rather than dissecting through the brachiocephalicus muscle (Figure 18.5). The superficial cervical artery and vein are ligated and divided. The facet and articular processes are identified by palpation of the transverse process of C6 and the first rib. The fascial plane between the longissimus capitis and complexus muscles is dissected. The tendinous attachments of the complexus and multifidus muscles to the articular facet is sharply transected. The muscles are then elevated from the laminae and the longissimus capitis muscle is sharply transected from the transverse processes. Care is taken to avoid the interspinous and interarcuate branches of the internal vertebral venous plexus. The serratus ventralis muscle fibers can be reapposed with simple interrupted sutures. The subcutaneous tissue and skin are closed according to the surgeon's preference.

Modified Dorsal Approach to Lateral Cervical Spine

The authors have performed numerous lateral cervical approaches using a modified dorsal approach. For this approach, the patient is placed in sternal recumbency. If exposure of the cranial cervical spine is desired, then the forelimbs are positioned in extension. If exposure of the caudal cervical spine is desired, the forelimbs are pulled cranially and secured with the elbows touching ventrally to allow for lateral retraction of the scapula during surgery.

A dorsal midline incision is made from C2 to T1. The incision is continued on the midline through the dorsal median raphe of the trapezius and rhomboideus muscles. The biventer cervicis muscle is not disturbed and the nuchal ligament is not visualized. At the level of the biventer cervicis the dissection is continued through the fascial plane lateral to the biventer muscle (Figure 18.6). This dissection is continued lateral to the complexus muscle and medial to the longissimus capitis muscle. The articular facet can be palpated in this plane and the spinous processes of the caudal cervical vertebrae and T1 are palpated to identify the appropriate site.

The most difficult aspect of the modified dorsal–lateral approach to the cervical spine is accurate intraoperative identification of the affected site. This can be particularly difficult in the region of C4–C5 since some of the facets of the spine are indistinct. During the procedure, the spinous processes are palpated and compared with lateral radiographs of the cervical spine. The articular facets are palpated along with the spinous processes. The authors have found that despite careful palpation, it can still be difficult to correctly identify the lesion. In some instances, postoperative CT has been performed to verify the site.

The complexus and multifidus muscles are subperiosteally elevated dorsally and their tendinous attachments to the articular facets are sharply transected to aid in elevation (Figure 18.7). The longissimus capitis muscle is carefully elevated with care taken to avoid the vertebral artery and foramen. Multiple Gelpi retractors are used to maintain retraction of the longissimus capitis and multifidus muscles to ensure visualization of the spine for drilling. Once the facet is exposed, a high-speed pneumatic burr is used to remove the bone. The laminectomy is completed using Kerrison rongeurs. In giant-breed dogs the bone can be very thick, and removal for adequate decompression requires extensive drilling. In order to maintain accurate anatomical location, the authors tend to follow the articular facet during drilling. The lamina and facet are removed and care is taken to control hemorrhage from the branches of the ventral vertebral venous plexus with the use of electrocautery or ligation. A hemilaminectomy or facetectomy can be performed (Figure 18.8). Depending on the underlying pathology, careful inspection of the spinal nerve as it exits the intervertebral foramen should be done. Degenerate disc material may be found in the sheath of connective tissue that surrounds the spinal nerve. Probing the nerve root with a nerve root retractor may be useful. Failure to remove this disc material may result in continued pain. The lateral and ventral aspects of the spinal canal are easily accessed following the hemilaminectomy. If neoplasia is suspected, a durotomy may be performed once the laminectomy is complete. This may be done by various techniques but the authors use a #12 scalpel blade to create the durotomy. This access allows for removal of neoplastic tissue that is located within the intradural space. For closure, the trapezius and rhomboideus muscles are reapposed along the median raphe using a simple continuous pattern. The subcutaneous tissue and skin are closed according to the surgeon's preference.

The most serious impediment to this procedure can be hemorrhage. Hemorrhage results from disruption of the vertebral arteries as well as the venous sinuses. This has also been reported in earlier reports for similar approaches [14]. Bleeding should be controlled with meticulous dissection, use of electrocautery, and hemostatic agents. In some instances hemorrhage can be difficult to control and suction must be used to visualize the lesion. This problem is most likely to occur during removal of a lateralized disc and can be quite problematic. In some instances a blood transfusion has been required [16].

Postoperative Care

Postoperative care of these patients is similar to that for other patients undergoing spine procedures. In the immediate postoperative period the patient should be monitored for discomfort and incisional complications. Multimodal pain management should be instituted immediately following surgery. A constant-rate infusion of an opioid, *N*-methyl-D-aspartate (NMDA) receptor antagonist,

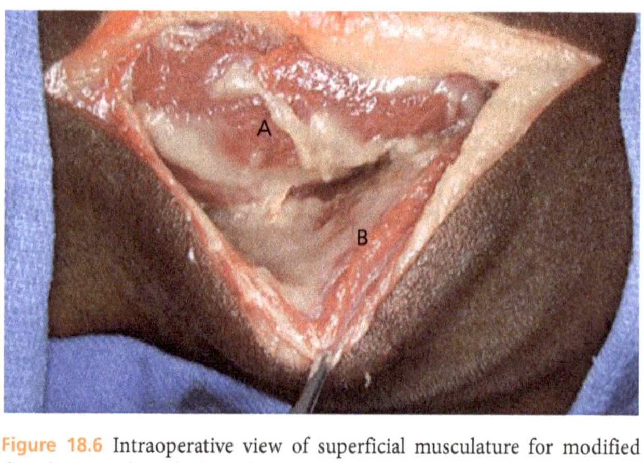

Figure 18.6 Intraoperative view of superficial musculature for modified dorsal approach to the lateral cervical spine: A, biventer cervicis muscle; B, splenius muscle. Note the fascial plane between these two muscles.

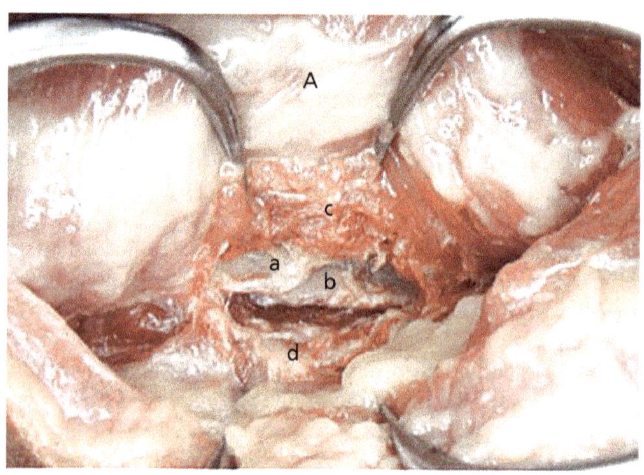

Figure 18.7 Intraoperative view of deep musculature for modified dorsal approach to lateral cervical spine: A, biventer cervicis muscle; a, cranial articular process; b, caudal articular process; c, elevated multifidus and complexus muscles; d, longissimus capitis muscle.

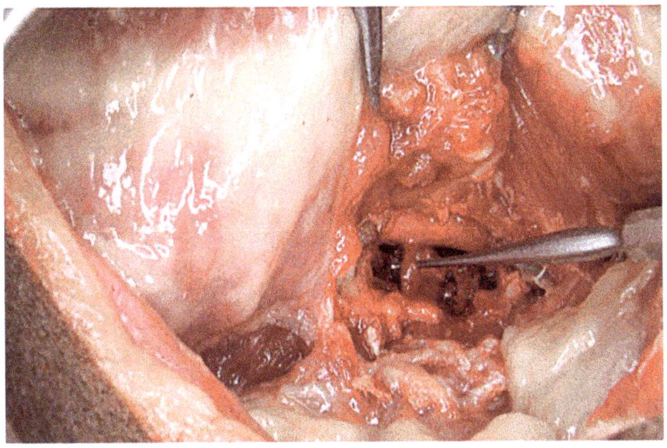

Figure 18.8 Intraoperative view of spinal canal following hemilaminectomy. The lateral and ventral spinal canal are easily accessible and the nerve root is well exposed.

and lidocaine can be started immediately following surgery. The patient can be weaned off the constant-rate infusion within 36–48 hours and oral pain medications can be started as the constant-rate infusion is being discontinued. Oral pain medications generally consist of an analgesic such as tramadol, an antiinflammatory drug such as prednisone, and other drugs such as gabapentin, when deemed necessary. The underlying disease or the manipulation of the nerve root may result in neuropathic pain. Gabapentin or pregabalin may be useful for a few weeks following surgery [17]. This type of pain management may help encourage movement during rehabilitation.

Depending on the preoperative neurological status, advanced nursing care for weak or recumbent patients will need to be diligently performed. The patient should be kept on clean and dry bedding with padding under bony prominences to avoid decubital ulceration. Passive range of motion exercises should be performed three to four times daily in nonambulatory patients.

While instability resulting in subluxation has not been reported, the disruption of the articular facet could create an increased risk of instability leading to pain or subluxation. Therefore, patients should be confined to an appropriately sized crate for 6 weeks following surgery. Neck leads should be avoided and it is often recommended for owners to switch to using a harness indefinitely to avoid putting pressure on the cervical spine.

Video clips to accompany this book can be found on the companion website at:
www.wiley.com/go/shores/neurosurgery

References

1 McDonnell JJ, Platt SR, Clayton LA. Neurologic conditions causing lameness in companion animals. *Vet Clin North Am Small Anim Pract* 2001;31:17–38.

2 Forterre F, Konar M, Tomek A et al. Accuracy of the withdrawal reflex for localization of the site of cervical disk herniation in dogs: 35 cases (2004–2007). *J Am Vet Med Assoc* 2008;232:559–563.

3 Chrisman CL. Electromyography in the localization of spinal cord and nerve root neoplasia in dogs and cats. *J Am Vet Med Assoc* 1975;166:1074–1079.

4 Somerville ME, Anderson SM, Gill PJ, Kantrowitz BJ, Stowater JL. Accuracy of localization of cervical intervertebral disk extrusion or protrusion using survey radiography in dogs. *J Am Anim Hosp Assoc* 2001;37:563–572.

5 Felts JF, Prata RG. Cervical disk disease in the dog: intraforaminal and lateral extrusions. *J Am Anim Hosp Assoc* 1983;19:755–760.

6 Olby NJ, Muñana KR, Sharp NJH, Thrall DE. The computed tomographic appearance of acute thoracolumbar intervertebral disc herniations in dogs. *Vet Radiol Ultrasound* 2000;41:396–402.

7 Drees R, Dennison SE, Keuler NS, Schwarz T. Computed tomographic imaging protocol for the canine cervical and lumbar spine. *Vet Radiol Ultrasound* 2009;50:74–79.

8 Petersen SA, Sturges BK, Dickinson PJ et al. Canine intraspinal meningiomas: imaging features, histopathologic classification, and long-term outcome in 34 dogs. *J Vet Intern Med* 2008;22:946–953.

9 Brehm DM, Vite CH, Steinberg HS, Haviland J, van Winkle T. A retrospective evaluation of 51 cases of peripheral nerve sheath tumors in the dog. *J Am Anim Hosp Assoc* 1995;31:349–359.

10 Kraft S, Ehrhart EJ, Gall D et al. Magnetic resonance imaging characteristics of peripheral nerve sheath tumors of the canine brachial plexus in 18 dogs. *Vet Radiol Ultrasound* 2007;48:1–7.

11 Da Costa RC, Samii VF. Advanced imaging of the spine in small animals. *Vet Clin North Am Small Anim Pract* 2010;40:765–790.

12 Lipsitz D, Bailey CS. Lateral approach for cervical spinal cord decompression. *Prog Vet Neurol* 1990;3:39–44.

13 Lipsitz D, Bailey CS. Clinical use of the lateral cervical approach for the cervical spinal cord and nerve root diseases: eight cases. *Prog Vet Neurol* 1995;6:60–65.

14 Rossmeisl JH Jr, Lanz OI, Inzana KD, Bergman RL. A modified lateral approach to the canine cervical spine: procedural description and clinical application in 16 dogs with lateralized compressive myelopathy or radiculopathy. *Vet Surg* 2005;34:436–444.

15 Tanaka H, Nakayama M, Takase K. Usefulness of hemilaminectomy for cervical intervertebral disk disease in small dogs. *J Vet Med Sci* 2005;67:679–683.

16 Schmied O, Golini L, Steffen F. Effectiveness of cervical hemilaminectomy in canine Hansen type I and type II disc disease: a retrospective study. *J Am Anim Hosp Assoc* 2011;47:342–350.

17 Grubb T. Chronic neuropathic pain in veterinary patients. *Top Companion Anim Med* 2010;25:45–52.

19 Cervical Distraction and Stabilization

Bianca Hettlich

Introduction

Cervical distraction and stabilization has become increasingly popular for the treatment of cervical spondylomyelopathy (CSM). The goal of surgery is to eliminate motion at the affected vertebral articulation, thereby decreasing tissue responses secondary to instability such as ligamentous or annular hypertrophy as well as articular facet proliferation. Distraction of the intervertebral disc space is beneficial for traction-responsive lesions such as soft tissue compression by thickened dorsal longitudinal ligament or ligamentum flavum. While distraction per se may not lead to improvement of bony compression by facet proliferation, the use of a disc spacer in a neutral or slightly distracted position is beneficial for load sharing between the affected vertebrae, thereby improving implant longevity. Interbody fusion is desired to provide long-term stability and prevent implant failure.

Preoperative Planning

Well-positioned orthogonal radiographs of the cervical vertebral column are obtained to gain a general idea of vertebral body and disc space dimensions. For plate fixation, radiographs help determine plate size and length and probable screw location. Computed tomography provides excellent bony detail and is considered the most useful modality for preoperative planning of vertebral column stabilization. Vertebral body dimensions, in particular height, should be determined via CT to assist with selection of screw lengths. If an intervertebral spacer is used, endplate height and width, and disc space depth need to be calculated to obtain an appropriately sized spacer. Disc space dimensions should be obtained from unaffected sites (if available) to determine "normal" dimensions. While MRI is considered the gold-standard imaging modality for spinal cord evaluation and invaluable for overall assessment of disease, the osseous detail it provides can be challenging for preoperative planning.

Anatomical Considerations

Cervical vertebral anatomy is challenging for rigid fixation, with limited compact bone stock and proximity of important neurovascular structures (Figure 19.1). Dorsal approaches for stabilization of the cervical vertebral column in large dogs are uncommon. The vertebral body offers the most bone for fixation and is easily approached via a standard ventral approach. However, even this part of the vertebra offers on average only 6–12 mm in bone depth in most large dogs until the vertebral canal is breached. The vertebral body is hourglass shaped and therefore the greatest bone depth is near the vertebral endplate and the thinnest portion over the mid-body. Intervertebral disc orientation is oblique in a craniodorsal to caudoventral direction; therefore most bone will be purchased if implants are directed parallel to the endplates. The presence of the sternum and the limited exposure of the caudal cervical vertebral column can make implant placement parallel to the endplate in C6 and C7 quite challenging. The transverse processes offer additional fixation sites; however, bone is quite thin and care must be taken to avoid the transverse foramen (present C1–C6). Advancing implants through the ventral aspect of the vertebral body in a laterodorsal direction toward the pedicle would provide increased bone purchase and also bicortical fixation. However, the pedicle is very narrow and pedicle width is not uniform throughout the span of a cervical vertebra, thus making it challenging to be engaged with a pin or screw.

Implant Selection

Evidence in the veterinary literature confirms that bicortical implant placement in the cervical vertebral bodies is associated with a high risk of injury to important neurovascular structures such as spinal cord, nerve roots, or vertebral vasculature (i.e., vertebral artery in transverse foramen) [1]. Therefore, bicortical vertebral body implants are not recommended for cervical fixation. Despite less bone purchase and concern for implant stiffness,

Current Techniques in Canine and Feline Neurosurgery, First Edition. Edited by Andy Shores and Brigitte A. Brisson.
© 2017 John Wiley & Sons, Inc. Published 2017 by John Wiley & Sons, Inc.
Companion website: www.wiley.com/go/shores/neurosurgery

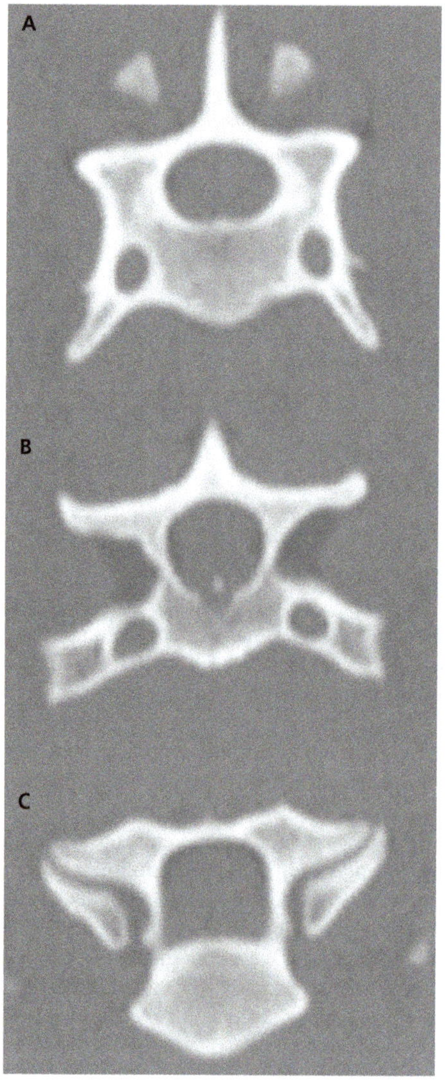

Figure 19.1 Axial CT at different levels of C5 vertebra in a large-breed dog. (A) Just caudal to the cranial endplate of C5. The pedicles and vertebral body dimensions are relatively large, and the transverse foramina are prominent. (B) Mid-body of C5. Pedicle dimensions are minute and the body depth has decreased significantly; note the limited space within the transverse processes when avoiding the transverse foramina. (C) Just cranial to the caudal endplate of C5. The vertebral body enlarges again, offering more bone for implant purchase; pedicle dimensions are minute.

monocortical screw fixation seems to compare favorably with bicortical pin fixation and eliminates the potential for major iatrogenic injury. Monocortical screw fixation has become the standard in current techniques [2–6].

The use of monocortical screws with polymethylmethacrylate (PMMA) provides the most freedom with regard to screw placement; however, presence of a large bulk of cement can interfere with adjacent soft tissues and also makes implant removal more time-consuming. Plate fixation eliminates bulky implants, and improves soft tissue closure and ease of implant removal if required. Depending on the surgeon's comfort with inventory, and its availability, locking plates with monocortical screws can be applied to the ventral vertebral bodies. Traditional nonlocking plates should be avoided as they are challenging to apply with appropriate contouring to produce excellent plate–bone contact and friction.

To date, most commonly used veterinary plate systems applied to the spine are made of stainless steel, prohibiting the use of immediate postoperative MRI. Titanium implants significantly reduce artifact development on MRI and are the preferred metal for vertebral instrumentation; however, human plate systems are expensive and few veterinary products are available. A simple and cost-efficient solution that allows postoperative spinal cord imaging is the use of titanium screws in conjunction with PMMA.

Positioning and Approach

The dog is placed in dorsal recumbency with thoracic limbs tied back caudally (Figure 19.2). The cervical vertebral column is supported with towels and a beanbag to level the spine horizontally in a neutral position. Placing a large roll of towels under the neck should be avoided as this overly extends the vertebral column and makes it more difficult to maintain the spine in alignment while traction is applied. Care must be taken to securely tie the dog's body to prevent displacement, especially if manual traction is applied for distraction. The dog's right side should be placed toward the edge of the surgery table to improve ease of access during a right-sided routine ventral approach. Both proximal humeri are included in the sterile field to allow harvesting of an autologous cancellous bone graft. Bone graft should be obtained as late as possible during the procedure and stored in a blood-soaked sponge until implantation to improve graft survival.

With the surgeon standing on the right side, a standard ventral midline or right paramedian approach is performed to the cervical vertebral column. With a paramedian approach, the insertion of the right sternocephalicus muscle can be partially tenotomized from the sternum. Rarely is it necessary to split the manubrium sterni. For a single-site distraction/stabilization, the ventral vertebral bodies adjacent to the affected disc space are exposed but dissection can usually spare the neighboring disc spaces. If PMMA fixation is used, part of the longus colli musculature can be resected to make room for the cement. Otherwise, soft tissues are preserved.

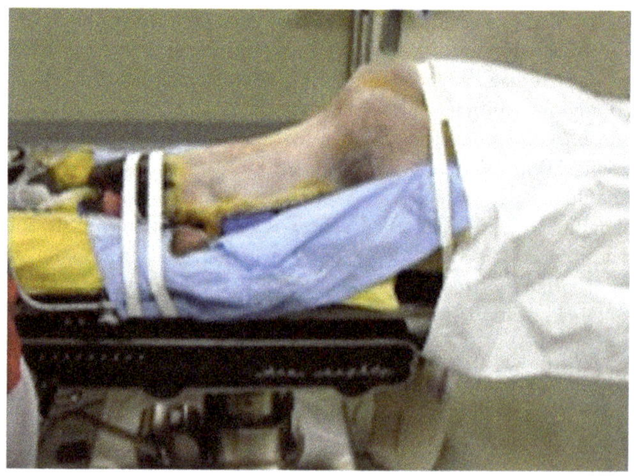

Figure 19.2 Positioning of a dog for cervical distraction and stabilization. The dog is in dorsal recumbency with the neck in neutral and the head extended. The sterile field includes both shoulder joints to allow for bone graft harvesting from the proximal humerus. Both forelimbs are tied back and the body is maintained in a straight position by using a vacuum bag. Tape is used to secure the dog to the table. During manual distraction, the tape holding the head will be removed.

Surgical Procedure

Vertebral Distraction

Distraction of the intervertebral space can be achieved via manual traction or vertebral distractors. Good distraction greatly facilitates discectomy and decompression of extruded material if present. For manual traction it is very important to secure the patient's body sufficiently to the surgical table without interfering with respiration or compromising circulation of blood flow to distal limbs. The pinnae and mandibular rami can be used as extra anchor points while gently pulling the dog's head rostrally. Manual traction usually leads to sufficient disc space distraction to perform discectomy, remove extruded disc material from the vertebral canal, and place a disc spacer. It avoids placement of distractors or distractor pins that can interfere with access to the affected disc space(s) and possibly compromise bone needed for fixation. However, manual traction is labor-intense and can often only be maintained for a few minutes without loosing distraction. The person applying traction must do so in a slow and deliberate way and avoid sudden collapse of the vertebral articulation with possible injury to the spinal cord. A variety of human vertebral distractors are available, with the most commonly used one in veterinary surgery being a Caspar-style distractor (Figure 19.3). This instrument uses two fixation pins placed perpendicularly into adjacent vertebral bodies. These pins are then connected to the distractor and the disc space is carefully distracted. If properly placed and assembled, distraction is easily achieved and greatly facilitates discectomy. However, over-distraction is also easily achieved and must be avoided to protect articular facet integrity and prevent nerve root injury. Also, since most distraction and stabilization techniques require implant placement along the ventral aspect of the vertebral bodies, distractor pins can obstruct and compromise valuable bone stock for instrumentation. A commonly used veterinary instrument to aid in disc space distraction is a modified Gelpi retractor, where the tips have been shortened to 2–3 mm length. The Gelpi retractor is placed into small holes that are drilled into the ventral vertebral bodies adjacent to the affected disc space. As with Caspar distractors, use of such a retractor, while beneficial for disc space distraction, will occupy and potentially compromise valuable bone needed for fixation. Therefore, benefits of a distractor need to be weighed against the potential disadvantages.

Discectomy

Discectomy is performed with the goal of ultimate arthrodesis between the affected vertebral bodies. Both endplates must be cleared of disc material to allow bone fusion, as remaining soft tissue will impede bony bridging. Sharp dissection of the ventral annulus fibrosus with a #11 blade will speed up disc removal. Lempert rongeurs are used to carefully remove the nucleus pulposus and as much of the lateral and dorsal annulus as possible. Distraction is required to allow rongeurs to be inserted sufficiently deep to remove enough disc. The goal is to remove approximately 90% of the disc, leaving a thin rim of annulus along the lateral and dorsal aspect (Figure 19.4). The remaining rim will prevent graft material and intervertebral spacer from protruding into the vertebral canal or dislodging laterally. Aggressive dorsal and lateral

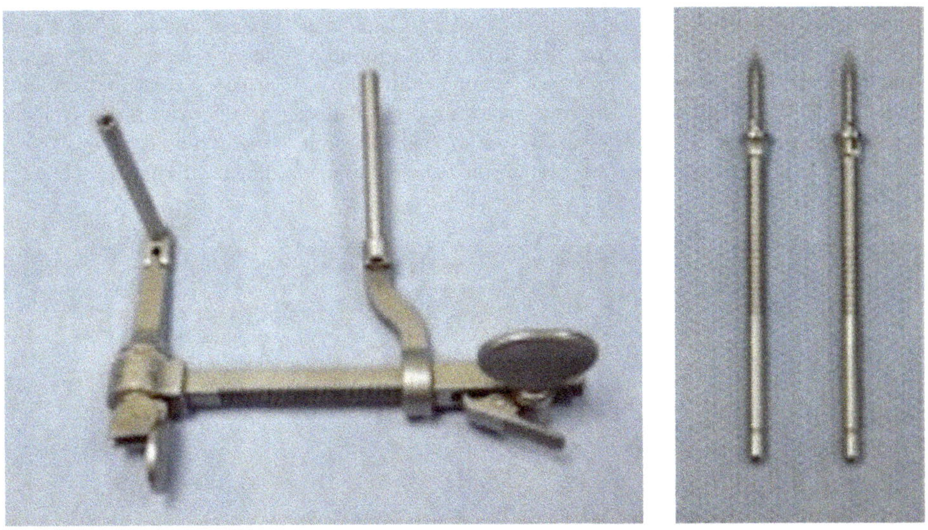

Figure 19.3 Caspar retractor with instrument-specific distraction pins. The pins are placed into the ventral aspect of adjacent vertebral bodies. Thereafter, the retractor arms are inserted over the pins. Distraction is then achieved by slowly turning the ratchet.

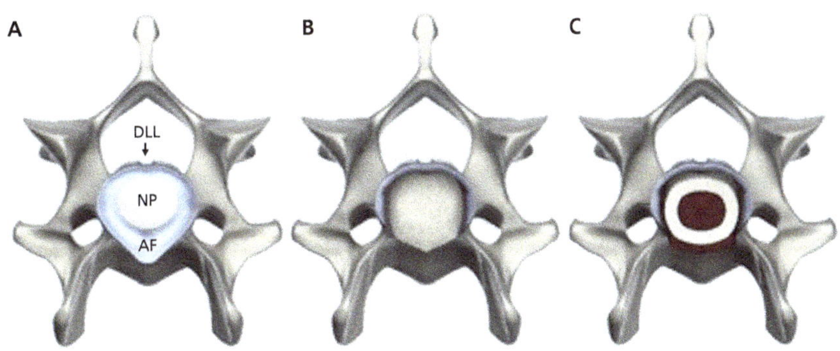

Figure 19.4 Illustration of an intervertebral disc in situ. (A) A partial discectomy with only a thin rim of annulus fibrosus (AF) remaining laterally and dorsally. (B) An intervertebral spacer using a cortical ring graft filled with cancellous bone (C). AF, annulus fibrosus; DLL, dorsal longitudinal ligament; NP, nucleus pulposus. *Source:* Reproduced with the permission of The Ohio State University.

annulus resection should be avoided to prevent inadvertent damage to the spinal cord as well as adjacent vasculature and nerve roots.

If a disc extrusion has occurred, the dorsal annulus must be partially removed to allow extraction of extruded material from the vertebral canal. Once as much disc material as possible has been removed by rongeurs, bone curettes are used to gently clear both vertebral endplates of remaining cartilaginous material. Careful use of a pneumatic drill can assist in clearing of the endplates; however, excessive removal of bone can weaken the endplates and lead to subsidence of the disc spacer (if used).

Intervertebral Spacer

Distraction of an intervertebral articulation ameliorates spinal cord compression by proliferated soft tissues and protruding dorsal annulus fibrosus. As there is no bone on bone contact between the affected vertebrae, vertebral implants must carry most of the load during normal movement of the cervical vertebral column. The goal of an intervertebral spacer is to maintain the desired disc space depth and provide load sharing between the affected vertebral bodies, thereby increased implant longevity.

Intervertebral spacers can range from simple cement plugs to carbon fiber reinforced polymer cages, cortical rings, and metal cages. While solid materials such as cement plugs will maintain distraction, they will not allow ingrowth of bone and fusion within the disc space. Cages or cortical ring allografts provide distraction while allowing placement of a fresh cancellous autogenous bone graft in the middle of the cage/ring to encourage bone fusion [3,5]. In the case of a cortical allograft, the ring will be resorbed and replaced with autogenous bone over time. Cortical allografts are commercially available in different length and diameters (Bergman block; Veterinary Transplant Services, Inc., Kent, WA). A round or slightly oval section of bone is preferred (femur or distal tibia). Patient-specific dimensions of a normal-appearing cervical disc space are measured. If all intervertebral discs are affected, the width and height of the vertebral endplates are obtained and disc space depth is estimated (traction may aid). Based on these measurements, a cortical allograft is ordered. Block segments are generally 2–5 cm long and several rings can be made from one length of bone for the same patient. Most large-breed dogs undergoing cervical distraction and stabilization have similar disc space dimensions, and if caseload is high enough several cortical ring allografts can be stored in hospital. At time of surgery, the allograft is thawed to room temperature in warm sterile saline. A sagittal saw is used to cut a cortical ring of sufficient depth (Figure 19.5). It is recommended to cut the ring slightly larger and do final adjustments by removing more bone with a bone rasp to avoid a ring that is of insufficient size. Fresh cancellous autograph is obtained from the proximal humerus just prior to placement of the disc spacer (Figure 19.6). The ring allograph is packed tightly with this fresh graft. The disc space is distracted and the ring allograph is inserted along the endplate orientation. Care must be taken to insert the ring sufficiently dorsal. The concavity in the endplate of the cranial vertebral body can act as a trap for the ring, preventing its full insertion, and leading to poor fit and inappropriate distraction of the disc space. If allograft ring dimensions fit with disc space dimensions and the discectomy has been performed appropriately, the ring allograft should be flush with the ventral aspect of the vertebral bodies. Any remaining cancellous graft is placed around the ventral aspect of the disc space and fixation of the affected vertebrae commences.

Indication for Additional Decompression

The two main indications for decompressive procedures in addition to cervical stabilization are compression by extruded nuclear material or severe dorsolateral compression by articular processes. In case of disc extrusion, removal of sequestered nuclear material can usually be achieved through the disc space after discectomy. If needed, a narrow ventral slot can be performed; however, any breach in vertebral endplate may compromise stability of a disc spacer if used. If no spacer is inserted, the ventral slot space can be filled with cancellous bone graft prior to closure to aid bony fusion.

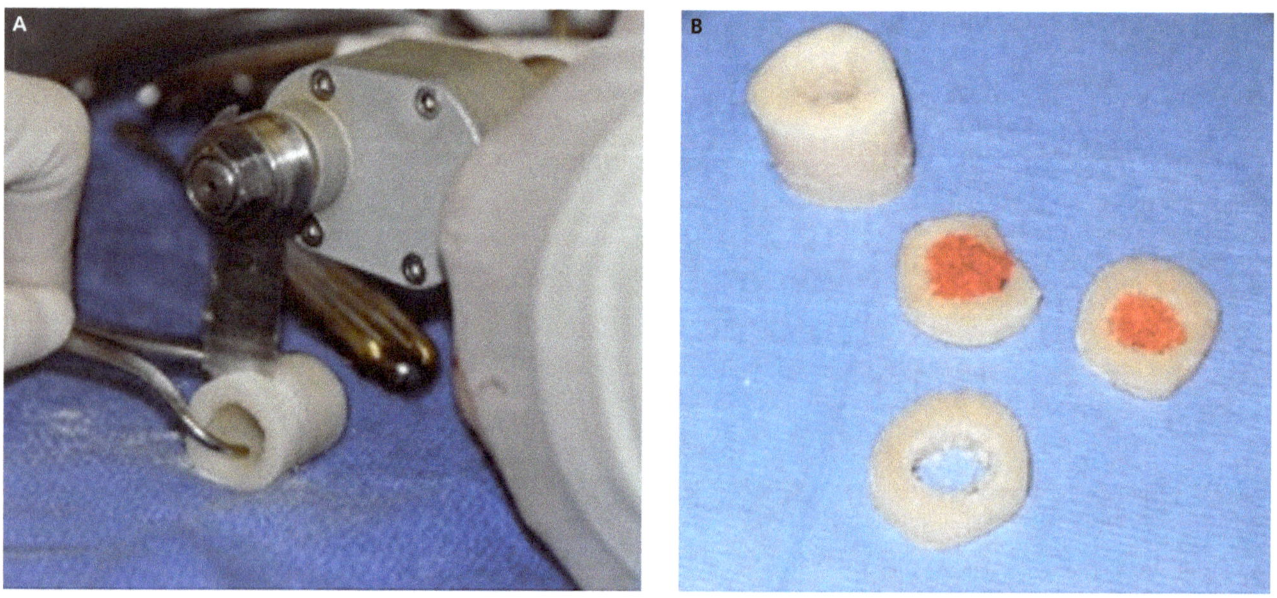

Figure 19.5 (A) A sagittal saw is used to cut a cortical allograft segment into a ring of appropriate depth to be used as an intervertebral spacer. (B) Several cortical rings have been cut and two are packed with fresh cancellous bone graft. One of the rings has been modified for improved fit by carefully cutting part the cortex. However, it is preferred to order a cortical segment that fits the patient-specific disc space dimensions rather than compromising the structure of the ring.

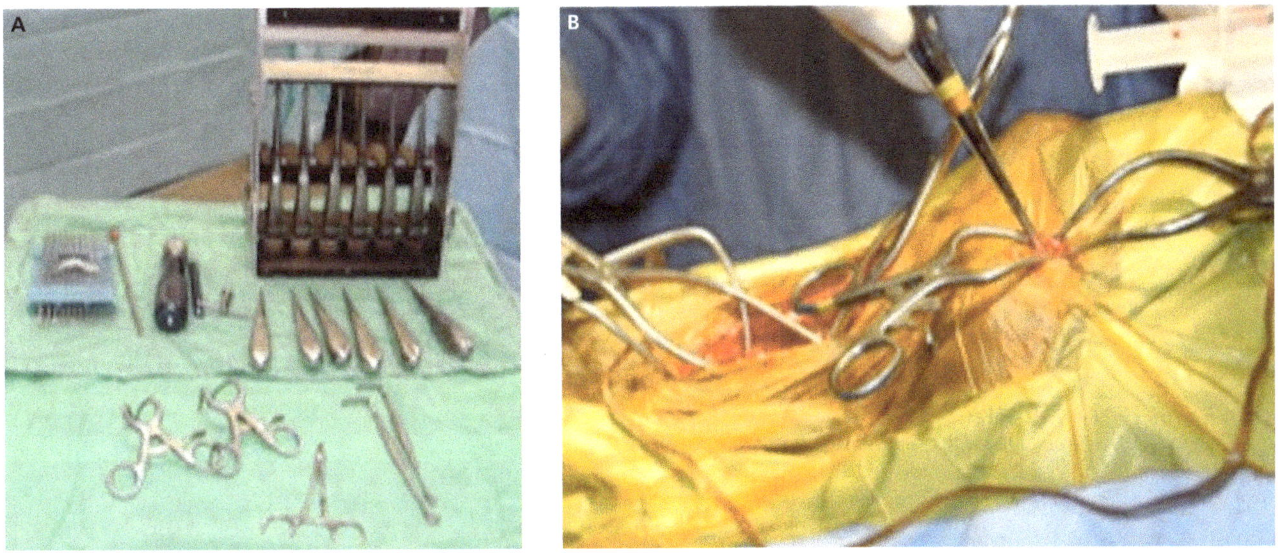

Figure 19.6 (A) Instrumentation used to obtain a fresh cancellous autograph from the proximal humerus. The greater tubercle is approached and a large Steinmann pin is used to create a hole in the cortical bone. Curettes of increasing size are used to remove cancellous bone that is collected in a sterile container. Graft should be obtained as late in the procedure as possible to increase graft survival. (B) Intraoperative photograph of a dog undergoing cervical distraction/stabilization. Both forelimbs are pulled caudally (toward the right) and both shoulder joints are included in the sterile preparation and drape. A standard approach to the caudal cervical spine has been performed and large drop-handle Gelpi retractors are in place. The right proximal humerus has also been approached and a cancellous bone graft is currently being harvested.

Care must be taken when filling the slot with bone graft to avoid displacement into the vertebral canal. A small piece of gel foam can be placed at the dorsal aspect of the slot, although usually sufficient dorsal longitudinal ligament remains to act as a natural barrier unless bone graft is too aggressively packed into the slot.

Of more clinical significance is the need for removal of dorsolateral compression by hypertrophied articular processes (Figure 19.7). While distraction/stabilization is aimed at alleviating compression by soft tissues as well as slowing or halting bony proliferation of articular facets, it does not actually remove current bony compression. While technically demanding, decompression is best achieved by removal of one of the hypertrophied facet joints via cervical hemilaminectomy. The affected site would first be distracted and stabilized via a ventral approach followed by repositioning and hemilaminectomy. As both procedures are considered major surgeries, they are sometimes performed separately with a few days of recovery between. Performing a dorsal laminectomy with removal of compressive articular process bone from within the vertebral canal carries a higher risk of iatrogenic spinal cord injury and is not as effective as direct decompression via hemilaminectomy. Rarely, a dorsal laminectomy is performed in addition to distraction/stabilization, if significant dorsal soft tissue compression is present that is not predictably improved by distraction.

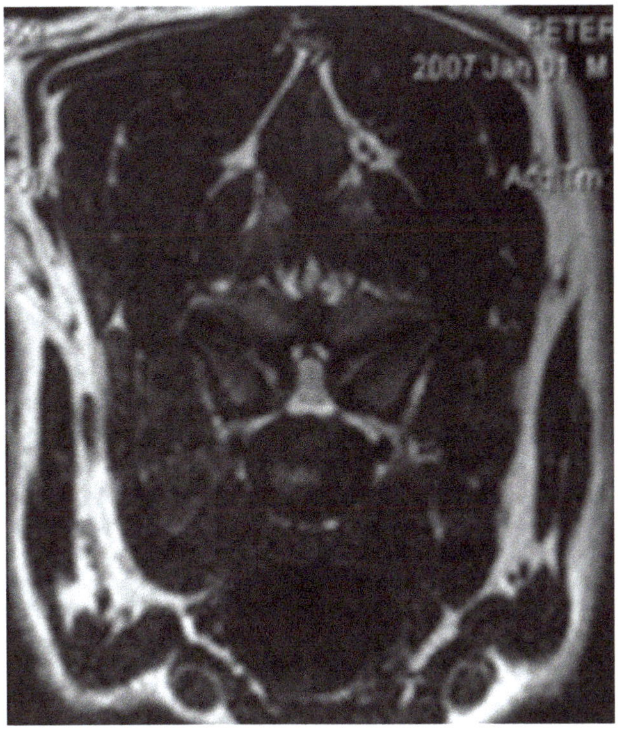

Figure 19.7 Axial MRI of a Great Dane affected with CSM. There is severe dorsolateral spinal cord compression by proliferated articular processes. In addition to stabilization to halt progression of proliferation, this dog requires direct decompression via cervical hemilaminectomy.

Surgical Stabilization

Monocortical Screw/PMMA Fixation

The vertebral body of large-breed dogs easily accommodates 3.5-mm cortical screws for monocortical implantation. Cancellous screws are not recommended due to their smaller core diameter and decreased stiffness compared with their cortical counterparts.

Nonself-tapping screws are preferred for this fixation as these screws have a larger area of threads at the screw tip. More importantly, self-tapping screws have the potential for inadvertent penetration of the trans-cortex into the vertebral canal. The use of titanium screws is advantageous over stainless steel as it allows postoperative spinal cord evaluation via MRI.

The fixation construct consists of six 3.5-mm cortical screws that are placed into the adjacent vertebrae of the affected vertebral articulation. In the cranially located vertebral body, one screw is positioned mid-body on the midline and two screws next to one another in the caudal metaphyseal region. In the caudally located vertebral

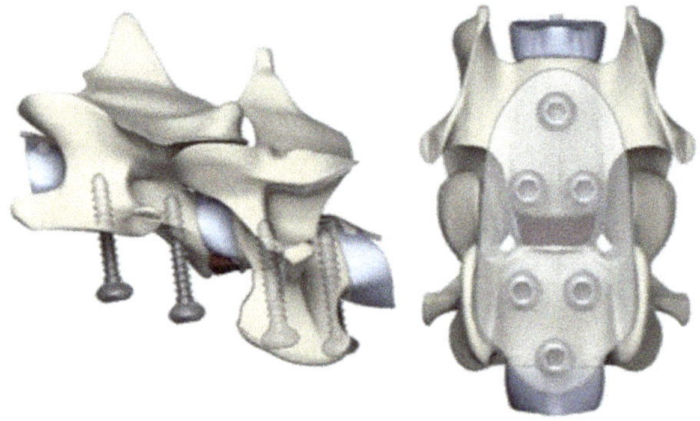

Figure 19.8 Illustration of the monocortical screw–PMMA construct. Three screws are placed per vertebra, with two screws in the metaphyseal bone closest to the endplates. Screws are placed parallel to the vertebral endplate orientation to avoid interference with the disc space. *Source:* Reproduced with the permission of The Ohio State University.

body, two screws are placed parallel to each other in the cranial metaphyseal region and one mid-body on the midline. This configuration allows for two screws in each vertebral body to engage the area of the bone with the most bone height (adjacent to the vertebral endplates) (Figure 19.8).

For each screw, a hole is drilled into the cis-cortex with a 2.5-mm drill bit. Drill bit orientation should be parallel to the vertebral endplates in a caudoventral to craniodorsal direction to engage the furthest depth of bone. Endplate angles can be reviewed on the lateral radiographic projection of the patient. The two screws positioned parallel to each other in the metaphysis can be slightly angled away from the midline to avoid interference of one screw with the other during placement. To prevent over-drilling into the trans-cortex, a drill stop (Animal Orthopaedics, Bishop Auckland, UK) or a depth-limiting drill guide (Synthes, West Chester, PA) can be used. Otherwise, drilling should be performed with careful pressure and attention to change in drill bit position once the cis-cortex is breached. A depth gauge or small blunt probe is then used to carefully evaluate the integrity of the trans-cortex prior to tapping and screw placement. Depth gauge measurement is also used for selection of screw length; 10–15 mm in length are added to allow for incorporation of the screw head into PMMA. An inventory of 3.5-mm screws of 18–24 mm length should be sufficient for this type of fixation in large- and giant-breed dogs. Screws are then carefully placed and advanced until increased resistance indicates that the screw tip is contacting the trans-cortex (Figure 19.9). If self-tapping screws are used, screws are placed after the drill hole is made without the need for tapping. Care must be taken to stop advancement of the screw once the trans-cortex is reached as self-tapping screws have an increased potential for breaking through into the vertebral canal. With the relatively small amount of available vertebral body bone, care is taken when drilling and tapping for screw placement as bone threads may strip. When using screws with PMMA, a stripped screw can be more easily replaced by a new screw with a different position compared with plate fixation.

The musculature around the monocortical screws needs to be sufficiently retracted to allow enough room for PMMA to fully engage all screw heads. If needed, musculature may be partially resected to accommodate the PMMA; however, overly aggressive resection should be avoided. Cement mantle height should be approximately 10–15 mm and should not exceed the ventral border of the longus colli muscles to prevent compression of adjacent soft tissues such as esophagus or trachea.

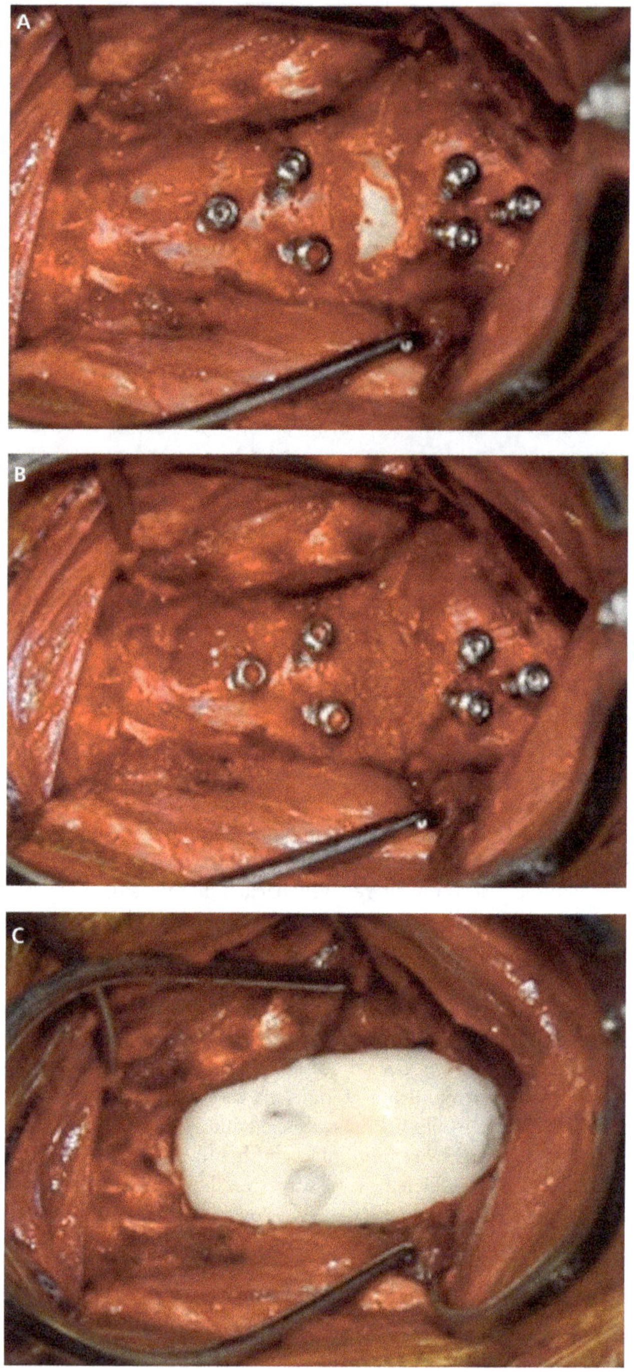

Figure 19.9 Intraoperative photographs of monocortical screw/PMMA fixation. (A) Three screws each have been placed into two adjacent vertebral bodies in a triangular pattern. Approximately 10 mm of screw is protruding to allow incorporation into PMMA. The intervertebral disc has been removed and a cortical ring allograft is in place. The graft is filled with fresh cancellous autograft and is flush with the ventral aspect of the endplates. (B) Remaining cancellous autograft is placed over the ring allograft. (C) PMMA (20 g) has been applied and covers all screw heads.

Vertebral Body Plates

Several locking plate systems have been reported in clinical use (Cervical Spine Locking Plate® and ComPact UniLock System® from Synthes, West Chester, PA; String of Pearls™ from Orthomed Ltd, Huddersfield, UK) and some have been evaluated

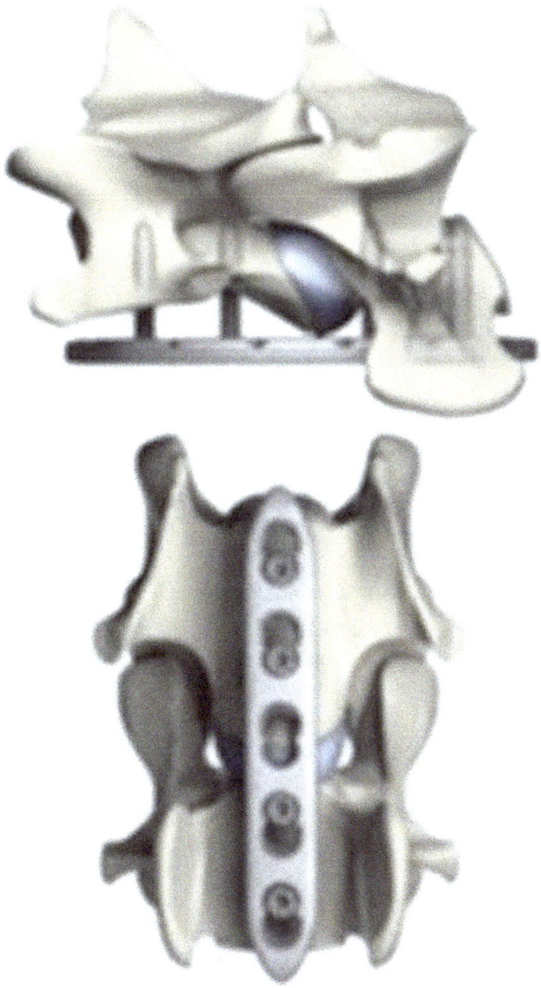

Figure 19.10 Synthes locking compression plate applied to C5–C6 vertebral bodies. Because of the locking mechanism, the plate does not require contouring and can sit proud on the bone. Screws engage the vertebral bodies in a monocortical fashion. Because of the dimensions of the plate, usually only two screws can be placed per vertebral body. *Source*: Reproduced with the permission of The Ohio State University.

biomechanically (Locking Compression Plate® from Synthes) [2,3,5]. Locking plates rigidly couple screws to the plate via a variety of locking mechanisms. To appropriately lock, most mechanisms require the screw to be inserted at a fixed angle trajectory, which dictates screw orientation (Figure 19.10). There are several important advantages of locking plates over traditional plates. Because screws are locked, plates do not need to be contoured to the undulating bone of the ventral vertebral bodies but can be laid on the bony surface with a potential offset of several millimeters. As any contouring would change the fixed angle screw trajectory, contouring should be avoided unless the change of screw orientation is desired. The second benefit is that locking plates can be used with monocortical screws because rigid fixation does not rely on friction between the implant and the bone. This greatly reduces potential damage to spinal cord, nerve roots, and vessels by bicortical implants.

Technical challenges with application of locking plates arise from the predetermined screw location based on hole position within the plate and the fixed screw trajectory. The dimensions of most plates allow two screws per vertebral body but care must be taken not to inadvertently violate the slanted intervertebral disc space. Monocortical drilling and careful tapping (unless self-tapping screws are used) commences as with regular screw placement. Measurement for screw length is performed prior to tapping and must be done through the locking plate, keeping in mind that many of these plates will sit proud on the bone and screws will traverse open space before engaging bone. The plate should be held as close to the bone with digital pressure while maintaining it in the desired position during screw application. Accurate placement of the first screw is paramount, as this single screw, once locked, will determine the path for all subsequent screws.

Other Techniques

As an alternative or augmentation to monocortical screw/PMMA fixation of the vertebral bodies, bicortical screws can be placed in the prominent transverse processes of the cervical vertebral column (Figure 19.11). For medium to large dogs, 3.5-mm cortical screws

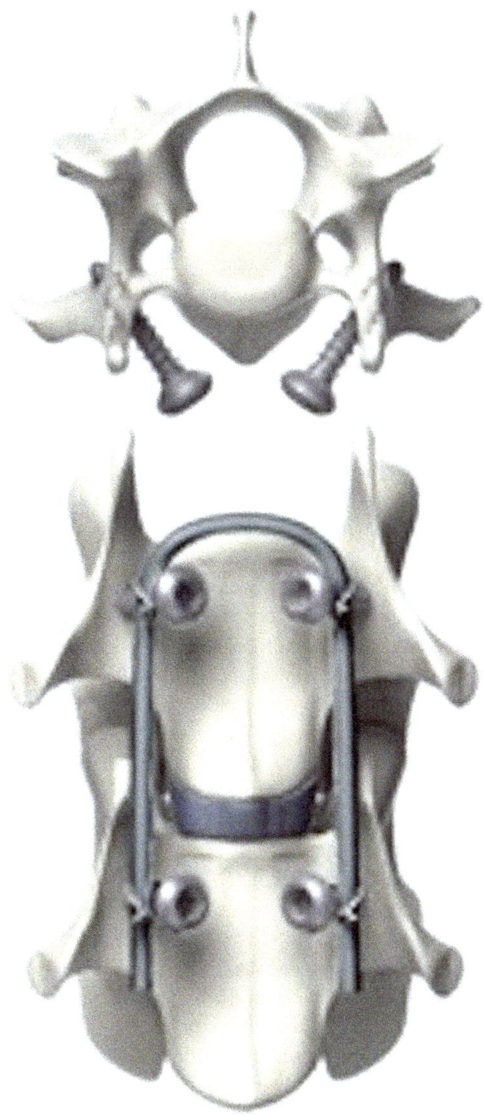

Figure 19.11 Bicortical transverse process screw and reinforcement bar fixation [7]. A Steinmann pin has been contoured to fit around the screws and is secured to the screws with cerclage wire to act as a reinforcement bar. The screws and bar are then incorporated into PMMA. *Source*: Reproduced with the permission of The Ohio State University.

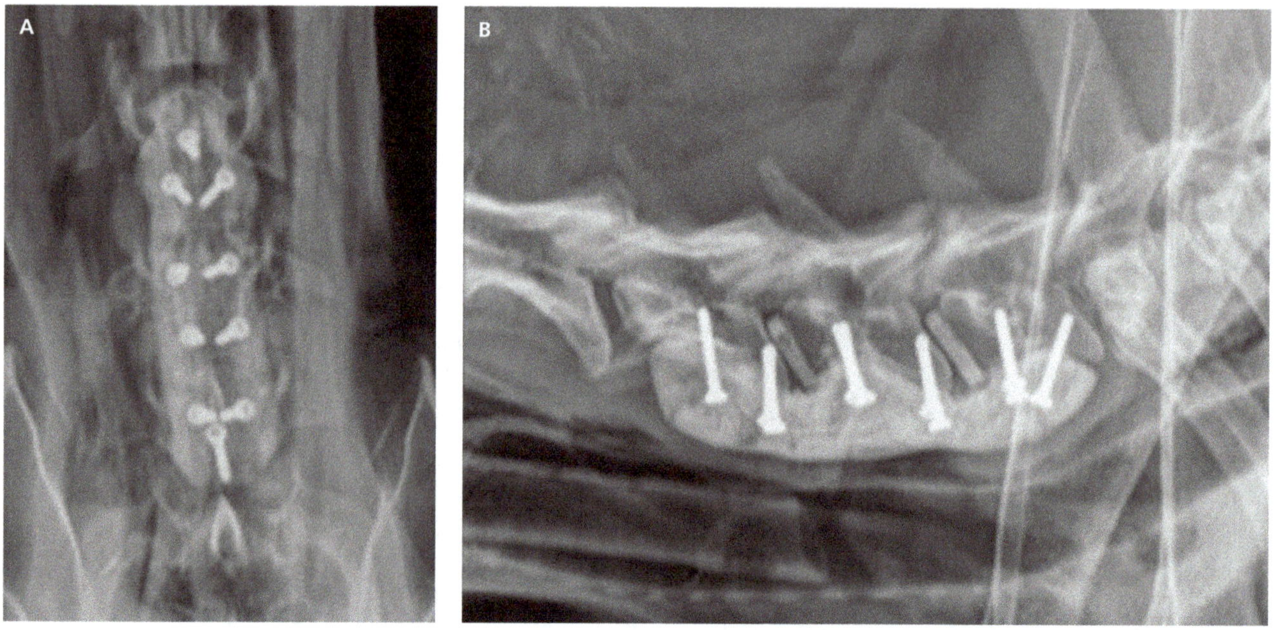

Figure 19.12 (A, B) Postoperative radiographs of a Great Dane with two-level cervical distraction and stabilization at C5, C6, and C7 using monocortical screws/PMMA and disc spacers. Three screws were placed into C5 and C7; four screws were placed into the cranial and caudal aspect of C6. The most caudal screw in C7 was angled caudally instead of parallel to the endplate due to interference with the sternum. Cortical ring allografts are well positioned within the two disc spaces; however, they appear to be slightly undersized (note the gap between ring and endplates).

are placed bilaterally perpendicular to the ventral surface into the center of each transverse process. Screws must be long enough to fully engage the trans-cortex while still protruding 10–15 mm toward the ventral midline to be incorporated into PMMA. Care must be taken to avoid screw placement near the base of the process to prevent injury to the transverse foramen and vertebral artery. Reinforcement of such screw fixation with a contoured Steinmann pin and cerclage wire has been reported and biomechanically assessed [7]. PMMA (20 g) is then placed around screws and reinforcement bar for fixation.

Stabilization of Multiple Spaces

CSM often affects multiple intervertebral articulations. Single space stabilization is generally appropriate for an individual site with obviously worse compression compared to adjacent spaces. However, sometimes there is no single space that would benefit the most from surgery but neighboring spaces are similarly compressed. Stabilization with or without distraction can be performed across multiple disc spaces with the techniques described in the preceding sections. If monocortical screws/PMMA fixation is used, the centrally located vertebral body can house four screws, with two each in the cranial and caudal metaphyseal bone (Figure 19.12). As a longer lever arm is created with the increased distance spanned by rigid internal fixation, concerns of implant failure become more prominent. In the screw–PMMA construct, failure would likely occur by fracturing of the cement, while plate fixation may fail by screw breakage through shear forces or failure of the screw–bone interface. Anecdotal reports indicate a decrease in cement breakage after multiple space fixation with the use of intervertebral spacers. It is likely that the increase in load sharing by the vertebral column via intervertebral spacers has a protective effect on implants and should improve implant longevity for both PMMA and plate fixations. As with single-site distraction/stabilization, adjacent segment disease can occur with fixation of multiple spaces; however, the implication of such is difficult to assess as severity may vary and may not contribute significantly to clinical signs.

Postoperative Assessment

To evaluate overall implant position and assess proper placement of the intervertebral spacer (if used), standard orthogonal radiographs should be obtained, centering over the stabilized vertebral motion units (VMUs). While radiographs have very low accuracy in predicting the position of bicortical cervical implants in relation to the vertebral canal, they are usually acceptable for monocortical implants. Monocortical screws should in theory not protrude beyond the floor of the vertebral canal on a lateral projection.

Postoperative CT is excellent in assessing implant position. Long term, radiographs can also be used to assess implant stability, overall vertebral alignment and, to some degree, bony fusion across the disc space; however, it is difficult to adequately judge the degree of arthrodesis on radiographs and even advanced imaging such as CT (Figure 19.13). Because of the common use of stainless steel implants in vertebral column stabilization, postoperative MRI is usually not possible. Titanium implants are compatible with MRI and are the implant material of choice to allow immediate and long-term follow-up with advanced imaging. This is particularly important for dogs with CSM to assess development or progression of signal changes within the spinal cord as the disease progresses.

Complications

The potential injury to immediately adjacent neurovascular structures is decreased by the use of monocortical implants. However, inadvertent drill bit advancement or screw penetration into the canal can still occur. Familiarization with the patient-specific vertebral body dimensions and use of a drill stop can help decrease overdrilling and subsequent screw placement into the canal. Damage to the vagosympathetic trunk, carotid artery, esophagus, or trachea

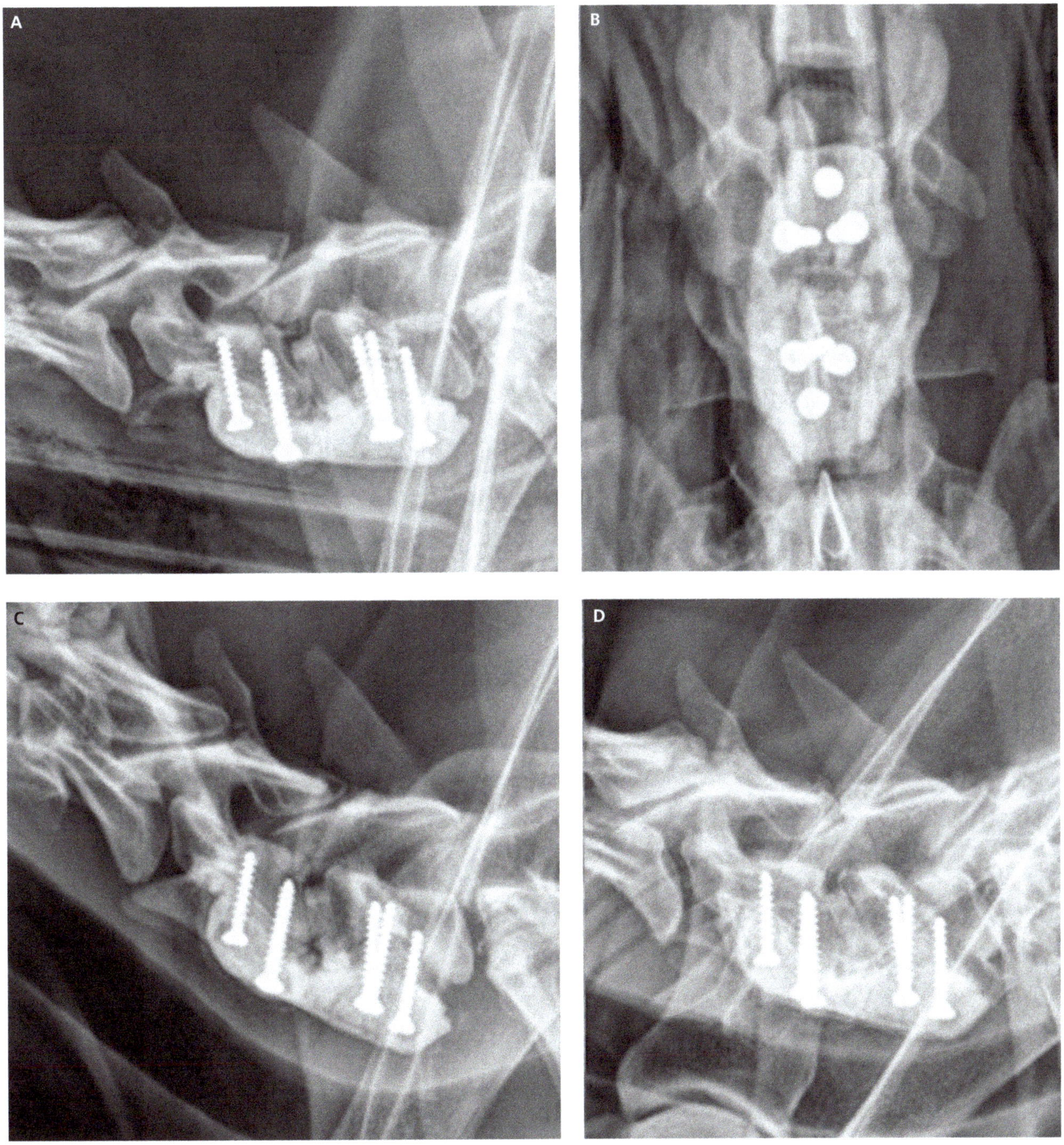

Figure 19.13 Radiographic follow-up of a Great Dane after distraction/stabilization at C6–C7 with monocortical screw/PMMA fixation and cortical ring allograft disc spacer. (A, B) Immediate postoperative orthogonal radiographs showing the fixation with triangular screw pattern and placement parallel to the endplates. (C) Lateral radiograph 2 months postoperatively. The cortical ring has shifted slightly within the disc space compared with (A); however, fit of the ring appears excellent at this time. (D) Lateral radiograph 2 year postoperatively. There is evidence of bony fusion across the mid to ventral aspect of the disc space. Implants are intact and appear stable.

can occur during aggressive approaches or negligent use of tissue retractors to access the ventral aspect of the vertebral column. Implant failure typically occurs by failure of the bone–screw interface, shearing of locking screws, or by cracking of the cement. It is unusual for screws to shear at the screw–cement interface. While an intervertebral spacer aids in maintaining disc space distraction and helps with load sharing, it can be improperly placed, leading to continued chronic pain and dysfunction, or it can acutely dislodge causing sudden-onset pain, radiculopathy, or myelopathy. Deep infection after surgical fixation is rare and would require implant removal. In case of screw/PMMA fixation, cement is removed around screws using a pneumatic drill. Filling screw heads with sterile bone wax prior to PMMA application will make screw removal easier. Postoperative seroma formation can occur if drill debris is not properly removed via flushing and dead space not carefully closed. Seromas are typically treated conservatively with warm compresses and time.

Long-term complications usually relate to chronic cycling and fatigue failure of implants when fusion of the stabilized VMU is delayed or does not occur. Subsidence of the disc spacer indicates subclinical implant failure and may be the cause of continued chronic pain and neurological deficits.

Finally, adjacent segment disease with degenerative disc changes, soft tissue hypertrophy, and bony changes can develop. Whether these changes occur due to progression of preexisting disease or secondary to biomechanical stress from the longer lever arm of the stabilized VMU is still debated.

Video clips to accompany this book can be found on the companion website at: www.wiley.com/go/shores/neurosurgery

References

1 Corlazzoli D. Bicortical implant insertion in caudal cervical spondylomyelopathy: a computed tomography simulation in affected Doberman Pinschers. *Vet Surg* 2008;37:178–185.
2 Agnello KA, Kapatkin AS, Garcia TC, Stover SM. Intervertebral biomechanics of locking compression plate monocortical fixation of the canine cervical spine. *Vet Surg* 2010;39:991–1000.
3 Bergman RL, Levine JM, Coates JR, Bahr A, Hettlich BF, Kerwin SC. Cervical spinal locking plate in combination with cortical ring allograft for a one level fusion in dogs with cervical spondylotic myelopathy. *Vet Surg* 2008;37:530–536.
4 Shamir MH, Chai O, Loeb E. A method for intervertebral space distraction before stabilization combined with complete ventral slot for treatment of disc-associated wobbler syndrome in dogs. *Vet Surg* 2008;37:186–192.
5 Steffen F, Voss K, Morgan JP. Distraction-fusion for caudal cervical spondylomyelopathy using an intervertebral cage and locking plates in 14 dogs. *Vet Surg* 2011;40:743–752.
6 Trotter EJ. Cervical spine locking plate fixation for treatment of cervical spondylotic myelopathy in large breed dogs. *Vet Surg* 2009;38:705–718.
7 Hicks DG, Pitts MJ, Bagley RS et al. In vitro biomechanical evaluations of screw-bar-polymethylmethacrylate and pin-polymethylmethacrylate internal fixation implants used to stabilize the vertebral motion unit of the fourth and fifth cervical vertebrae in vertebral column specimens from dogs. *Am J Vet Res* 2009;70:719–726.

20 Thoracolumbar Hemilaminectomy

Andy Shores

Introduction

A dorsolateral [1–4] or a lateral [5] approach to the thoracolumbar spine is used for the hemilaminectomy procedure. The dorsolateral approach provides the best exposure [2,6] and is the more commonly used approach [3]. Decompression of the thoracolumbar spine is defined as the removal of the dorsal or lateral components of the vertebral arch to relieve pressure on the spinal cord. The thoracolumbar hemilaminectomy is indicated for intervertebral disc (IVD) extrusions or protrusions, for decompression in association with spinal trauma and vertebral fracture/luxations, for exposure of tumors located on the lateral aspect of the spinal cord, for decompression and removal of inflammatory material associated with vertebral osteomyelitis/discospondylitis, for excision or marsupialization of laterally located subarachnoid diverticula, and for removal of projectiles or foreign bodies that have entered the spinal canal. Modifications of this procedure include the pediculectomy, lateral corpectomy, and the mini-hemilaminectomy [7] and are discussed in other chapters of this book.

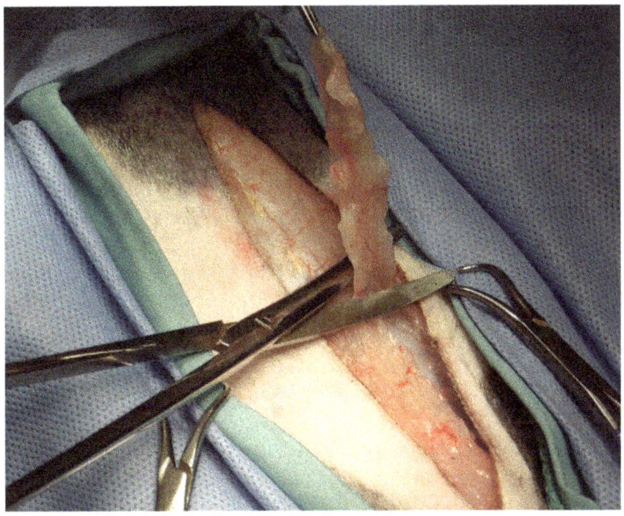

Figure 20.1 An approximately 3-cm long by 2-cm wide by 0.3-cm thick portion of the thoracolumbar subcutaneous adipose tissue is excised at the *beginning* of surgery, then wrapped in a moistened gauze sponge and stored for use at the end of the procedure.

Surgical Approach

The patient is placed in sternal recumbency. A sandbag or rolled towel can be placed under the abdomen to slightly arch the spine and facilitate surgical exposure. An area 7–10 cm on either side of the dorsal midline and from T7 to approximately L5 is clipped and prepared for surgery. The midline skin incision usually extends three vertebrae cranial and three caudal to the lesion. The thin cutaneous trunci muscle is usually incised with the skin. Next, the subcutaneous tissue and fat are incised. A small, moderately thin section of fat (about 3 cm long and 2 cm wide) is excised, wrapped in a moistened gauze sponge, and stored for use at the end of the procedure (Figure 20.1) [4].

With the thick thoracolumbar fascia exposed, the midline is identified by palpating the spinous processes of the thoracolumbar vertebrae. The fascia is incised with a #10 or #15 scalpel blade or an electroscalpel in an undulating or scalloped fashion, beginning at the dorsal midline between the first two spinous processes, hugging the near lateral aspect of the spinous process, returning to midline between each vertebra, then going around the next spinous process (Figure 20.2). This is continued in the same scalloped fashion for the length of the incision. This exposes the underlying multifidus muscle. The multifidus is dissected from the lateral aspect of the vertebrae on the side nearest the surgeon. The dissection begins at the caudal-most vertebrae and continues cranially until the planned exposure is completed. The blunt end of a scalpel handle or periosteal elevator (Freer or Adson) is used to reflect the musculature laterally from the spinous processes. The tendinous attachments to the spinous processes are severed at each vertebra (with Mayo scissors, #10 or #15 scalpel blade, or electroscalpel) as the dissection is carried cranially [4].

Current Techniques in Canine and Feline Neurosurgery, First Edition. Edited by Andy Shores and Brigitte A. Brisson.
© 2017 John Wiley & Sons, Inc. Published 2017 by John Wiley & Sons, Inc.
Companion website: www.wiley.com/go/shores/neurosurgery

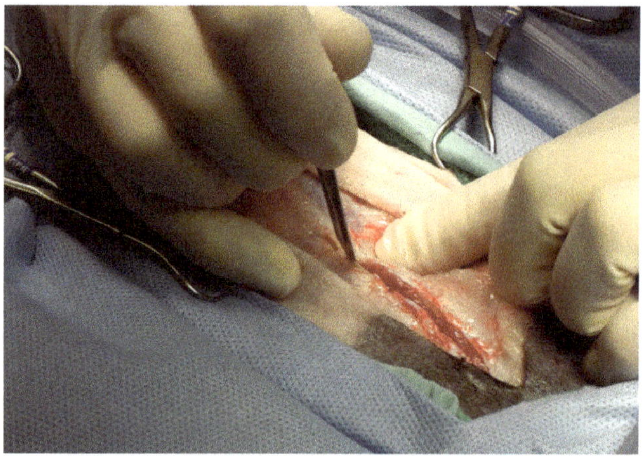

Figure 20.2 The thoracolumbar fascia is incised in a scalloped fashion, beginning at the dorsal midline between the first two spinous processes, hugging the near lateral aspect of the spinous process, and returning to the midline between each vertebra.

Multifidus muscle is next dissected from the articular facets. The periosteal elevation begins at the junction of the caudal aspect of the articular process and the lamina. Using a Senn retractor and a Freer elevator, elevation of the muscle continues around the articular process, exposing the tendinous attachments, which are severed close to the bone to minimize hemorrhage. When the dissection is completed at the cranial extent of the exposure, Gelpi retractors are placed to increase exposure. The author often uses a dry gauze sponge over the exposed vertebrae to then remove any remaining muscular attachments [4].

Hemilaminectomy

Thoracolumbar hemilaminectomies are generally performed at a site between the ninth thoracic and fourth lumbar vertebrae. After completing the muscle dissection, a Senn retractor and Freer elevator are used to slightly lift the longissimus muscle and identify the short transverse process of L1 and the thirteenth rib for orientation. The site of the suspected IVD protrusion is identified and the hemilaminectomy begun by removing the articular processes directly over the involved IVD with a bone rongeur or surgical drill (Figure 20.3A) [1,2,4].

The spinal canal is entered by one of two methods.

- The spinous process of the vertebra just cranial to the IVD is clamped with Backhaus towel forceps and gently elevated by an assistant (Figures 20.3C and 20.4). This increases the space between the vertebrae at their articulation. A 3-mm Lempert rongeur is used to widen the space and expose the spinal cord [2,6]. This method is used most effectively in dogs weighing less than 10 kg [2]. With the rongeur grasped in the surgeon's dominant hand, the tip is positioned in the small separation, always with a finger from the opposite hand pulling against the shaft of the rongeur to prevent inadvertent slipping of the instrument toward the canal (Figures 20.3C and 20.5; Video 20.1, Part I).
- A surgical drill is used to create the hemilaminectomy (Video 20.1, Part II) [2,8]. This is the preferred method in larger dogs. The drill is placed initially at the caudal or cranial aspect of the planned opening as the drilling begins, progressing toward the foramina, then continued on the opposite side of the foramina, removing the outer cortical layer of bone. The surgeon will note reaching the softer cancellous layer as a reddish-brown color change. Drilling is frequently interrupted to allow irrigation of the drill site with a normal saline flush. This is necessary to dissipate heat from the drill and to remove bony debris. The surgeon should keep the depth of the drilling even on each side of the foramina. Continued drilling will remove the cancellous bone and reveal the thin inner cortical bone. This level is identified as a return to a whitish cortical bone color. At this juncture, a small probe, ear curette, or tartar scraper is used to feel the remaining thickness of the bone. A very thin layer of cortical bone or exposure of the thick inner periosteum evenly

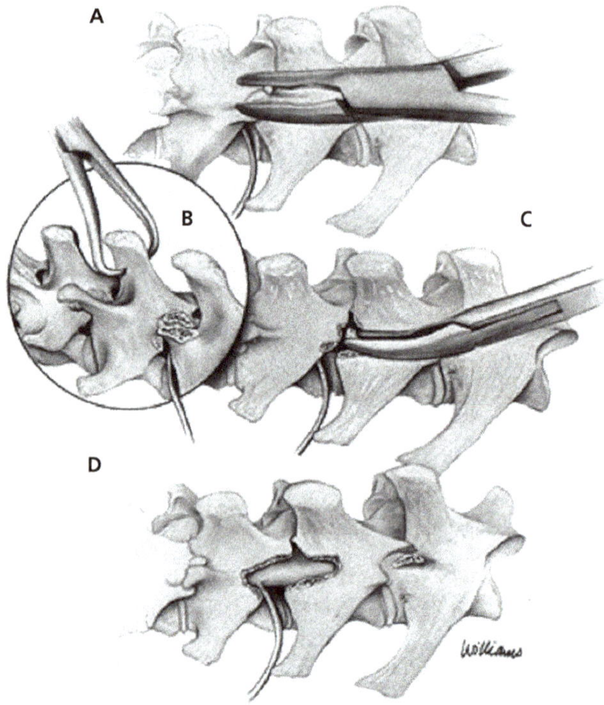

Figure 20.3 The hemilaminectomy. (A) Removal of the articular processes with rongeurs. (B) Elevation of the vertebra with a towel clamp to widen the articular space. (C) Performing the hemilaminectomy with Lempert rongeurs. (D) The completed hemilaminectomy. *Source*: Adapted from Shores [6].

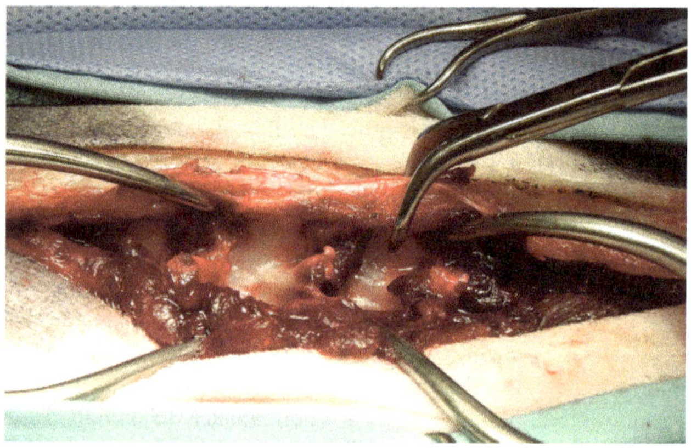

Figure 20.4 Intraoperative photo demonstrating placement of Backhaus towel forceps through the spinous process of the vertebra just cranial to the offending IVD. An assistant gently elevates the forceps to open the vertebral articulation, expanding the surgeon's access for placement of the Lempert rongeurs used to perform the hemilaminectomy.

distributed along the length and height of the lamina is a stopping point. Lempert (3 mm) or Kerrison (1 or 2 mm, 40°) rongeurs are used to complete the laminectomy [4].

The hemilaminectomy should be at least one vertebral body length cranial and caudal to the affected IVD (Figures 20.3D and 20.6). The final length of the hemilaminectomy defect is governed by the appearance of the spinal cord and adjacent tissue within the canal. The length is extended until normal-appearing tissue is encountered (presence of epidural fat; absence of IVD material or cord swelling). Lempert rongeurs, Kerrison rongeurs, or the surgical drill can be used to lengthen the hemilaminectomy when necessary [9]. Of critical importance is assuring the opening extends ventrally to the floor of the spinal canal. Failure to do this often results in failure to visualize and remove portions of the extruded disc material or in undue trauma when sweeping underneath the spinal cord to remove disc material.

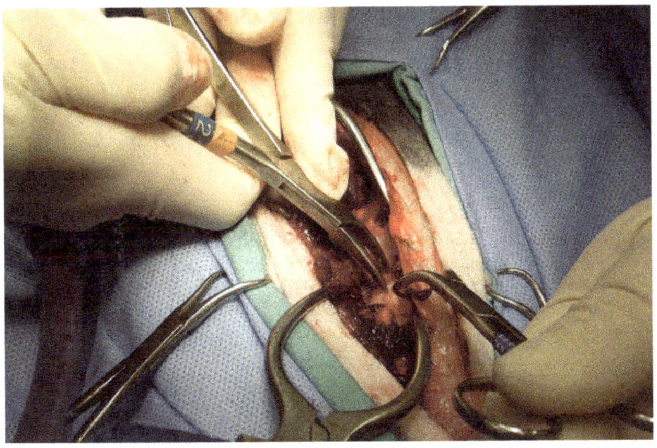

Figure 20.5 Intraoperative photo demonstrating placement of the Lempert rongeur tips in the small separation between the articular facets to begin the hemilaminectomy. Note that the surgeon places the index finger from the opposite hand against the shaft of the rongeur to prevent inadvertent slipping of the instrument toward the canal as the cut is made.

After creating the hemilaminectomy defect, if the thin tough layer of inner periosteum is encountered, a dural hook, tartar scraper, or similar instrument is used to penetrate it, allowing visualization of the spinal canal. The site of the IVD protrusion often contains necrotic epidural fat and hemorrhage that is often associated with the extruded IVD material.

The extruded IVD material is removed at the hemilaminectomy site with a small curved blunt probe (e.g., ophthalmic strabismus hook or small ear curette) or a thin, flattened and curved tartar scraper. The probe is carefully passed under and above the spinal cord to dislodge the extruded material [6]. This portion of the surgery is performed with extreme care to avoid damage to the spinal cord. If the IVD material is hardened or adhered to the dura, it may be especially difficult to dislodge. The IVD material can be adhered to the ventral venous sinuses, and removal results in hemorrhage from these vessels. Application of an absorbable gelatin sponge over the hemilaminectomy site for a few minutes will often control the hemorrhage [2,9].

The hemilaminectomy exposes only one side of the spinal cord, and therefore disc material on the contralateral side may be inaccessible. A bilateral hemilaminectomy can be performed in such instances if the surgeon deems it necessary [10]. The advent of advanced imaging (CT, MRI) has helped to alleviate the necessity of many bilateral hemilaminectomies as the transverse images correctly identify the location of the herniated IVD material.

The majority of the extruded IVD material is removed with the small probe. The remaining small amounts of material are removed through irrigation with sterile normal saline or Ringer's solution and careful suctioning. The suction tip should never contact the spinal cord [2,6].

A durotomy can be performed to allow direct visualization of the spinal cord. The author feels very strongly that as a diagnostic procedure (identification of a malacic spinal cord and therefore a grave prognosis for recovery of ambulation), a durotomy and visual inspection of the cord is very subjective and therefore unwarranted.

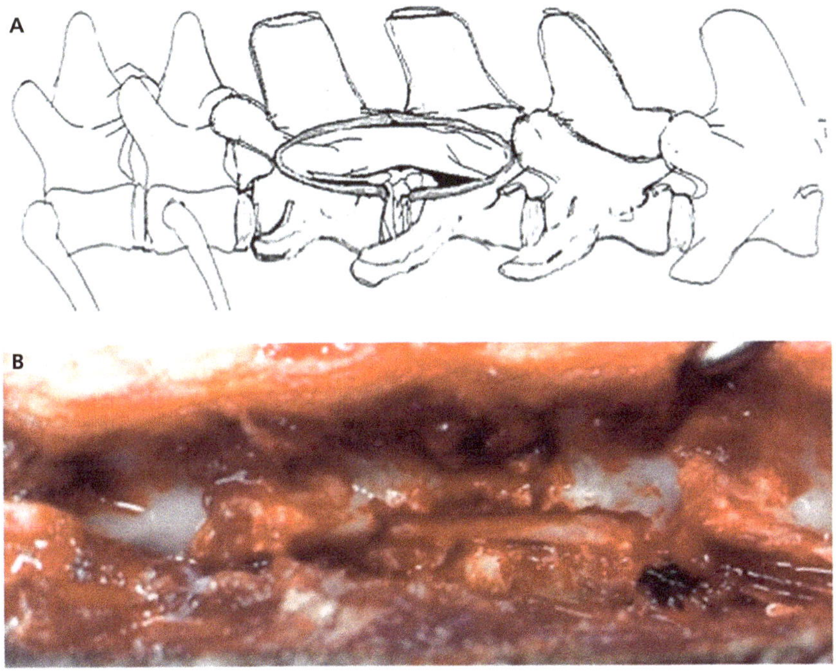

Figure 20.6 (A) Illustration and (B) intraoperative photo of the completed hemilaminectomy. Note the ventral extent of the opening to the floor of the spinal canal. Failure to do this often results in failure to visualize and remove portions of the extruded disc material or in undue trauma when sweeping underneath the spinal cord to remove disc material.

The durotomy does not provide significant additional decompression in the majority of cases [11]. A durotomy is often necessary if removing a suspected mass or marsupializing a subarachnoid diverticulum. If a durotomy is performed, a #12 scalpel blade is used. The cutting edge of the scalpel blade is directed upward to protect the spinal cord [2,9]. The durotomy is extended by tenting the dura with small tissue forceps (microsurgical, ophthalmic) or a 5-0 silk suture and using small tenotomy scissors or Potts scissors.

Closure

Several applications of irrigation solution are applied to the decompression site to remove any remaining blood clots, tissue debris, or small bone fragments. Complete hemostasis is achieved before closure and may require application of a gelatin sponge for a period of time to eliminate hemorrhage from the venous sinus. The exposed spinal cord is protected with a layer of sublumbar fat or absorbable gelatin sponge [2,12]. The stored fat is rinsed with warm saline before placing it over the decompression site.

The incision is closed in three layers. The thoracolumbar fascia is closed with 2-0 absorbable sutures in an interrupted cruciate mattress pattern. The thoracolumbar muscle should be completely covered with the fascia. The subcutaneous layer is closed with 3-0 absorbable suture, and the skin is closed in a routine manner.

Discussion

Prophylactic fenestrations of IVDs from T11–T12 through L3–L4 are often performed in association with the hemilaminectomy [2]. The benefits of prophylactic fenestration have been debated over many years and many investigations; however, recent evidence seems to indicate it is strongly warranted in the chondrodystrophic dog. When performing a hemilaminectomy in a chondrodystrophic dog, because it is known that the offending IVD already has a tear in the dorsal annulus, it would be poor surgical judgment to not at least fenestrate the offending IVD.

The hemilaminectomy provides good decompression and visualization of the spinal cord and nerve roots, it allows removal of IVD material from the spinal canal without excessive spinal cord manipulation and, when necessary, a durotomy can be performed with the exposure provided. This procedure is easily combined with prophylactic fenestration from a dorsolateral or lateral approach [4,13].

Video clips to accompany this book can be found on the companion website at: www.wiley.com/go/shores/neurosurgery

References

1 Gage ED. Modifications in dorsolateral hemilaminectomy and disc fenestration in the dog. *J Am Anim Hosp Assoc* 1975;11:407–411.
2 Hoerlein BF. Intervertebral disks. In: Hoerlein BF (ed.) *Canine Neurology*, 3rd edn. Philadelphia, PA: WB Saunders, 1978:470–560.
3 Toombs JP, Waters DJ. Intervertebral disc disease. In: Slatter D (ed.) *Textbook of Small Animal Surgery*, 3rd edn. Philadelphia, PA: WB Saunders, 2003: 1193–1209.
4 Shores A. Intervertebral disk disease. In: Newton CD, Nunamaker DM (eds) *Textbook of Small Animal Orthopaedics*. Philadelphia, PA: JB Lippincott, 1985: 739–764.
5 Braund KG, Taylor TKF, Ghosh P, Sherwood AA. Lateral spinal decompression in the dog. *J Small Anim Pract* 1976;17:583–592.
6 Shores A. The intervertebral disk syndrome in the dog: Part III. Thoracolumbar disk surgery. *Compend Contin Educ Pract Vet* 1982;4:24–31.
7 Huska JL, Gaitero L, Brisson BA, Nykamp S, Thomason J, Sears WC. Comparison of the access window created by hemilaminectomy and mini-hemilaminectomy in the thoracolumbar vertebral canal using computed tomography. *Can Vet J* 2014;55:449–455.
8 Swaim SF. Use of pneumatic surgical instruments in neurosurgery. I. Spinal surgery. *Vet Med Small Anim Clin* 1973;68:1275–1280.
9 Gage ED. Practical management of thoracolumbar disc disease. *Proc Am Anim Hosp Assoc* 1980;47:283.
10 Swaim SF. Bilateral hemilaminectomy: a technique for extensive spinal decompression. *Auburn Vet* 1976;32:62–65.
11 Parker AJ, Smith CW. Functional recovery from spinal cord trauma following delayed incision of the spinal meninges in dogs. *Res Vet Sci* 1975;18:110–112.
12 Prata RG. Neurosurgical treatment of thoracolumbar disks: the rationale and value of laminectomy with concomitant disk removal. *J Am Anim Hosp Assoc* 1981; 17:17–26.
13 Hoerlein BF. Various surgical methods for repair of intervertebral disc protrusions. *Anim Hosp* 1968;4:12.

21 Pediculectomy/Mini-Hemilaminectomy

Brigitte A. Brisson

Indications

Surgical decompression of thoracolumbar intervertebral disc (IVD) herniation has traditionally been accomplished by dorsal laminectomy [1–3] or hemilaminectomy [4]. Dorsal laminectomy is no longer in favor to treat thoracolumbar IVD herniation since removal of the extruded disc material located ventral to the spinal cord is not possible using this approach or requires significant spinal cord manipulation [5]. Lateral and modified lateral decompression techniques [5–8], also known as mini-hemilaminectomy [9], pediculectomy or extended foraminotomy [10–12], along with the partial pediculectomy procedure [13] have aimed to achieve spinal cord decompression through less invasive approaches that preserve the zygapophyseal joint and remove less vertebral bone [5–7,9,10] (Figure 21.1). These procedures are reportedly quicker to perform, create less tissue trauma and less vertebral instability, and lead to a more rapid postoperative recovery [5,9,10,13,14]. Although there are discrepancies in the literature, pediculectomy and mini-hemilaminectomy are considered by the author as the same procedure and the terms are used interchangeably in this chapter.

Procedure

Pediculectomy (or mini-hemilaminectomy) consists of removing a portion of the pedicle bone of two adjacent vertebrae to essentially enlarge the intervertebral foramen while preserving the articular processes [5–10] (Figure 21.1B) Although the partial pediculectomy technique described by McCartney [13] spares the accessory process (Figure 21.1C), the pediculectomy procedure removes the accessory process to form the dorsal margin of the laminectomy [5,9,10]. As shown in two recent studies [15,16] the removal of the accessory process results in mild to moderate invasion of the ventral aspect of the articular processes in most dogs.

The window provided by the pediculectomy or mini-hemilaminectomy is adequate for visualizing the ventrolateral aspect of the vertebral canal and provides excellent access for retrieving ventrally or laterally extruded disc material while limiting intraoperative spinal cord manipulation [5,6,15,16]. Direct access to the dorsal aspect of the canal may be limited compared with hemilaminectomy, as was demonstrated in a recent study [15], but this was not shown to have an impact on the ability to retrieve disc material in clinical patients [16]. This surgical approach offers good visualization of the dorsal nerve root and ganglia and of the venous sinus located on the floor of the spinal canal [5,15]. Preservation of the majority of the articular processes reduces postoperative vertebral instability compared with the hemilaminectomy procedure [14]. Effective spinal cord decompression can be achieved from T10 to L6 using this procedure [5]. The dorsolateral and lateral approaches used for pediculectomy also allow direct access to the IVD for fenestration [5,6,13]. Like the hemilaminectomy procedure, the pediculectomy window is created close to the vertebral venous plexus (sinus) and foraminal structures, requiring care to prevent hemorrhage and nerve root damage [5,16]. The partial pediculectomy procedure (Figure 21.1C) creates a window that is limited to the pedicle bone of one vertebra and does not invade the intervertebral foramen, thus reducing the risk of hemorrhage from the vertebral vessels [13]. However, it may provide too small a window to adequately decompress extensive lesions or ensure that all the extruded disc material is removed. In fact, one study reported that 8 of 27 dogs (29%) undergoing partial pediculectomy required extension of the partial pediculectomy into a mini-hemilaminectomy in order to retrieve the extruded disc material located within the intervertebral foramen [13]. In addition, blind probing of the vertebral canal is typically performed during partial pediculectomy to ensure that the extruded disc material has been removed and this can increase the risk of venous sinus hemorrhage [13].

A pediculectomy or mini-hemilaminectomy can easily be converted into a hemilaminectomy (Figure 21.1A) or be extended over several adjacent vertebrae if required [5]. The author has performed continuous pediculectomies over as many as five contiguous vertebrae without complication. Because the pediculectomy does not significantly invade the articular processes, it can also be performed bilaterally without causing vertebral instability. However, this is

Current Techniques in Canine and Feline Neurosurgery, First Edition. Edited by Andy Shores and Brigitte A. Brisson.
© 2017 John Wiley & Sons, Inc. Published 2017 by John Wiley & Sons, Inc.
Companion website: www.wiley.com/go/shores/neurosurgery

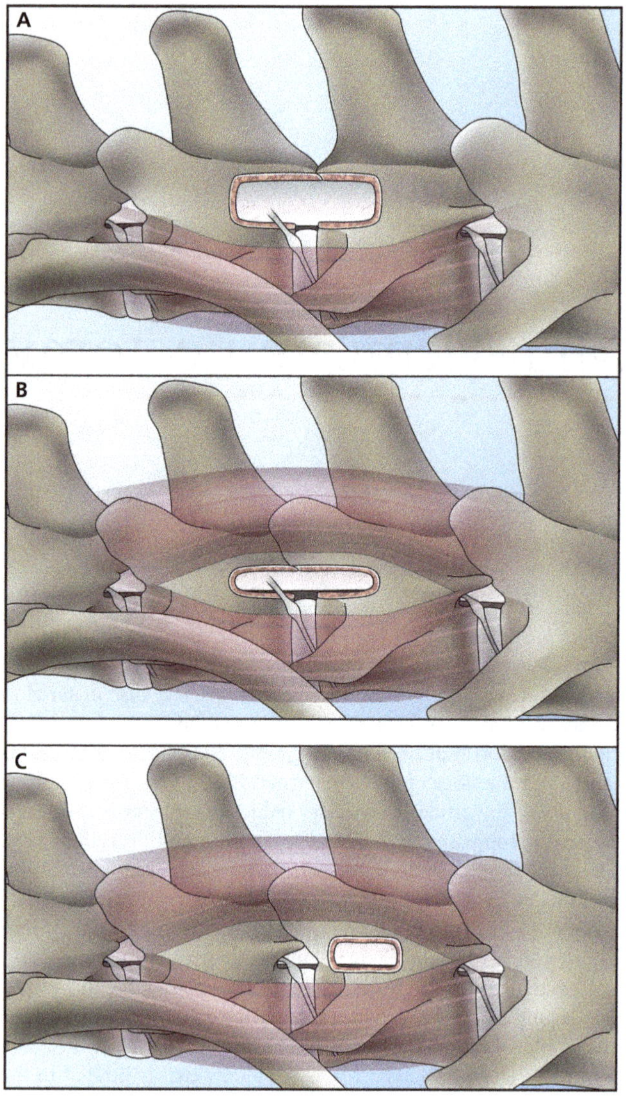

Figure 21.1 Illustrations depicting the approach and bony defect of (A) hemilaminectomy, (B) mini-hemilaminectomy or pediculectomy or foraminotomy, and (C) partial pediculectomy.

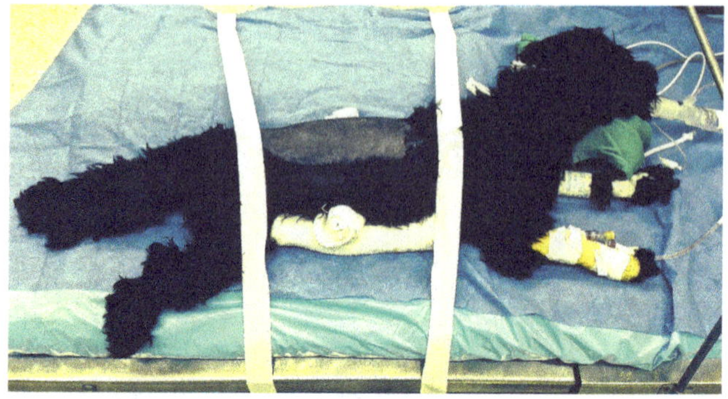

Figure 21.2 Oblique patient positioning (midway between sternal and lateral) with the spine rotated away from the surgeon and with the affected side facing up. A sandbag is placed behind the patient and under the table cover to maintain the oblique position. A rolled towel of appropriate size is placed under the patient's spine at the level of the lesion to open the disc space and facilitate fenestration of the affected disc. In some patients, as shown here, a small sandbag or towel can be tucked under the abdomen in order to straighten the spine and further stabilize the patient.

dependent on a portion of the pedicle being left intact (cranial and/or caudal to the pediculectomy window) to prevent disconnecting the dorsal lamina from the vertebral body [17]. A dorsal laminar subluxation was reported in a dog following bilateral mini-hemilaminectomy and fenestration of T12–T13 with bilateral (partial) pediculectomy at T13 [18].

Pediculectomy or mini-hemilaminectomy is indicated for cases of disc herniation that are lateralized or ventral [5]. Although this procedure can be used to retrieve dorsally extruded disc material, access to the dorsal spinal canal can appear limited depending on the size of the dog and window created [15,16] and could also possibly depend on patient positioning.

Technique: Surgical Approach (Video 21.1)

Mini-hemilaminectomy can be performed through a lateral or dorsolateral approach. An area caudal to the scapula and cranial to the wing of the ilium is clipped bilaterally but more so on the side of the lesion and is prepared for aseptic surgery. The patient is positioned in lateral (limbs toward the surgeon) [5,13,19,20] or oblique (midway between sternal and lateral recumbency with the spine rotated away from the surgeon and with the affected side facing up) recumbency for a lateral approach [21], and in sternal [19,20] or oblique [15,16,22] recumbency for a dorsolateral approach [21]. The author positions the patient obliquely for pediculectomy, and uses a dorsolateral approach as it appears to provide the best surgical field and access under the facet joints (Figure 21.2).

With the lateral and oblique position, the front limbs are tied cranially and the hind limbs are tied caudally with tape or ties. A rolled towel of appropriate size is placed under the patient's spine at the level of the lesion to open the disc space and facilitate fenestration of the affected disc. In some patients, a small sandbag or towel is tucked under the abdomen in order to straighten the spine and further stabilize the patient. When performing surgery in a sternal position, the hind limbs are flexed cranially to maintain the normal curvature of the spine.

An alternate position used by some surgeons for the lateral approach to the thoracolumbar spine involves placing the patient in lateral recumbency with the spine (lesion side up) towards the surgeon. With this position, the surgeon effectively works upside down along the spine (Figure 21.3).

The surgeon should review the diagnostic images prior to surgery to ensure there are no missing ribs or unusually shaped transverse processes that could confuse localization of the surgical site.

Dorsolateral Approach [19–22] (Video 21.2)

The thoracolumbar area is palpated to identify the last rib and grossly determine the site of herniation. With the dorsolateral approach, a skin incision is made toward the affected side, approximately 1–2 cm lateral to the dorsal midline over the area of interest and extending over one to two vertebrae cranial and caudal to the lesion. The incision is carried through the subcutaneous fat and fascia to identify the thick lumbodorsal fascia. Although some descriptions recommend undermining the fat on either side of the proposed incision through the lumbodorsal fascia to facilitate closure [19,22], this is not necessary as it creates dead space and increases the risk of postoperative seroma formation. An incision through the thoracolumbar fascia exposes a second layer of fat of variable thickness. In the caudal thoracic region, the caudal border

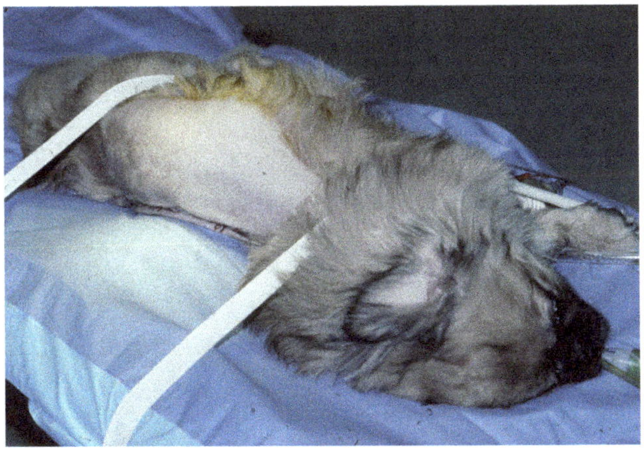

Figure 21.3 An alternate position used by some surgeons for a dorsolateral approach to the thoracolumbar vertebrae for pediculectomy/mini-hemilaminectomy involves placing the patient in lateral recumbency with the spine (lesion side up) towards the surgeon, who effectively works upside down.

of the spinalis and semispinalis thoracis muscles must also be incised. Focal blunt dissection between the fascicles of the iliocostalis musculature allows the surgeon to palpate and count the ribs and transverse processes for orientation. The last rib and first transverse process are landmarks used to identify the surgical site. Once the desired space is identified, the intermuscular plane between the multifidus and longissimus lumborum musculature is identified and bluntly dissected leaving the attachments of the multifidus muscle along the articular processes intact. Once the bone of the pedicle is identified, the longissimus muscle is elevated with a periosteal elevator to expose the pedicle and the attachment of the tendon of the longissiumus muscle to the accessory process. This tendon is transected using a blade or Mayo scissors; the author typically uses bipolar cautery to separate this attachment. Gelpi and/or Weitlaner self-retaining retractors are used to provide retraction of the multifidus muscle dorsomedially and the longissimus muscle ventrally.

Variation

Bitetto and Thacher [6] described a modified lateral decompression technique that used a dorsal midline approach like that described for hemilaminectomy. This approach has since been used and reported on by others [8–10]. While the dorsal approach would allow easy conversion to a hemilaminectomy or dorsal laminectomy if this was required, it lengthens the procedure time and increases tissue dissection and trauma and is not considered the approach of choice by the author.

Lateral Approach [19]

With the lateral approach, the incision overlies the rib heads and transverse processes and extends over one to two vertebral bodies cranial and caudal to the lesion. When performing a decompressive procedure accompanied by multiple disc fenestrations, the incision extends from the dorsal spine of T9 towards the ventral aspect of the wing of the ilium [23]. The incision is carried through the subcutaneous fat and lumbodorsal fascia. As described for the dorsolateral approach, the surgeon should identify and bluntly dissect between the muscle fascicles of the iliocostalis lumborum muscle focally to palpate and count the ribs or transverse processes [5]. The 13th rib and first transverse process (L1) are landmarks used to identify the surgical site. Once the desired space is identified, a portion of the iliocostalis lumborum and the longissimus muscles are elevated dorsally using a periosteal elevator to expose the vertebral pedicle and the tendinous attachment of the longissimus muscle to the accessory process, which is separated as described above [5].

Modified Dorsolateral Approach

The author uses a modified dorsolateral approach that incises through the longissimus muscle fibers, directly over the area of the intervertebral foramen of interest. This previously described approach [17] has also been published as a case series [24]. As for the other approaches, focal blunt dissection between the fascicles of the iliocostalis musculature allows the surgeon to palpate and count the ribs and transverse processes for orientation. After exposing the epaxial musculature through a dorsolateral approach made 1–2 cm lateral to the dorsal midline on the side of the lesion, a #15 blade is used to create a focal incision and dissection plane along and through the fibers of the musculus longissimus thoracis et lumborum. The incision is made midway between the articular processes and the rib heads or transverse processes (Figure 21.4 and see Video 21.2). Through this small incision, the pedicle bone is identified focally and the incision is extended as required cranially and caudally using a combination of sharp dissection, periosteal elevation, and muscle retraction. The attachment of the tendon of the longissimus muscle to the accessory process is transected using a blade, Mayo scissors, or preferably bipolar cautery. Gelpi and/or Weitlaner retractors are used to provide retraction of the dorsal portion of the longissimus muscle dorsally and of the remainder of the longissimus and iliocostalis muscles ventrally. With this approach, only the base of the ribs and/or transverse processes and the adjacent vertebral pedicles are exposed. Although this approach traumatizes the fibers of the longissimus muscle focally, it reduces the overall amount of muscle dissection required for exposure and leads to a smaller mass of muscle that must be elevated and retracted either ventrally or dorsally compared with the other approaches. This results in an overall smaller incision and is especially helpful in the lumbar area of larger dogs where dorsal retraction of the bulky iliocostalis and longissimus muscles can be challenging [7]. By providing direct access to the site of surgery, this modified dorsolateral approach also facilitates ventral drilling for pediculectomy and provides direct access to the IVD for fenestration.

Technique: Pediculectomy Procedure (Video 21.3)

With either approach, once the lateral pedicles of the two vertebrae of interest are identified, they are cleared of soft tissues using a periosteal elevator until the tendinous attachment of the longissimus muscle is visualized inserting on the accessory process of the cranial-most vertebra (Figure 21.5). The tendon is cauterized using bipolar cautery and then sharply transected at the level of its insertion on the accessory process, which exposes the desired intervertebral foramen. The self-retaining retractors are adjusted to provide further exposure of the bony structures. When exposure seems limited, muscle retraction and visualization can sometimes be facilitated by "blindly" (using palpation) transecting the tendon of the longissimus muscle attachment to the vertebra cranial to the decompression site without having to extend the skin incision. Any remaining soft tissue attachments along the pedicles of the two vertebrae of interest are cleared off using a periosteal elevator and retraction continues to be maintained with self-retaining retractors, typically two one-inch right angle Gelpi retractors. The surgical exposure spans a space dorsal to the level of the rib head or transverse

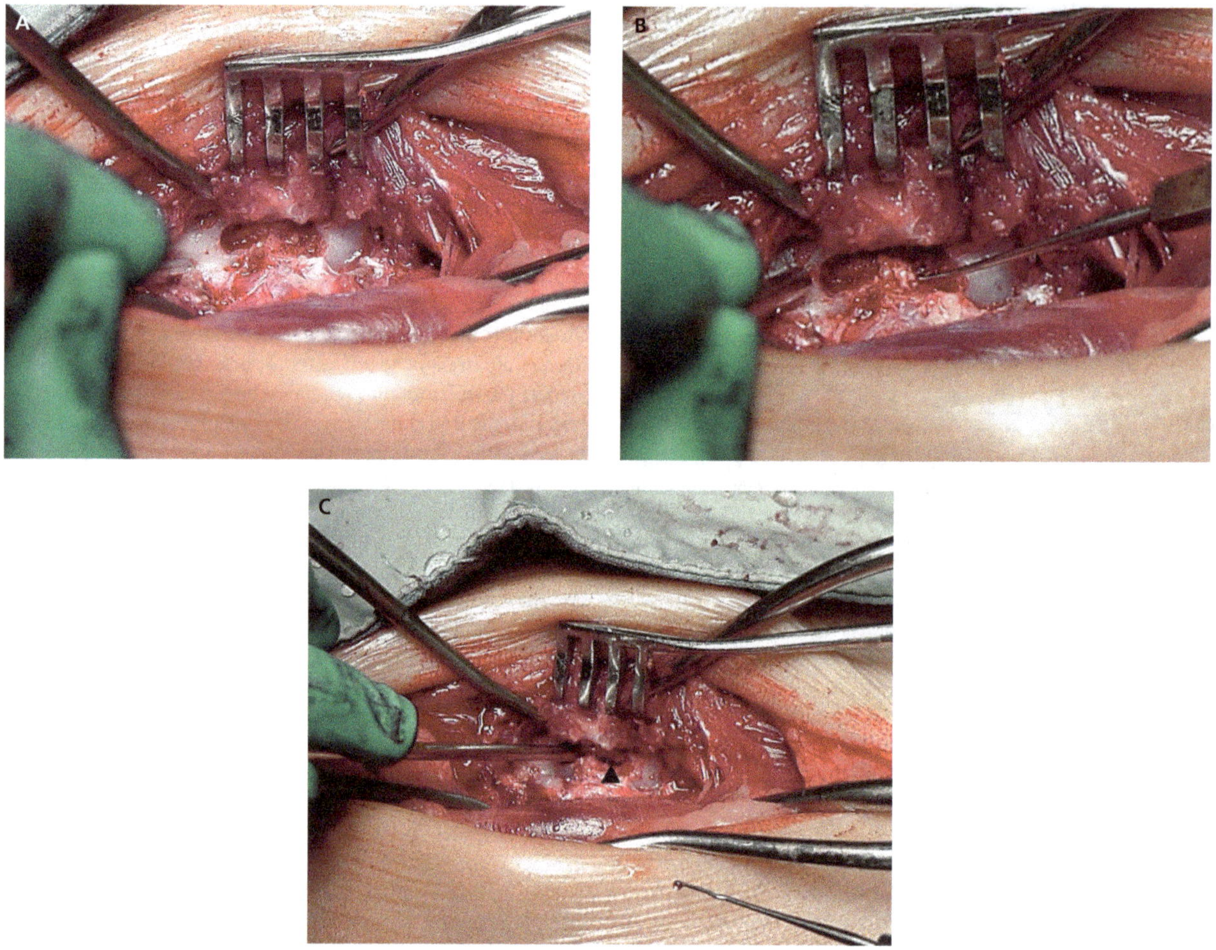

Figure 21.4 Mini-hemilaminectomy/pediculectomy to remove extruded disc material in a 5.5-kg dog using a modified dorsolateral approach that separates the longissimus lomborum muscle fibers: (A) before, (B) during and (C) after removal of extruded disc material. Note that the spinal cord (arrowhead) has returned to its normal position within the spinal canal and is clearly visible after removal of the extruded disc material (C).

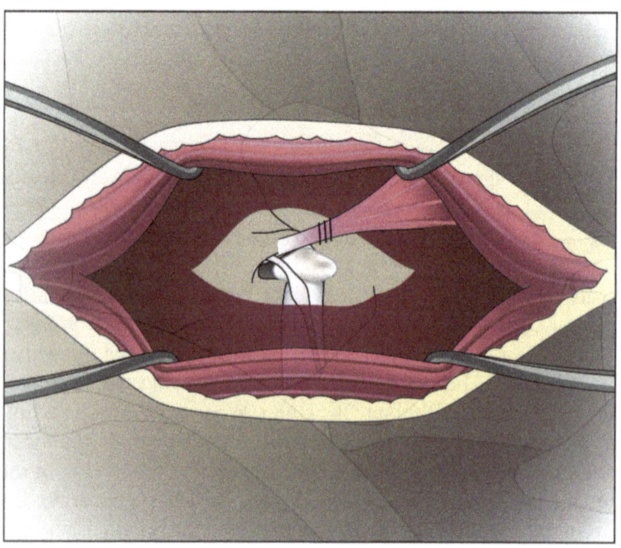

Figure 21.5 The lateral pedicles of interest are identified, they are cleared of soft tissues using a periosteal elevator, and the tendinous attachment of the longissimus musculature is cauterized and then sharply transected at the level of its insertion on the accessory process exposing the desired intervertebral foramen.

process, and ventral to the base of the articular processes, without exposing the articular processes. Cranially and caudally, the dissection extends to, but does not expose, the adjacent intervertebral foramina (Figure 21.4).

Mini-hemilaminectomy is performed using a drill. Some surgeons use magnification for this portion of the procedure, especially in smaller dogs. The accessory process that overlies the dorsal aspect of the foramen is first removed using rongeurs or preferably a drill and this forms the dorsal-most extent of the mini-hemilaminectomy, thus leaving the zygapophyseal joint intact [5,9]. The small artery located just medial to the accessory process is coagulated with bipolar cautery [9]. Ventral to this, the pedicle is thinned cranially and caudally to essentially enlarge the intervertebral foramen over approximately half to two-thirds of the length of each vertebra, or longer if extruded disc extends beyond [5,15,16]. The ventral extent of the mini-hemilaminectomy is as much as possible the ventral aspect of the intervertebral foramen/spinal canal [5]. The cranial and caudal aspects of the laminectomy extend until normal epidural fat is identified or until the surgeon believes all extruded disc material has been removed [5,15,16].

The pedicle bone is drilled using a high-speed air or electric drill, taking notice of the change from cortical (white) to more spongy (red) cancellous bone (Figure 21.6 and Video 21.4). As much as possible, the bone should be thinned evenly, preventing focal

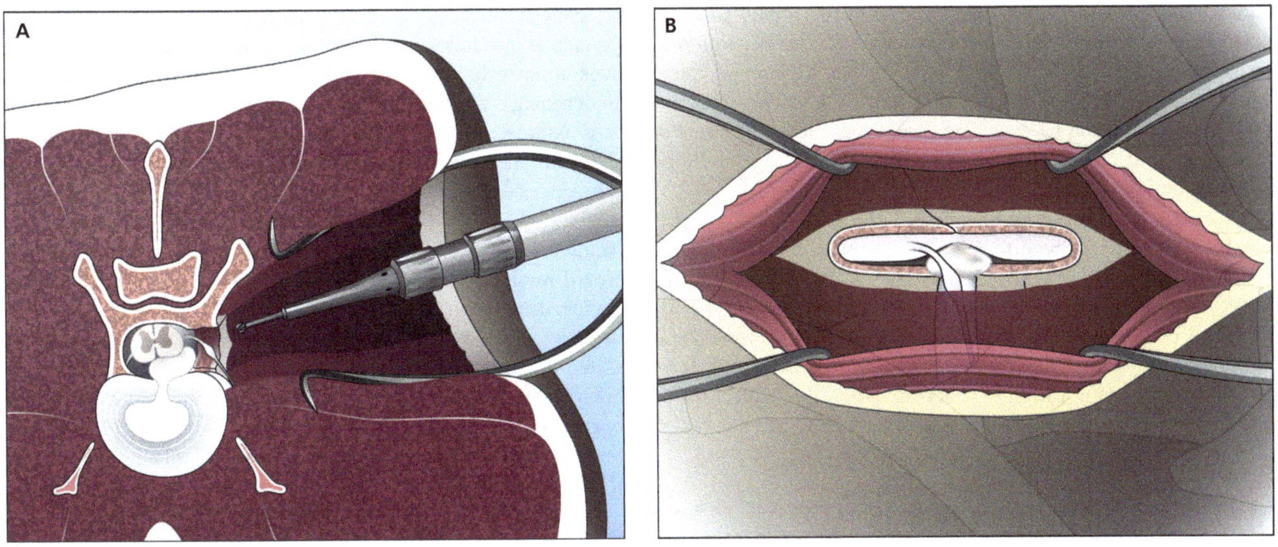

Figure 21.6 Cross-section (A) and sagittal (B) views of the vertebral spine depicting the bone window provided by the pediculectomy approach. This procedure provides direct access to the lateral and ventral spinal canal for removal of extruded disc material while leaving the articular facets intact.

penetration in one area of the canal. Sterile saline lavage and suction is performed regularly to remove bony debris and cool the bone. Cancellous bone hemorrhage can be controlled using small amounts of bone wax. Note that cancellous bone will not be present at the edge of the foramen and that the bony edge will also be thinner in this area. The surgeon should assess bony thickness visually and by palpating with a small blunt probe (e.g., iris spatula or small curette) as often as needed. Once the cancellous bone is removed and the inner cortical bone is thinned out to a moveable thin layer of periosteum, it can be penetrated using a 22G needle with the tip bent at 90° and a #11 scalpel blade (Figure 21.7 and Video 21.5), exposing the spinal canal over the entire length of the laminectomy. Some surgeons prefer to use a house curette or Kerrison rongeur to remove the inner periosteal edges. Should the laminectomy site need to be extended ventrally or craniocaudally, it is best done before removing the extruded disc material because this will allow the displaced spinal cord to return to a more normal position within the laminectomy site possibly leading to iatrogenic trauma.

Necrotic fat, hemorrhage, and soft and hard disc material are retrieved using a blunt probe, iris spatula, small curette, or suction (the suction tip should never be allowed to contact the dura) while avoiding manipulation of the spinal cord and trauma to the dorsal nerve root (Video 21.6). After removal of the disc material located lateral to the spinal cord, sweeping extends ventrally and then dorsally to ensure as much disc material as possible is removed. When sweeping the canal, care should be taken to retrieve disc material rather than push it towards the opposite side or beyond the pediculectomy site. The author prefers to use a bent iris spatula that moves from craniodorsal and from dorsocaudal towards the mid section of the pediculectomy ventrally (Video 21.7). Hard or adherent disc material may also be removed with a scalpel blade [7,22,25]. Chronically extruded disc material may form adhesions to the venous sinus, the nerve root and vascular bundle, or the dura mater and could result in laceration of the venous sinus and hemorrhage during removal. Venous sinus hemorrhage can be controlled by applying direct pressure using an iris spatula or placing a small block of gelatin sponge directly at the site of hemorrhage [25]. Although the gelatin sponge can be left in place if required [25], it should be removed, if possible, prior to closing the surgical defect.

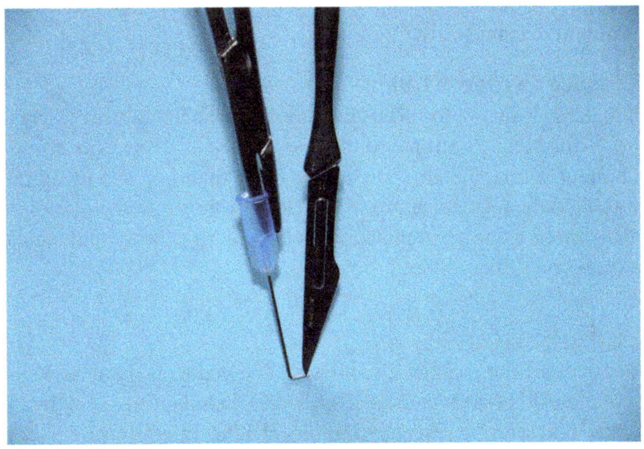

Figure 21.7 Bent needle (90°) and #11 blade used to enter the spinal canal after drilling the pedicle bone to a paper-thin layer of inner cortical bone/periosteum.

An alternative is to fill the entire laminectomy defect with a precut piece of gelatin sponge and to fill the surgical site with cool or room temperature saline to increase pressure at the laminectomy site and promote clotting without direct contact between the gelatin sponge and the vascular defect. After 5 min, the saline can be suctioned and the gelatin sponge gently removed without peeling away a blood clot at the level of the vascular defect. Hemorrhage caused by a laceration of the spinal artery or vein is controlled using bipolar cautery.

Once the extruded disc material is removed the spinal cord should return to a normal position within the spinal canal. In instances where the spinal cord remains displaced, the surgeon should consider that additional disc material might be present cranially, caudally, or on the contralateral side requiring extension of the laminectomy in either direction or that a contralateral procedure be performed. Indentation of the spinal cord at the site of extrusion is possible and most common in chronic cases and does not require treatment as long as the compressive mass is removed.

If sufficient disc material is not found, the surgeon should verify that the correct site and side was approached surgically. If the correct site/side was approached, the surgeon might consider extending the mini-hemilaminectomy cranially (most common), or caudally to find disc that extruded further within the spinal canal. High-impact, low-volume disc extrusion or an incorrect diagnosis should also be considered when significant amounts of disc material are not recovered. In such cases, imaging should be reviewed and possibly repeated.

If desired, fenestration of the affected and adjacent disc spaces can be performed through these approaches (see Chapter 22 and see Video 22.1).

Although Braund et al. [5] described placing gelatin sponge over the decompression site prior to closure to prevent dural adhesions in the first description of this procedure, fat graft or gelatin sponge are not used to cover the surgical site after mini-hemilaminectomy [7,16].

Procedure Variations

Partial pediculectomy (Figure 21.1C) has been described as a less invasive and faster surgical procedure [13]. This procedure requires adequate knowledge of the lesion location such that the bony window is created specifically over the site of lesion and to allow adequate decompression by removal of the extruded disc material. For these reasons, partial pediculectomy is not recommended as the standard decompression technique.

Closure (Video 21.8)

Standard closure of the deep and superficial thoracolumbar fascia is performed using a simple continuous pattern of absorbable monofilament suture. When approaching more than one site using the modified dorsolateral approach, the longissimus muscle incision is also closed using a simple continuous pattern. The subcutaneous tissues and skin are closed routinely.

Complications

The presence of residual disc material is noted in as many as 100% of patients that recover satisfactorily after hemilaminectomy but is rarely found to be clinically significant [26]. In contrast, residual disc material (7.7%, range 0–27.3%) was found in 44% of nine patients undergoing mini-hemilaminectomy when preoperative and postoperative MRI were compared [16]. Delayed recovery or lack of postoperative improvement has been associated with the presence of large amounts of residual disc material related to the wrong approach, shifting of disc material during surgery, and to the herniation of additional disc material within the spinal canal requiring further imaging and surgery [27–29]. Failure to retrieve any disc material requiring extension to a different disc space or a bilateral procedure is considered a major complication [7]. A disadvantage of mini-hemilaminectomy is that the lateral or oblique positioning of the dog requires that the surgical site be closed and the patient be repositioned if the wrong side was initially approached surgically [7]. This is less likely to occur with the routine use of advanced imaging such as CT and MRI to identify and localize the lesion [27]. When lateralization is not evident, the surgeon chooses the side of surgery based on preference; most right-handed surgeons prefer approaching the left side [30]. An advantage of the pediculectomy over the hemilaminectomy is that it can be performed bilaterally without compromise to the bony support or soft tissues [30].

Hemorrhage is typically minor and in most instances is easily controlled but in cases where severe hemorrhage is encountered it can hinder visualization and prevent adequate spinal decompression or lead to marked blood loss [12].

Scoliosis and lateral abdominal wall weakness are reported complications following fenestration by the dorsolateral muscle separating technique [31] and have also been reported in dogs undergoing lateral decompression techniques with fenestration [7]. It is assumed that these are caused by trauma to the lateral and medial branches of the thoracic and lumbar ventral spinal nerves and are related to the fenestration but this cannot be confirmed [7]. The muscle weakness typically resolves within a few weeks [7]. Transection of the nerve root (dorsal, or both dorsal and ventral) would result in some deficits that would be more evident if they occurred caudal to L3.

Late recurrent disc herniation is possible at a previously unaffected disc space or at the site of surgery if residual disc material contained within the annulus herniates into the spinal canal postoperatively [11,12,28,32–35]. Fenestration of the surgical site with or without fenestration of adjacent disc spaces is believed to reduce the rate of recurrence [11,12,35].

Postoperative Care

Following pediculectomy, dogs are hospitalized on intravenous fluids and injectable analgesics until sufficiently comfortable to receive oral medications (typically 24 hours). Discharge is most commonly within 48 hours of surgery in patients that retain motor function. Dogs with loss of motor function are typically discharged once voluntary urinary control is confirmed or when the owner is comfortable expressing the bladder at home. Postoperative rehabilitation is recommended in most cases (see Chapter 29). For general postoperative recommendations, see Chapter 28.

As for hemilaminectomy, overall, recovery rates of greater than 90% have been reported following mini-hemilaminectomy with or without prophylactic fenestration [6–12].

Video clips to accompany this book can be found on the companion website at:
www.wiley.com/go/shores/neurosurgery

References

1 Funkquist B. Thoracolumbar disk protrusion with severe cord compression in the dog. III. Treatment by decompressive laminectomy. *Acta Vet Scand* 1962;3:344–366.
2 Funkquist B. Decompressive laminectomy in thoraco-lumbar disc protrusion with paraplegia in the dog. *J Small Anim Pract* 1970;11:445–451.
3 Trotter EJ, Brasmer TH, deLahunta A. Modified deep dorsal laminectomy in the dog. *Cornell Vet* 1975;65:402–427.
4 Hoerlein BF. The status of the various intervertebral disc surgeries for the dog in 1978. *J Am Anim Hosp Assoc* 1978;14:563–570.
5 Braund KG, Taylor TKF, Ghosh P, Sherwood AA. Lateral spinal decompression in the dog. *J Small Anim Pract* 1976;17:583–592.
6 Bitetto WV, Thacher C. A modified lateral decompression technique for treatment of canine intervertebral disk disease. *J Am Anim Hosp Assoc* 1987;23:409–413.
7 Black AP. Lateral spinal decompression in the dog: a review of 39 cases. *J Small Anim Pract* 1988;29:581–588.
8 Yovich JC, Read R, Eger C. Modified lateral spinal decompression in 61 dogs with thoracolumbar disc protrusion. *J Small Anim Pract* 1994;35:351–356.
9 Jeffery ND. Treatment of acute and chronic thoracolumbar disc disease by "mini hemilaminectomy". *J Small Anim Pract* 1988;29:611–616.
10 Lubbe AM, Kirberger RM, Verstraete FJM. Pediculectomy for thoracolumbar spinal decompression in the dachshund. *J Am Anim Hosp Assoc* 1994;30:233–238.
11 Brisson BA, Moffatt SL, Swayne SL, Parent J. Recurrence of thoracolumbar intervertebral disk extrusion in chondrodystrophic dogs after surgical decompression with or without prophylactic fenestration: 265 cases (1995–1999). *J Am Vet Med Assoc* 2004;224:1808–1814.

12 Brisson BA, Holmberg DL, Parent J, Sears WC, Wick SE. Comparison of the effect of single-site and multiple-site disk fenestration on the rate of recurrence of thoracolumbar intervertebral disk herniation in dogs. *J Am Vet Med Assoc* 2011;238: 1593–1600.

13 McCartney W. Partial pediculectomy for the treatment of thoracolumbar disc disease. *Vet Comp Orthop Traumatol* 1997;10:117–121.

14 Hill TP, Lubbe AM, Guthrie AJ. Lumbar spine stability following hemilaminectomy, pediculectomy, and fenestration. *Vet Comp Orthop Traumatol* 2000;13:165–171.

15 Huska JL, Gaitero L, Brisson BA, Nykamp S, Thomason J, Sears WC. Comparison of the access window created by hemilaminectomy and mini-hemilaminectomy in the thoracolumbar vertebral canal using computed tomography. *Can Vet J* 2014;55: 449–455.

16 Huska JL, Gaitero L, Brisson BA, Nykamp S, Thomason J, Sears WC. Presence of residual material following mini-hemilaminectomy in dogs with thoracolumbar intervertebral disc extrusion. *Can Vet J* 2014;55:975–980.

17 Slocum B, Slocum TD. Thoracolumbar spine: pediculotomy in the thoracolumbar vertebra. In: Bojrab MJ, Ellison GW, Slocum B (eds) *Current Techniques in Small Animal Surgery*, 4th edn. Baltimore, MD: Williams & Wilkins, 1998: 835–858.

18 Arthurs G. Spinal instability resulting from bilateral mini-hemilaminectomy and pediculectomy. *Vet Comp Orthop Traumatol* 2009;22:422–426.

19 Piermattei DL, Johnson KA. The vertebral column. In: *An Atlas of Surgical Approaches to the Bones and Joints of the Dog and Cat*, 4th edn. Philadelphia, PA: WB Saunders, 2004: 47–105.

20 Kerwin SC, Levine JM, Hicks DG. Thoracolumbar spine. In: Tobias KM, Johnston SA (eds) *Veterinary Surgery: Small Animal*. St Louis, MO: Elsevier Saunders, 2012: 449–475.

21 Dewey C. Surgery of the thoracolumbar spine. In: Fossum TW (ed.) *Small Animal Surgery*, 4th edn. St Louis, MO: Elsevier Mosby, 2013: 1508–1528.

22 Sharp N, Wheeler S. Thoracolumbar disc disease. In: *Small Animal Spinal Disorders: Diagnosis and Surgery*, 2nd edn. Philadelphia, PA: Elsevier Mosby, 2005: 121–159.

23 Flo GL, Brinker WO. Lateral fenestration of thoracolumbar discs. *J Am Anim Hosp Assoc* 1975;11:619–626.

24 Tanaka N, Kitagawa M, Ito D, Watari T. A modified lateral muscle-separation approach for mini-hemilaminectomy. *Vet Rec* 2013;173:296.

25 Bitetto WV, Kapatkin AS. Intraoperative problems associated with intervertebral disc disease. *Probl Vet Med* 1989;1:434–444.

26 Roach WJ, Thomas M, Weh JM, Bleedorn JA, Wells K. Residual herniated disc material following hemilaminectomy in chondrodystrophic dogs with thoracolumbar intervertebral disc disease. *Vet Comp Orthop Traumatol* 2012;25:109–115.

27 Forterre F, Gorgas D, Dickomeit M, Jaggy A, Lang J, Spreng D. Incidence of spinal compressive lesions in chondrodystrophic dogs with abnormal recovery after hemilaminectomy for treatment of thoracolumbar disc disease: a prospective magnetic resonance imaging study. *Vet Surg* 2010;39:165–172.

28 Stigen O. Early recurrence of thoracolumbar intervertebral disc extrusion after surgical decompression: a report of three cases. *Acta Vet Scand* 2010; 52:10.

29 Hettlich BF, Kerwin SC, Levine JM. Early reherniation of disk material in eleven dogs with surgically treated thoracolumbar intervertebral disk extrusion. *Vet Surg* 2012;41:215–219.

30 Simpson ST. Thoracolumbar spine: hemilaminectomy of the caudal thoracic and lumbar spine. In: Bojrab MJ, Ellison GW, Slocum B (eds) *Current Techniques in Small Animal Surgery*, 4th edn. Baltimore, MD: Williams & Wilkins, 1998: 844–849.

31 Bartels KE, Creed JE, Yturraspe DJ. Complications associated with the dorsolateral muscle-separating approach for thoracolumbar disk fenestration in the dog. *J Am Vet Med Assoc* 1983;183:1081–1083.

32 Dhupa S, Glickman N, Waters DJ. Reoperative neurosurgery in dogs with thoracolumbar disc disease. *Vet Surg* 1999;28:421–428.

33 Necas A. Clinical aspects of surgical treatment of thoracolumbar disc disease in dogs. A retrospective study of 300 cases. *Acta Vet Brno* 1999;68:121–130.

34 Mayhew PD, McLear RC, Ziemer LS et al. Risk factors for recurrence of clinical signs associated with thoracolumbar intervertebral disk herniation in dogs: 229 cases (1994–2000). *J Am Vet Med Assoc* 2004;225:1231–1236.

35 Forterre F, Konar M, Spreng D, Jaggy A, Lang J. Influence of intervertebral disc fenestration at the herniation site in association with hemilaminectomy on recurrence in chondrodystrophic dogs with thoracolumbar disc disease: a prospective MRI study. *Vet Surg* 2008;37:399–405.

22 Intervertebral Disc Fenestration

Brigitte A. Brisson

Introduction

Intervertebral disc (IVD) fenestration involves the mechanical removal of the nucleus pulposus (NP) through a window, or fenestration, created in the annulus fibrosus (AF). Fenestration can be performed using an air drill and burr, known as power-assisted fenestration, or with a scalpel blade, known as blade fenestration (Figure 22.1) [1,2]. The simple creation of a window within the lateral AF does not result in a path for any remaining disc material to herniate, nor does postoperative chiropractic bending maneuvers result in disc material being expelled through the fenestration site [1–4]. Studies assessing the fate of the NP following surgical disc fenestration have failed to document a significant inflammatory reaction which would verify that the remaining disc material is subsequently dissolved preventing recurrence, nor has it confirmed that the window remains open to offer an alternate path for future disc extrusion since fibrocartilage fills the void created by fenestration soon after surgery [3,5]. Rather, the effectiveness of fenestration is thought to be governed by the amount of NP removed at the time of surgery [3] and is directly related to the skill and experience of the operator [6]. Despite skill, complete removal of the remaining NP is not expected when performing fenestration [2]. This is supported by a recent study that found some residual disc material in all fenestrated discs even after power-assisted fenestration through a lateral approach [7]. A previous cadaver study comparing blade and power-assisted fenestration documented that power-assisted fenestration removed on average 65% of the NP compared with approximately 41% of the NP being removed with blade fenestration [2]. However, the author believes that either technique can

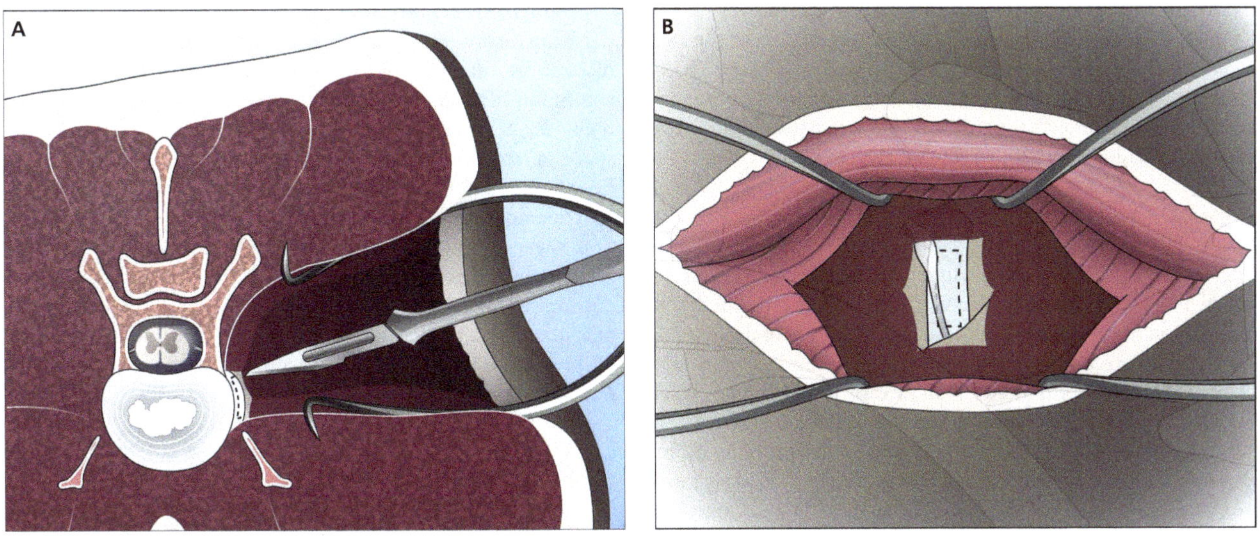

Figure 22.1 Illustration of a transverse section through a canine lumbar intervertebral disc (A) and sagittal view (B) depicting blade fenestration performed through a lateral approach.

Current Techniques in Canine and Feline Neurosurgery, First Edition. Edited by Andy Shores and Brigitte A. Brisson.
© 2017 John Wiley & Sons, Inc. Published 2017 by John Wiley & Sons, Inc.
Companion website: www.wiley.com/go/shores/neurosurgery

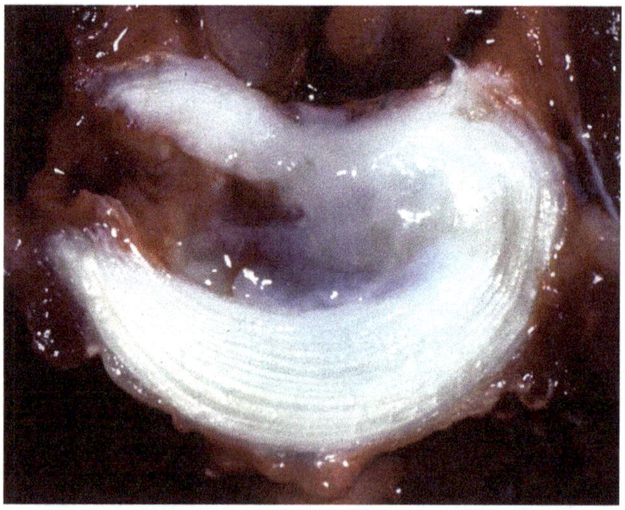

Figure 22.2 Transverse section through an intervertebral disc after fenestration was performed showing that some nucleus remains within the annulus, mostly on the side contralateral to the fenestration.

effectively remove large amounts of disc material as long as the surgeon is comfortable with the technique chosen.

A study evaluating the effect of surgical approach to the spine determined that using the lateral approach for IVD fenestration may increase the efficiency of the procedure compared with the dorsal or dorsolateral surgical approaches by providing a better angle and working depth for fenestration [8]. Despite the increased efficiency and depth obtained through a lateral approach, it is likely to result in removal of more NP from the ipsilateral side and less from the contralateral side of the IVD being fenestrated [9] (Figure 22.2). It is also likely that much of the residual nonherniated NP still present within the affected disc space is located on the contralateral side to a lateralized extrusion and will be difficult to remove from the side approached for decompressive surgery [8].

Other reported techniques for prophylactic ablation of the IVD in dogs include percutaneous laser disc ablation [10–13], CUSA aspiration [9], vacuum aspiration [14], chemonucleolysis using collagenase [15], chymopapain [16] and, most recently, discolysis by injection of radiopaque gelified ethanol [17].

Indications

Fenestration has been advocated to reduce the rate of early and late recurrence of disc herniation in dogs affected by this condition. Fenestration of the herniated disc space at the time of decompressive surgery is recommended to prevent further extrusion of disc material through the ruptured AF in the early postoperative period [4,7,18–23]. Reports documenting early recurrent disc extrusion at a decompressed site [4,7,24] do not support the previous claims suggesting that recurrent herniated disc material would likely move spontaneously outside of the canal through the laminectomy site and not cause clinical deterioration. However, it is possible that the previously made laminectomy offers some relief from spinal cord or nerve root compression which could explain why some dogs documented as having recurrent herniated material do not develop neurological deficits [7].

The benefit of fenestration should increase with increasing amounts of degenerative NP material remaining within the disc after the initial extrusion [4,7]. The amount of NP remaining within the disc space and its exact location cannot be determined using imaging nor can it be anticipated based on how much extruded disc material is retrieved from the surgical site [7]. However, radiographic evidence of mineralization at the herniated IVD space is thought to be indicative of residual degenerated NP material and to support fenestration of the affected disc space at the time of decompressive surgery [4].

Although controversial for decades, prophylactic fenestration of unaffected adjacent thoracolumbar discs has prospectively been shown to significantly reduce (7.45% vs. 17.89%) the rate of late recurrence in dogs undergoing disc fenestration between T11–T12 and L3–L4 compared to those fenestrated only at the site of herniation [23]. A recent retrospective study followed 662 chondrodystrophic dogs that recovered from hemilaminectomy and prophylactic disc fenestration of at least three thoracolumbar IVD spaces and showed a 2.3% rate of recurrence confirmed with repeat surgery [25]. Most recently, percutaneous laser disc ablation (PLDA) was reported as a safe and minimally invasive procedure associated with a low rate of recurrence of disc herniation [13]. In this study, 60 of 303 dogs (19.8%) had an episode of suspected or confirmed IVD herniation after undergoing PLDA, but only 11 of 303 (3.6%) had a recurrence of IVD herniation confirmed by means of CT or MRI and hemilaminectomy [13].

Recurrence of signs consistent with cervical disc herniation after ventral slot has been reported to be between 0 and 17% [26–29]. Since removal of the affected disc is integral to performing a ventral slot procedure, fenestration of the affected disc space is always performed. Ventral fenestration of the adjacent disc spaces has been advocated to prevent repeat herniation at another disc space but has also been reported to result in a significant increase in range of motion during flexion–extension which could contribute to the development of "domino" lesions, especially in larger-breed dogs [30,31]. Cervical disc fenestration has also been recommended in cases where IVD compression is not evident on imaging and discogenic pain is suspected [32,33].

Prophylactic fenestration of the cervical region is typically performed between C2–C3 and C5–C6 [33] because the C6–C7 disc can be difficult to access surgically. While C2–C3 is the most commonly affected disc space in the cervical spine of small-breed dogs [27,28,34–36], C6–C7 is the most commonly affected disc space in large-breed dogs [27]. Recent studies have also reported C5–C6 [29] and C6–C7 [36] as the most commonly affected disc spaces among all dog breeds presenting for cervical IVD herniation, suggesting that if fenestration is performed it should probably include these disc spaces. Fenestration of a ruptured disc without decompression can lead to neurological deterioration if further disc material herniates into the spinal canal during the procedure [37] so fenestration alone is not recommended to treat known herniated discs.

Technique

Cervical disc fenestration is typically performed through a ventral approach [38,39]. Thoracolumbar disc fenestration has been described using a dorsal, dorsolateral [19,38–41], lateral [1,42], ventrolateral [38,39,43,44], and ventral approach [45–48]. A study that compared various surgical approaches used for thoracolumbar fenestration found that using the lateral approach for IVD fenestration may increase the efficiency of the procedure compared with the dorsal or dorsolateral surgical approaches by providing a better angle and working depth for fenestration [8].

Cervical Disc Fenestration

Patient preparation, patient positioning, surgical approach, and surgical closure are identical to those described for the ventral slot procedure (see Chapter 17). Identification of the disc space of interest is facilitated by palpation of the large and prominent transverse processes of C6 and the ventral process of C1. The C5–C6 disc space lies on the midline just cranial to the most cranial aspect of the transverse processes of C6. Once exposed the origin of the paired tendons of the longus colli muscles overlying the disc are separated or transected with bipolar cautery, a #15 scalpel blade, or Mayo scissors and the muscles are elevated using a periosteal elevator. Retraction is maintained using Gelpi retractors. Once exposed, the ventral AF is fenestrated using a #11 scalpel blade. First, a rectangular window of no more than 50% of the width of the vertebral body is created through the annulus [30]. The window is created by puncturing the disc with the blade on the side opposite the surgeon and advancing it through the AF from endplate to endplate. Then the blade follows each of the cranial and caudal endplates over no more than half the width of the endplate. Finally, the rectangle is completed by advancing the blade from endplate to endplate at the opposite end of the rectangle. In small dogs, care is taken not to penetrate the spinal canal located deep to the dorsal annulus. The excised annulus is then removed using small curved mosquito forceps or rongeurs and the exposed NP is removed using curettes, spatulas, or dental scrapers. The instruments are carefully directed within the disc space in a dorsocranial direction following the orientation of the disc space while being mindful of the location/depth of the spinal canal. If performing fenestration at a site of herniation without concurrent decompression, care is taken that additional material is not forced dorsally into the spinal canal [49].

Thoracolumbar Disc Fenestration

Preparation/Positioning

Right-handed surgeons typically find that thoracolumbar fenestration is more easily performed on the left side of the spine [50] but since fenestration is most commonly performed with concurrent decompression, the approach will depend on the side of the lesion. An appropriate area of the thoracolumbar region relative to the location of the lesion and/or location of proposed fenestrations is clipped and prepared aseptically. The patient is positioned in sternal recumbency or oblique recumbency (sternal recumbency with 45° rotation away from the surgeon using a sandbag or towel and tape) for the dorsal and dorsolateral approaches (see Figure 21.2). The lateral approach can be performed in lateral or oblique recumbency with the surgical side facing up. The front limbs are tied cranially and the hind limbs tied caudally. A towel roll is frequently inserted under the thoracolumbar region to open the disc spaces on the side of surgery and to facilitate fenestration. The surgeon should review the anatomy to ensure there are no missing or unusually shaped ribs or transverse processes in the area of interest.

Approach

Lateral Approach [1,8,42,51]

The animal is placed in lateral or oblique recumbency to visualize the left or right side of the spine. Placing a sandbag or rolled towel under the thoracolumbar area (perpendicular to the spine) opens the disc spaces on the side of surgery and allows a larger annular window to be created, facilitating curettage of the disc spaces. For fenestration of all disc spaces between T11 and L4, the skin incision is made obliquely from the lateral aspect of the dorsal vertebral spines in the thoracic region (T9) towards the ventral aspect of the wing of the ilium, stopping at about L5 [1,51]. Alternatively, an incision that follows the transverse processes of the vertebrae of interest is appropriate and should extend over one to two vertebrae cranial and caudal to the intended fenestration sites. When fenestrating only a few disc spaces on either side of the herniated disc, the surgical incision made for decompression can be enlarged accordingly.

For fenestration, the skin incision extends through the subcutaneous fat layer and the lumbodorsal fascia allowing its retraction. A deep layer of fat of variable thickness is encountered and is incised to reveal the epaxial musculature. Using deep digital palpation, the appropriate disc spaces are located and exposed by identifying the rib head or the tip of the transverse process caudal to the disc of interest. Metzembaum scissors or Kelly forceps are used to split the iliocostalis thoracis and lumborum muscles in an oblique direction along the muscle fibers (dorsal to the tip of the transverse process or just cranial to the rib head) allowing the area of the disc space to be digitally palpated (Figure 22.3). In the lumbar region, a periosteal elevator is then used to elevate the loose layer of fascia that covers the lateral annulus from the edge of the transverse process. Dissection should proceed from the base of the transverse process in a cranial direction exposing the fibers of the AF. Retraction of the deep muscle is most easily maintained using small-tipped, right-angled Gelpi retractors (Figure 22.4). The exposure obtained is small but allows excellent visualization of the lateral annulus for fenestration.

Fenestration of thoracic discs is slightly more challenging and offers less visualization. After separating the fibers of the iliocostalis lumborum muscle which attach to the 13th, 12th, 11th and 10th ribs, an index finger is used to follow the rib to the level where it articulates with the vertebral body. Alternatively, the iliocostalis lumborum muscles can be transected close to their insertion on the associated ribs [51]. The levator costae muscles originate on the transverse processes of T1–T12 and insert on the anterior surface of the rib caudal to each process. This muscle is separated using a blade or periosteal elevator and is retracted ventrally. Retraction of the epaxial muscles dorsally and of the levator costae muscle ventrally is best achieved using a Gelpi retractor or hand-held retractors.

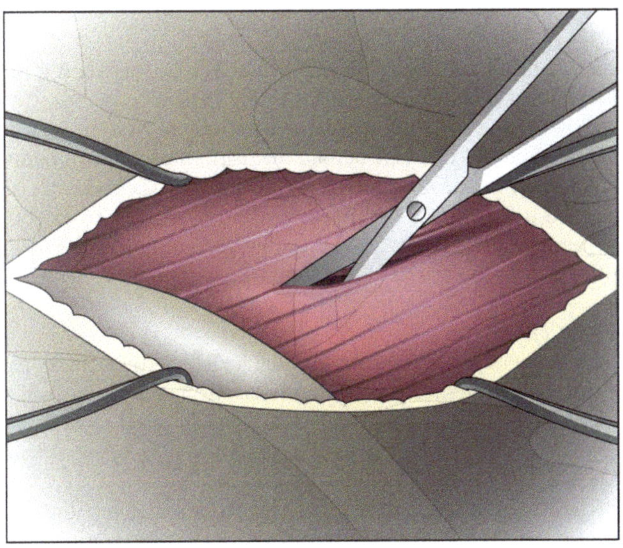

Figure 22.3 Metzembaum scissors are used to split the iliocostalis lumborum muscle in the direction of its muscle fibers (dorsal to the tip of the transverse process of L1) to expose the annulus fibrosus.

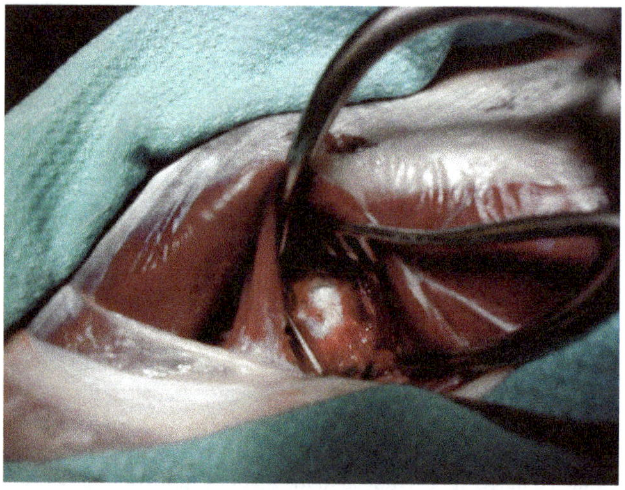

Figure 22.4 Approach for disc fenestration in a cadaver. Note that Gelpi and Weitlaner retractors are used to maintain muscle retraction.

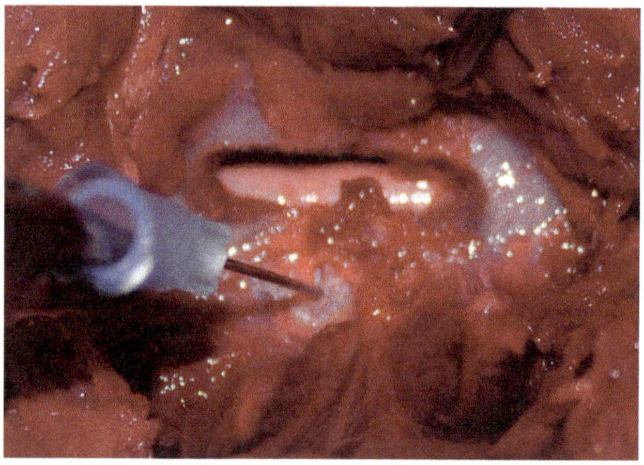

Figure 22.5 A hypodermic needle is used to palpate each of the vertebral endplates and to penetrate the annulus fibrosus identifying the disc space for fenestration. Note that the exposure gained for mini-hemilaminectomy was sufficient for fenestration at this site.

Care is taken to prevent pleural puncture while separating the levator costae muscle and while inserting retractors.

Fenestration of the affected disc space does not typically require much additional exposure beyond that performed for mini-hemilaminectomy or hemilaminectomy (Figure 22.5). The incision may need to be extended cranially or caudally if fenestration extends beyond the affected disc space. The disc spaces of interest are identified as described above.

Variations

Morelius et al. [8] describe an approach for lateral fenestration that dissects along the plane between the longissimus and iliocostalis muscles rather than through the fibers of the iliocostalis muscle.

Dorsal Approach [8,52]

Because of the amount of muscle dissection required for this approach, it is typically used for fenestration when decompression is performed through a dorsal approach. The animal is positioned in sternal recumbency. A longitudinal skin and fascial incision is made along one side of the spinous processes followed by blunt dissection and elevation of the multifidus muscle from the spinous processes of interest. The tendinous attachments of the multifidus muscle are then sharply transected from the mammillary processes and the multifidus and longissimus muscle are elevated and retracted ventrolaterally to expose the pedicle and IVD [8]. The attachment of the longissimus muscle to the accessory process is transected to increase exposure for laminectomy. The intervertebral foramen is located ventral to the articular process and the disc space is located below this, immediately cranial to the rib head or the base of the transverse process. The loose connective tissues containing the spinal nerves and vessels that overlie the disc space are retracted cranially to expose the glistening annulus for fenestration.

Dorsolateral Approach [8,40,41,53]

The animal is positioned in sternal recumbency or slight oblique away from the affected side. A longitudinal skin and fascial incision is made over the articular processes of the area of interest or 1–2 cm lateral to the spinous processes towards the affected side [41]. In the caudal thoracic region, the caudal border of the spinalis and semispinalis thoracis muscles must also be incised. Blunt dissection is performed along the intermuscular plane between the multifidus (thoracic and lumborum) and longissimus (thoracis and lomborum) muscles revealing the articular process that are easily palpable. Dissection extends ventrally as described above to the level of the rib head or the base of the transverse process, retracting the longissimus muscle ventrolaterally.

Procedure/Variations

With experience, the surgeon can "tunnel" down [53] or create a keyhole access [54] to each disc space by palpating the transverse process or rib head to avoid excessive tissue dissection and trauma.

Fenestration Procedure (Video 22.1)

The lateral annulus is covered by a loose fascia that contains the spinal nerve and associated vessels. A #11 blade is used to transect the soft tissue attachments along the cranial border of the rib head or transverse process and a periosteal elevator is then used to elevate these soft tissue structures in a cranial direction. Care must be taken not to injure the spinal nerve; this is especially important in the caudal lumbar region. The ventral branches of the spinal nerves run along the ventrolateral aspect of the disc and can be damaged by dissecting too low along the lateral annulus [53]. If hemorrhage is encountered during dissection, pressure or bipolar cautery is typically effective for control. The lateral annulus is visualized as a white, glistening, fibrous sheath. Puncture with a straight hypodermic needle (22G) can confirm the exact location of the disc space and of the vertebral endplates on either side [55] (Figure 22.5). Ensure that the needle is inserted as perpendicular as possible to the annulus (the required angle varies depending on patient position and surgical approach) and that it does not inadvertently penetrate the intervertebral foramen and spinal canal. Fenestration can be performed using a blade or a drill.

Blade fenestration. Once the surgeon has identified the annulus, a #11 scalpel blade is used to create a rectangular window within it (Figure 22.6). The blade is oriented such that its cutting edge is directed away from the spinal cord (located dorsally) and away from the neurovascular structures (located cranially). Cranial retraction of the nerve and vessel is maintained using a periosteal elevator or suction tip during fenestration. Four adjoining cuts are made within the annulus and the rectangular piece of annulus (approximately 2 × 4–5 mm in a small dog) [2,8] is removed using a small curved hemostatic forceps or a rongeur to expose the NP for curettage (Figure 22.7). In the thoracolumbar spine, as large a window as possible (slightly larger than the instrument used to retrieve disc material) is created to facilitate removal of NP.

Power fenestration. This is performed through the same approach as described above but the window is created using a high-speed pneumatic drill (Hall's drill) and a 4-mm burr [2].

After creating the fenestration or opening into the annulus, instruments such as a curved spatula, small curettes, or dental curettes are used to remove as much of the abnormal nucleus as possible from the disc space (Figure 22.8). The curettage is never directed dorsally towards the spinal cord but rather uses a circular pattern that begins with entering the fenestration at the top of the window and moving in a downward and "in and out" motion. Surgeons should avoid rotating curettes along their long axis within the disc space as this may result in fracture at the neck of the curette. The largest curette possible should also be used to allow effective removal of the disc material (Figure 22.9). Smaller curettes are ineffective and are more likely to fracture within the disc space, making it difficult to retrieve the metal foreign body. Once fenestrated, the disc space should look and feel empty and might appear to collapse (Figure 22.10).

Post-fenestration chiropractic maneuvers aiming to loosen up disc material for more complete fenestration have been described [1] but are not performed or recommended.

Prior to closing and after fenestrating the site of decompression, the surgeon should verify that disc material has not been pushed through the damaged annulus and within the spinal canal during fenestration.

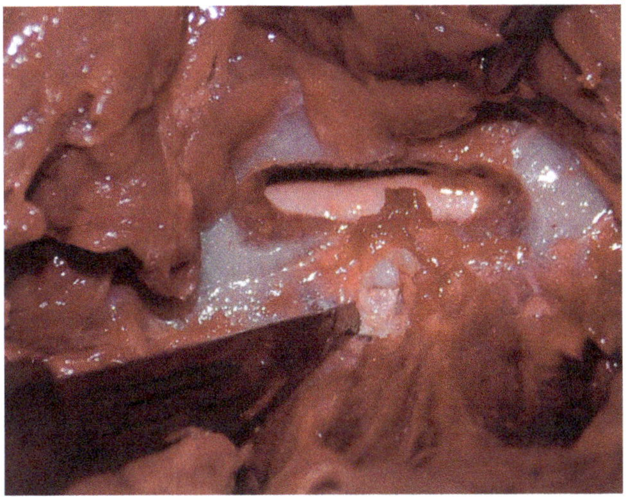

Figure 22.6 A #11 scalpel blade is used to remove a rectangular section of the lateral annulus. Alternatively, a drill and 4-mm burr could be used to create the fenestration.

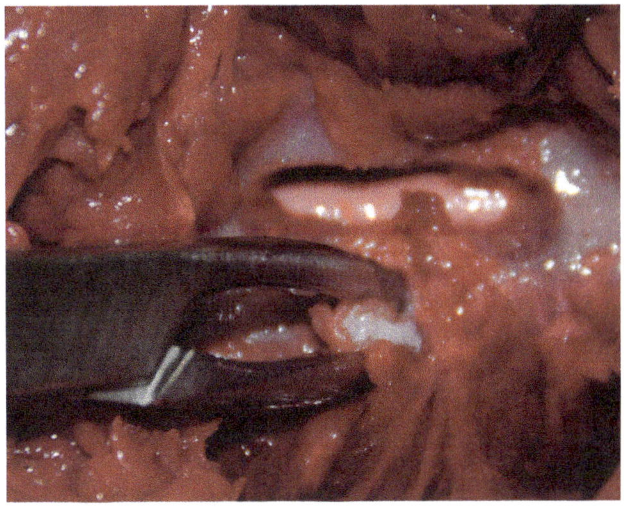

Figure 22.7 A rongeur is used to remove the fenestrated section of lateral annulus.

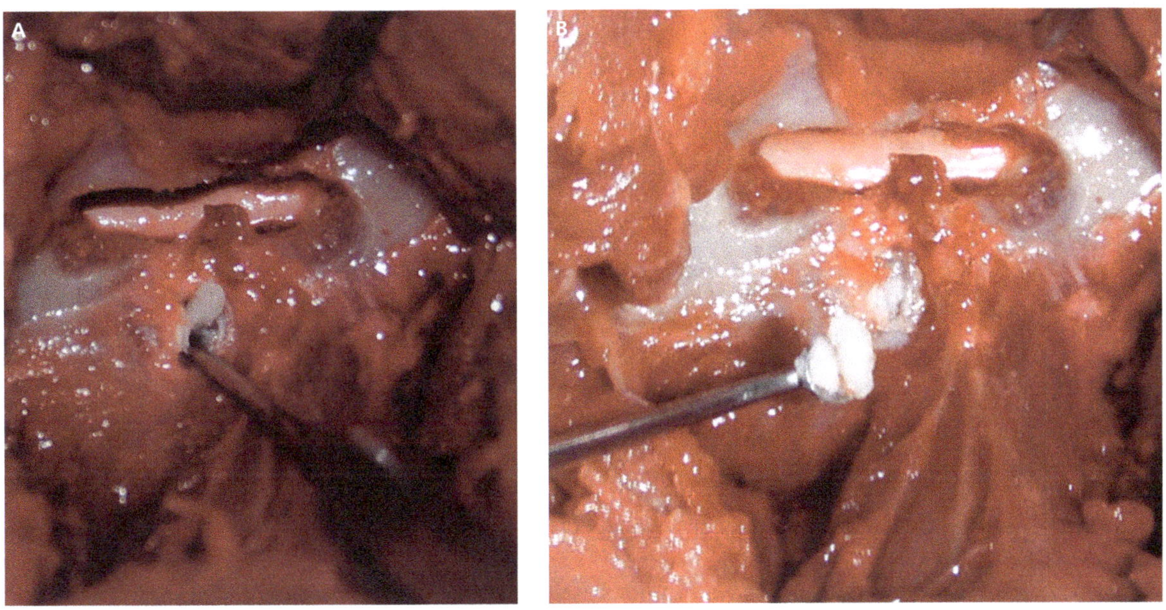

Figure 22.8 (A, B) A curette is used to retrieve the nucleus pulposus from the disc. The curette with the largest diameter that will fit the disc space should be used. The curette is inserted and moved in a dorsoventral and in-and-out motion without turning within the disc space. Alternatively, a curved spatula or dental scraper can be used to retrieve the nucleus pulposus.

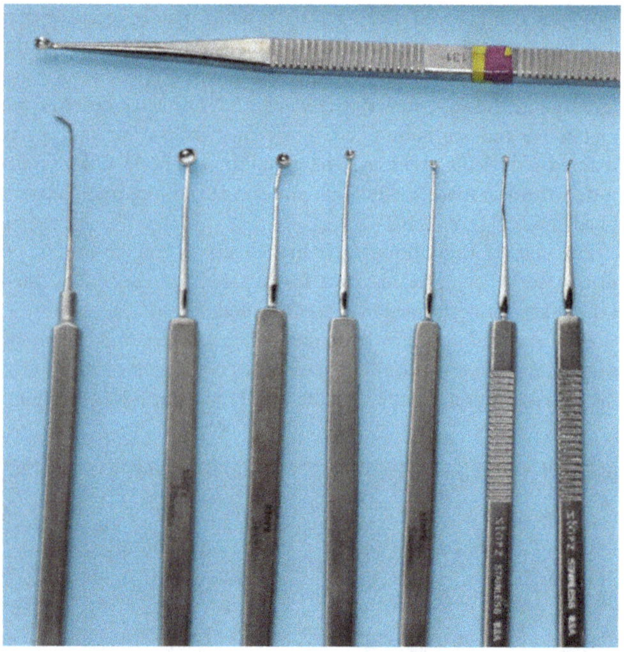

Figure 22.9 A variety of neurological currettes. The largest curette possible should be used to allow effective removal of the disc material during fenestration. Smaller curettes are ineffective and are more likely to fracture within the disc space, making it difficult to retrieve the metal foreign body.

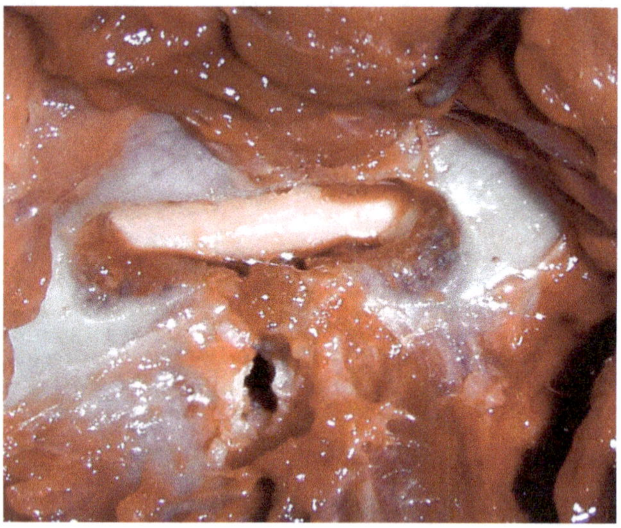

Figure 22.10 The disc space of a cadaver appears empty after fenestration has been completed. Fenestration in a live patient typically results in collapse of the disc space.

Procedure/Variations

A ventrolateral approach to T13–L1 through L6–L7 discs has been described [44] but is not commonly used because it is a more complicated and invasive approach that requires the severing of several muscle attachments and lumbar nerves. A ventral approach for fenestration of T9–T10 to L5–L6 has also been described [45–47] but has the disadvantage of requiring a thoracotomy and/or laparotomy and not allowing decompression to be performed through the same approach.

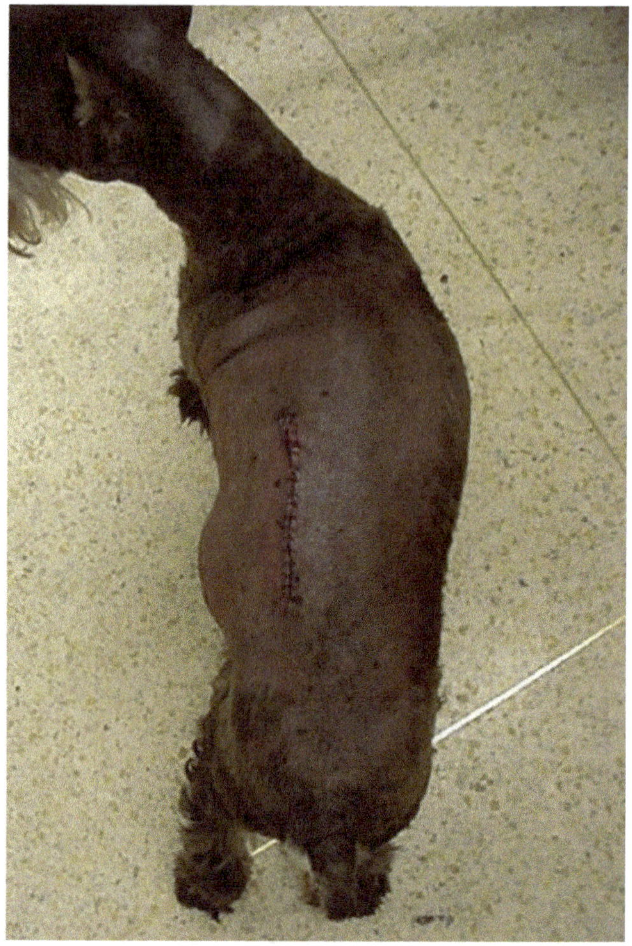

Figure 22.11 Postoperative view of a Miniature Schnauzer with abdominal wall weakness following decompression for IVD herniation and fenestration of all discs between T11–T12 and L3–L4.

Other Requirements

Positive-pressure ventilation is ideal during fenestration in the thoracic region to prevent pneumothorax should the parietal pleura be punctured during fenestration. If puncture of the pleura is suspected, one can confirm it by filling the surgical site with sterile saline and observing for air bubbles during ventilation (hand bagging or mechanical ventilation).

Closure

The muscle separation planes do not require closure. Closure is standard for a laminectomy and consists of apposing the lumbar fascia, subcutaneous tissues, and skin in separate layers using simple continuous patterns for the fascia and subcutaneous fat followed by routine skin closure.

Complications

Reported complications associated with fenestration include increased anesthetic and surgical times [18], displacement of disc material into the vertebral canal and/or spinal cord trauma causing worsening of neurological grade [10,25,37,41,54,56], hemorrhage [21,23], pleural puncture or pneumothorax when fenestrating thoracic discs [21,41,54], soft-tissue and nerve-root trauma leading to postoperative pain, scoliosis and abdominal wall weakness [6,23,54] (Figure 22.11), bone damage (Figure 22.12), lysis and discospondylitis,

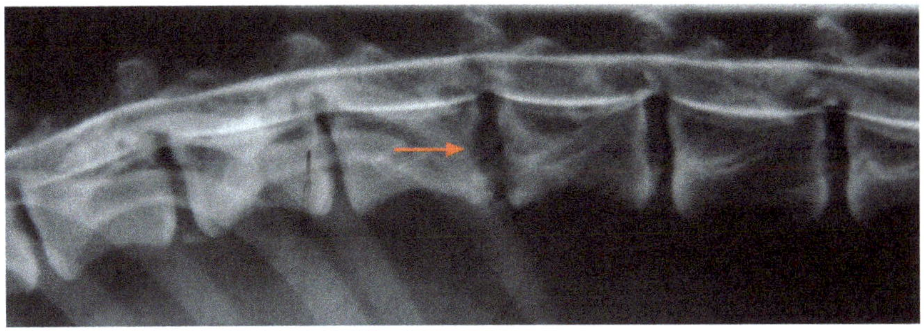

Figure 22.12 Lateral radiograph showing burr damage (arrow) along the vertebral endplates of T13–L1 caused by power fenestration.

especially related to power fenestration [41,57], difficulty identifying one or more disc spaces for fenestration [21,23,25], and most recently vertebral subluxation and instability which developed weeks to months after hemilaminectomy and prophylactic fenestration [25]. Most reported complications are minor and have no long-term negative effects [6,21,23,25,54]. However, increased cost associated with longer surgical and anesthetic times, increased surgical incision length, and possibly postoperative morbidity related to additional tissue dissection and trauma should be considered. Recurrent disc herniation at a previously fenestrated disc space is possible and has been reported but is rare [4,21,23].

Postoperative Care

There are no additional postoperative considerations following fenestration than those required for other surgeries of the spine. Dogs that undergo fenestration of all discs between T11–T12 and L3–L4 (or more) are subjectively more painful in the initial postoperative period and require more analgesics than those undergoing decompression with single-site fenestration. Application of a soft padded bandage and cold compresses for the initial 24–36 hours can reduce swelling and appears to increase patient comfort.

Video clips to accompany this book can be found on the companion website at:
www.wiley.com/go/shores/neurosurgery

References

1 Flo GL, Brinker WO. Lateral fenestration of thoracolumbar discs. *J Am Anim Hosp Assoc* 1975;11:619–626.
2 Holmberg DL, Palmer NC, VanPelt D, Willan AR. A comparison of manual and power assisted thoracolumbar disc fenestration in dogs. *Vet Surg* 1990;19:323–327.
3 Shores A, Cechner PE, Cantwell HD, Wheaton LG, Carlton WW. Structural changes in thoracolumbar disks following lateral fenestration. A study of radiographic, histologic and histochemical changes in the chondrodystrophic dog. *Vet Surg* 1985;14:117–123.
4 Stigen O, Ottesen N, Jaderlund KH. Early recurrence of thoracolumbar intervertebral disc extrusion after surgical decompression: a report of three cases. *Acta Vet Scand* 2010;52:10.
5 Wagner SD, Ferguson HR, Leipold H, Guffy MM, Butler HC. Radiographic and histologic changes after thoracolumbar disc curettage. *Vet Surg* 1987;16:65–69.
6 Black AP. Lateral spinal decompression in the dog: a review of 39 cases. *J Small Anim Pract* 1988;29:581–588.
7 Forterre F, Konar M, Spreng D, Jaggy A, Lang J. Influence of intervertebral disc fenestration at the herniation site in association with hemilaminectomy on recurrence in chondrodystrophic dogs with thoracolumbar disc disease: a prospective MRI study. *Vet Surg* 2008;37:399–405.
8 Morelius M, Bergadano A, Spreng D, Schawalder P, Doherr M, Forterre F. Influence of surgical approach on the efficacy of the intervertebral disk fenestration: a cadaveric study. *J Small Anim Pract* 2007;48:87–92.
9 Forterre F, Dickomeit M, Senn D, Gorgas D, Spreng D. Microfenestration using the CUSA Excel ultrasonic aspiration system in chondrodystrophic dogs with thoracolumbar disk extrusion: a descriptive cadaveric and clinical study. *Vet Surg* 2011;40:34–39.
10 Dickey DT, Bartels KE, Henry GA et al. Use of the holmium yttrium aluminum garnet laser for percutaneous thoracolumbar intervertebral disc ablation in dogs. *J Am Vet Med Assoc* 1996;208:1263–1267.
11 Nerubay J, Caspi I, Levinkopf M, Tadmor A, Bubis JJ. Percutaneous laser nucleolysis of the intervertebral lumbar disc. An experimental study. *Clin Orthop Relat Res* 1997;337:42–44.
12 Bartels KE, Higbee RG, Bahr RJ, Galloway DS, Healey TS, Arnold C. Outcome of and complications associated with prophylactic percutaneous laser disk ablation in dogs with thoracolumbar disk disease: 277 cases (1992–2001). *J Am Vet Med Assoc* 2003;222:1733–1739.
13 Dugat DR, Bartels KE, Payton ME. Recurrence of disk herniation following percutaneous laser disk ablation in dogs with a history of thoracolumbar intervertebral disk herniation: 303 cases (1994–2011). *J Am Vet Med Assoc* 2016;249:1393–1400.
14 Thomovsky SA, Packer RA, Lambrechts NE, Moore GE. Canine intervertebral disc fenestration using a vacuum-assisted tissue resection device. *Vet Surg* 2012;41:1011–1017.
15 Miyabayashi T, Lord PF, Dubielzig RR, Biller DS, Manley PA. Chemonucleolysis with collagenase. A radiographic and pathologic study in dogs. *Vet Surg* 1992;21:189–194.
16 Bradford DS, Cooper KM, Oegema TR Jr. Chymopapain, chemonucleolysis and nucleus pulposus regeneration. *J Bone Join Surg Am* 1983;65:1220–1231.
17 MacKenzie SD, Brisson BA, Gaitero L et al. Distribution and short- and long-term effects of injected gelified ethanol into the lumbosacral intervertebral disc in healthy dogs. *Vet Radiol Ultrasound* 2016;57:180–190.
18 Scott HW. Hemilaminectomy for the treatment of thoracolumbar disc disease in the dog: a follow-up study of 40 cases. *J Small Anim Pract* 1997;38:488–494.
19 Funkquist B. Decompressive laminectomy in thoraco-lumbar disc protrusion with paraplegia in the dog. *J Small Anim Pract* 1970;11:445–451.
20 Colter SB. Fenestration, decompression, or both? Symposium on Controversial Problems in Clinical Practice. *Vet Clin North Am* 1978;8:379–383.
21 Brisson BA, Moffatt SL, Swayne SL, Parent JM. Recurrence of thoracolumbar intervertebral disk extrusion in chondrodystrophic dogs after surgical decompression with or without prophylactic fenestration: 265 cases (1995–1999). *J Am Vet Med Assoc* 2004;224:1808–1814.
22 Fingeroth JM. Fenestration. Pros and cons. *Probl Vet Med* 1989;1:445–466.
23 Brisson BA, Holmberg DL, Parent J, Sears WC, Wick SE. Comparison of the effect of single-site and multiple-site disk fenestration on the rate of recurrence of thoracolumbar intervertebral disk herniation in dogs. *J Am Vet Med Assoc* 2011;238:1593–1600.
24 Hettlich BF, Kerwin SC, Levine JM. Early reherniation of disk material in eleven dogs with surgically treated thoracolumbar intervertebral disk extrusion. *Vet Surg* 2012;41:215–219.
25 Aikawa T, Fujita H, Shibata M, Takahashi T. Recurrent thoracolumbar intervertebral disc extrusion after hemilaminectomy and concomitant prophylactic fenestration in 662 chondrodystrophic dogs. *Vet Surg* 2012;41:381–390.
26 Russel SW, Griffiths RC. Recurrence of cervical disc syndrome in surgically and conservatively treated dogs. *J Am Vet Med Assoc* 1968;153:1412–1417.
27 Cherrone KL, Dewey CW, Coates JR, Bergman RL. A retrospective comparison of cervical intervertebral disk disease in nonchondrodystrophic large dogs vs small dogs. *J Am Anim Hosp Assoc* 2004;40:316–320.
28 Seim HB III, Prata RG. Ventral decompression for the treatment of cervical disk disease in the dog: a review of 54 cases. *J Am Anim Hosp Assoc* 1982;18:233–240.
29 Hillman RB, Kengeri SS, Waters DJ. Reevaluation of predictive factors for complete recovery in dogs with nonambulatory tetraparesis secondary to cervical disk herniation. *J Am Anim Hosp Assoc* 2009;45:155–163.
30 Fauber AE, Wade JA, Lipka AE, McCabe GE, Aper RL. Effect of width of disk fenestration and ventral slot on biomechanics of the canine C5–6 vertebral motion unit. *Am J Vet Res* 2006;67:1844–1848.
31 Macy NB, Les CM, Stover SM, Kass PH. Effect of disk fenestration on sagittal kinematics of the canine C5–6 intervertebral space. *Vet Surg* 1999;28:171–179.

32 Morgan PW, Parent J, Holmberg DL. Cervical pain secondary to intervertebral disc disease in dogs: radiographic findings and surgical implications. *Prog Vet Neurol* 1993;4:76–80.
33 Bojrab MJ, Constantinescu GM. Cervical spine: cervical disc fenestration. In: Bojrab MJ, Ellison GW, Slocum B (eds) *Current Techniques in Small Animal Surgery*, 4th edn. Baltimore, MD: Williams & Wilkins, 1998: 822–823.
34 Gage ED. Incidence of clinical disc disease in the dog. *J Am Anim Hosp Assoc* 1975;11:135–138.
35 Tartarelli CL, Baroni M, Borghi M. Thoracolumbar disc extrusion associated with extensive epidural haemorrhage: a retrospective study of 23 dogs. *J Small Anim Pract* 2005;46:485–490.
36 Ryan TM. Detection of spinal cord compression in dogs with cervical intervertebral disc disease by magnetic resonance imaging. *Vet Rec* 2008;163:11–15.
37 Tomlinson J. Tetraparesis following cervical disc fenestration in two dogs. *J Am Vet Med Assoc* 1985;14:240–246.
38 Olsson SE. Observations concerning disc fenestration in dogs. *Acta Orthop Scand* 1951;20:349–356.
39 Olsson SE. Surgical treatment with special reference to the value of disc fenestration. *Acta Orthop Scand Suppl* 1951;8:51–70.
40 Yturraspe DJ. A dorsolateral muscle-separating approach for thoracolumbar intervertebral disc fenestration in the dog. *J Am Vet Med Assoc* 1973;162:1037–1040.
41 Funkquist B. Investigations of the therapeutic and prophylactic effects of disc evacuation in cases of thoraco-lumbar herniated discs in dogs. *Acta Vet Scand* 1978;19:441–457.
42 Seeman CW. A lateral approach for thoracolumbar disc fenestration. *Mod Vet Pract* 1968;49:73–74.
43 Leonard EP. Intervertebral disc disease (enchondrosis intervertebralis). In: *Orthopedic Surgery of the Dog and Cat*. Philadelphia, PA: WB Saunders, 1960: 251–271.
44 Northway RB. A ventrolateral approach to lumbar intervertebral disc fenestration. *Vet Med Small Anim Clin* 1965;60:884–893.
45 Bojrab MJ, Constantinescu GM. Thoracolumbar spine: prophylactic thoracolumbar disc fenestration. In: Bojrab MJ, Ellison GW, Slocum B (eds) *Current Techniques in Small Animal Surgery*, 4th edn. Baltimore, MD: Williams & Wilkins, 1998: 839–842.
46 Leonard EP. Intervertebral disc disease. In: *Orthopedic Surgery of the Dog and Cat*, 2nd edn. Philadelphia, PA: WB Saunders, 1971: 288–312.
47 Shores A. Intervertebral disk syndrome in the dog. Part III. Thoracolumbar disk surgery. *Compend Contin Educ Pract Vet* 1982;4:24–31.
48 Knapp DW. A retrospective study of thoracolumbar disk fenestration in dogs using a ventral approach: 160 cases (1976 to 1986). *J Am An Hosp Assoc* 1990;26:543–549.
49 Bruecker KA. Cervical spine: ventral slot decompression of the herniated cervical disc. In: Bojrab MJ, Ellison GW, Slocum B (eds) *Current Techniques in Small Animal Surgery*, 4th edn. Baltimore, MD: Williams & Wilkins, 1998: 823–826.
50 Simpson ST. Thoracolumbar spine: hemilaminectomy of the caudal thoracic and lumbar spine. In: Bojrab MJ, Ellison GW, Slocum B (eds) *Current Techniques in Small Animal Surgery*, 4th edn. Baltimore, MD: Williams & Wilkins, 1998: 844–849.
51 Denny HR. The surgical management of cervical disc protrusions in the dog: a review of 40 cases. *J Small Anim Pract* 1978;19:251–257.
52 Piermattei DL, Johnson KA. The vertebral column. In: *An Atlas of Surgical Approaches to the Bones and Joints of the Dog and Cat*, 4th edn. Philadelphia, PA: WB Saunders, 2004: 47–105.
53 Creed JE, Yturraspe. Thoracolumbar spine: intervertebral disc fenestration. In: Bojrab MJ, Ellison GW, Slocum B (eds) *Current Techniques in Small Animal Surgery*, 4th edn. Baltimore, MD: Williams & Wilkins, 1998: 835–839.
54 Bartels KE, Creed JE, Yturraspe DJ. Complications associated with the dorsolateral muscle-separating approach for thoracolumbar disk fenestration in the dog. *J Am Vet Med Assoc* 1983;183:1081–1083.
55 Hoerlein BF. Further evaluation of the treatment of disk protrusion paraplegia in the dog. *J Am Vet Med Assoc* 1956;129;495–502.
56 Sterna J, Burzykowski T. Assessment of the usefulness of the fenestration method in cases of disc extrusion in the cervical and thoraco-lumbar spine in chondrodystrophic dogs. *Pol J Vet Sci* 2008;11:55–62.
57 Hoerlein BF. The treatment of intervertebral disc protrusion in the dog. *Proc Am Vet Med Assoc* 1952;89:206–212.

23 Thoracolumbar Lateral Corpectomy

Pierre Moissonnier

Definition and Initial Description

The goal of surgical management of disc herniation is to decompress the spinal cord by complete removal of herniated disc material [1,2]. The ideal surgical technique should provide adequate exposure to allow removal of the disc material without trauma to the spinal cord and without significant postoperative intervertebral instability [3]. In the thoracolumbar region, laminectomy [4–6], hemilaminectomy [7,8], mini-hemilaminectomy/pediculectomy [9,10], and partial pediculectomy [11] allow exposure of the dorsolateral to lateroventral aspects of the vertebral canal, which correspond to the usual location of acute extruded disc material. In patients with a chronic history and patients with disc protrusion, disc removal is technically demanding because of its hard encapsulated nature, ventral (or ventrolateral) location, and adhesion to the dura mater or to the venous sinus. In these instances, the disc is often wrapped laterally around the spinal cord, precluding direct visualization or access to the disc material via standard hemilaminectomy. Inadequate exposure can lead to incomplete removal of extruded material or protruding annulus and carries a high risk of iatrogenic spinal cord trauma while attempting to remove the herniated disc, possibly worsening the patient's neurological status. Hemilaminectomy did not initially result in a better outcome compared with conservative treatment in 36 large-breed dogs with type II (annular) disc protrusion; however, nearly half of the dogs treated conservatively deteriorated within a year [12]. In fact, 9 of 36 dogs treated conservatively were euthanized due to progressive hindlimb paresis, while long-term deterioration of the neurological grade was not observed in dogs treated surgically [12]. This suggests that although neurological deficits may remain, surgical decompression is useful in the management of degenerative annular protrusion [12].

In order to limit the surgical approach to disc material and to limit the iatrogenic trauma associated with its removal, the thoracolumbar lateral corpectomy (TLLC) technique was developed [13]. TLLC involves the partial removal of adjacent thoracic and/or lumbar vertebral bodies that support the extruded/protruded disc material inside the vertebral canal. As such, some authors refer to it as a partial lateral corpectomy [14]. TLLC provides access to most of the floor of the vertebral canal at the approached site, enabling the removal of extruded/protruded disc material with minimal manipulation of the spinal cord [13,14]. During the procedure, a power-assisted disc fenestration [15] is also performed to prevent further postoperative disc extrusion [16–19] (see Chapter 22).

Lateral corpectomy was initially described in 15 dogs [13]. Since then, studies assessing neurological outcome [16,17] as well as the degree of decompression and the biomechanical effects of TLLC on vertebral column motion [20,21] have provided a better understanding of the technique and its indications. TLLC can also be performed in cats to treat chronic (or subacute), ventrally located disc herniations or when adhesions are present between the disc material and the dura mater [22,23].

Technical Aspects

Surgical Approaches for Lateral Corpectomy

In the thoracolumbar area, both dorsolateral [24] and ventrolateral [25] approaches for TLLC have been described. Since the objective of TLLC is to remove the floor of the vertebral canal via the vertebral body, a ventrolateral approach seems most appropriate. This conclusion was reached in a 2007 study [26] that evaluated the completeness of thoracolumbar disc fenestration. Through a dorsal approach, the paraspinal musculature limits access to the vertebral bodies and limits the dorsomedial angle needed by the instrumentation to complete the corpectomy. In contrast, the ventrolateral approach is made ventral to the paraspinal muscles and dorsal to the ribs and/or transverse process, establishing direct access to the lateral annulus and adjacent vertebral bodies. The transverse processes and/or the rib heads may be partially removed to improve access to the vertebral body if desired.

In the thoracic region, TLLC can be used as part of the surgical treatment for spinal deformities to obtain ventral decompression before realignment of the vertebra [27]. An intercostal thoracotomy provides access to the thoracic vertebral bodies but requires the transection of the vertebral segmental arteries. Although it is an infrequent site for disc herniation, this approach has been used by

Current Techniques in Canine and Feline Neurosurgery, First Edition. Edited by Andy Shores and Brigitte A. Brisson.
© 2017 John Wiley & Sons, Inc. Published 2017 by John Wiley & Sons, Inc.
Companion website: www.wiley.com/go/shores/neurosurgery

the author as cranial as the T2–T3 disc space (after release of the scapulum and with internal rotation of the limb), and this compared favorably to the dorsal approach that is very deep at this level (Pierre Moissonnier, personal observation).

At the level of the lumbar intumescence (L4–S1), particular care must be taken to identify the ventral branches of the spinal nerves and protect them with a nerve retractor to avoid lower motor neuron deficits. A transiliac approach to the L7–S1 intervertebral disc space was described to allow lateral corpectomy in this particular location [28].

Lateralization of the disc material within the canal on preoperative imaging determines the side of the approach; when purely ventral compression exists, a right-handed surgeon is typically more comfortable with a left-sided approach.

Instrumentation

A general instrumentation pack, standard neurosurgical instruments (e.g., Freer dissector-elevator, Lempert rongeurs, Kerrison rongeurs), and a high-speed drill are necessary. Appropriate self-retaining retractors are essential to allow adequate exposure of the surgical site.

Surgical Technique

In the preliminary description of the technique, the following theoretical landmarks were described. The slot should extend (Figure 23.1):

- one-quarter of the length of each vertebral body (craniocaudally);
- half the height of the vertebral body;
- half (50%) to two-thirds (66%) of the vertebral canal diameter width.

From a more practical point of view, and since extruded disc material can migrate cranial and/or caudal within the vertebral canal, these limits are defined in each individual case based on the location of the extruded/protruded disc material on advanced imaging. The surgeon must also keep in mind that the cranial and caudal attachments of the annulus fibrosus are located cranial and caudal to the vertebral endplates. Caudal to T10, the dorsal limit of the intervertebral foramina is approximately at the level of the accessory process (Figures 23.2 and 23.3). The spinal nerve is identified and a nerve retractor is positioned over the ventral branch during lateral corpectomy (Figure 23.4). In some instances, this nerve can be transected (rhizotomy) to facilitate the surgical approach; this is not recommended caudal to L3.

The slot is created perpendicular to the long axis of the spine. Patient positioning is particularly important in order to limit the risk of inadvertently entering the vertebral canal. The surgical burr initially penetrates the cortical bone of the lateral aspect of the vertebral body followed by cancellous bone (Figures 23.1 and 23.5). Hemorrhage from the cancellous bone is controlled with bone wax

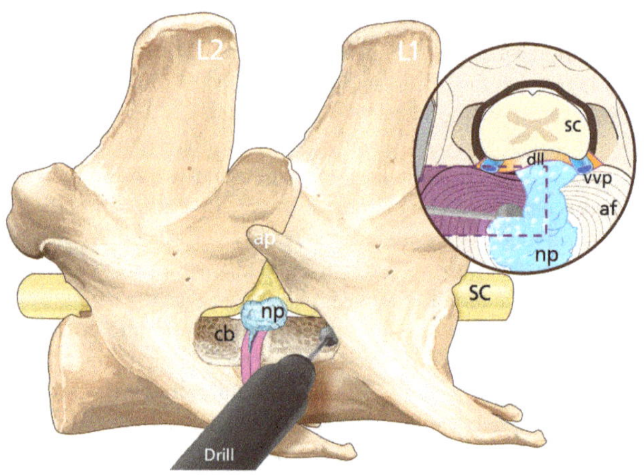

Figure 23.1 Schematic representation of lateral corpectomy at L1–L2 in a dog with chronic disc protrusion (left lateral view and cross-section [*inset*]). L1, first lumbar vertebra; L2, second lumbar vertebra; ap, accessory process of L1; cb, cancellous bone; sc, spinal cord (yellow); np, nucleus pulposus (blue); af, annulus fibrosus (white) and its removal (purple); drill, high-speed air drill; dll, dorsal longitudinal ligament (orange); vvp, ventral venous plexus (vein in blue). Dashed line indicates limits of corpectomy in the frontal plane; standard limits are half of vertebral body height, two-thirds of vertebral body width, one-quarter of each vertebral body length.

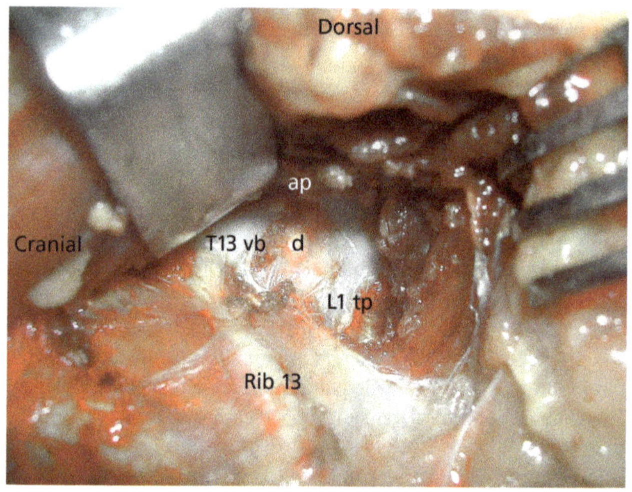

Figure 23.2 Ventrolateral surgical approach of T13–L1 (left side) for corpectomy. Rib 13, 13th rib; T13 vb, vertebral body of T13; L1 tp, transverse process of L1; d, lateral aspect of intervertebral annulus fibrosus (disc); ap, accessory process.

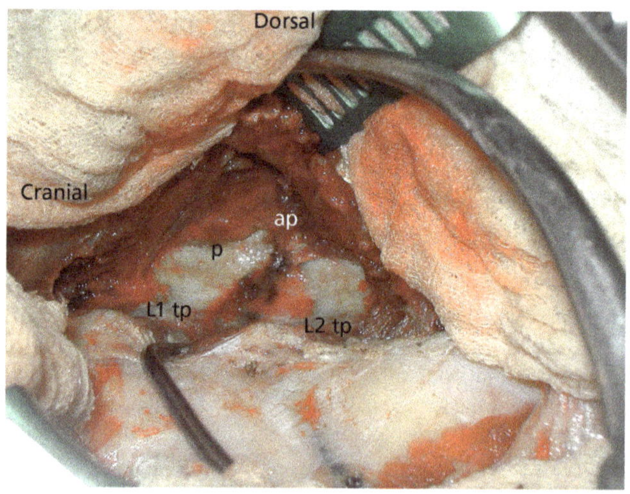

Figure 23.3 Ventrolateral surgical approach of L1–L2 (left side) for corpectomy. L1 tp, transverse process of L1; L2 tp, transverse process of L2; p, pedicle of the vertebral arch of L1; ap, accessory process.

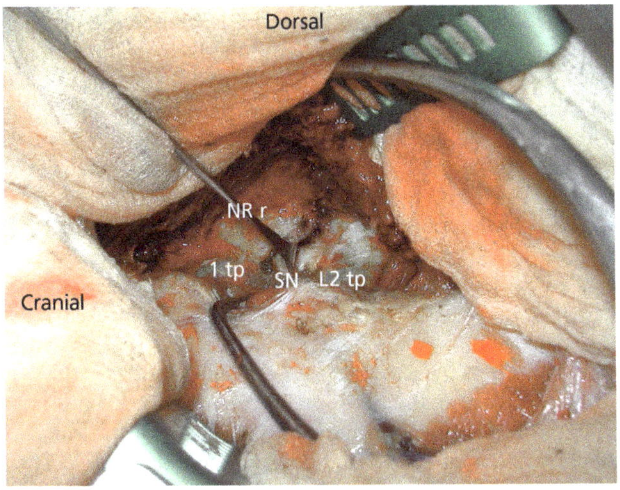

Figure 23.4 Ventrolateral surgical approach of L1–L2 (left side) for corpectomy. Spinal nerve L1 is retracted cranially to provide access to the lateral aspect of the annulus fibrosus. 1 tp, transverse process of L1; L2 tp, transverse process of L2; NR r, nerve root retractor; SN, spinal nerve L1.

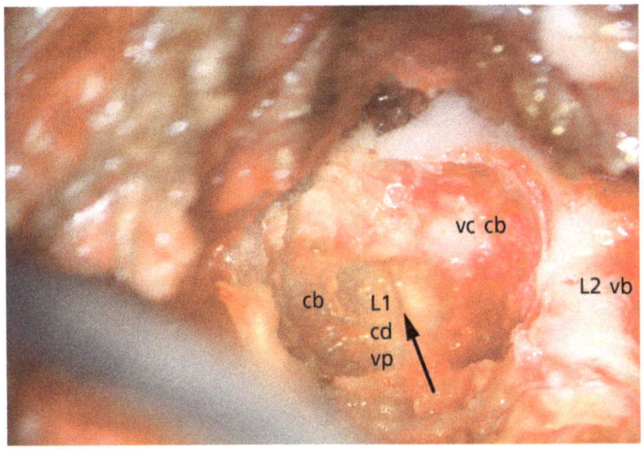

Figure 23.6 Ventrolateral surgical approach of L1–L2 (left side) for corpectomy: close-up view of the corpectomy. The slot provides access to the inner cortex along the ventrolateral aspect of the vertebral canal. L2 vb, L2 vertebral body; cb, cancellous bone of L1; L1 cd vp, caudal vertebral plateau of L1 (arrow; note the collapse between L1 and L2 vertebral plateau); vc cb, cortical bone of the vertebral canal.

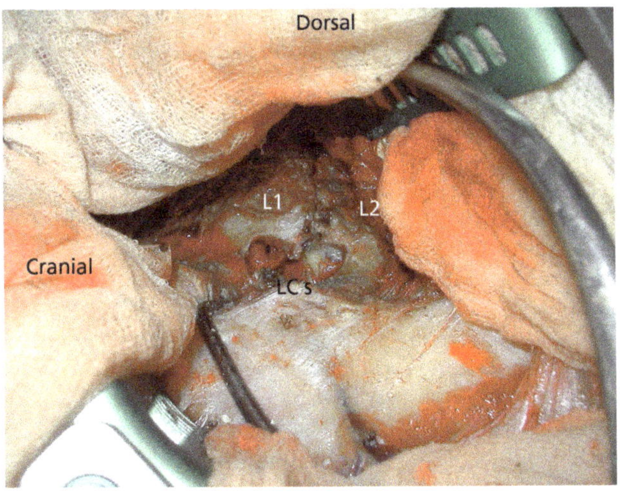

Figure 23.5 Ventrolateral surgical approach of L1–L2 (left side) for corpectomy. L1, lumbar vertebra 1; L2, lumbar vertebra 2; LC s, lateral corpectomy slot.

as necessary. In the frontal plane, the slot can extend about two-thirds of the vertebral canal diameter. The burr is continuously irrigated with a saline solution and the site kept free of debris by suction. The surgeon should frequently assess the thickness/resistance of the remaining cortical bone along the ventral aspect of the vertebral canal (Figure 23.6). Once the cortical bone of the floor of the vertebral canal is sufficiently thin, the vertebral canal is entered.

When treating disc protrusion, dorsal drilling stops when the dorsal longitudinal ligament is exposed in order to avoid contact of the burr with the vertebral sinus and/or spinal cord (Figure 21.1). If encountered, hemorrhage from the venous sinus is controlled using hemostatic sponge, bipolar coagulation, or direct compression of the sinus along the vertebral canal floor. When treating disc extrusion, the dorsal longitudinal ligament is excised to retrieve the extruded disc material from the spinal canal.

The protruding annulus is progressively resected with the burr, and when thin enough is gently retracted ventrally into the slot in a dorsoventral direction using rongeurs or other grasping instruments (Figure 23.7). Excision of the protrusion is considered complete when annulus and/or disc material is no longer retrieved from the vertebral canal and when exploration of the vertebral canal floor is flat.

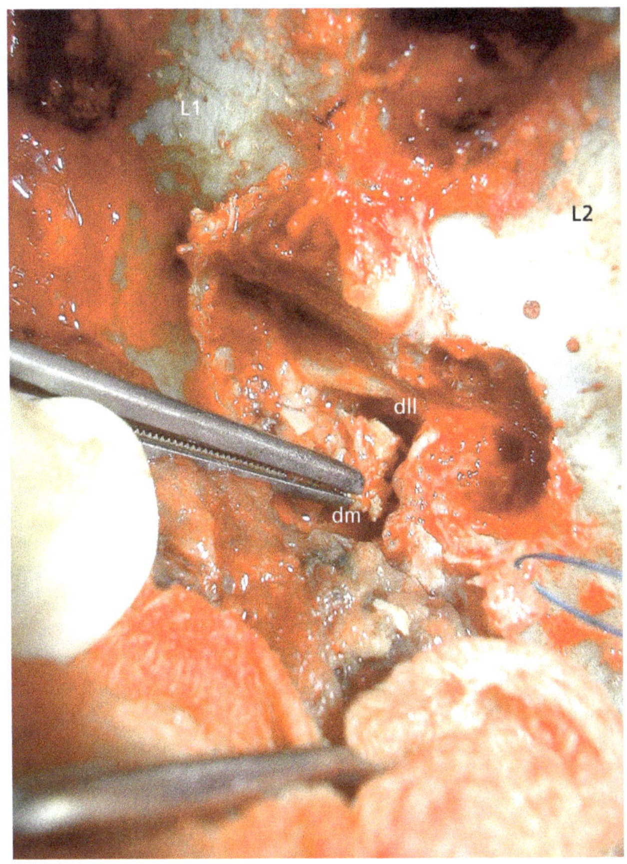

Figure 23.7 Ventrolateral surgical approach of L1–L2 (left side): magnified view of the corpectomy site. The slot provides access for removal of degenerative disc material (in the forceps). L1, lumbar vertebra 1; L2, lumbar vertebra 2; dm, disc material; dll, dorsal longitudinal ligament.

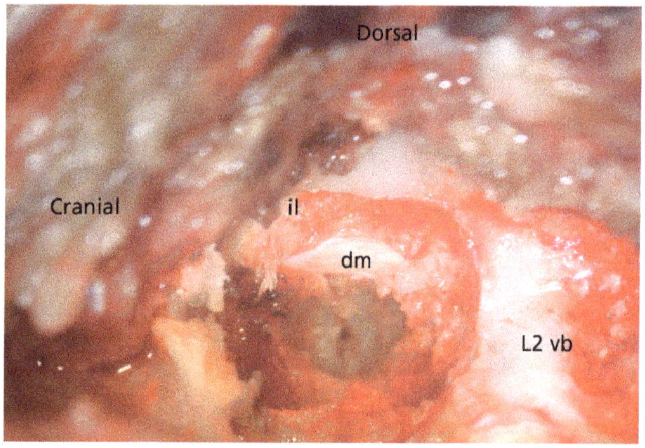

Figure 23.8 Ventrolateral surgical approach of L1–L2 (left side) for corpectomy. Magnified view of the corpectomy site after removal of the remaining inner cortical bone which provides access to the protruded or extruded disc material as well as direct visualization of the dura mater and ventral portion of the interarcuate ligament. L2 vb, L2 vertebral body; dm, dura mater; il, interarcuate ligament (ventral portion).

Once completed, the dura mater should be visible at the top of the slot (Figure 23.8). Magnification using an operating microscope improves visualization of the spinal cord and the venous sinus, limiting the risk of iatrogenic injury.

There is no specific reconstruction to be performed after TLLC, except in extremely rare cases of suspected postoperative intervertebral instability.

Combining TLLC with Other Techniques

Using the same surgical approach (especially with the lateral approach), it is technically possible to combine the TLLC procedure with a pediculectomy, foraminotomy, mini-hemilaminectomy, or hemilaminectomy. Combined procedures offer improved visualization of the spinal cord and degree of spinal cord decompression achieved but could, in some cases, lead to vertebral column instability [20,21].

Minimally Invasive TLLC

In order to limit the surgical trauma associated with TLLC, an endoscope-assisted minimally invasive approach was developed [27]. Based on the results obtained in six fresh cadavers [29] and 23 client-owned dogs [30], the authors concluded that adequate spinal cord decompression was possible using a minimally invasive, 2-cm long skin incision with blunt dissection of the underlying muscle planes. An additional advantage to using an endoscope for spinal surgery is the magnification it provides, which may reduce the risk of iatrogenic trauma to the spinal cord and hemorrhage of the venous sinus [29,30]. Clinical results obtained by this approach were similar to those obtained with a conventional approach [30].

Experimental and Clinical Results

Stability of the Vertebral Column after Lateral Corpectomy Alone and in Association with Other Techniques

Postoperative instability has been documented 1 year after TLLC in a dog that presented with reluctance to walk because of pain (Pierre Moissonnier, personal observation). In this patient, spinal radiographs revealed a collapse of the intervertebral space with a step between the adjacent vertebrae along the floor of the vertebral canal. Using the three-compartment theory [31–33], TLLC could theoretically affect two of three vertebral compartments unilaterally and, as such, it is possible that transient, lateralized, postoperative instability might exist similar to that demonstrated after dorsal decompression techniques [34,35].

In vitro biomechanical studies assessing the stability of L1–L2 [20] and T13–L1 [21] canine vertebral segments after TLLC alone revealed a 30% increase in range of motion during lateral bending on the corpectomy side. Spinal instability worsened significantly when TLLC was combined with hemilaminectomy, with a 57% increase in range of motion in a ventral direction [20], but this increased instability was not observed when mini-hemilaminectomy was combined with TLLC [20]. Accordingly, a recommendation is made to combine TLLC with a mini-hemilaminectomy when required but to avoid hemilaminectomy without spinal stabilization.

Adjacent Lateral Corpectomies

Multiple consecutive lateral corpectomies can be performed in the same patient. Flegel et al. [17] reported that 12 dogs had two adjacent TLLC and one had three adjacent TLLC procedures performed. We have performed TLLC along as many as five adjacent sites unilaterally without complication [13,16].

Overall Results

The first published case of corpectomy was performed in 1991. Three retrospective studies assessing the clinical results of this technique have since been published [13,14,16]. In the initial report on 15 clinical patients [13], neurological status was seen to improve by one grade (3 dogs), two grades (8 dogs), three grades (2 dogs), or four grades (2 dogs). Eleven dogs were found to be free of neurological signs at the end of the survey. The same team [16] designed a 14-year retrospective study to assess the long-term effects of TLLC for chronic thoracolumbar intervertebral disc disease among 107 dogs in two veterinary teaching hospitals. In this study, mean follow-up time was 19.6 months and mean duration of clinical signs prior to surgery was 6.7 months (range 0.2–78 months, median 3 months). At the end of one survey, 91.4% of dogs were ambulatory and had voluntary control of micturition, 69.1% of dogs were neurologically improved, 27.2% were stable, and 3.7% were worsened [16]. Final neurological improvement was significantly influenced by presurgical grade, with dogs with higher presurgical grades showing more improvement [14,16]. Neurological improvement was negatively influenced by the duration of clinical signs prior to surgery [14,16]. Based on these results, TLLC appears to be a good surgical option for the treatment of chronic disc herniation in dogs while limiting the risks of postoperative deterioration.

Complications

Hemorrhage of the venous sinus, wound infection, nerve root injury, incomplete spinal cord decompression, postoperative spinal instability, and other complications have been described following TLLC [13,14,16]. Between 0% [13] and 6% [16] of dogs died or were euthanized postoperatively because of complications related to TLLC surgery; more specifically, secondary to worsening of their neurological status.

Hemorrhage of the venous sinus is the most commonly encountered complication during TLLC surgery and occurred in 25% of cases in one study [14]. This complication is likely related to the anatomical proximity of the venous sinus and its adhesion to the chronically protruded/extruded disc. Unobstructed visualization of the vascular structures is essential to reduce the risk of hemorrhage and is best achieved using magnification such as that provided by an operating microscope. Combining the corpectomy with another lateral decompressive procedure (e.g., hemilaminectomy or mini-hemilaminectomy) does not reduce the risk of intraoperative hemorrhage since a branch of the venous sinus exits through the intervertebral foramen and is more easily damaged when approaching the vertebral canal laterally. The author believes it is safer to gain access to the vertebral canal by drilling from the ventral aspect of the slot in a sagittal direction rather than from the lateral aspect of the vertebra inward to avoid entering the venous sinuses. As for any surgery, the TLLC procedure is associated with a learning curve, and in the early stage it may be beneficial to also perform a mini-hemilaminectomy to identify the exact location of the vertebral canal while accepting the additional risk of encountering hemorrhage.

Wound complications such as infection, inflammation, or delayed healing were reported in 15.9% of cases in one study [16] and seroma which resolved with drainage was reported in one case in another study [13]. Other complications were reported in 9.3% of cases in one study [16] and included respiratory infection, abdominal hernia, fecal incontinence, fecal and urinary incontinence, megaesophagus, stomach dilatation, and crossed-extensor reflex.

Nerve root injury occurred in 8.3% of dogs in one study [14] and was also encountered in the first report of the technique [13]. In these cases, abdominal wall paralysis resulting in a bulge was presumably caused by the iatrogenic damage to two (or more) spinal nerves during the surgical approach (Figure 23.9). In the author's experience, abdominal wall paralysis typically resolves within 1–3 months, and rhizotomy (L3 or above) is best performed preventively in cases where the nerve root is not mobile enough to protect it with a nerve retractor during drilling.

Revision surgery could be necessary if insufficient decompression is obtained or when postoperative instability is suspected. In one study, six dogs (8%) underwent repeat surgery for instability or residual disc material identified on postoperative imaging [14]. In another study [16], four dogs (3.7%) were found to have significant residual disc material and two dogs (1.8%) demonstrated excessive postoperative pain with a step along the canal floor supporting vertebral instability. Stabilization must be performed as soon as a diagnosis of instability is made. In the initial report, none of the 15 dogs treated with TLLC developed postoperative worsening of their neurological status [13], and all dogs that were nonambulatory regained ambulatory function. More recently, two studies [14,16] reported that approximately 10% of patients demonstrated a transient worsening of their neurological status (one neurological grade) in the immediate postoperative period. Reported hospitalization times for TLLC are on average 3.5 days [13,16] and are short compared to those reported after hemilaminectomy for disc disease in large nonchondrodystrophic dogs [12,36].

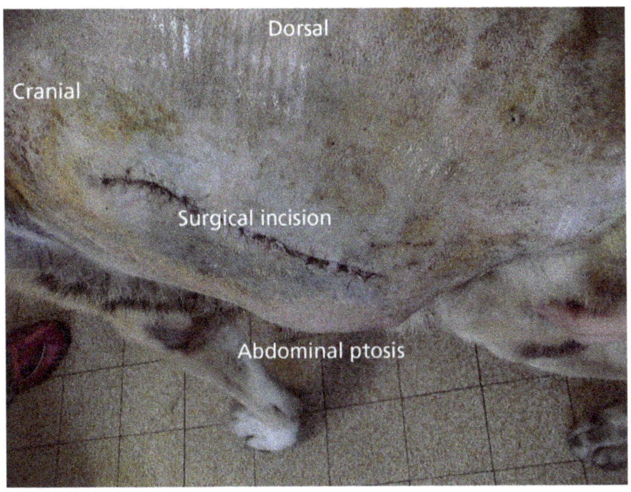

Figure 23.9 Abdominal wall weakness (ptosis) observed following corpectomy at three adjacent sites.

Assessment of Degree of Decompression and Outcome

Nine client-owned dogs that underwent MRI evaluation before and twice (immediately and 6 weeks) after TLLC showed clinical improvement even in cases of incomplete decompression (Frank Forterre, personal communication). Of nine dogs with initial spinal cord compression greater than 50%, decompression by TLLC achieved decompression to less than 20% in three dogs and between 20 and 50% in six dogs immediately postoperatively. Eight of these dogs showed less than 20% spinal cord compression at 6 weeks after decompression. A likely feature of corpectomy is that it provides a ventral dead space that could allow for progressive decompression of remaining disc material within the canal.

Fifty-one dogs with mild (<20%) to severe (>50%) spinal cord compression were assessed after TLLC by CT, myelogram, or MRI, and this revealed satisfactory spinal cord decompression in 90% of patients [14]. Decompression was deemed complete in 58% of cases and good (<15% reduction in spinal cord diameter) in 32% of cases. Decompression was considered unsatisfactory (>15% reduction in spinal cord diameter) in 9% of cases (five discs) [17]. In this study mean slot depth was 64.1% of vertebral body width and 43% of vertebral body height. Mean cranial and caudal extension were respectively 29.5% and 22% of vertebral body length [17]. There were no known complications related to slot dimensions, which verified that the initial recommendations [13] for slot dimensions (25% of body length, 50% of body height, and 50–66% of body width) do not appear to lead to clinical vertebral instability. This is also consistent with published in-vitro biomechanical studies [20,21]. Slot depth tended to influence complete decompression, while none of the other factors assessed (age, weight, breed) seemed to influence the result of the surgery [17].

Conclusion

TLLC is a relatively new procedure that offers an alternative to dorsal decompressive procedures. TLLC appears to be the technique of choice for treating chronic lateralized thoracolumbar disc disease in the dog but may also be of interest for patients with chronic disc extrusion. TLLC can be performed anywhere from the cranial thoracic to the lumbosacral junction and is associated with good spinal cord decompression, a low rate of complications, and a short median hospitalization. TLLC does not require vertebral stabilization unless it is combined with hemilaminectomy.

Video clips to accompany this book can be found on the companion website at:
www.wiley.com/go/shores/neurosurgery

References

1 McKee WM. A comparison of hemilaminectomy (with concomitant disc fenestration) and dorsal laminectomy for the treatment of thoracolumbar disc protrusion in dogs. *Vet Rec* 1992;130:296–300.

2 Coates JR. Intervertebral disc disease. *Vet Clin North Am Small Anim Pract* 2000;30:77–110.

3 Corse M, Renberg W, Friis E. In vitro evaluation of biomechanical effects of multiple hemilaminectomies on the canine lumbar vertebral column. *Am J Vet Res* 2003;64:1139–1145.

4 Redding RW. Laminectomy in the dog. *Am J Vet Res* 1951;12:123–128.

5 Henry WB. Dorsal decompressive laminectomy in the treatment of thoracolumbar disc disease. *J Am Anim Hosp Assoc* 1975;11:627–635.

6 Forterre F, Spreng D, Rytz U, Jaggy A, Schawalder P. Thoracolumbar dorsolateral laminectomy with osteotomy of the spinous process in fourteen dogs. *Vet Surg* 2007;36:458–463.

7 Schulman A, Lippincott CL. Dorsolateral hemilaminectomy in the treatment of thoracolumbar intervertebral disc disease in dogs. *Compend Contin Educ Pract Vet* 1987;9:305–310.

8 Scott H. Hemilaminectomy for the treatment of thoracolumbar disc disease in the dog: a follow-up studv of 40 cases. *J Small Anim Pract* 1997;38:488–494.

9 Jeffery N. Treatment of acute and chronic thoracolumbar disc disease by mini hemilaminectomy. *J Small Anim Pract* 1988;29:611–616.

10 Lubbe AM, Kirberger RM, Verstraete FJM. Pediculectomy for thoracolumbar spinal decompression in the dachshund. *J Am Anim Hosp Assoc* 1994;30:233–238.

11 McCartney W. Partial pediculectomy for the treatment of thoracolumbar disc disease. *Vet Comp Orthop Traumatol* 1997;10:117–121.

12 Macias C, McKee WM, May C, Innes JF. Thoracolumbar disc disease in large dogs: a study of 99 cases. *J Small Anim Pract* 2002;43:439–446.

13 Moissonnier P, Meheust P, Carozzo C. Thoracolumbar lateral corpectomy for treatment of chronic disc herniation. *Vet Surg* 2004;33:620–628.

14 Salger F, Ziegler L, Boettcher IC, Oechtering G, Böttcher P, Flegel T. Neurologic outcome after thoracolumbar partial lateral corpectomy for intervertebral disc disease in 72 dogs. *Vet Surg* 2014;43:581–588.

15 Holmberg D, Palmer N, Vanpelt D, Willan A. A comparison of manual and power-assisted thoracolumbar disc fenestration in dogs. *Vet Surg* 1990;19:323–327.

16 Filleur A, Moissonnier P, Cachon T, Fau D, Genevois JP, Carozzo C. Benefits of thoracolumbar lateral corpectomy for chronic intervertebral disc disease treatment in dogs. Results of a 14 years retrospective study among 107 dogs in two veterinary teaching hospitals. Poster presented at the Annual Scientific Meeting of the ECVS, July 5–7, 2012, Barcelona, Spain.

17 Flegel T, Boettcher IC, Ludewig E, Kiefer I, Oechtering G, Böttcher P. Partial lateral corpectomy of the thoracolumbar spine in 51 dogs: Assessment of the slot morphometry and spinal cord decompression. *Vet Surg* 2011;40:14–21.

18 Brisson B, Moffatt SL, Swayne SL, Parent J. Recurrence of thoracolumbar intervertebral disc extrusion in chondrodystrophic dogs after surgical decompression with or without prophylactic fenestration: 265 cases (1995–1999). *J Am Vet Med Assoc* 2004;224:1808–1814.

19 Forterre F, Konar M, Spreng D, Jaggy A, Lang J. Influence of intervertebral disc fenestration at the herniation site in association with hemilaminectomy on recurrence in chondrodystrophic dogs with thoracolumbar disc disease: a prospective MRI study. *Vet Surg* 2008;37:399–405.

20 De Vincente F, Bernard F, Fitzpatrick D, Moissonnier P. In vitro radiographic characteristics and biomechanical properties of the canine lumbar vertebral motion unit after lateral corpectomy, after lateral corpectomy, minihemilaminectomy and hemilaminectomy. *Vet Comp Orthop Traumatol* 2013;26:19–26.

21 Vizcaíno-Revés N, Bürki A, Ferguson S, Geissbühler U, Stahl C, Forterre F. Influence of partial lateral corpectomy with and without hemilaminectomy on canine thoracolumbar stability: a biomechanichal study. *Vet Surg* 2012;41:228–234.

22 Böttcher P, Flegel T, Böttcher IC, Grevel V, Oechtering G. Partial lateral corpectomy for ventral extradural thoracic spinal cord compression in a cat. *J Feline Med Surg* 2008;10:291–295.

23 Malik Y, Konar M, Wernick M, Howard J, Forterre F. Chronic intervertebral disc herniation associated with fused vertebrae treated by vertebral lateral corpectomy in a cat. *Vet Comp Orthop Traumatol* 2009;22:170–173.

24 Yturraspe DJ, Lumb WV. A dorsolateral muscle separating approach for thoracolumbar intervertebral disc fenestration in the dog. *J Am Vet Med Assoc* 1973;162:1037–1040.

25 Seeman CW. A lateral approach for thoracolumbar disc fenestration. *Mod Vet Pract* 1968;49:73–74.

26 Morelius M, Bergadano A, Spreng D, Schawalder P, Doherr M, Forterre F. Influence of surgical approach on the efficacy of the intervertebral disc fenestration: a cadaveric study. *J Small Anim Pract* 2007;48:87–92.

27 Gossot P, Scotti S, Klein A et al. Thoracic hemivertebra surgical realignment and stabilisation: radiographic study in 41 asymptomatic French bulldogs and results in 4 operated dogs. Poster presented at the 16th Annual Scientific Meeting of the ECVS, Dublin, Ireland, 2007.

28 Carozzo C, Cachon T, Genevois J-P et al. Transiliac approach for exposure of lumbosacral intervertebral disk and foramen: technique description. *Vet Surg* 2008;37: 27–31.

29 Carozzo C, Maitre P, Genevois JP, Gabanou PA, Fau D, Viguier E. Endoscope-assisted thoracolumbar lateral corpectomy. *Vet Surg* 2011;40:738–742.

30 Carozzo C, Gabanou P, Viguier E. Endoscope-assisted minimally invasive approach in the treatment of thoracolumbar chronic disc herniae. Technical considerations and first applications. Poster presented at the ACVS Veterinary Symposium, San Diego, USA, October 27–29, 2005. Available at http://onlinelibrary.wiley.com/doi/10.1111/j.1532-950X.2005.00082.x/full

31 Shores A. Spinal trauma: pathophysiology and management of traumatic spinal injuries. *Vet Clin North Am Small Animal Pract* 1992;22:859–888.

32 Panjabi M. The stabilizing system of the spine. Part I. Function, dysfunction, adaptation, and enhancement. *J Spinal Disord* 1992;5:383–389.

33 Panjabi M. The stabilizing system of the spine. Part II. Neutral zone and instability hypothesis. *J Spinal Disord* 1992;5:390–396.

34 Hill T, Lubbe A, Guthrie A. Lumbar spine stability following hemilaminectomy, pediculectomy, and fenestration. *Vet Comp Orthop Traumatol* 2000;13:165–171.

35 Arthurs G. Spinal instability resulting from bilateral mini-hemilaminectomy and pediculectomy. *Vet Comp Orthop Traumatol* 2009;22:422–426.

36 Cudia SP, Duval JM. Thoracolumbar intervertebral disc disease in large, non chondrodystrophic dogs: a retrospective study. *J Am Anim Hosp Assoc* 1997;33: 456–460.

24 Dorsal Laminectomy in the Thoracolumbar Region

Cory Fisher and Andy Shores

Introduction

Dorsal laminectomy of the thoracolumbar region has been described for treatment of intervertebral disc disease [1–17], fractures [12–16], neoplastic processes [12–16,18,19], cysts causing compression to spinal cord [20–22], and other disease processes that cause spinal cord compression [23,24]. Dorsal laminectomy is used to access dorsal, lateral and ventral aspects of the spinal canal depending on the type of dorsal laminectomy appropriate to the disease process [13,14]. Numerous modifications to the dorsal laminectomy procedure have been described since Greene's first report in 1951 [17]. Dorsal laminectomies are classified by the extent of the vertebrae removed. The four types of dorsal laminectomies described in veterinary neurosurgery are (listed in order from the least amount of bone removed to the most) Funkquist B, modified dorsal laminectomy, Funkquist A, and deep dorsal laminectomy [13–15]. The two most commonly used are the Funkquist B and modified dorsal laminectomy [3]. An osteotomy of the spinous process instead of the traditional ostectomy has also been reported [25]. Unilateral excision of the vertebral arch, including the articular processes (facetectomy), accessory process (foramenotomy) and pedicle (pediculectomy), have been performed after osteotomy of the spinous process [25].

The type of dorsal laminectomy performed is based on the disease process causing neurological dysfunction. Advanced diagnostic imaging (myelography, CT, CT with myelography, or MRI) is used to determine the extent of the disease process. Once the extent of the disease process is recognized and classified, the type of dorsal laminectomy is chosen.

Surgical Approach (Video 24.1)

The patient is clipped and aseptically prepared for surgery then positioned in sternal recumbency with the spinous processes perpendicular to the surgery table. A rolled towel or sandbag may be placed in the mid-abdominal region to help elevate the area of interest. Once positioned to the surgeon's discretion, the animal is secured in this position using tape. A dorsal midline skin incision is made for a distance of a minimum of two vertebrae cranial and caudal to the affected intervertebral disc space. The subcutaneous fat and fascia are incised using blunt/sharp dissection with Metzenbaum scissors until the deep lumbodorsal fascia is reached. A continuous scalloped incision is made bilaterally around each spinous process in the superficial and deep external fasciae of the trunk. Using periosteal elevators, the epaxial musculature is reflected laterally on both sides to the level of the accessory process. Gelpi retractors are used to retract the epaxial musculature for better visualization of the dorsal and lateral aspect of the vertebral column [12,13,19,26]. The spinous processes of the vertebrae cranial and caudal to the affected disc space are removed with bone rongeurs [12–14,19]. A laminectomy is performed using a high-speed surgical air drill [12–14,19]. Because the dorsal lamina is thinner than the lateral lamina, frequent pausing of the drilling is necessary to assess bone depth at the drilling site [3]. The outer cortex of the lamina normally has a whitish tint. The medullary bone is recognized by its reddish-brown color. The inner cortex of the lamina is very thin and also whitish in color [12–14,19]. Small Lempert or Kerrison ronguers are used to expand the laminectomy after entering the canal [3,13, 14]. The extent of bone removal is dictated by the lesion of interest and amount of accessibility of the vertebral canal needed (Funkquist A, Funkquist B, or modified dorsal laminectomy).

After completing the decompression and the remainder of an indicated procedure (tumor excision, opening of a subarachnoid diverticulum, removal of scar tissue, etc.), the surgical site is thoroughly lavaged with warm physiological saline and either gelatin sponge or autogenous fat graft is placed over the laminectomy site to prevent dural adhesions [3, 12]. Synthetic nonabsorbable suture can then be used to span over the laminectomy site or the

Current Techniques in Canine and Feline Neurosurgery, First Edition. Edited by Andy Shores and Brigitte A. Brisson.
© 2017 John Wiley & Sons, Inc. Published 2017 by John Wiley & Sons, Inc.
Companion website: www.wiley.com/go/shores/neurosurgery

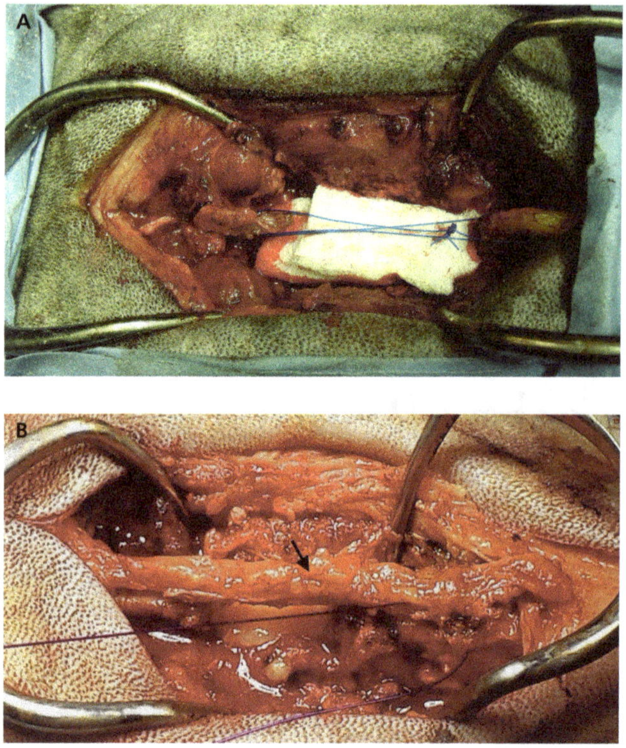

Figure 24.1 To limit the possibility of a laminectomy membrane, (A) synthetic nonabsorbable #1 or #2 suture material in a figure-of-eight pattern or (B) a preserved supraspinous ligament (arrow) is used to span the length of the dorsal laminectomy by attachment to the nearest cranial and caudal spinous processes. The muscle is sutured over the figure-of-eight suture or ligament. In (A) the spinal cord is protected with sheets of a gelatin sponge, and in (B) with an autogenous free fat graft.

supraspinous ligament can be preserved and reattached at the end of the procedure to span the defect (Figure 24.1). The suture is placed either around the spinous processes or through a small hole that is made in the spinous processes cranial and caudal to the laminectomy site [3,12]. The fascia and epaxial muscles are closed with absorbable suture in a simple continuous pattern over the spanning suture [3,12]. Closure of the subcutaneous tissue and skin is in routine fashion.

Classification of Dorsal Laminectomies

Funkquist A Method

Funkquist A dorsal laminectomy involves removal of the spinous process, cranial and caudal articular processes, dorsal laminae, and pedicle to the appropriate height, usually to the level of the spinal cord (Figure 24.2A) [13–15].

Funkquist B Method

Funkquist B dorsal laminectomy involves removal of the spinous process and dorsal lamina. Both cranial and caudal articular processes are preserved. This technique allows limited access to the vertebral canal (Figure 24.2B) [13–15].

Modified Dorsal Laminectomy

The modified dorsal laminectomy, the most commonly used technique, involves the removal of an amount of lamina intermediate between Funkquist A and Funkquist B, with preservation of the

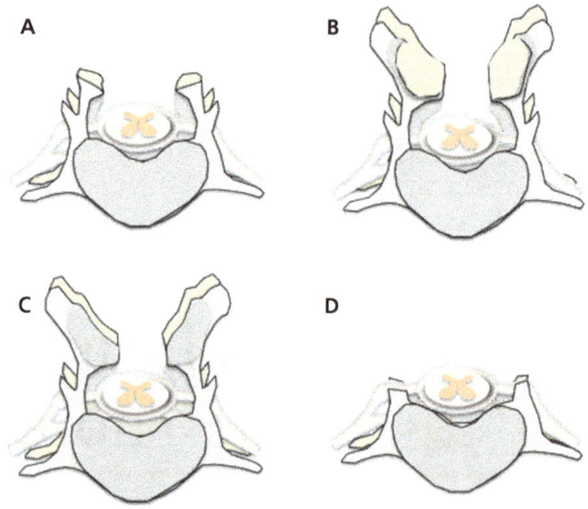

Figure 24.2 Illustration of (A) Funkquist A, (B) Funkquist B, (C) modified, and (D) deep dorsal laminectomies. See text for details. *Source*: illustration by Andy Shores.

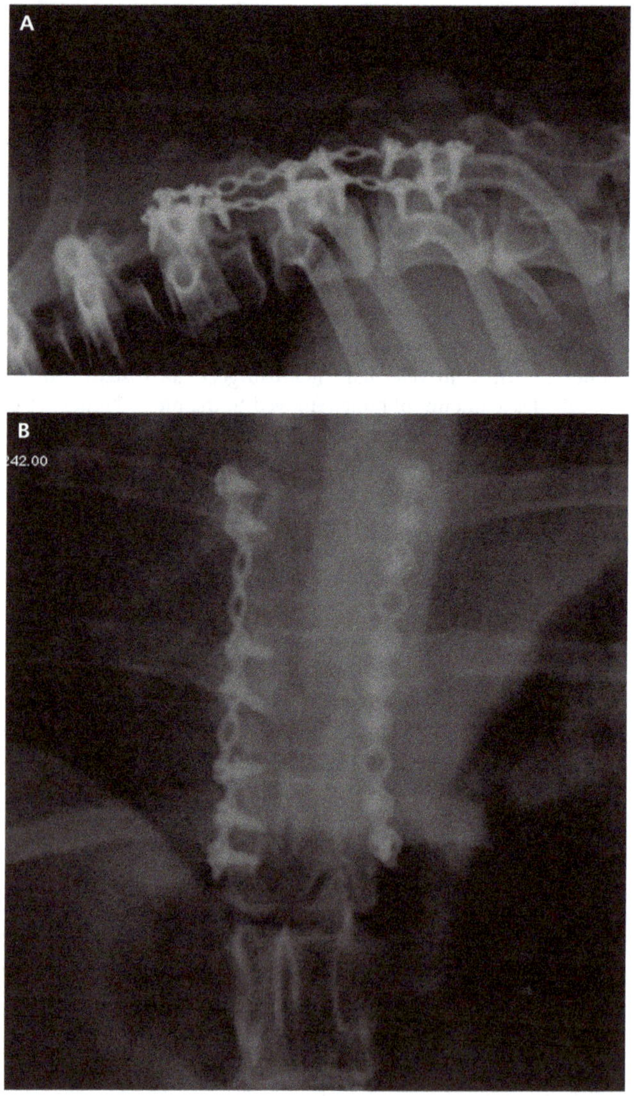

Figure 24.3 (A) Lateral and (B) ventrodorsal radiographs after T11–T12 dorsal laminectomy with stabilization in a Chinese Pug with constrictive myelopathy.

cranial articular processes but removal of the caudal articular processes (Figures 24.2C and 24.3) [3,12–16].

Deep Dorsal Laminectomy

A deep dorsal laminectomy is performed by removing articular processes, dorsal lamina, and pedicles to the ventral aspect of the vertebral canal. This procedure is rarely performed and not recommended because of the instability created and constrictive laminectomy membrane formation (Figure 24.2D) [8,13].

Video clips to accompany this book can be found on the companion website at:
www.wiley.com/go/shores/neurosurgery

References

1 Brisson B. Intervertebral disc disease in dogs. *Vet Clin North Am Small Anim Pract* 2010;40:829–858.

2 Shores A. Intervertebral disk syndrome in the dog. Part III. Thoracolumbar disk surgery. *Compend Contin Educ Vet* 1982;4:24–31.

3 Shores A. Intervertebral disk disease. In: Newton CD, Nunamaker DM (eds) *Textbook of Small Animal Orthopaedics*. New York: Lippincott Williams and Wilkins, 1985.

4 Swaim SF, Vandevelde M. Clinical and histologic evaluation of bilateral hemilaminectomy and deep dorsal laminectomy for extensive spinal cord decompression in the dog. *J Am Vet Med Assoc* 1977;170:407–413.

5 Muir P, Johnson KA, Manley PA, Dueland RT. Comparison of hemilaminectomy and dorsal laminectomy for thoracolumbar intervertebral disc extrusion in dachshunds. *J Small Anim Pract* 1995;36:360–367.

6 Griffin JF, Levine JM, Kerwin SC, Cole R. Canine thoracolumbar intervertebral disk disease: diagnosis, prognosis, and treatment. *Compend Contin Educ Vet* 2009;31:E1–E14.

7 McKee WM. A comparison of hemilaminectomy (with concomitant disc fenestration) and dorsal laminectomy for the treatment of thoracolumbar disc protrusion in dogs. *Vet Rec* 1992;130:296–300.

8 Horne TR, Power RD, Swaim SF. Dorsal laminectomy techniques in the dog. *J Am Vet Med Assoc* 1977;171:742–749.

9 Gage ED, Hoerlein BF. Hemilaminectomy and dorsal laminectomy for relieving compression of the spinal cord in the dog. *J Am Vet Med Assoc* 1968;152: 351–359.

10 Henry WB Jr. Dorsal decompressive laminectomy in the treatment of thoraco-lumbar disc disease. *J Am Anim Hosp Assoc* 1975;11:627–635.

11 Davis GJ, Brown DC. Prognostic indicators for time to ambulation after surgical decompression in nonambulatory dogs with acute thoracolumbar disk extrusions: 112 cases. *Vet Surg* 2002;31:513–518.

12 Trotter EJ. Modified dorsal laminectomy for thoracolumbar disease. In: Bojrab MJ, Ellison GW, Slocum B (eds) *Current Techniques in Small Animal Surgery*, 4th edn. Baltimore, MD: Williams and Wilkins, 1998: 849–853.

13 Seim HB III. Surgery of thoracolumbar spine. In: Fossum TW (ed.) *Small Animal Surgery*, 3rd edn. St Louis, MO: Mosby Elsevier, 2007: 1460–1464.

14 Kerwin SC, Levine JM, Hicks DG. Thoracolumbar spine. Dorsal laminectomy. In: Tobias KM, Johnston SA (eds) *Veterinary Surgery: Small Animal*. St Louis, MO: Elsevier Saunders, 2012: 456–457.

15 Toombs JP, Waters DJ. Intervertebral disc disease. Dorsal laminectomy. In: Slatter D (ed.) *Textbook of Small Animal Surgery*, 3rd edn. Philadelphia, PA: WB Saunders, 1993: 1205–1206.

16 Trotter EJ, Brasmer TH, deLahunta A. Modified deep dorsal laminectomy in the dog. *Cornell Vet* 1975;65:402–427.

17 Greene JE. Surgical intervention for paraplegia due to herniation of the nucleus pulposus. *North Am Vet* 1951;32:411–412.

18 Levy MS, Kapatkin AS, Patnaik AK, Mauldin GN, Mauldin GE. Spinal tumors in 37 dogs: clinical outcome and long-term survival (1987–1994). *J Am Anim Hosp Assoc* 1997;33:307–312.

19 Sharp NJH, Wheeler SJ. Neoplasia. In: *Small Animal Spinal Disorders: Diagnosis and Surgery*, 2nd edn. Edinburgh: Elsevier Mosby, 2005: 247–280.

20 Skeen TM, Olby NJ, Muñana KR, Sharp NJ. Spinal arachnoid cysts in 17 dogs. *J Am Anim Hosp Assoc* 2003;39:271–282.

21 Oxley W, Pink J. Amelioration of caudal thoracic syringohydromelia following surgical management of an adjacent arachnoid cyst. *J Small Anim Pract* 2012;53:67–72.

22 Shamir MH, Lichovsky D, Alzenberg I, Chrisman CL. Partial surgical removal of an intramedullary epidermoid cyst from the spinal cord of a dog. *J Small Anim Pract* 1999;40:439–442.

23 Jeffery ND, Smith PM, Talbot CE. Imaging findings and surgical treatment of hemivertebrae in three dogs. *J Am Vet Med Assoc* 2007;230:532–536.

24 Fisher SC, Shores A, Simpson ST. Constrictive myelopathy secondary to hypoplasia or aplasia of thoracolumbar caudal articular processes in the Pug: 11 cases (1993–2009). *J Am Vet Med Assoc* 2013;242:223–229.

25 Forterre F, Spreng D, Rytz U, Jaggy A, Schawalder P. Thoracolumbar dorsolateral laminectomy with ostectomy of the spinous process in fourteen dogs. *Vet Surg* 2007;36:458–463.

26 Piermattei DL, Johnson KA. Approach to the thoracolumbar vertebrae through a dorsal incision. In: Piermattei DL, Johnson KA (eds) *An Atlas of Surgical Approaches to the Bones and Joints of the Dog and Cat*, 4th edn. Philadelphia, PA: Saunders, 2004: 78–83.

25 Vertebral Fracture and Luxation Repair

Bianca Hettlich

Introduction

Vertebral column injuries are typically the result of high-impact trauma such as vehicular accidents or falls from heights. While trauma can be sustained via bite wounds, projectiles and crushing injuries, fractures and luxations most often occur due to tremendous compression forces, rotation, hyperflexion or hyperextension (Figure 25.1). The need for surgical stabilization is based on the degree of vertebral column instability and spinal cord compression. Injury to the intervertebral disc, articular processes, vertebral body, and associated ligamentous structures will have differing impact on the stability of the spine.

The three-compartment concept can be applied to guide decision-making after vertebral trauma [1]. With this concept the vertebra is divided into dorsal, middle and ventral compartments that comprise (i) spinous process, dorsal ligamentous structures, lamina, articular processes, and pedicles; (ii) dorsal longitudinal ligament, dorsal annulus fibrosus, dorsal aspect of the vertebral body, and transverse processes; and (iii) remaining vertebral body and annulus fibrosus, nucleus pulposus, and ventral longitudinal ligament (Figure 25.2). Injury to two or more compartments is generally considered unstable. Apart from assessing stability and spinal cord compression, the decision to pursue vertebral column stabilization has to consider the patient's neurological status, chronicity of injury, and concurrent injuries.

Preoperative Planning

Preoperatively, standard orthogonal radiographic views of the affected vertebral column are used to assess the type and location of the vertebral column injury. Radiographs will help determine whether the immediate vertebrae can be utilized for fixation (i.e., in case of vertebral column luxation) or if instrumentation needs to be applied to adjacent vertebrae (i.e., in case of vertebral fracture). A preoperative CT scan should be performed to better identify the extent of injury and allow familiarization with the anatomy around the injury and patient-specific landmarks. Decisions must be made regarding the type of implant, number of implants, and unilateral or bilateral placement. If the type of implant allows, individual implant insertion angles should be measured for each vertebra and each implant to allow for maximum bone purchase, while assuring a safe implant corridor (Figure 25.3).

Decompression in Addition to Stabilization

At times, it is necessary to access the vertebral canal to address compression by hematomas, traumatic disc extrusions, and displaced bone fragments. The type of approach depends on the location of the inciting compression. For the cervical spine, a ventral slot can be performed through the same approach as for ventral stabilization; however, it is limited in the amount of exposure to the vertebral canal it provides. A separate approach for a dorsal laminectomy is possible, but must be carefully considered due to the need for a second major surgical approach. For thoracolumbar trauma, it is common to perform a hemilaminectomy, mini-hemilaminectomy (sparing the articular processes), or partial pediculectomy in conjunction with vertebral column stabilization if compression is located ventrally or ventrolaterally. If a dorsal laminectomy is required for dorsal compression, articular processes should be spared if possible to avoid further destabilization of the affected vertebral articulation.

Lumbosacral fractures or luxations can be decompressed via dorsal laminectomy while sparing the articular facets and because these can be challenging to reduce, a concurrent dorsal laminectomy may be of benefit to offset compression secondary to malalignment.

Protection of exposed spinal cord or nerve roots during application of polymethylmethacrylate (PMMA) can be achieved by using celluloid sponges and molding cement away from the laminectomy site with Freer elevators. While accessing the vertebral canal in such

Current Techniques in Canine and Feline Neurosurgery, First Edition. Edited by Andy Shores and Brigitte A. Brisson.
© 2017 John Wiley & Sons, Inc. Published 2017 by John Wiley & Sons, Inc.
Companion website: www.wiley.com/go/shores/neurosurgery

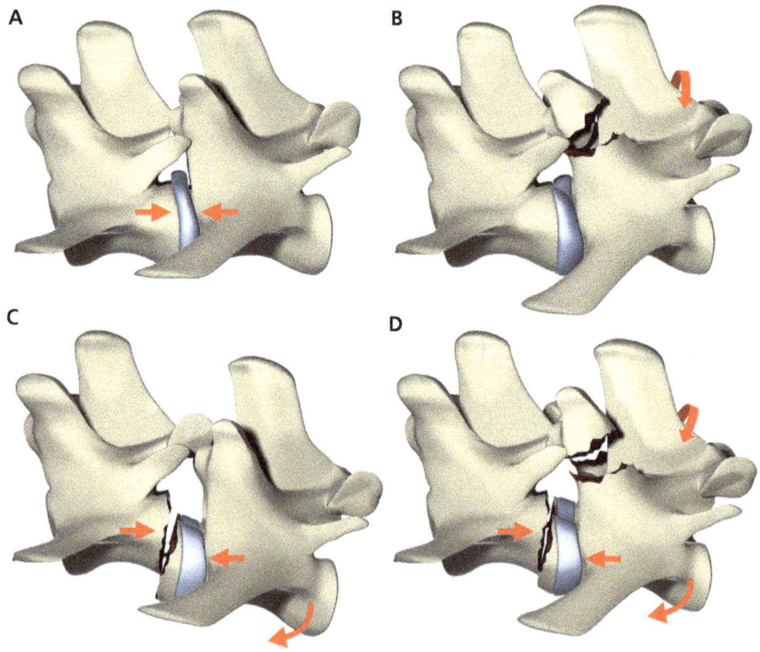

Figure 25.1 Examples of different types of vertebral column injuries due to different forces. (A) Axial compression injury leading to traumatic disc extrusion. (B) Rotational forces leading to fracture of the articular processes; disc integrity can also be compromised. (C) Hyperflexion and compression injury leading to vertebral endplate fracture and ventral subluxation. (D) Hyperflexion, compression and rotational injury leading to endplate fracture, ventral subluxation and fracture of the articular processes.

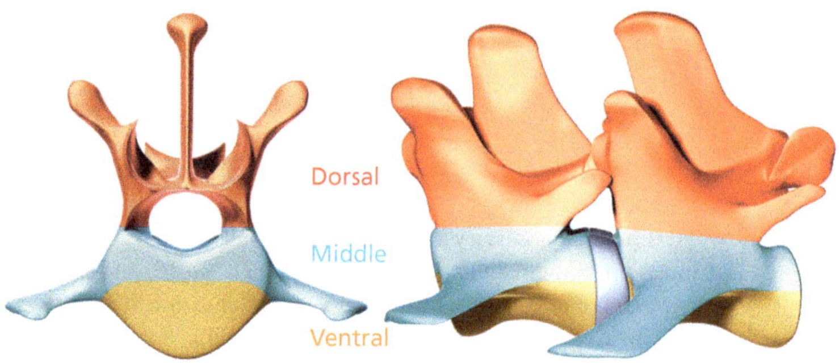

Figure 25.2 The three compartments in two adjacent lumbar vertebrae. The dorsal compartment (red) consists of spinous process, dorsal ligamentous structures, lamina, articular processes, and pedicles. The middle compartment (blue) consists of dorsal longitudinal ligament, dorsal annulus fibrosus, dorsal aspect of the vertebral body, and transverse processes. The ventral compartment (yellow) consists of the remaining vertebral body and annulus fibrosus, nucleus pulposus, and ventral longitudinal ligament.

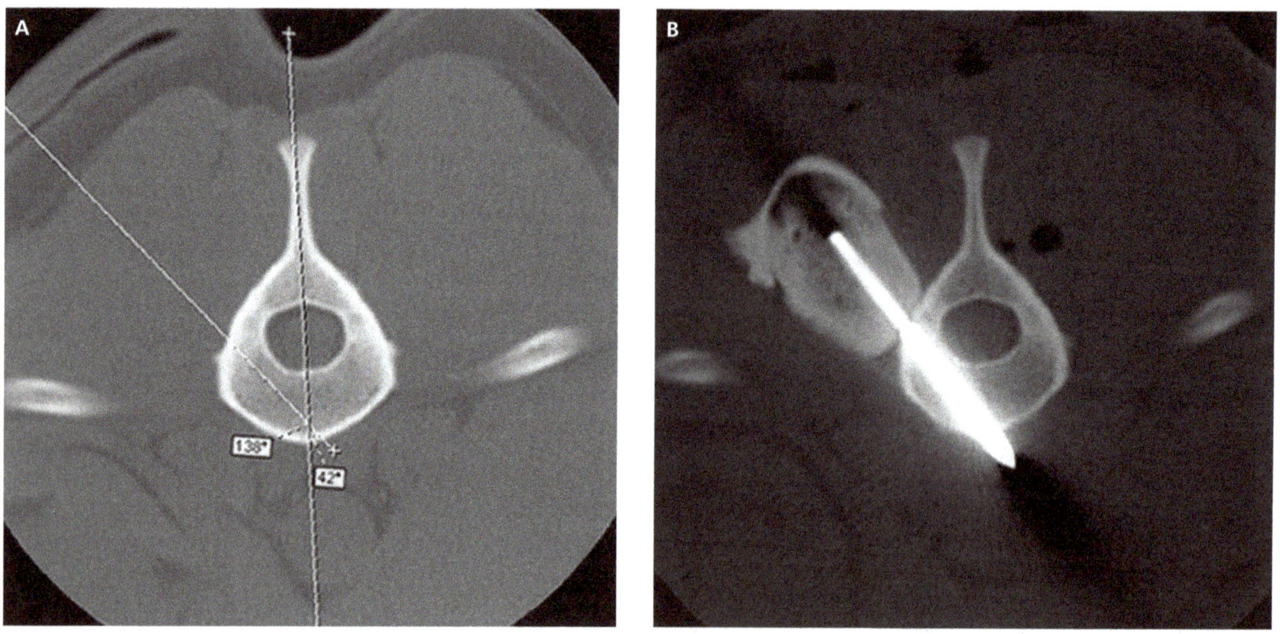

Figure 25.3 Preoperative axial CT with planned pin insertion angle and location (A) and postoperative axial CT of the same dog with a bicortical pin in place (B).

approaches allows familiarization of location and dimension of the canal in relation to implants at the opened site, they should only be performed if compression is deemed sufficiently significant.

Cervical Injuries

Cervical fractures or luxations generally require substantial force as the surrounding musculature provides relative protection during trauma. Unstable vertebral body fractures are the most common indication for cervical stabilization.

Anatomical Considerations

The vertebral bodies offer the most substantial amount of bone and can easily be exposed via a ventral approach. Pedicle dimensions are small and the presence of the transverse foramen, which houses the vertebral artery, makes safe transpedicular implant passage challenging. Articular processes extend more laterally than dorsal and are in close proximity to the exiting nerve roots via the intervertebral foramina. More challenging muscular coverage and the lack of easily palpable landmarks hinders lateral approaches. Dorsal access to the vertebral canal requires an approach through what is oftentimes massive dorsal cervical musculature with the potential for increased postoperative morbidity.

Positioning and Approach

Careful positioning of the anesthetized dog in dorsal recumbency with the cervical spine in relative extension helps with alignment and reduction of some fractures/luxations. A standard ventral midline or paramedian approach will provide access to the ventral aspect of the vertebral column. For caudal cervical trauma, partial myotomy at the insertion of the sternocephalicus muscle from the sternum may provide a somewhat improved access. Bony landmarks for a ventral approach include the wings of C1, the increased spacing between the ventral processes of C2 and C3 compared with other vertebrae, the prominent transverse processes of C6, and the first pair of ribs. Surgical stabilization generally requires instrumentation of vertebrae adjacent to the site of trauma; therefore, the approach often exposes most of the cervical vertebral bodies.

Implant Selection

Bicortical pin fixation with smooth or positive-profile end-threaded fixation pins has long been the standard for cervical vertebral fixation. Unfortunately, it carries an unacceptably high risk of injury to neurovascular structures as pins, even at recommended insertion angles (30–40°) and landmarks (ventral midline), may violate the vertebral canal, transverse foramen, or intervertebral foramen. Therefore, bicortical cervical implants are no longer recommended. Monocortical implants significantly decrease the risk of such injury. While either cortical or cancellous screws can be utilized for monocortical fixation, cortical screws may offer improved resistance to shear forces due to their larger core diameter. Biomechanical studies are supporting the use of monocortical screw constructs in the canine cervical spine [2,3].

Reduction

Gentle manipulation for reduction of the unstable cervical vertebral column can be achieved in several ways. Point-to-point reduction forceps can be placed carefully around the mid-vertebral body to manipulate the vertebra. Screws or small positive-profile end-threaded pins can used for manipulation if they are inserted in an area that does not jeopardize bony purchase for surgical fixation. In small-breed dogs, reduction can sometimes be achieved with thumb forceps alone.

Monocortical Screw and PMMA Fixation

The ventral aspect of the vertebral bodies is utilized for monocortical screw fixation with PMMA. Since bone near the vertebral endplates has the largest dimensions, screw position should be as cranial or caudal in relation to the vertebral body as possible. Care must be taken not to perforate the vertebral endplate and the screw should be oriented parallel to the caudoventral/craniodorsally angled disc space. Medium- to large-breed dogs can usually accommodate 3.5-mm cortical screws, while 2.0-mm or 2.7-mm screws are more appropriate for smaller dogs and cats. The use of titanium screws allows for improved postoperative advanced imaging, especially MRI. Nonself-tapping screws are preferred to avoid inadvertent perforation of the transcortex into the vertebral canal. When drilling, a drill stop is advantageous to help prevent penetration into the vertebral canal. Screw-on drill stops (e.g., Positive Drill Stop by Animal Orthopedics) are positioned along the drill bit based on preoperative measurements of the height of the vertebral body. Alternatively, drilling can commence without a stop, relying on the change in drill bit pressure to indicate penetration of the cis-cortex into the narrow medullary space of the vertebral body. An appropriate size depth gauge or blunt straight probe can be used to carefully determine integrity of the trans-cortex. Two to four screws can be placed into each vertebral body as necessary depending on the size of the bone and the degree of instability. Screw length must be sufficient to allow about 10–15 mm of screw protruding that will be incorporated into the PMMA. If screws are placed parallel to one another near an endplate, they may be angled slightly toward the midline to prevent interference of implants during drilling and placement of the second screw. Transverse processes offer an additional location for screw placement (Figure 25.4). While these processes do not provide a large amount of bony purchase, bicortical screw placement is possible,

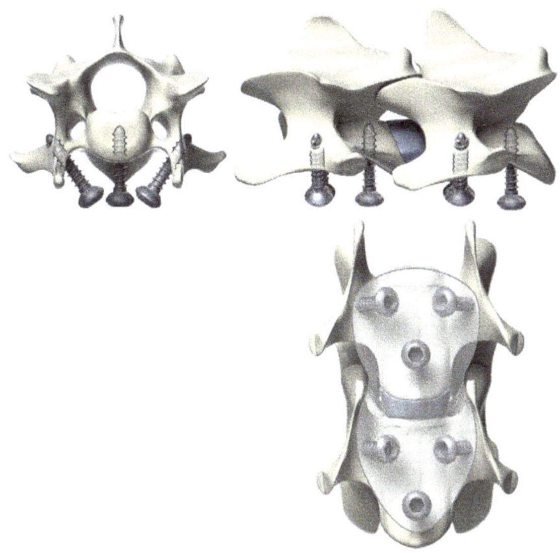

Figure 25.4 Monocortical vertebral body and bicortical transverse process screw fixation with PMMA in the cervical spine. Note how the transverse process screws avoid the transverse foramen. Vertebral body screws can be placed anywhere along the ventral aspect to accommodate the injury, affording a high degree of freedom in application. For fixation of two adjacent vertebrae, 20 g PMMA is usually sufficient.

offering another point of fixation in cases where good vertebral body bone stock is not available. Screw orientation must take into consideration the path of the transverse foramen.

In the case of cervical vertebral luxation, fixation of the adjacent vertebrae is often sufficient. In the case of cervical vertebral fracture, fixation may need to span the affected vertebra.

Prior to application of PMMA, local resection of part of the longus colli musculature improves ease of cement application. If multiple vertebrae are spanned, Kirschner wires can be used to reinforce the PMMA by gently bending them around screws or connecting them with small-gauge cerclage wire. Twenty grams of PMMA is often sufficient to create a uniform cement bar around protruding screw heads and proximal threads if fixation spans two vertebrae. The cement mantle should be 1–1.5 cm thick. Increasing the height of the PMMA bar beyond the level of the longus colli muscles is not recommended as protruding cement can apply pressure on esophagus or trachea and may lead to difficulty in swallowing and respiratory signs.

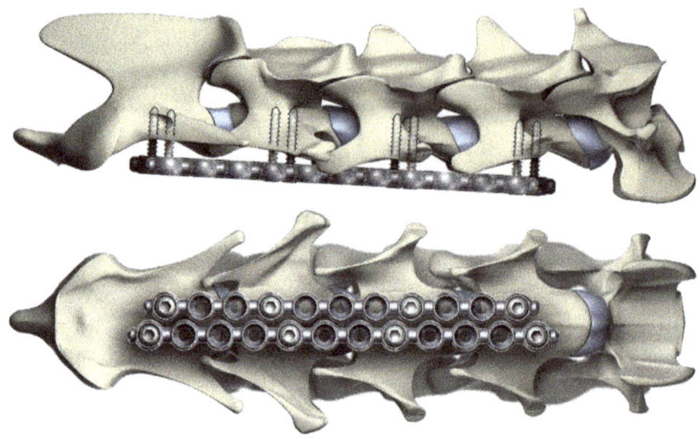

Figure 25.5 Two String of Pearl (SOP) plates are applied to the ventral aspect of the cervical spine with monocortical screw fixation. Note how the plates are not contoured to the vertebral bodies but are locked in place by the locking screw mechanism.

Vertebral Body Plates

The main benefit of plate fixation of the vertebral column is the decrease in implant profile and ease of closure after instrumentation. However, traditional plate fixation can be challenging in the cervical vertebral column. Implant stability of nonlocking plates relies on friction between the plate and bone; this is provided by screw tension on a well-contoured plate with excellent bone contact. Good contouring with appropriate bone contact is difficult to achieve along the vertebral column due to the complex vertebral anatomy. In addition, with regular plates bicortical screw purchase is preferred to prevent premature loosening of screws, which poses a problem in light of the high risk of possible injury with bicortical implant placement. Monocortical screw placement can be performed with regular plates; however, any loosening of screws would lead to implant failure, as friction would be lost.

The development of locking plates offers a solution to using monocortical screw placement in traditional plates that rely on friction [2,4]. Different locking mechanisms rigidly couple screws to the plate, thereby eliminating the potential for loosening of the plate–screw interface. Failure of locking plates typically occurs by shearing of the screws or by pull-out of the plate–screw construct from the bone. Because of the locking mechanism, perfect contouring of the plate to bone is unnecessary (provided that the gap between bone and plate is restricted to a few millimeters) allowing for application of a straight plate over the uneven vertebral body surface.

Two commonly used locking plate systems for vertebral fixation in veterinary medicine are String of Pearls™ (SOP; Orthomed UK Ltd, Halifax, West Yorkshire, UK) and Locking Compression Plate (LCP; DePuy Synthes, West Chester, PA). Both plate types have a fixed screw trajectory to ensure proper engagement of the locking mechanism; this trajectory places screws perpendicularly to the plate. This can pose technical challenges when gaining experience with such an implant type as plates are fixed in position as soon as the first screw is engaged and locked, making subsequent screw trajectory changes difficult. Planning, positioning and exact screw placement are extremely important to avoid a malpositioned locking plate with inappropriately placed screws.

SOP Plate Application

Because of its round core, the SOP plate can be contoured in every direction, making this a very versatile implant. However, with every contouring, screw trajectories change, especially toward each end of the plate. As a general rule, SOP plates should be applied with the least contouring possible. Multiple vertebral bodies can be spanned with the SOP plate and two plates can be placed next to one another to increase freedom with screw placement and strengthen the fixation construct (Figure 25.5).

The ventral aspect of the affected cervical vertebral bodies is exposed and the appropriate size and length of SOP plate is selected (3.5 mm for large, 2.0–2.7 mm for small to medium-sized dogs). Care must be taken to avoid inadvertent screw placement into an intervertebral disc. If screw hole spacing does not fit as desired, a different size SOP can be considered or a second SOP plate can be applied adjacent to the first. Dedicated drill guides are required for proper screw placement to engage the locking mechanism. This will place screws perpendicularly to the plate into bone. Monocortical screw purchase is sufficient and length of screw is determined via depth gauge. During depth measurement, the SOP plate must be held securely, with some pressure and in proper position, since once engaged in the plate screws will not pull the plate toward the bone. Once a screw is placed cranially and caudally, the plate is fixed in position and all subsequent screws must follow the fixed trajectory to be properly locked.

LCP Application

The LCP has hybrid holes allowing for placement of traditional cortical screws as well as locking screws. For use along the vertebral column, only locking screws should be used. The locking portion of the LCP screw holes have threads into which the threaded head of locking screws lock. Special threaded drill guides are used to ensure proper position of the drill hole and subsequent screw and avoid cross-threading. The locking screws specific to the LCP are self-tapping and have a larger core than regular cortical screws. It is therefore important to use the appropriate diameter drill bit for the specific size plate used. Since locking screws are used, there is no need for a high degree of contact between plate and bone. The locking screws in the LCP are fixed trajectory and are placed perpendicularly to the plate. Careful preoperative planning and choosing the appropriate implant size and length are important to avoid malpositioned screws (Figure 25.6).

Other Locking Plates

Other veterinary locking plate systems can be applied abiding by the same principles of application. Human spinal locking plates can be utilized in veterinary medicine but are unfortunately prohibitively expensive. The design of these plates allows for two screws to be

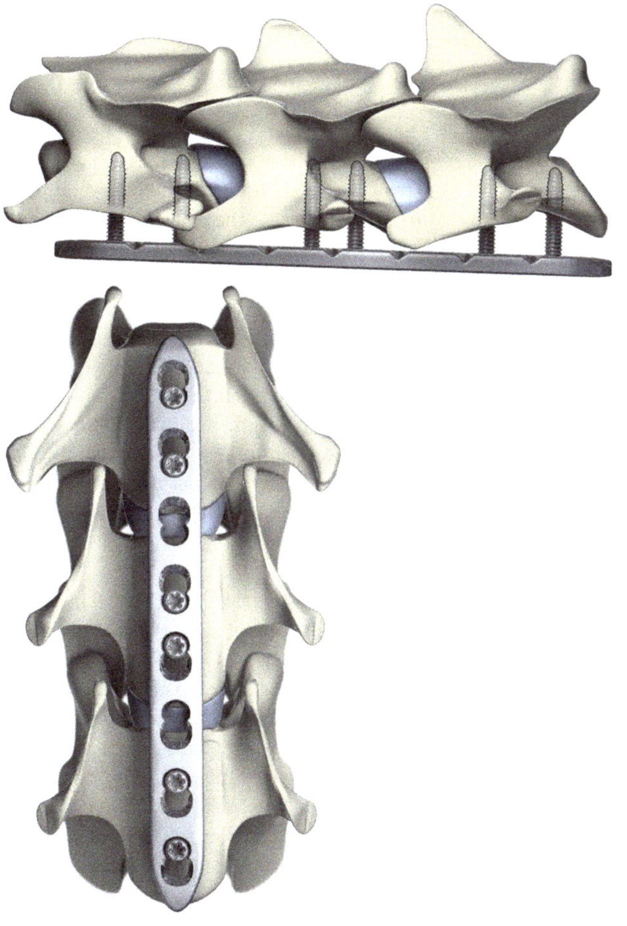

Figure 25.6 A locking compression plate (LCP) is applied to the ventral aspect of the cervical spine with monocortical screw fixation.

placed into the bone near the endplate on both sides of a disc space. While they are available in different lengths and sizes, their primary application has been for cervical spondylomyelopathy rather than cervical vertebral column trauma.

Thoracolumbar Injury

Vertebral column trauma most commonly affects the thoracolumbar spine, with a high incidence of injury at the thoracolumbar junction. Fractures or luxations of the cranial thoracic spine are rare due to the inherent stability and protection afforded by the musculature of thoracic limbs and rib cage. The natural lever arm of the lumbar spine against the less mobile thoracic spine creates a stress riser at the thoracolumbar junction.

Hyperflexion injuries are overrepresented, leading to caudal endplate fractures and luxations at the affected disc space. Rotational forces can lead to articular process fractures, while hyperextension can cause fractures of the vertebral lamina. Fractures of ribs and spinous and transverse processes, while not affecting the spinal cord directly, must be taken as evidence of significant trauma and initiate a thorough evaluation of the integrity of the affected vertebral column.

Anatomical Considerations

The anatomy of thoracic vertebrae poses several challenges to instrumentation. The articular processes become less distinct in the cranial thoracic vertebrae and rib head articulations obscure

Table 25.1 Recommended insertion angles and landmarks for bicortical spinal implants.

Location	Insertion angle from vertical	Landmarks for insertion
T10	22° (20–25°)	Tubercle of ribs and base of accessory process
T11	28° (25–35°)	
T12	30.5° (25–35°)	
T13	44.5° (40–45°)	
L1–L6	60° (55–65°)	Junction between pedicle and transverse process

Source: Watine et al. [5].

part of the lamina. Bone stock for implants is limited to the generally small and narrow vertebral body. Rib head disarticulation can be performed if needed for improved implant position. Alternatively, ribs may be utilized for certain types of fixation methods such as cerclage wiring to augment spinal stapling. The approach has to consider the thoracic cavity and the possible creation of an iatrogenic pneumothorax. If the pleural space is opened, air can often be evacuated in conjunction with closure of the surgical site via a large-gauge over-the-needle catheter or temporary chest tube. Lumbar vertebrae have distinct articular, transverse, and accessory processes, which provide helpful anatomical landmarks for implantation. General guidelines for insertion angles and landmarks for traditional bicortical implants are available (Table 25.1) but should be supplemented with CT images of the individual patient [5]. While the larger insertion angle for lumbar vertebrae (60° from vertical) provide maximum bone purchase based on imaging studies, this angle is challenging to achieve with a standard open approach due to soft tissue interference. Often the angle is reduced to 30–45° to accommodate musculature without dramatic loss of bone purchase.

Positioning and Approach

For a standard dorsal approach, the patient is positioned in ventral recumbency and a bean bag and suction are used to maintain a straight body position. Additionally, tape can be used to further improve patient stability. It is important to maintain the spine as straight as possible to allow proper angling of pins into the vertebral column. A liberal standard dorsal approach to the affected thoracic or lumbar segments is performed. If the integrity of the vertebral canal has been compromised, extra caution must be employed to avoid inadvertent iatrogenic injury during elevation of the musculature. The approach must reach ventral enough to expose the rib heads of the thoracic vertebrae or the base of the transverse processes of the lumbar vertebrae to observe pertinent landmarks and aid in implant placement.

Implant Selection

Implant size is based on vertebral pedicle width and vertebral body dimensions. Vertebrae of large dogs typically accept 3.5 mm screws or ⅛ inch pins, while smaller dogs usually require 2.7 mm screws or 3/32 inch pins. Depending on the implant type, the surgeon has a certain degree of freedom with implant sizes, for example when using a pin–PMMA construct in a large-breed dog, ⅛ inch pins can be placed for the main fixation with additional 3/32 inch pins. In screw constructs, cortical screws are preferred over cancellous screws owing to their larger core and increased stiffness. In the PMMA construct, positive-profile end-threaded pins are recommended for improved pull-out resistance [6]. Pins with a blunt tip may reduce the risk of injury to adjacent soft tissues. Fixation pins are preferred over screws in a PMMA construct as their larger core diameter affords them increased stiffness [7]. The pin–PMMA construct also offers more insertion freedom in areas of challenging anatomy that may not lend themselves well to implants with fixed insertion angle such as locking plates. Conversely, plate fixation has a much lower implant profile, eliminating the need for soft tissue resection to accommodate PMMA and allowing normal closure of the surgical site. Also, removal of implants is significantly easier when PMMA is not used.

Depending on the type of injury (luxation versus fracture) and degree of instability, fixation may be limited to one adjacent vertebra cranially and caudally (inherently stable fracture or luxation) or include two on each side of the injury (unstable fracture or luxation). Fixation can be performed unilaterally or bilaterally depending on desired degree of stiffness, anatomical considerations, or the selected implant type (i.e., the use of a locking plate with predetermined screw holes may require bilateral plate placement to engage a sufficient number of screws per segment).

Reduction

Thoracolumbar fractures caused by hyperextension typically present with ventral and possibly cranial subluxation of the affected caudal vertebral segment. Reduction is aimed at reducing the subluxation and improving alignment. Point-to-point reduction forceps can be clamped on spinous processes to apply careful dorsal and slight caudal traction of the caudal segment until alignment appears normal. Manipulation must be performed with care so as not to further damage the spinal cord. Chronic injuries tend to be challenging to reduce and one has to weigh the benefits of reduction against the potential for further spinal cord damage. In a patient with mild subluxation on preoperative imaging, manipulation can aid in assessing overall stability of the injured intervertebral articulation. If articular processes are intact, a small K-wire can be placed transarticularly across the dorsal lamina into both facet joints to help maintain reduction and offer additional anchorage if PMMA fixation is used. Landmarks for transarticular pin insertion should be determined on preoperative CT to ensure that the K-wire is positioned in the dorsal lamina and does not violate the vertebral canal. The ends of this K-wire are gently bent to avoid migration. If embedded into PMMA the ends should protrude far enough to allow incorporation into cement. If reduction is not easily achieved by gentle manipulation, a transarticular K-wire may not suffice to maintain reduction throughout the procedure; manual reduction with forceps may be required until implants have been applied.

Bicortical Pin and PMMA Fixation

Based on preoperative CT planning, insertion points for each pin are confirmed using recognizable landmarks and other measurements. A goniometer is used to measure the predetermined angle of pin insertion for that particular pin. Once location and angle are satisfactory, a drill bit of appropriate size is used to predrill for subsequent pin placement. Predrilling is essential to avoid thermal bone necrosis and premature pin loosening. During drilling attention is paid to maintaining the desired angle of insertion, while both cortices are drilled (Figure 25.7). A drill bit with a sharp point at the tip (StickTite™; IMEX Vet Inc., Longview, TX) can be beneficial to avoid drill bit slippage on the often steep outer cortical surface during initial drilling. In larger dogs, once the cis-cortex has been drilled, a small K-wire or other straight probe can be used as a pedicle feeler to probe the pin path within vertebral pedicle. The angle of the probe should reflect the planned insertion angle as long as presurgical planning for insertion landmark and angle were done appropriately. Because of the proximity of major vessels ventrolaterally to the thoracolumbar spine, the drill bit should not be advanced further once the trans-cortex has been penetrated. A drill stop can be used to avoid over-penetration. The length of the fixation pin is determined by measuring the length of the drill hole with a depth gauge (Figure 25.7). Depth gauge length should be similar to depth measure on preoperative CT images as long as pin location and insertion angles are similar. The depth gauge can also be used to probe the walls of the drill hole. Intact bone should be felt in every direction when probing. Pins can be marked with sterile marker or carefully notched to identify to which point they will be inserted. Large dogs may require extended-length positive-profile pins to allow threads to engage along the entire length of vertebral body bone. Slow-power insertion of the pin is then performed to the predetermined depth. The entire trocar or blunt tip of the pin should be advanced to ensure full engagement of the threaded portion within the trans-cortex (Figure 25.7).

The remaining pins are planned, predrilled, and placed in a similar manner. Each pin will have its individual insertion landmarks and angles, and insertion depth may vary. Orientation of pins can center around the injury (cranial pins inserted in a caudal to cranial direction, caudal pins inserted in a cranial to caudal direction) to decrease the overall area of cement coverage. Pins do not need to be bent unless incorporation into bone cement is difficult due to the insertion angle. Bending pins can be challenging due to limited space and has the potential for pin loosening and iatrogenic bone damage; it should be considered carefully prior to performing. Pins are cut short, with 15–20 mm of pin protruding from the bone to be incorporated into bone cement. Notching of the protruding pin ends is often not necessary as pins are generally placed in slightly different angles, making cement loosening around the pins unlikely. Notching can otherwise be carefully performed with pin cutters. In cases where the threaded portion of the pin extends into the PMMA, notching is not necessary. Muscles must be sufficiently reflected and Gelpi retractors adjusted to allow removal after PMMA has been applied. At times, some muscle may have to be resected to allow room for PMMA. Reduction forceps can be used to maintain the unstable intervertebral articulation in proper position while PMMA is applied and has hardened. If intact, transarticular K-wires can aid with reduction (Figure 25.8).

Twenty grams of PMMA are mixed to a smooth, slightly runny liquid and poured into a 35-mL catheter tip syringe to facilitate application around the pins. The PMMA is then applied around the base of each pin, building upwards to cover the pin ends. Ideally the PMMA should be in the putty phase when applied around the pins when it is still soft but will not spread and leak easily. During application Freer elevators are used to keep the PMMA in the desired location. PMMA is applied in uniform thickness around and between all pins. Application has to be done efficiently to avoid hardening of cement in the syringe; however, if PMMA is applied when too liquid, it is challenging to maintain cement around the pin ends appropriately. If a bilateral configuration is chosen, two rows of PMMA are applied (depending on the size of the animal, 40 mg of PMMA may need to be utilized). Antimicrobials are not routinely added to PMMA used for vertebral column fixation.

During curing of PMMA the surgical site is lavaged to decrease thermal injury to soft tissues. Gelpi retractors are carefully removed. The fascial layer is closed where apposition is possible. Typically,

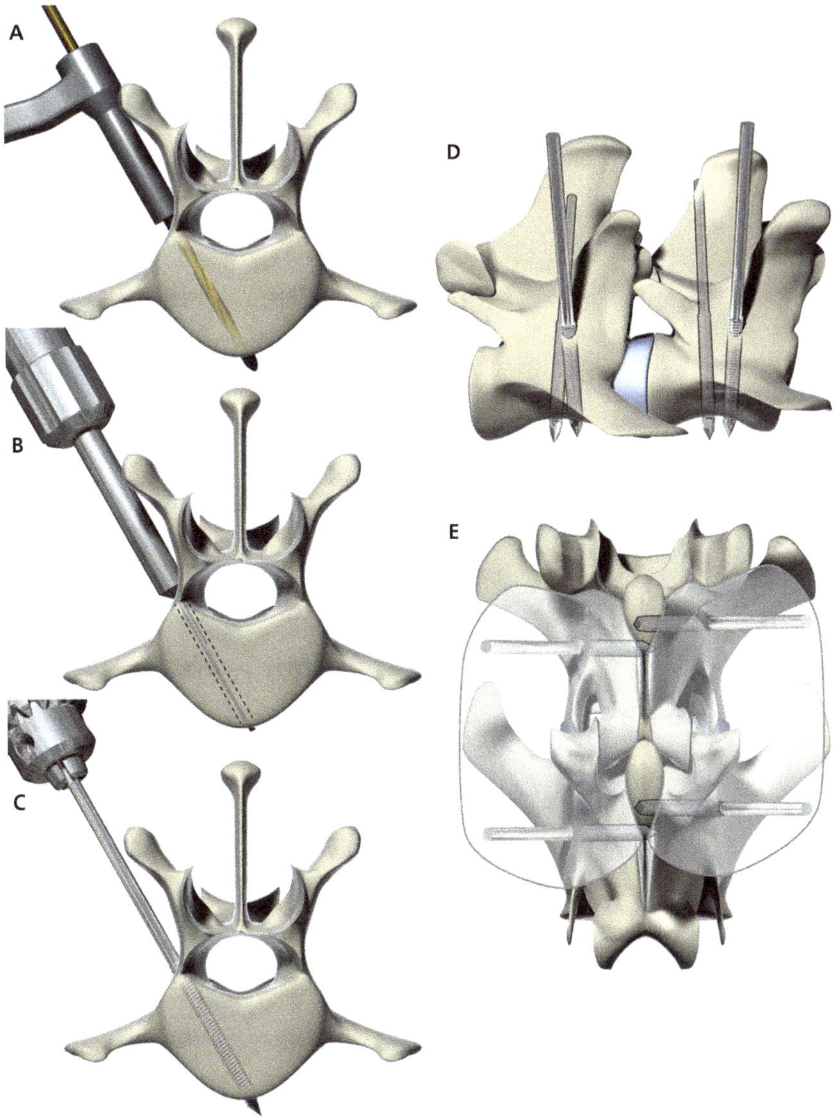

Figure 25.7 Proper application of a positive-profile pin in bicortical fashion in a lumbar vertebra. (A) The vertebral body is predrilled using predetermined anatomical landmarks and insertion angle. Care must be taken to avoid excessive advancement of the drill bit once the trans-cortex has been perforated. (B) A depth gauge is used to determine corridor length and to probe the integrity of the drilled canal. (C) A positive-profile fixation pin with sufficient thread length is placed using slow-speed power insertion. Insertion depth is based on previous depth-gauge measurements. (D) Four bicortical pins have been placed. The number and location of pins can vary depending on the type and degree of injury. (E) Protruding pins on each side of the vertebral column have been incorporated into PMMA.

muscle closure is not possible over the PMMA. Subcutaneous layers are closed diligently to provide soft tissue coverage of PMMA.

Vertebral Plate Fixation

Locking plates such as the SOP plate or the LCP do not require excessive plate contouring in order to ensure sufficient plate-bone contact for friction. Instead the locking mechanism allows these plates to be applied relatively straight along the vertebral column with acceptable distance between the bone and the plate (Figure 25.9). Failure of these implants generally occurs via shearing of the screws or by screw pull-out rather than by plate failure. Small dogs and cats usually accept 2.7 mm screws and plates, whereas medium and larger dogs require 3.5 mm implants. Screw insertion angle and implant corridor are the same as for pin fixation. Because of the predetermined screw hole locations within the plate, the plate size and type will determine the number of screws that can be placed per vertebra. Most plates are placed across two cranial and two caudal vertebrae in relation to the injury to provide sufficient screw numbers and avoid screw placement into the intervertebral disc space or near the intervertebral foramen. Bilateral plate fixation is also common to allow more freedom with screw placement and increase construct stiffness [8].

External Skeletal Fixation

Application of external skeletal fixation (ESF) to the vertebral column can be performed via an open approach or closed approach with fluoroscopic guidance. Closed pin application has been shown to lead to improved bone purchase and decreased injury to paravertebral vasculature [9]. Insertion angles can be adjusted more horizontally with closed application as pins are not placed in the confines of an open approach with impeding musculature. Pins are placed bilaterally, typically one pin per vertebra and spanning two vertebrae cranial and caudal to the injury. Externally, pins are connected to carbon fiber arches, which are interconnected to form a stable framework. One of the main benefits of vertebral column ESF is the ability of implant removal without a second large surgery. On the downside, ESF requires good owner compliance and daily care, and may put limitations on certain aspects of postoperative rehabilitation.

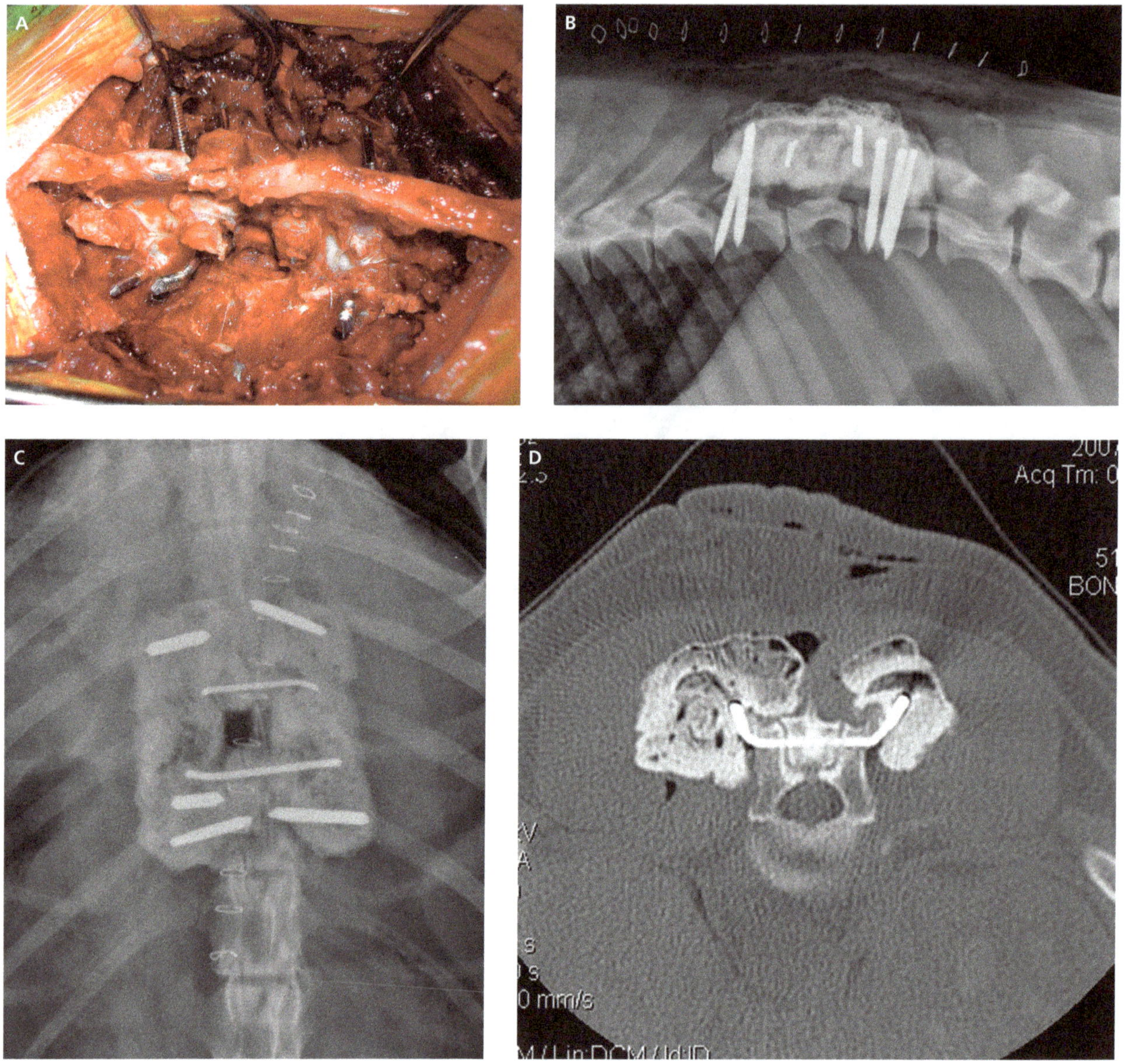

Figure 25.8 Case example: a 3-year-old female Dalmatian suffered from an unstable T11 fracture/luxation after running into a tree. (A) Intraoperative image showing a right-sided T11 partial pediculectomy performed; transarticular pins have been placed across the T10–T11 and T11–T12 articular facets and positive-profile fixation pins are in place. (B, C) Postoperative lateral (B) and dorsoventral (C) radiographs of the same Dalmatian showing the bicortical pin/PMMA fixation and two transarticular K-wires. (D) Axial CT showing one of the transarticular K-wires. Both ends of the wire were bent and incorporated into the PMMA.

Spinal Stapling

This construct is only used in small dogs and cats with vertebral column injuries that are inherently stable and are expected to heal relatively quickly [10]. A K-wire or Steinmann pin of appropriate size for the patient is contoured to act as a staple around spinous processes spanning the site of injury. Typically, three vertebrae cranial and caudal to the injury are included in the staple. The Steinmann pin or K-wire acts as an internal splint and prevents excessive range of motion; however, it does not eliminate motion at the affected space. In smaller patients, a single K-wire can be anchored directly through the base of the most caudal spinous process and bent acutely to incorporate the remaining processes cranially. In most patients, however, either one or two Steinmann pins are applied around the base of the spinous processes. With two pins, each end is contoured with an acute angle to hook around a spinous process. Fixation of the Steinmann pins is achieved by drilling small holes through the base of the spinous processes, feeding individual loops of cerclage wire through each hole, and tightening these around the Steinmann pins. While the use of two pins makes application easier, it also allows the pins to be distracted with flexion of the spine as they are not rigidly connected. Distraction can be avoided if a single Steinmann pin can be contoured at both ends to fit snugly around both the cranial and caudal spinous processes (Figure 25.10). While precontouring is essential and time-saving, intraoperative adjustments are often needed to perfect the tight fit of the Steinmann staple.

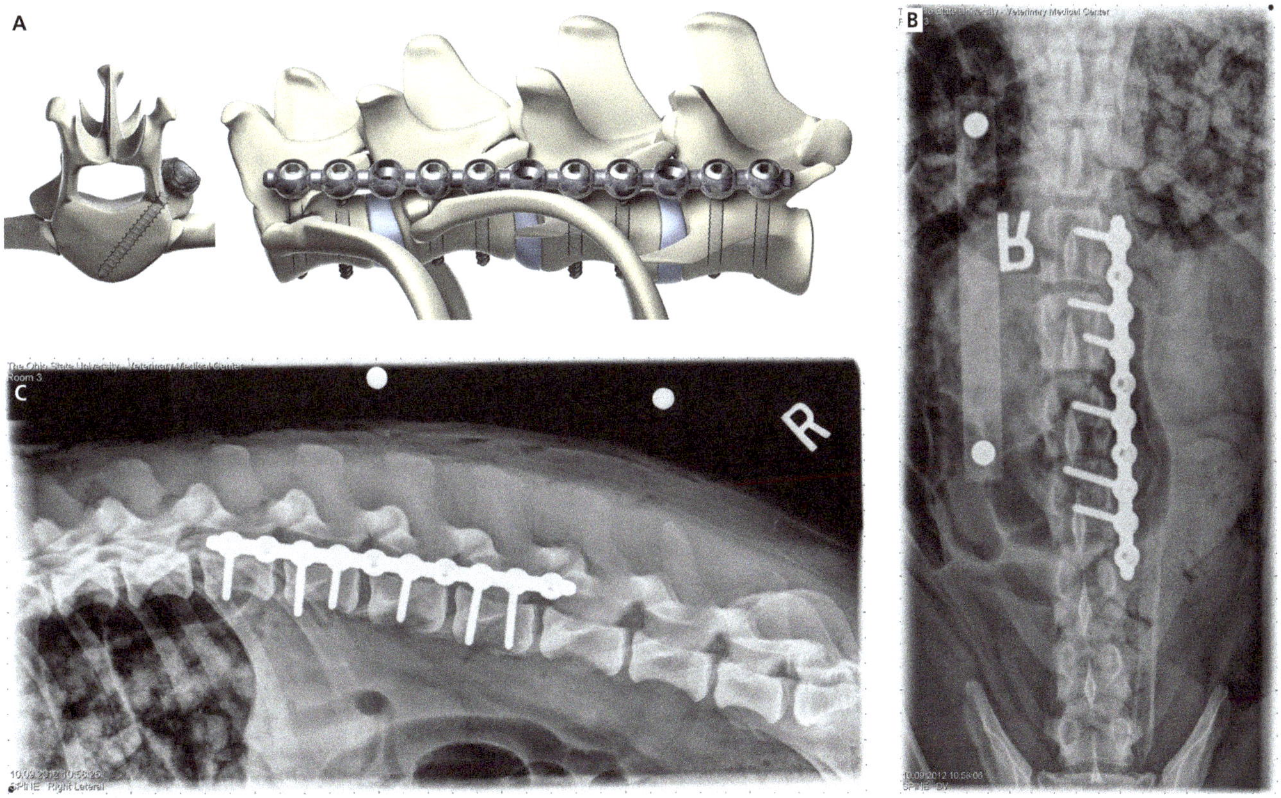

Figure 25.9 (A) Unilateral String of Pearls (SOP) plate application to the thoracolumbar spine. Note that the position of the plate depends on the insertion angle of the screws as these plates have an angle-fixed screw locking mechanism. To avoid placement of screws into the intervertebral disc space, not all plate holes are filled with screws. (B, C) Orthogonal radiographs of a dog with a lumbar SOP plate fixation.

Additional fixation can be achieved by carefully looping cerclage wire around rib heads or the base of transverse processes and connecting to the staple (Figure 25.11).

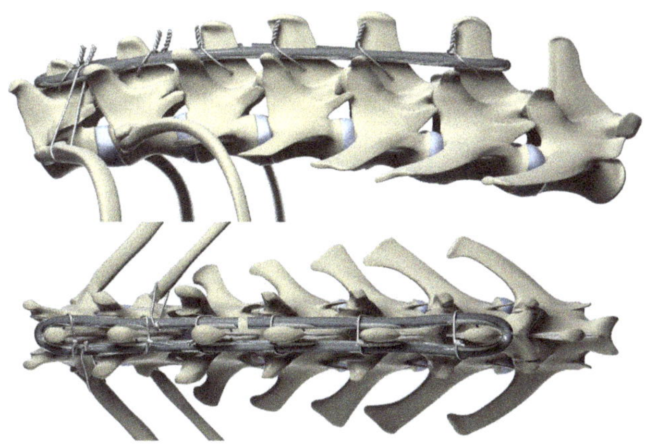

Figure 25.10 Application of a spinal staple to the thoracolumbar spine. A single Steinmann pin is contoured to snugly fit around the most cranial and caudal spinous processes of six vertebrae. Cerclage wires through the base of the spinous processes anchor the Steinmann pin in location. Additional cerclage wires around adjacent rib heads help maintain stability of the staple.

Lumbosacral Injuries

Fracture of the caudal endplate of L7 with ventral subluxation of the sacrum is the most common injury affecting the lumbosacral articulation in the dog. This injury is the result of severe hyperflexion and compression forces, typically due to a high-energy vehicular trauma. Concurrent injuries such as pelvic fractures and abdominal organ trauma are common. Vertebral column injury may also not be restricted to the lower lumbar spine and lumbosacral space but additional trauma can be present at the sacrococcygeal joint or tail.

Anatomical Considerations

Approaches are limited to dorsal and dorsolateral due to the presence of the ilial wings and sacroiliac joints. The articular processes at the lumbosacral articulation are very large and important stabilizers of this portion of the spine. The pedicle of L7 is also wider than that of the other lumbar vertebrae, allowing for more perpendicular implant placement with sufficient bone purchase. The sacrum is wide and flat with limited target bone for rigid fixation. Care must be taken to avoid injury to the cauda equina within the vertebral canal and exiting nerve roots within the intervertebral foramina. Insertion angles for L7 and S1 range between 0 and 20° from vertical. Insertion landmark for L7 is just caudal to the base of the cranial articular process. If pins are angled, insertion should begin more lateral to the base of the cranial articular process. Insertion landmark for S1 is the fossa just caudal to the cranial articular process.

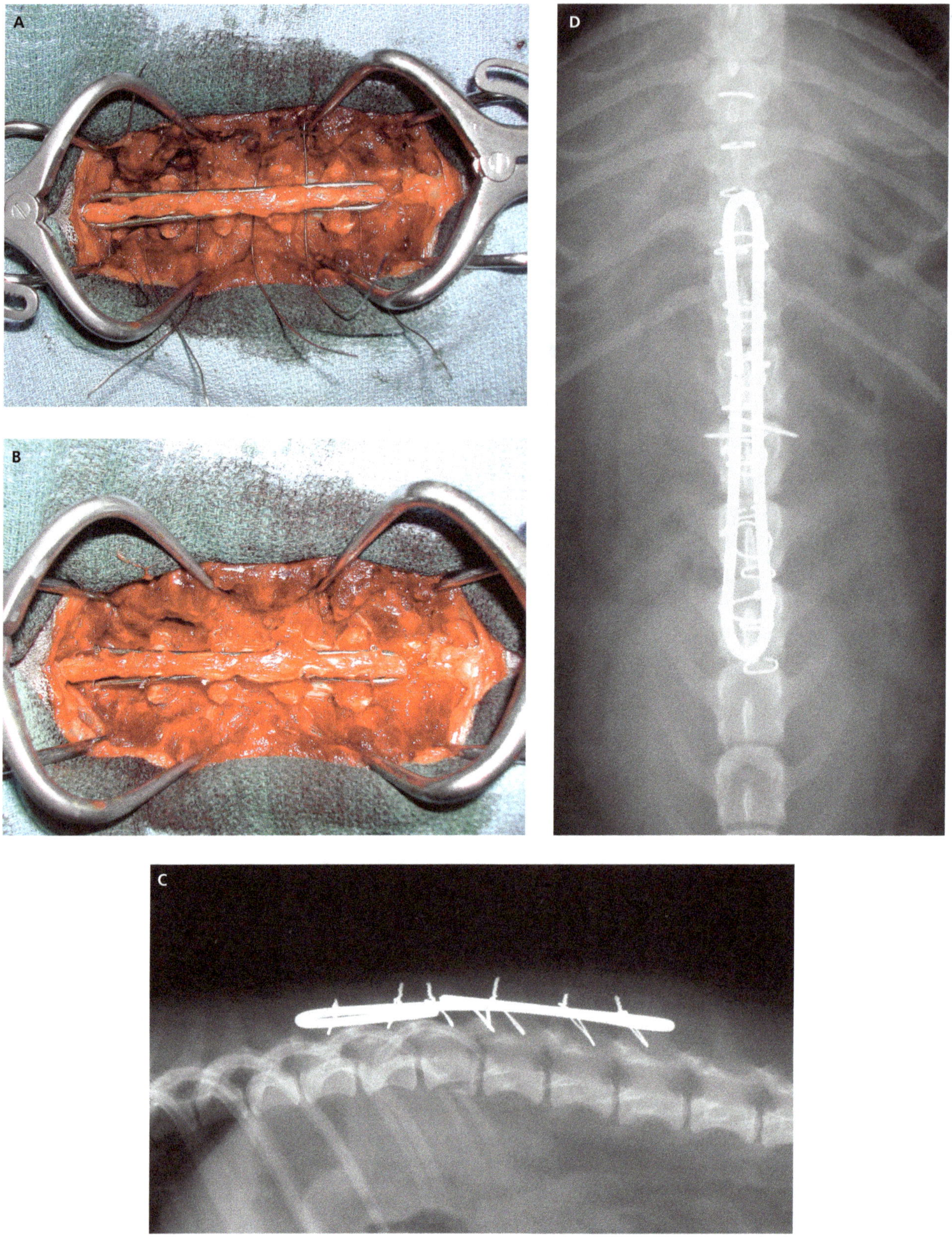

Figure 25.11 Case example: an 8-year-old male neutered Chihuahua presented for a fracture/luxation of L1–L2. (A, B) Intraoperative photographs of the Steinmann pin fitted around six spinous processes. Fixation cerclage wires have been placed through the base of the spinous processes (A) and are tightened around the Steinmann pin (B). (C, D) Postoperative radiographs showing the spinal staple in place. Additionally, two small K-wires have been placed transarticularly at L1–L2 to aid temporary reduction while the spinal staple was placed.

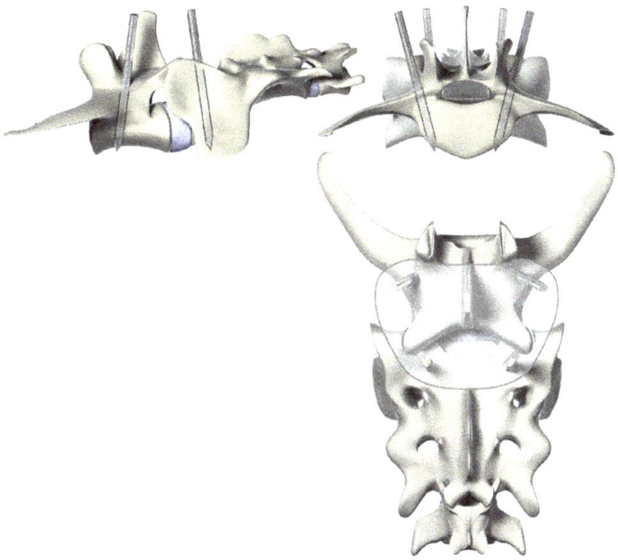

Figure 25.12 Pin and PMMA fixation of the lumbosacral articulation. Bicortical positive-profile fixation pins have been placed into L7 and S1. Note the insertion landmark for L7 caudal and a little lateral to the base of the cranial articular process; the insertion landmark for S1 is within the slight fossa just caudal to the cranial sacral articular process.

Positioning and Approach

The patient is positioned in sternal recumbency and the lumbosacral vertebral column is maintained in a neutral position. Towels are used to elevate and support the pelvis, allowing the pelvic limbs to be positioned in flexion with less extreme abduction of the coxofemoral joints. It is beneficial to place the animal's tail at the end of the surgical table to allow access caudal to the spine as well as on each side. Tape and additional bean bags can be used to maintain the patient in a straight position. A liberal standard dorsal approach to the lumbosacral space is performed.

Implant Selection

The lumbosacral joint is considered a high motion joint within the confines of vertebral column mobility. A large fulcrum is created between the lumbar spine and the pelvis. Implants must be strong enough to counteract this motion, especially flexion. Many implants ultimately fail by shearing of screws or pins or loosening/breaking out of bone, although fracture healing and successful outcome are usually not affected by implant failure. The amount of instability and length of time required for healing must guide the decision-making about implant strength. Transarticular fixation, while the least technically demanding, provides limited stability and often fails by screw loosening or fracture of the processes. Pins or screws and PMMA are more versatile and can incorporate transarticular fixation and even fixation points within the ilial wings. Positive-profile pins are preferred over screws as their larger core diameter affords increased stiffness. Regular fixation plates are disadvantageous as they must be contoured perfectly and are being increasingly replaced by locking plates.

Reduction

Bone reduction forceps can be anchored to the spinous processes and used to improve alignment of the lumbosacral injury. Chronic fracture/subluxations are difficult to reduce and sometimes stabilization has to be performed in light of poor alignment. If reduction can be achieved, temporary or permanent transarticular pins or screws can be placed to help maintain position and free up space for definitive stabilization. If reduction cannot be achieved and subluxation causes compression of the cauda equina by the sacral lamina, a partial dorsal laminectomy can be carefully performed to remove the compressing bone.

Another anchor point for reduction forceps are the ilial wings, which can provide a larger area for instruments to attach to and manipulate the sacrum.

Pins or Screws and PMMA

Insertion angle and landmarks are reviewed and adjusted based on patient-specific anatomy. Positive-profile pins are preferred over cortical screws due to their superior stiffness. Most medium to large dogs will accept ⅛ inch pins or 3.5 mm cortical screws. Principles of application are the same as for thoracolumbar implants. L7 and S1 pins can be slightly angled in a cranial and caudal direction to bring the protruding pin portions into closer proximity for PMMA application (Figure 25.12). If needed, pins can be bent carefully toward the L7–S1 disc space to improve pin incorporation into the cement; however, great care should be taken during bending to avoid damage to the pin–bone interface. To further augment the fixation, pins can be added into the ilium and incorporated into the PMMA. Ilial body pins have been used instead of sacral pins for L7–S1 injuries [11]. Likewise, transarticular fixation or pins in L6 can be added to the construct if indicated.

Transarticular Fixation

Transarticular pins or screws at the lumbosacral joint can provide some degree of stability but are prone to loosening or failure. Long-term stability can be improved by achieving arthrodesis between the articulations. For this, cartilage is removed by pneumatic drill or curettage and fresh cancellous bone graft or substitute is placed into the articulation. Insertion point on L7 is the mid-body of the caudal articular process with direction across the facet joint into the sacral articular process. The sacroiliac joint is not included. Most screws are oriented approximately 45° in the craniodorsal to caudoventral and 30° in the dorsomedial to ventrolateral plane (Figure 25.13).

Locking Plates

Contouring plates to conform to the anatomy of the vertebral column is challenging. Locking plates allow screw heads to be locked into the plate and do not rely on perfect contouring and friction with the bone to sustain stable implants. Because of the locking mechanism, these plates can also be used with monocortical screw fixation.

Another benefit is their low profile, allowing for improved soft tissue closure. Locking screws are angle fixed and adjustment of screw position can only be achieved by changing the contour of the plate. Generally, the less these plates are contoured, the better. Safe implant corridors are the same as for other lumbosacral fixation methods. To ensure sufficient number of fixation points, two plates are used, one on each side of the spinous processes, with each plate having one screw in L7 and one screw in S1 (Figure 25.14).

Postoperative Imaging Assessment

Standard orthogonal radiographs are obtained to assess alignment of the vertebral column and general implant placement. While radiographs have been found inadequate to assess implant violation

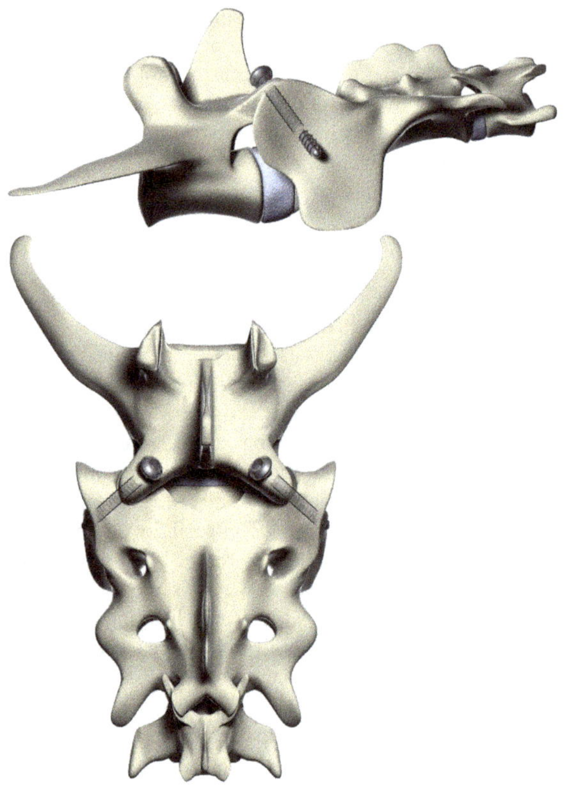

Figure 25.13 Transarticular screws have been placed across the large L7–S1 articular facets. Prior to instrumentation the articular cartilage would be debrided and a bone graft placed to encourage arthrodesis. Note that the ideal screw orientation for maximal purchase is 45° in the craniodorsal to caudoventral plane and 30° in the dorsomedial to ventrolateral plane.

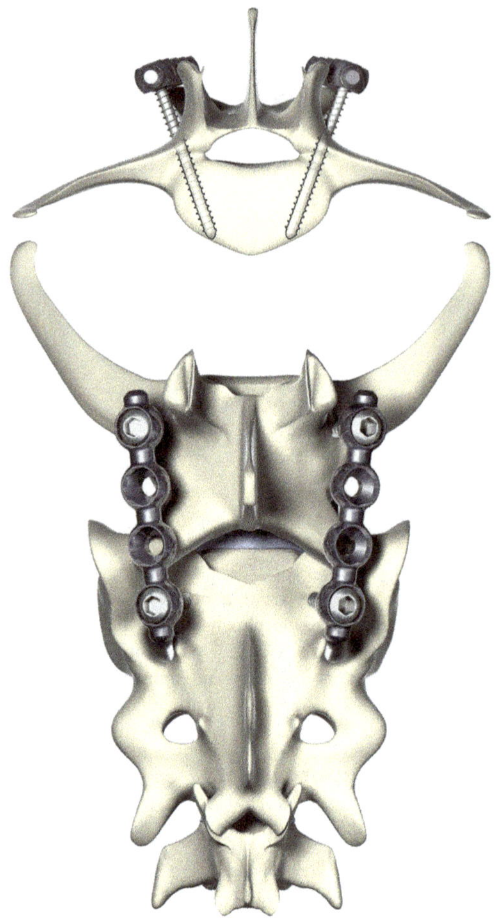

Figure 25.14 Two String of Pearls™ (SOP) plates have been applied to the dorsal surface of L7–S1 with one screw of each plate engaging L7 and S1. Insertion landmarks and angles are the same as for pin fixation.

into the canal, they serve an important role as a baseline evaluation tool for long-term follow-up [12]. Postoperative CT is performed to determine the actual position of implants in relation to the vertebral canal and length of screw or pin penetration past the trans-cortex. Accuracy of CT in determining canal violation is excellent, allowing prompt identification of inappropriately placed pins or screws (i.e., violating the canal or intervertebral foramen, or insufficient bone purchase due to lateralization of implant). While it is uncommon to replace mildly malpositioned implants once identified on CT, the knowledge gained is beneficial for future stabilization procedures. Stainless steel implants, which are to date the most commonly used, create prohibitive artifacts on MRI, eliminating this modality for postoperative evaluation of the instrumented site.

Complications

Because of the proximity of important neurovascular structures and the anatomical restrictions of the vertebral column, iatrogenic injury to spinal cord, nerve roots, vascular supply, and intervertebral discs are possible. Thorough and precise preoperative planning with proper translation at the surgical table should decrease the potential for catastrophic complications. Postoperative imaging, while not preventing iatrogenic damage, is a valuable tool for subsequent surgeries as it provides immediate feedback about what went well and not so well during a recent procedure.

If implant placement is appropriate, and bony alignment and apposition are acceptable, postoperative complications are most often due to implant failure or infection. Implant loosening and failure may be due to inappropriately sized or placed fixation, poor bone-holding properties, or excess patient mobility after surgery. Catastrophic implant failure is usually due to poor decision-making regarding type and size of fixation. Infection is less likely due to intraoperative contamination but more to hematogenous spread of bacteria. Appropriate perioperative antimicrobials should be administered to decrease risk of contamination from the skin. Providing a course of therapeutic antimicrobials after a clean surgery is controversial and should be decided on a case-by-case basis.

Seroma formation can occur despite meticulous dead-space closure. Warm compresses and time are usually sufficient to resolve these and repeated aspiration should be avoided due to the risk of iatrogenic contamination. Because of the resection of lumbar musculature and possible muscle atrophy around the PMMA fixation of thoracolumbar injuries, the PMMA can often be palpated and may be displeasing to owners who should be educated about this possibility.

Appropriate stabilization of vertebral column injuries should lead to fracture healing and stable fibrosis of luxations. Long-term complications may include stable nonunion, malalignment, granuloma formation, and chronic pain from low subclinical implant loosening or infection. When stability is deemed appropriate, implants can be removed if necessary. With the exception of external skeletal vertebral column fixation, implants generally remain in place if they are not causing problems.

Video clips to accompany this book can be found on the companion website at:
www.wiley.com/go/shores/neurosurgery

References

1 Shores A. Spinal trauma. Pathophysiology and management of traumatic spinal injuries. *Vet Clin North Am Small Anim Pract* 1992;22:859–888.

2 Agnello KA, Kapatkin AS, Garcia TC, Hayashi K, Welihozkiy AT, Stover SM. Intervertebral biomechanics of locking compression plate monocortical fixation of the canine cervical spine. *Vet Surg* 2010;39:991–1000.

3 Hettlich BF, Allen MJ, Pascetta D, Fosgate GT, Litsky TS. Biomechanical comparison between bicortical pin and monocortical screw/polymethymethacrylate constructs in the cadaveric canine cervical vertebral column. *Vet Surg* 2013;42:693–700.

4 Voss K, Steffen F, Montavon PM. Use of the ComPact UniLock System for ventral stabilization procedures of the cervical spine: a retrospective study. *Vet Comp Orthop Traumatol* 2006;19:21–28.

5 Watine S, Cabassu JP, Catheland S, Brochier L, Ivanoff S. Computed tomography study of implantation corridors in canine vertebrae. *J Small Anim Pract* 2006;47: 651–657.

6 Sandman KM, Smith CW, Harari J, Manfra Marretta S, Pijanowski GJ, Schaeffer DJ. Comparison of pull-out resistance of Kirschner wires and Imex (TM) miniature interface fixation half pins in polyurethane foam. *Vet Comp Orthop Traumatol* 2002;15:18–22.

7 Garcia JNP, Milthorpe BK, Russell D, Johnson KA, et al., Biomechanical study of canine spinal fracture fixation using pins or bone screws with polymethylmethacrylate. *Vet Surg* 1994;23:322–329.

8 Mckee WM, Downes CJ. Vertebral stabilisation and selective decompression for the management of triple thoracolumbar disc protrusions. *J Small Animal Pract* 2008;49:536–539.

9 Wheeler JL, Lewis DD, Cross AR, Sereda CW. Closed fluoroscopic-assisted spinal arch external skeletal fixation for the stabilization of vertebral column injuries in five dogs. *Vet Surg* 2007;36:442–448.

10 Voss K, Montavon PM. Tension band stabilization of fractures and luxations of the thoracolumbar vertebrae in dogs and cats: 38 cases (1993–2002). *J Am Vet Med Assoc* 2004;225:78–83.

11 Weh JM, Kraus KH. Use of a four pin and methylmethacrylate fixation in L7 and the iliac body to stabilize lumbosacral fracture-luxations: a clinical and anatomic study. *Vet Surg* 2007;36:775–782.

12 Hettlich BF, Fosgate GT, Levine JM et al. Accuracy of conventional radiography and computed tomography in predicting implant position in relation to the vertebral canal in dogs. *Vet Surg* 2010;39:680–687.

26 Lumbosacral Decompression and Foraminotomy

Trevor Bebchuk

Pathophysiology

Degenerative lumbosacral stenosis (DLSS), also known as cauda equina disease or syndrome and lumbosacral compression, is a common cause of pain and pelvic limb dysfunction in dogs [1–5]. It may be especially prevalent among military working dogs [6]. The clinical signs, including difficulty rising and going up and down stairs, reluctance to jump and, in some cases, neurological deficiencies of the pelvic limb(s), are primarily a result of compression of the cauda equina, the seventh lumbar nerve (L7), and vascular supply to the cauda equina and nerve roots [1–5,7]. The disease occurs secondary to the high mobility at the lumbosacral joint primarily in dorsoventral flexion and extension but also in lateral flexion, extension and rotation. This mobility places a large amount of stress on the lumbosacral disc space as this is the connection between the relatively flexible lumbar spine and the rigid sacrum and pelvis. These forces are complex and concentrated on the connectors and stabilizers of the joint: the intervertebral disc (IVD), facetal synovial joints, dorsal and ventral longitudinal ligaments, interarcuate ligaments, interspinous ligaments, and perispinal fascia and muscles (Figure 26.1) [1–5,7–9]. In addition, the presence of anatomical malformations of the structures in the lumbosacral region (e.g., sacralization of the seventh lumbar vertebrae, lumborization of the first sacral vertebrae, malarticulation of the diarthrodial joints at the L7–S1 junction) can contribute to changes in the three-dimensional motion pattern of the lumbosacral junction. Even without these changes, there may be certain breeds that have an inherent abnormal motion pattern at L7–S1 [10,11]. While the exact pathophysiology and progression that leads to DLSS is unknown, it is thought to follow a specific sequence of events. Chronic repetitive microtrauma and aging causes the nucleus pulposus to desiccate, altering the shock-absorbing biomechanics of the IVD and leading to greater forces being absorbed by the annulus fibrosus. The annulus fibrosus subsequently weakens and develops small tears in the dorsal portion, allowing it to bulge within the spinal canal at L7 and S1, also known as IVD protrusion or Hansen type II disc disease [1–5,7–9,11–14]. These changes lead to or add to the instability at the lumbosacral space, resulting in subluxation of the vertebral endplates and facetal joints between L7 and S1. As a response to instability, the dorsal longitudinal ligament, the interarcuate ligaments, and the facetal synovial capsules hypertrophy. This instability also leads to new bone formation (spondylosis deformans) along the ventral aspect of the L7 and S1 vertebral endplates and facetal joints. Together, these changes cause compression of the

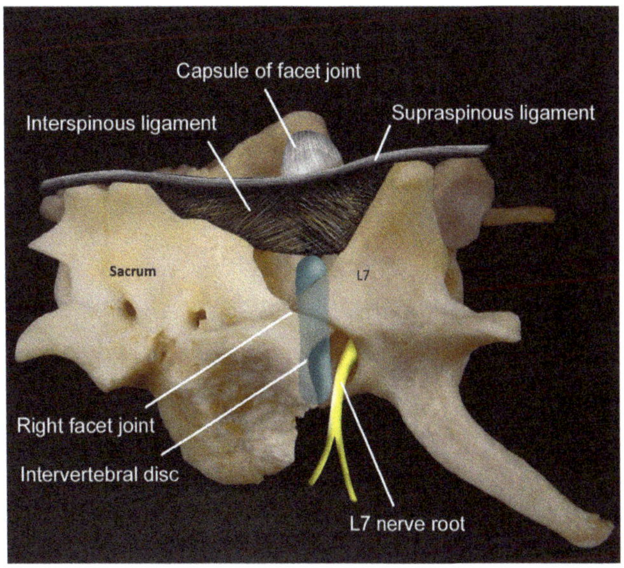

Figure 26.1 Schematic of the lumbosacral joint. Note the L7 nerve root exiting the intervertebral foramen and the proximity to both the intervertebral disc and the facetal joint. *Source*: Smith et al. [58].

Current Techniques in Canine and Feline Neurosurgery, First Edition. Edited by Andy Shores and Brigitte A. Brisson.
© 2017 John Wiley & Sons, Inc. Published 2017 by John Wiley & Sons, Inc.
Companion website: www.wiley.com/go/shores/neurosurgery

cauda equina and foraminal stenosis. The foramina are narrowed by facetal joint hypertrophy and spondylosis and the vertebral canal is narrowed ventrally by the bulging annulus and dorsal longitudinal ligament, and dorsally by the interarcuate ligaments [1–5,7,9,10]. As such, the compression of vascular and neural structures seen in DLSS can be caused by any or a number of the following: transitional and asymmetric vertebra, or hemivertebra at L7 or S1 [15–20]; sacral osteochondrosis [21–23]; subluxation of the sacral vertebral endplate relative to L7 [1–5]; subluxation of the L7–S1 facetal joints [1–5]; narrowing of the intervertebral foramen secondary to facetal joint hypertrophy [1–5], osteophytosis and ligamentous hypertrophy [5,7]; synovial cysts [5]; IVD protrusion [1–5]; narrowing of the spinal canal secondary to proliferation of the ligamentous structures such as the dorsal longitudinal ligament and interarcuate ligaments [1–5,7].

Diagnosis

The diagnosis of DLSS begins with a thorough history, and physical, orthopedic and neurological examinations. Electrodiagnostics [24,25], radiographic imaging, possibly with contrast studies and advanced imaging are also typically performed (see Chapter 7). Survey radiographs are useful but do not provide the information necessary for definitive diagnosis and treatment planning.

History and Clinical Signs

Pain is the most common sign of DLSS, resulting in varying degrees of pelvic limb gait abnormalities. Neurological signs generally occur as the condition progresses and can include proprioceptive deficits, mild paresis, loss of tail function, and incontinence [1–5,7,21]. Neurological deficits related to the sciatic nerve are most common and involve the caudal thigh muscles and those distal to the stifle. Compression of the pelvic and pudendal nerves can lead to urinary incontinence (lower motor neuron) and fecal incontinence secondary to poor anal sphincter tone [1–5,7].

Physical Examination Findings

A thorough orthopedic examination is essential to rule out hip dysplasia and cranial cruciate ligament rupture, which are common in breeds prone to DLSS. Some dogs have more than one disorder, which can complicate diagnosis. In addition, the neurological deficits seen with DLSS can resemble those seen with degenerative myelopathy. Genetic testing for degenerative myelopathy is advised before proceeding with an invasive treatment procedure since both conditions may exist concurrently.

Physical examination findings specific to DLSS include pain with extension of the pelvic limbs either individually or concurrently, pain with dorsiflexion of the tail until it is perpendicular to the lumbar spine or beyond (tail jack), pain elicited during the lordosis test, pain with rotation of the lumbosacral spine, and pain with direct palpation of the lumbosacral spine while the dog is supported or in lateral recumbency [1,7].

Radiography and Contrast Studies

While the ligamentous structures and the IVD are not visible on routine radiographs, these can demonstrate changes such as sacral subluxation, osteophyte formation at the facetal joints, ventral and lateral spondylosis deformans, and evidence of discospondylitis that support a diagnosis of DLSS (Figure 26.2) [26–30]. However, the presence of radiographic changes consistent with DLSS do not always correlate with clinical signs [31,32]. In contrast, the absence

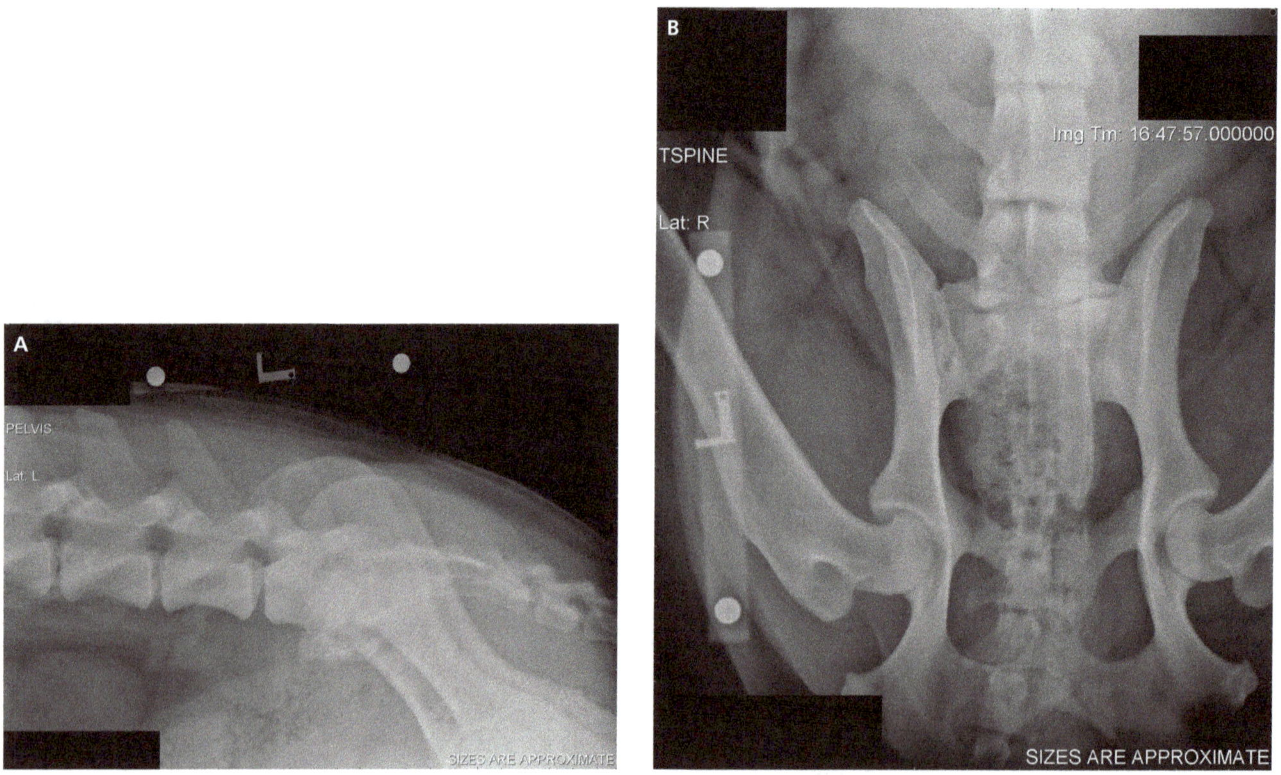

Figure 26.2 Lateral (A) and ventrodorsal (B) radiographic projections of a dog with DLSS showing facetal joint osteophytes, ventral spondylosis deformans, sclerosis of the vertebral endplates, and narrowing of the lumbosacral intervertebral space. *Source*: Courtesy of Dr. N. Fitzpatrick.

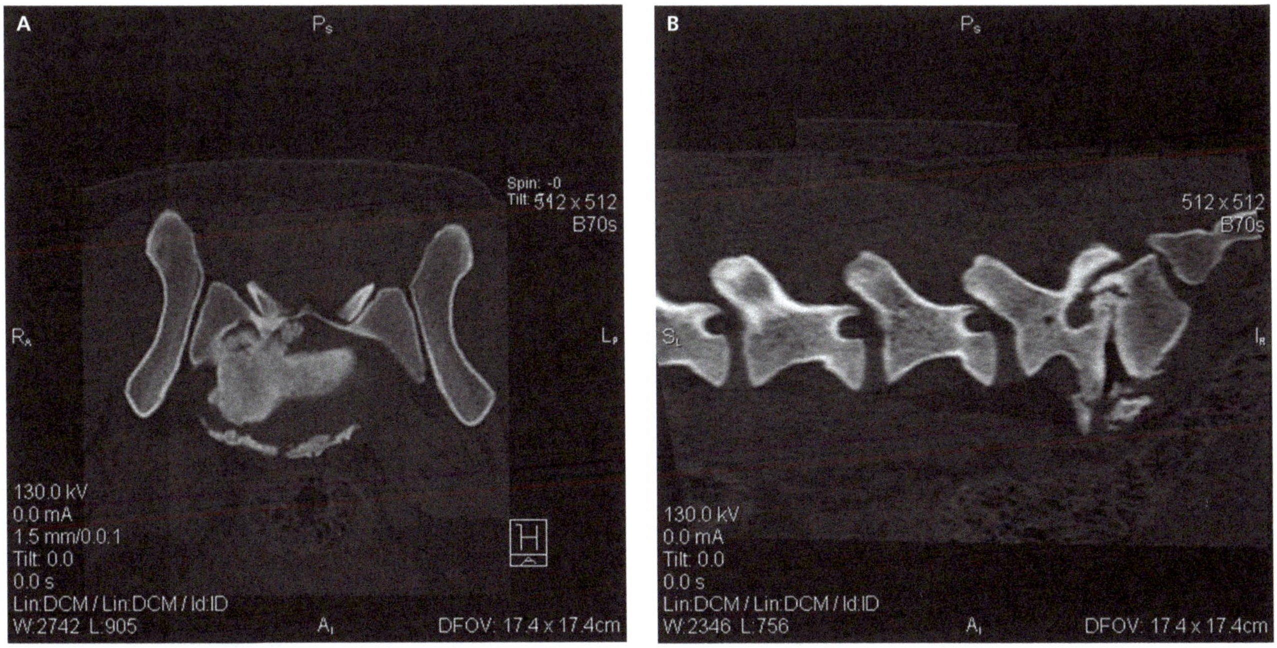

Figure 26.3 Axial (A) and sagittal (B) CT of a dog with DLSS showing intervertebral disc space collapse, intervertebral disc protruding into the vertebral canal and lateral recess of L7, as well as ventral spondylosis deformans and facetal joint osteophytes. Note the excellent bony definition and ability to evaluate disc protrusion but poor detail for evaluating the individual nerves of the cauda equina and other soft tissue structures. *Source*: Courtesy of Dr. N. Fitzpatrick.

of abnormality on routine radiographs does not preclude a diagnosis of DLSS as instability and stenosis can occur without bony changes. Routine radiography is also helpful in screening for other orthopedic abnormalities such as canine hip dysplasia.

Radiographic contrast studies are of little use in the diagnosis of DLSS. Myelography can provide a diagnosis in dogs with a dural sac that extends beyond the lumbosacral space but does not provide information regarding compression of the cauda equina [1–5,7,33–35]. Flexion-extension myelography can in some cases help to discern dynamic lesions [33]. Discography and epidurography have been described but they can be difficult to perform and interpret [33,35,36]. CT and MRI have become the gold standard for the diagnosis of DLSS.

Computed Tomography

CT allows visualization of sacral and facetal joint subluxation, vertebral canal stenosis, IVD hypertrophy, and dorsal longitudinal ligament hypertrophy. The L7 nerve root lateral recess and the L7–S1 intervertebral foramen are also visible on CT (Figure 26.3) [37–41]. Compared with MRI, CT is more readily available, requires a shorter anesthetic, and allows visualization of bone and mineralized soft tissues [41].

Magnetic Resonance Imaging

Soft tissues, both within and surrounding the spinal canal, are more discernible on MRI than CT [41]. Like CT, MRI allows for the collection of images in multiple planes but has distinct advantages over CT for assessing IVD degeneration and visualizing the cauda equina and L7 nerve roots. Using MRI, the L7 nerve root can be followed for its entire path out of the lateral recess and through the intervertebral foramen. Images obtained in flexion and extension are useful for demonstrating the changes in the soft tissue and intermittent stenosis that can occur with dynamic lesions (Figure 26.4) [41–46].

MRI and CT findings must be carefully correlated with patient history and physical examination findings to prevent over-diagnosis since imaging abnormalities have been documented to increase with age in asymptomatic human and canine patients [47,48].

Treatment

Conservative and Medical Therapy

Epidural infiltration of methylprednisolone acetate with fluoroscopic guidance has been advocated as therapy for DLSS. In one study, 79% of dogs showed improvement after single or multiple infusions and 53% were judged as cured by owner questionnaire [49]. More conservative treatment of DLSS can consist of rest and antiinflammatory medications such as nonsteroidal antiinflammatory drugs (NSAIDs) or corticosteroids as well as physical therapy. Other modalities (electrical stimulation, ultrasound therapy, laser therapy, and acupuncture) have been employed, but there are few clinical data to support their use. Conservative therapy is not typically appropriate for working or performance dogs since return to function after conservative or medical therapy often leads to recurrence of clinical signs [4,6,7].

Surgery

Surgery is indicated in dogs with DLSS that have not responded to pain management and conservative therapy, or in dogs with neurological deficits. Surgery may also be the best option for performance or working dogs that need to return to activity. The primary goals of surgery for DLSS include decompression of the cauda equina, release of entrapped nerve roots and, in some cases, stabilization to prevent further collapse and degenerative disease.

The most commonly performed decompressive procedure is dorsal laminectomy, which can be combined with disc fenestration or discectomy. Foraminotomy, and in some cases partial or complete facetectomy, can also be performed to achieve additional

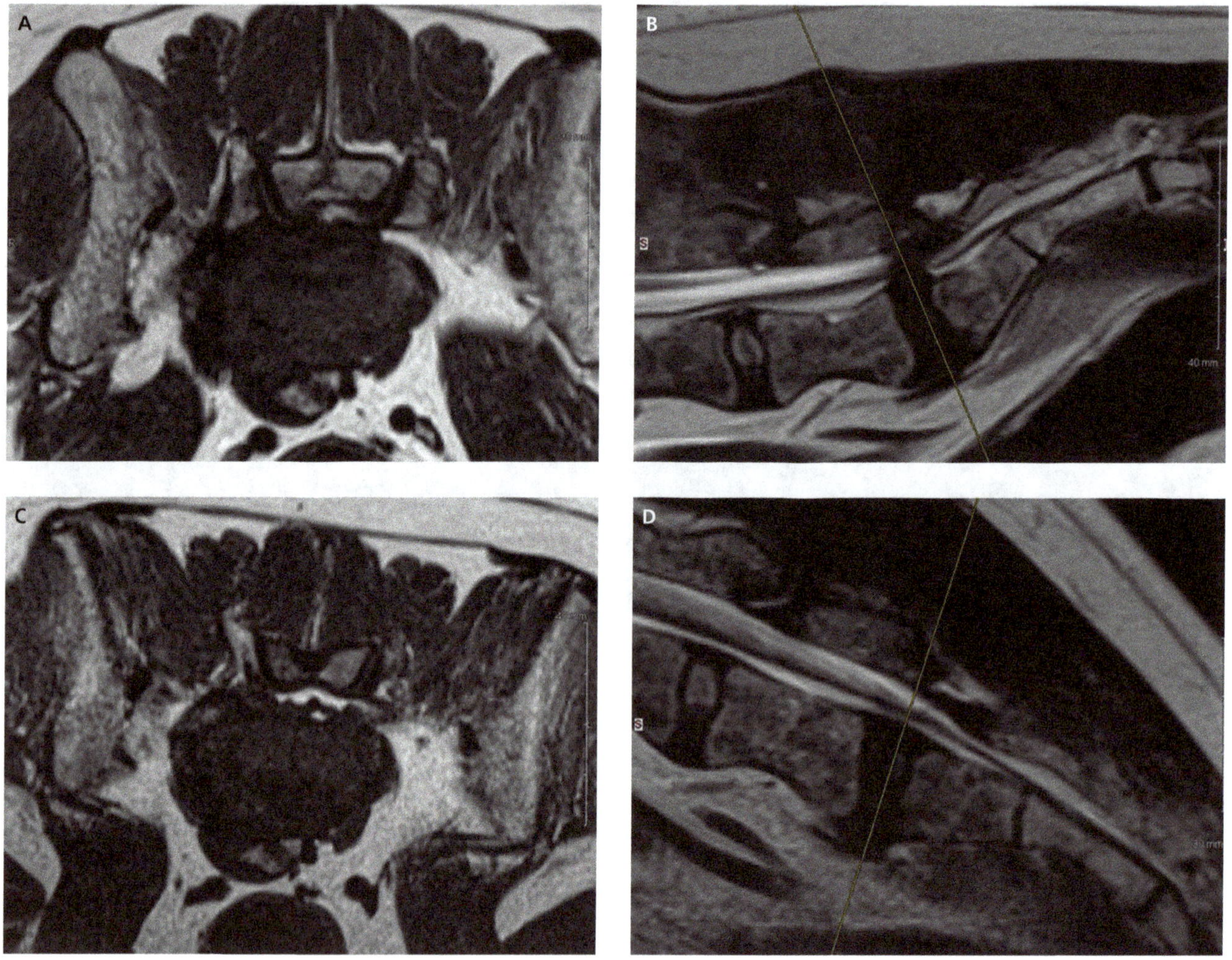

Figure 26.4 MRI of a dog with DLSS. (A) Transverse and (B) sagittal images with the pelvic limbs extended causing dorsiflexion of the lumbosacral space. (C) Transverse and (D) sagittal images taken with the pelvic limbs pulled forward. Note the dramatic difference in the bulge of the disc and compression of the nerves of the cauda equina, illustrating the dynamic nature of the lesion. *Source*: Courtesy of Dr. Laurent Guiot.

decompression. Intervertebral stabilization techniques may also be performed in cases with preexisting instability or those where postoperative instability is a concern. For some dogs foraminotomy alone may be recommended.

Surgical Anatomy

It is crucial that the anatomy of the lumbosacral region be well understood to maximize the effectiveness of surgery and to prevent complications.

The spinal cord ends in the caudal half of L6 and the cranial half of L7 in the majority of large-breed dogs, though it may extend more caudally in some small-breed dogs [50]. The cauda equina arises from the conus medullaris and is composed of the L6, L7, S1–S3 and Cd1–Cd5 nerve roots. It is bordered dorsally by the interarcuate ligament and laminae of L7 and S1, ventrally by the dorsal longitudinal ligament, IVD and vertebral bodies of L7 and S1, and laterally by the vertebral foramina and pedicles of L7 and S1. The connection between L7 and S1 is formed by the facetal joints and the IVD [12]. This articulation is further stabilized by the dorsal and ventral longitudinal ligaments, interarcuate ligament, the interspinous ligament, and the surrounding spinal musculature and fascia.

One of the most important anatomical features for adequate decompression of the lumbosacral disc space is that the L7 nerve root arises just cranial to the intervertebral foramen (Figure 26.5) and travels through a lateral recess prior to exiting the foramen. Adequate decompression of the nerve root through the limited approach offered by a dorsal laminectomy may not be possible (Figure 26.6) [2]. A partial or complete facetectomy, which carries a risk of destabilizing the lumbosacral space, or foraminotomy may therefore be required [2].

Dorsal Laminectomy

Patient Preparation and Positioning

The dog is positioned in sternal recumbency with the pelvic limbs either drawn forward or in a neutral frog-leg position. The pubis can be supported with a sandbag or rolled towel to further open the intervertebral space for decompressive surgery.

Surgical Technique

The landmarks for surgical approach include the wings of the ilium and the spinous process of L6. The spinous process of L7 is short and can be difficult to palpate. A midline skin incision is made from

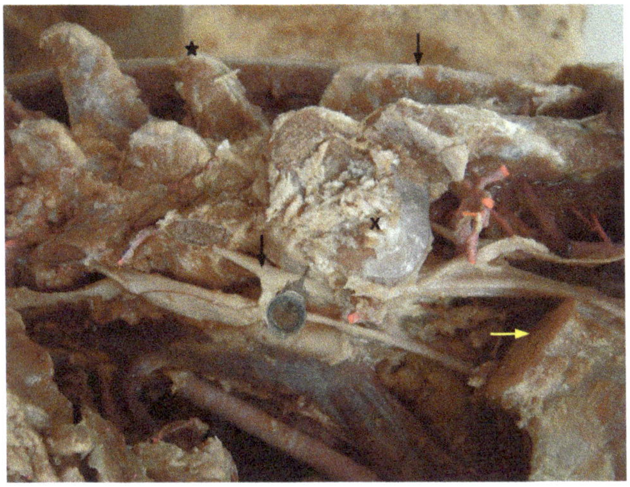

Figure 26.5 This dissected anatomical specimen shows the relationship of the L7 nerve root (black arrows) to the intervertebral disc (hypodermic needle). The spinous process of L7 (asterisk), median crest of the sacrum (arrowhead), sacral wing (cross), and cut edge of the ilial wing (yellow arrow) facilitate orientation. *Source*: Courtesy of Dr. Laurent Guiot.

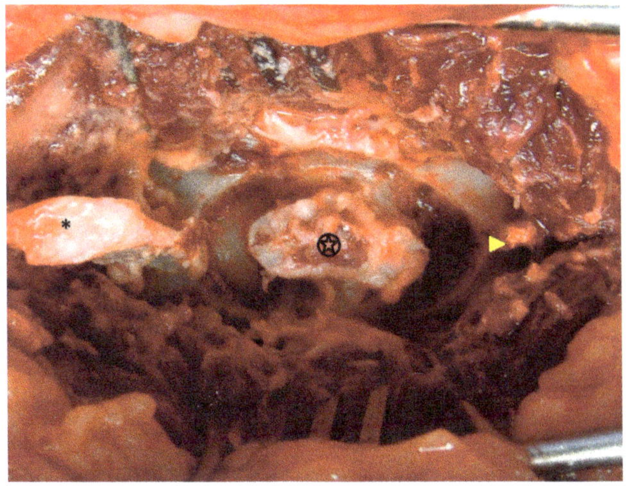

Figure 26.7 Intraoperative image showing the initial steps for standard dorsal laminectomy. The borders of the laminectomy have been burred using a high-speed drill. The spinous process of L6 is cranial to the laminectomy (asterisk), the remnant of the spinous process of L7 (circled star) is visible within the laminectomy, and the sacral crest is also visible (yellow arrowhead). *Source*: Courtesy of Dr. Laurent Guiot.

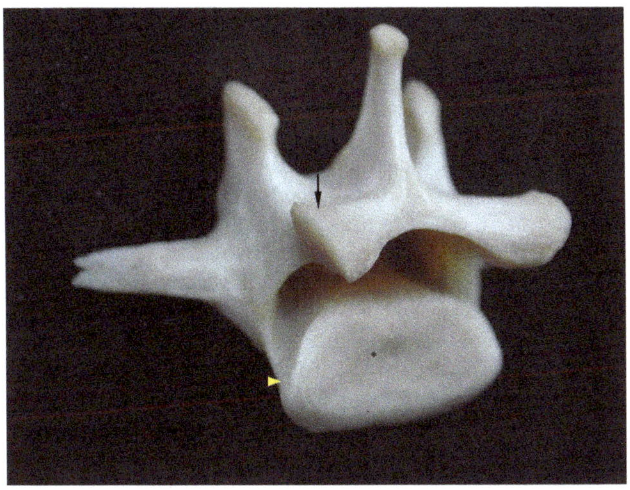

Figure 26.6 A skeletal specimen of the L7 vertebral body showing the lateral recess through which the L7 nerve root exits the spine (yellow arrowhead), vertebral endplate (asterisk), vertebral foramen, and facetal joint (black arrow).

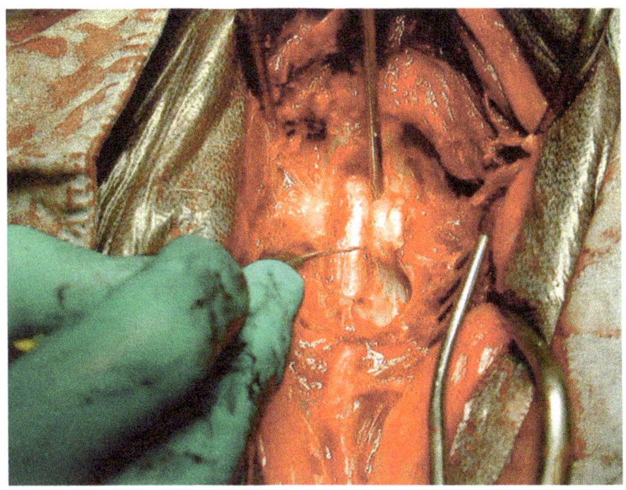

Figure 26.8 Intraoperative image of a dorsal laminectomy showing the thin layer of inner cortical bone being carefully peeled away with an iris spatula providing access to the spinal canal. *Source*: Courtesy of Dr. B. Brisson.

the spinous process of L5 to the caudal median eminence of the sacrum. The subcutaneous fat and superficial fascia are incised along the midline to expose the deep gluteal and caudal fascia. The fascia is incised around each of the spinal processes. This allows for the elevation of the multifidus lumborum muscles (L6) and the sacrocaudalis dorsal medialis epaxial muscles (L7) from the spinous processes and along the midline in between the processes. Soft tissue elevation is continued laterally to expose the L6–L7 and L7–S1 articular processes, and the median sacral crests caudally [51,52]. The fascia between the spinous processes can be very thick and difficult to elevate. The spinous processes of L7 and S1 are removed with double-action rongeurs. The dorsal laminectomy is performed using a high-speed surgical drill including at least the caudal half of L7 and most of the sacrum. The lateral extent of the laminectomy is generally the caudal facets of L7 and the cranial facets of S1 (Figure 26.7). Once through the outer cortical bone, the laminectomy continues in the red cancellous bone layer until the white inner cortical bone is reached. At this point the ligamentum flavum is resected, exposing the epidural fat of the lumbosacral space. When removing the ligamentum flavum it is important the dissection does not extend deeper than the remaining bony lamina to avoid damage to the cauda equina [7]. The inner cortical bone is then thinned with the burr until it can be peeled using elevators and forceps or removed with Kerrison rongeurs (Figure 26.8) to expose the cauda equina (Figure 26.9).

The S1 nerve root is visible through this approach and runs lateral to the dural sac. In contrast, the L7 nerve root is located more laterally and runs through the lateral recess prior to emerging from the foramen; this allows only a portion of the L7 nerve root to be visualized through this approach. The laminectomy site can be enlarged to the medial limit of the facetal joint capsule [51,52] and

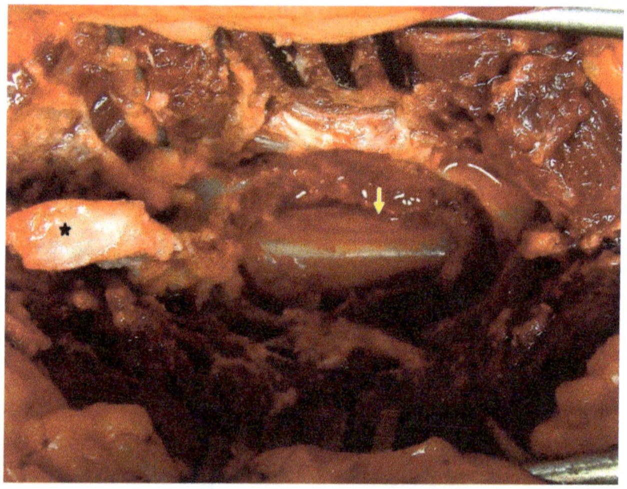

Figure 26.9 Intraoperative image of a completed dorsal laminectomy providing visualization of the cauda equina (yellow arrow). The L6 spinous process is cranial to the laminectomy (asterisk) and the facetal joints are located laterally. The laminectomy can be carefully widened as required using Kerrison rongeurs. *Source*: Courtesy of Dr. Laurent Guiot.

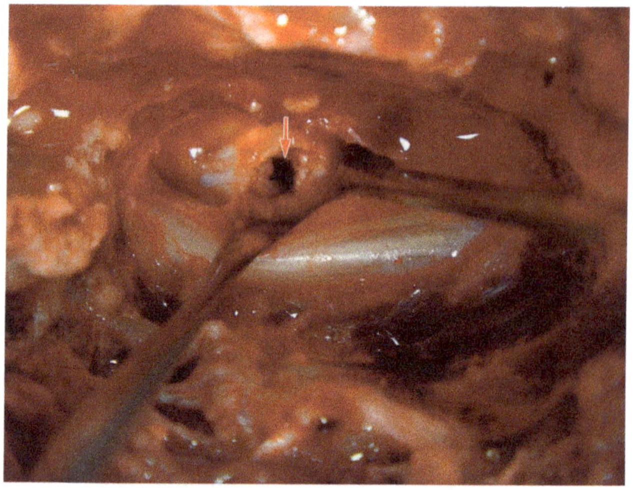

Figure 26.11 Intraoperative image of a dorsal laminectomy. The cauda equina is gently retracted while the dorsal annulus is incised (arrow) and discectomy is performed by removing the contents of the disc using curettes or a high-speed burr. *Source*: Courtesy of Dr. Laurent Guiot.

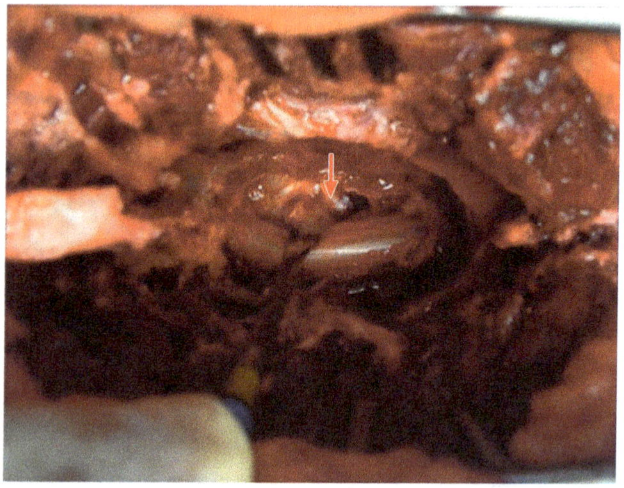

Figure 26.10 Intraoperative image of a dorsal laminectomy showing gentle retraction of the cauda equina to expose the bulging dorsal annulus of the intervertebral disc (arrow). *Source*: Courtesy of Dr. Laurent Guiot.

the L7 nerve root examined using a probe. The L7 nerve root should move a few millimeters with minimal traction [7]; if this is not possible, further decompression (partial or complete facetectomy, or foraminotomy) is indicated.

The IVD is often visualized as protruding dorsally within the spinal canal and can otherwise be palpated by running a nerve retractor, ball-end probe, or other blunt instrument gently under the cauda equina (Figure 26.10). Patient positioning (pelvic limbs forward/flexed spine) can distract the dorsal annulus and may artificially decrease intraoperative annular protrusion compared with preoperative advanced imaging; this is especially true in dogs with dynamic lesions. With the cauda equina gently retracted using a nerve retractor or smooth blunt probe, the dorsal annulus can be visualized and excised. This allows for fenestration or partial discectomy to relieve the compression caused by a protruding IVD. When the dorsal annulus and the dorsal longitudinal ligament are excised the patient often develops hyperpnea, tachycardia, and elevated mean arterial blood pressure [53]; these changes may support the concept of discogenic pain in DLSS. Discectomy can be accomplished using curettes but some surgeons prefer to use a high-speed drill (power fenestration). In either instance the cauda equina must be carefully protected. Half of the disc can be resected while retracting the cauda equina to one side, then it can be retracted to the opposite side to resect the other half of the disc (Figure 26.11) [6].

Following adequate decompression, the cauda equina is generally covered with an autogenous fat graft to prevent the formation of a laminectomy membrane that may cause recurrence of compression [54].

Variation

In order to decrease the amount of instability created by the dorsal laminectomy procedure, a partial laminectomy approach has been described [55]. This limited laminectomy approach involves removal of the ligamentum flavum and a laminectomy of only S1. As a result the exposure to the cauda equina is more limited but there is no expected loss of stability. Biomechanical testing of this laminectomy in conjunction with discectomy has not been done but one would expect it to be more stable than a standard dorsal laminectomy. One study of 86 dogs treated with this procedure reported very good outcomes [55].

Foraminotomy and Facetectomy

Foraminotomy is an additional procedure that is commonly performed to enlarge the L7–S1 foramen in order to decompress the L7 nerve root at the point of exit from the vertebral canal. This procedure attempts to preserve stability by undercutting rather than removing the articular processes [2,7,56,57]. If foraminotomy does not adequately decompress the L7 nerve root, a facetectomy can also be considered. Facetectomy consists of extending a standard dorsal laminectomy laterally (dorsal to the foramen) by removing a portion of the articular facets. Unlike foraminotomy, the facetectomy procedure has been shown to cause significant instability in normal canine cadaver spines in vitro [58].

Surgical Approach

The L7–S1 foraminotomy has been described using a lateral approach, a transiliac approach, and an endoscopic-assisted approach [56,57,59]. The lateral approach can be performed bilaterally, combined with a dorsal laminectomy or partial dorsal laminectomy and is performed using the same patient positioning and initial approach as the dorsal laminectomy [56]. Once the superficial fascia has been incised, dissection continues about midway between the spinous processes and the ilial wing. A combination of blunt and sharp dissection is used to separate the multifidus and sacrocaudalis muscles, exposing the transverse process and intervertebral foramen. The quadratus lumborum and longissimus muscles are then partially elevated with periosteal elevators to allow exposure of the transverse process and pedicle of L7. The L7–S1 foramen can only be accessed from a dorsal-oblique approach because of the ilial wing. The foraminotomy is initiated using a high-speed drill and extended with fine burs or Kerrison rongeurs [56].

The transiliac approach to the L7 foramen involves a dorsal approach to the wing of the ilium followed by the creation of an 18 mm window through the iliac wing using a surgical drill. Through this approach, endoscopic exploration of the L7 nerve root, the intervertebral foramen, and the IVD can be performed [57]. This technique was performed on cadavers and has not yet been reported in clinical patients with follow-up [56].

An alternative technique described in normal dogs involves the use of a modified mini-dorsal laminectomy with endoscopic-assisted foraminotomy. CT follow-up demonstrated that it is possible to enlarge the foramen using this approach, and that although it decreased in size by the 12th postoperative week it remained larger than preoperatively. Further clinical research is necessary to determine if this technique can effectively treat dogs with DLSS and foraminal stenosis [59].

Distraction and Stabilization/Fusion

Instability and subluxation are considered by some as integral to the pathological processes that result in DLSS [60,61]. In contrast, others report the process is associated with abnormal motion rather than true instability [10,11]. Partial discectomy or facetectomy may further exacerbate any existing instability [58,60,61]. Results of one study suggest that recurrence of clinical signs in dogs with DLSS following successful surgical decompression is associated with ongoing instability. In-vitro testing of lumbosacral spines taken from normal dogs revealed that while dorsal laminectomy does not result in a significant loss of stiffness in the dorsoventral plane, the addition of discectomy caused a significant decrease in stiffness in ventroflexion [58]. Combined facetectomy and dorsal laminectomy decreased stiffness in both dorsiflexion and ventroflexion and combined dorsal laminectomy, discectomy and facetectomy resulted in a significantly less stable lumbosacral unit than any of the other combinations [58].

Some authors recommend stabilization following lumbosacral decompression. Stabilization techniques include the placement of screws through the L7–S1 facetal joints with bone graft for fusion, the use of pins or screws and polymethylmethacrylate (PMMA), and the use of pedicle screw-rod constructs designed for applications in the human spine [61–66]. A biomechanical study of canine lumbosacral spinal segments that were stabilized with pedicle screw–rod fixation following dorsal laminectomy and discectomy found that the pedicle screw–rod construct effectively stabilized the lumbosacral spine [60]. Another study determined the safe corridors for pedicle screw placement for lumbosacral stabilization [67]. To date, there are no long-term clinical studies that conclusively demonstrate an advantage of stabilization techniques over dorsal decompression and foraminotomy alone.

Dorsal distraction/stabilization has been advocated in order to increase the opening of the intervertebral foramina, essentially decompressing the L7 nerve roots and correcting any preexisting instability. Following dorsal laminectomy or partial dorsal laminectomy, distraction is achieved using a laminectomy spreader [6] and any of the previously mentioned stabilization options. If screw fixation of the facetal joints is employed, the screws should be placed in the approximate center of the facetal joint and directed at a 30–45° angle from the sagittal plane to prevent injury to the lumbosacral trunk and entry into the sacroiliac joint [61–63]. Stabilization can also be achieved by inserting pins or screws into the body of L7 and the sacral wings and then embedding the pin ends or screw heads in PMMA to act as an internal fixator [64,65]. Fusion of the joints is promoted by the removal of the articular cartilage prior to fixation and placing an autogenous cancellous or commercially available bone graft. Pedicle screw fixation is achieved with four pedicle screws, two each in L7 and S1, much like the screw and rod fixation described for the spacer screw technique (Figure 26.12) [60,66–69]. Surgical techniques including dorsal laminectomy and lumbosacral stabilization using pins or screws and PMMA have also been employed to treat DLSS in cats with good results [70,71].

Variation

A more novel approach to distraction/fusion involves distracting the lumbosacral space with a permanent intervertebral device. A threaded titanium intervertebral spacer is placed into the L7–S1 intervertebral space following dorsal laminectomy, annulectomy and discectomy [68,69] and is stabilized with a 2.7-mm screw placed dorsoventrally from the vertebral body of S1, through a slot in the spacer screw, and into the vertebral body of L7. The L7–S1 region can be further stabilized by using threaded pins and PMMA or 4.5-mm pedicle screws placed bilaterally into the base of the transverse processes of L7 and the alar wings of the sacrum. The screws are then connected by two rods with spherical stopper ends abutting slotted polyhedral screw fixation clamps (Figures 26.12 and 26.13) [68,69].

Postoperative Management

Depending on the procedure (degree of laminectomy and whether distraction/stabilization procedures were performed), a 4–8 week period of rest is recommended following surgery. Following this, a gradual return to activity is recommended over a 4–6 week period. This period may need to be longer for working dogs. Rehabilitation including swimming and underwater treadmill may also help recovery. It is very important that any rehabilitation program be designed by the surgeon and a qualified animal physiotherapist working in tandem [1,7].

Postoperative Outcomes

A summary of the recent studies reporting on outcome in dogs with DLSS is presented in Table 26.1. Following surgery, dogs with DLSS have good overall prognosis for improvement;

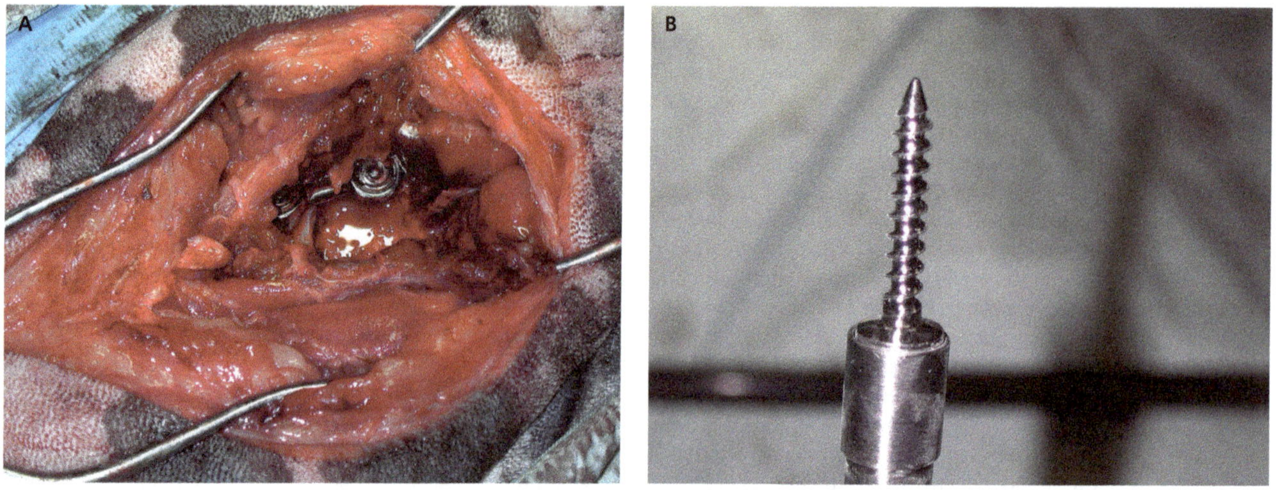

Figure 26.12 Intraoperative image of a dog treated by dorsal laminectomy and stabilized using pedicle screws. Two pedicle screws were implanted and connected with a rod held by fixation clamps (A). A pedicle screw can be seen prior to insertion within the insertion device (B).

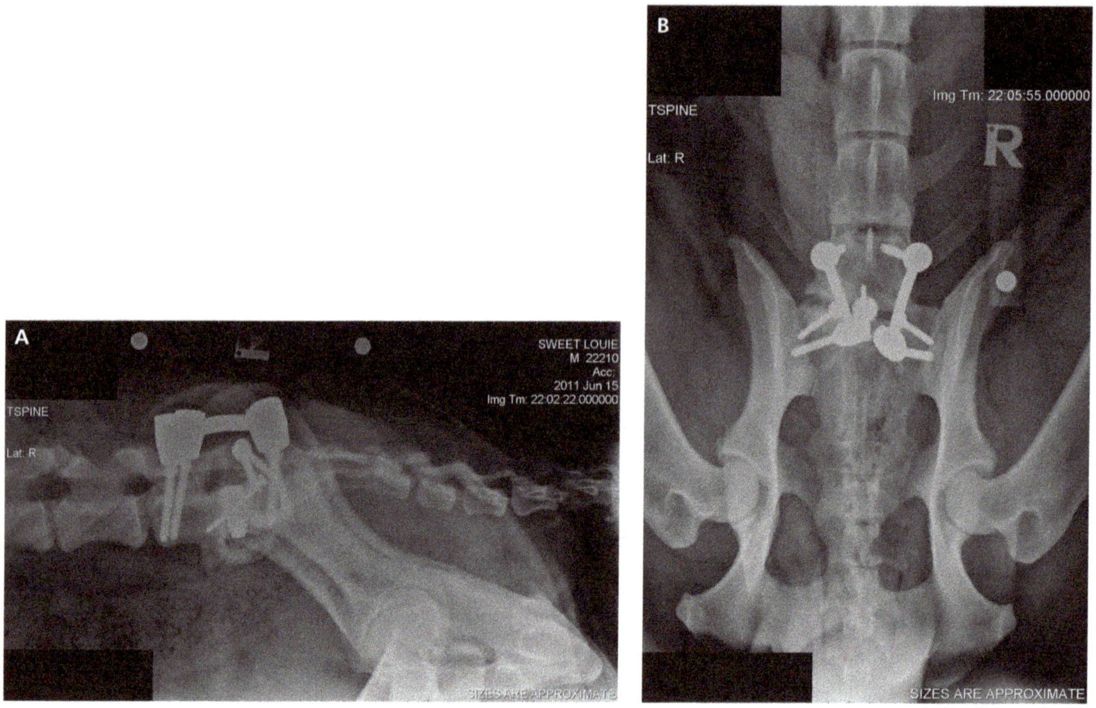

Figure 26.13 Lateral (A) and ventrodorsal (B) radiographic projections of a dog treated by dorsal laminectomy, annulectomy, and discectomy followed by stabilization with an intervertebral spacer screw and pedicle screws. Note the enlargement of the intervertebral foramina and spreading of the intervertebral disc space compared with the preoperative radiographs seen in Figure 26.2. *Source*: Courtesy of Dr. N. Fitzpatrick.

75–90% of dogs reportedly achieve good to excellent function postoperatively [42,53,55,56,72–80]. Recurrence rates are quite variable between studies (2.4–27%). This range may be due to the length and type of follow-up achieved but may also vary depending whether the animals are pets or working dogs. It would be expected that military working dogs may have a higher recurrence rate if returned to active duty [72]. Dogs with more severe preoperative neurological deficits, and especially dogs with signs of urinary incontinence, seem to carry a worse prognosis [53,75,79,80]. One study reported a decreased prognosis for older dogs, particularly working dogs [73]. Overall, most dogs improve postoperatively but only 50% return to full function, and this number may be lower for working dogs. Recurrence of clinical signs may be related to residual compression, instability, or laminectomy membrane formation, which can occur months to years after surgery [53,73–75].

Video clips to accompany this book can be found on the companion website at:
www.wiley.com/go/shores/neurosurgery

Table 26.1 Summary of the recent studies evaluating surgical outcomes in dogs with DLSS.

Study	Danielsson & Sjöström (1999) [53]	Janssens et al. (2000) [77]	Jones et al. (2000) [42]	De Risio et al. (2001) [75]	Linn et al. (2003) [72]	Kinzel et al. (2004) [55]	Van Klaveren et al. (2005) [73]	Gödde & Steffen (2007) [56]	Suwankong et al. (2007) [76]	Suwankong et al. (2008) [74]
Design	Retrospective	Retrospective	Prospective	Retrospective	Retrospective	Retrospective	Prospective	Retrospective	Prospective	Retrospective
Outcome assessment	Medical records and telephone interview	Questionnaire	Standardized obstacle course 6 months after surgery	Reevaluation at VTH, by rDVM and owner questionnaire	Medical records	Medical records	Force plate analysis	Medical records, follow-up examinations and owner telephone interviews	Force plate and owner questionnaire	Medical records (MR) and owner questionnaire (OQ)
Technique	Dorsal laminectomy/ discectomy ± foraminotomy	Dorsal laminectomy, annulectomy and discectomy	Dorsal laminectomy ± foraminotomy and facetectomy	Dorsal laminectomy/ discectomy/ foraminotomy	Dorsal laminectomy ± facetectomy, foraminotomy, discectomy, traction-fusion	Partial dorsal laminectomy	Dorsal laminectomy ± fenestration and discectomy	Lateral foraminotomy ± partial dorsal laminectomy ± annulectomy	Dorsal laminectomy and discectomy	Dorsal laminectomy ± discectomy, facetectomy, foraminotomy
Number of dogs	131	35	12 military working dogs	69	29 military working dogs	86	12	20	31	156
Normal	78.6%	53%	8 fit for full duty	38%	41%		3 propulsive force = control dogs	40%	50%	NA
Improved	18%	32%	3 not fit for full duty but could do reduced duty	40%	38%, but 54.5% of this group recurred	96.5%	7 propulsive force improved	55%	36%	79% MR 76% OQ
Not improved	3.1%	15%	1	22%	21%	1.2%	2 propulsive force decreased	1	9%	21% MR 24% OQ
Recurrence	18%	16%	NA	3%	17%	2.4%	NA	NA	27%	NA

References

1 Indrieri RJ. Lumbosacral stenosis and injury of the cauda equina. *Vet Clin North Am Small Anim Pract* 1988;18:697–710.

2 De Risio L, Thomas WB, Sharp NJ. Degenerative lumbosacral stenosis. *Vet Clin North Am Small Anim Pract* 2000;30:111–132.

3 Tarvin G, Prata RG. Lumbosacral stenosis in dogs. *J Am Vet Med Assoc* 1980;177:154–159.

4 Palmer RH, Chambers JN. Canine lumbosacral diseases. Part I. Anatomy, pathophysiology, and clinical presentation. *Compend Contin Educ Pract Vet* 1991;13:61–68.

5 Meij BP, Bergknut N. Degenerative lumbosacral stenosis in dogs. *Vet Clin North Am Small Anim Pract* 2010;40:983–1009.

6 Moore GE, Burkman KD, Carter MN, Peterson MR. Causes of death or reasons for euthanasia in military working dogs: 927 cases (1993–1996). *J Am Vet Med Assoc* 2001;219:209–214.

7 Sharp NJH, Wheeler SJ. Lumbosacral disease. In: *Small Animal Spinal Disorders*, 2nd edn. Edinburgh: Elsevier Mosby, 2005: 181–209.

8 Braund KG, Taylor TK, Ghosh P, Sherwood AA. Spinal mobility in the dog. A study in chondrodystrophoid and non-chondrodystrophoid animals. *Res Vet Sci* 1977;22:78–82.

9 Hediger KU, Ferguson SJ, Gedet P et al. Biomechanical analysis of torsion and shear forces in lumbar and lumbosacral spine segments of nonchondrodystrophic dogs. *Vet Surg* 2009;38:874–880.

10 Benninger MI, Seiler GS, Robinson LE et al. Three-dimensional motion pattern of the caudal lumbar and lumbosacral portions of the vertebral column of dogs. *Am J Vet Res* 2004;65:544–551.

11 Benninger MI, Seiler GS, Robinson LE et al. Effects of anatomic conformation on three-dimensional motion of the caudal lumbar and lumbosacral portions of the vertebral column of dogs. *Am J Vet Res* 2006;67:43–50.

12 Bray JP, Burbidge HM. The canine intervertebral disk. Part one: structure and function. *J Am Anim Hosp Assoc* 1998;34:55–63.

13 Bray JP, Burbidge HM. The canine intervertebral disk. Part two: degenerative changes in nonchondrodystrophoid versus chondrodystrophoid disks. *J Am Anim Hosp Assoc* 1998;34:135–144.

14 Zimmerman MC, Vuono-Hawkins M, Parsons JR et al. The mechanical properties of the canine lumbar disc and motion segment. *Spine* 1992;17:213–220.

15 Oliver JE Jr, Selcer RR, Simpson S. Cauda equina compression from lumbosacral malarticulation and malformation in the dog. *J Am Vet Med Assoc* 1978;173: 207–214.

16 Steffen F, Berger M, Morgan JP. Asymmetrical, transitional, lumbosacral vertebral segments in six dogs: a characteristic spinal syndrome. *J Am Anim Hosp Assoc* 2004;40:338–344.

17 Morgan JP. Transitional lumbosacral vertebral anomaly in the dog: a radiographic study. *J Small Anim Pract* 1999;40:167–172.

18 Aihara T, Takahashi K, Ogasawara A, Itadera E, Moriya H. Intervertebral disc degeneration associated with lumbosacral transitional vertebrae: a clinical and anatomical study. *J Bone Joint Surg Br* 2005;87:687–691.

19 Flückiger MA, Damur-Djuric N, Hassig M, Morgan JP, Steffen F. A lumbosacral transitional vertebra in the dog predisposes to cauda equina syndrome. *Vet Radiol Ultrasound* 2006;47:39–44.

20 Damur-Djuric N, Steffen F, Hassig M, Morgan JP, Flückiger MA. Lumbosacral transitional vertebrae in dogs: classification, prevalence, and association with sacroiliac morphology. *Vet Radiol Ultrasound* 2006;47:32–38.

21 Mathis KR, Havlicek M, Beck JB, Eaton-Wells RD, Park FM. Sacral osteochondrosis in two German Shepherd dogs. *Aust Vet J* 2009;87:249–252.

22 Hanna FY. Lumbosacral osteochondrosis: radiological features and surgical management in 34 dogs. *J Small Anim Pract* 2001;42:272–278.

23 Lang J, Häni H, Schawalder P. A sacral lesion resembling osteochondrosis in the German Shepherd dog. *Vet Radiol Ultrasound* 1992;33:69–76.

24 Meij BP, Suwankong N, van den Brom WE, Venker-van Haagen AJ, Hazewinkel HA. Tibial nerve somatosensory evoked potentials in dogs with degenerative lumbosacral stenosis. *Vet Surg* 2006;35:168–175.

25 Sisson AF, LeCouteur RA, Ingram JT, Park RD, Child G. Diagnosis of cauda equina abnormalities by using electromyography, discography, and epidurography in dogs. *J Vet Intern Med* 1992;6:253–263.

26 Ramirez O III, Thrall DE. A review of imaging techniques for canine cauda equina syndrome. *Vet Radiol Ultrasound* 1998;39:283–296.

27 Morgan J, Bailey C. Cauda equina syndrome in the dog: radiographic evaluation. *J Small Anim Pract* 1990;31:69–76.

28 Sande RD. Radiography, myelography, computed tomography, and magnetic resonance imaging of the spine. *Vet Clin North Am Small Anim Pract* 1992;22: 811–831.

29 Steffen F, Hunold K, Scharf G, Roos M, Flückiger M. A follow-up study of neurologic and radiographic findings in working German Shepherd dogs with and without degenerative lumbosacral stenosis. *J Am Vet Med Assoc* 2007;231:1529–1533.

30 Scharf G, Steffen F, Grünenfelder F, Morgan JP, Flückiger M. The lumbosacral junction in working German shepherd dogs: neurological and radiological evaluation. *J Vet Med A Physiol Pathol Clin Med* 2004;51:27–32.

31 Schmid V, Lang J. Measurements on the lumbosacral junction in normal dogs and those with cauda-equina compression. *J Small Anim Pract* 1993;34:437–442.

32 Gradner G, Bockstahler B, Peham C, Henninger W, Podbregar I. Kinematic study of back movement in clinically sound Malinois dogs with consideration of the effect of radiographic changes in the lumbosacral junction. *Vet Surg* 2007;36:472–481.

33 Lang J. Flexion–extension myelography of the canine cauda equina. *Vet Radiol Ultrasound* 1988;29:242–257.

34 Hachcock JT, Pechmanm RD, Dillon AR, Knecht CD, Braund KG. Comparison of three radiographic contrast procedures in the evaluation of the canine lumbosacral spinal canal. *Vet Radiol Ultrasound* 1988;29:4–15.

35 Robert RE, Selcer BA. Diagnostic imaging: myelography and epidurography. *Vet Clin North Am Small Anim Pract* 1993;23:307–329.

36 Barthez PY, Morgan JP, Lipsitz D. Discography and epidurography for evaluation of the lumbosacral junction in dogs with cauda equina syndrome. *Vet Radiol Ultrasound* 1994;35:152–157.

37 Jones JC, Wilson ME, Bartels JE. A review of high resolution computed tomography and a proposed technique for regional examination of the canine lumbosacral spine. *Vet Radiol Ultrasound* 1994;35:339–346.

38 Jones JC, Sorjonen DC, Simpson ST et al. Comparison between computed tomographic and surgical findings in nine large-breed dogs with lumbosacral stenosis. *Vet Radiol Ultrasound* 1996;37:247–256.

39 Jones JC, Inzana KD. Subclinical CT abnormalities in the lumbosacral spine of older large-breed dogs. *Vet Radiol Ultrasound* 2000;41:19–26.

40 Jones JC, Shires PK, Inzana KD, Mosby AD, Sponenberg DP, Lanz OI. Use of computed tomographic densitometry to quantify contrast enhancement of compressive soft tissues in the canine lumbosacral vertebral canal. *Am J Vet Res* 2002;63: 733–737.

41 Suwankong N, Voorhout G, Hazewinkel HA, Meij BP. Agreement between computed tomography, magnetic resonance imaging, and surgical findings in dogs with degenerative lumbosacral stenosis. *J Am Vet Med Assoc* 2006;229:1924–1929.

42 Jones JC, Banfield CM, Ward DL. Association between postoperative outcome and results of magnetic resonance imaging and computed tomography in working dogs with degenerative lumbosacral stenosis. *J Am Vet Med Assoc* 2000;216: 1769–1774.

43 Adams WH, Daniel GB, Pardo AD, Selcer RR. Magnetic resonance imaging of the caudal lumbar and lumbosacral spine in 13 dogs (1990–1993). *Vet Radiol Ultrasound* 1995;36:3–13.

44 de Haan JJ, Shelton SB, Ackerman N. Magnetic resonance imaging in the diagnosis of degenerative lumbosacral stenosis in four dogs. *Vet Surg* 1993;22:1–4.

45 Karkkainen M, Punto LU, Tulamo RM. Magnetic resonance imaging of canine degenerative lumbar spine diseases. *Vet Radiol Ultrasound* 1993;34:399–404.

46 Mayhew PD, Kapatkin AS, Wortman JA, Vite CH. Association of cauda equina compression on magnetic resonance images and clinical signs in dogs with degenerative lumbosacral stenosis. *J Am Anim Hosp Assoc* 2002;38:555–562.

47 Jones JC, Inzana KD. Subclinical CT abnormalities in the lumbosacral spine of older large breed dogs. *Vet Radiol Ultrasound* 2000;41:19–26.

48 Jensen MC, Brandt-Zawadzki MN, Obuchowski N, Modic MT, Malkasian D, Ross JS. Magnetic resonance imaging of the lumbar spine in people without back pain. *N Engl J Med* 1994;331:69–73.

49 Janssens L, Beosier Y, Daems R. Lumbosacral degenerative stenosis in the dog. The results of epidural infiltration with methylprednisolone acetate: a retrospective study. *Vet Comp Orthop Traumatol* 2009;22:486–491.

50 Fletcher TF, Kitchell RL. Anatomical studies on the spinal cord segments of the dog. *Am J Vet Res* 1966;27:1759–1767.

51 Piermattei DL, Johnson KA. The vertebral column: approach to lumbar vertebra 7 and the sacrum through a dorsal incision. In: *An Atlas of Surgical Approaches to the Bones and Joints of the Dog and Cat*, 4th edn. Philadelphia, PA: Saunders, 2004: 92–95.

52 Johnson KA. The vertebral column: approach to lumbar vertebra 7 and the sacrum through a dorsal incision. In: *Piermattei's Atlas of Surgical Approaches to the Bones and Joints of the Dog and Cat*, 5th edn. St Louis, MO: Elsevier Saunders, 2014: 94–97.

53 Danielsson F, Sjöström L. Surgical treatment of degenerative lumbosacral stenosis in dogs. *Vet Surg* 1999;28:91–98.

54 Trevor PB, Martin RA, Saunders GK, Trotter EJ. Healing characteristics of free and pedicle fat grafts after dorsal laminectomy and durotomy in dogs. *Vet Surg* 1991;20:282–290.

55 Kinzel S, Koch J, Stopinski T et al. [Cauda equina compression syndrome (CECS): retrospective study of surgical treatment with partial dorsal laminectomy in 86 dogs with lumbosacral stenosis.] *Berl Munch Tierarztl Wochenschr* 2004;117: 334–340.

56 Gödde T, Steffen F. Surgical treatment of lumbosacral foraminal stenosis using a lateral approach in twenty dogs with degenerative lumbosacral stenosis. *Vet Surg* 2007;36:705–713.
57 Carozzo C, Cachon T, Genevois JP et al. Transiliac approach for exposure of lumbosacral intervertebral disk and foramen: technique description. *Vet Surg* 2008;37:27–31.
58 Smith MEH, Bebchuk TN, Schmon CL, Watson LG, Steinmetz H. An in vitro biomechanical study of the effects of surgical modification upon the canine lumbosacral spine. *Vet Comp Orthop Traumatol* 2004;17:17–24.
59 Wood BC, Lanz OI, Jones JC, Shires PK. Endoscopic-assisted lumbosacral foraminotomy in the dog. *Vet Surg* 2004;33:221–231.
60 Meij BP, Suwankong N, Van der Veen AJ et al. Biomechanical flexion–extension forces in normal canine lumbosacral cadaver specimens before and after dorsal laminectomy-discectomy and pedicle screw-rod fixation. *Vet Surg* 2007;36:742–751.
61 Hankin EJ, Jerram RM, Walker AM, King MD, Warman GA. Transarticular facet screw stabilization and dorsal laminectomy in 26 dogs with degenerative lumbosacral stenosis with instability. *Vet Surg* 2012;41:611–619.
62 Golini L, Kircher PR, Lewis FI, Steffen F. Transarticular fixation with cortical screws combined with dorsal laminectomy and partial discectomy as surgical treatment of degenerative lumbosacral stenosis in 17 dogs: clinical and computed tomography follow-up. *Vet Surg* 2014;43:405–413.
63 Bagley R. Surgical stabilization of the lumbosacral joint. In: Slatter D (ed.) *Textbook of Small Animal Surgery*, 3rd edn. Philadelphia, PA: Elsevier Science, 2003: 1238–1243.
64 Slocum B, Devine T. L7–S1 fixation–fusion for treatment of cauda equina compression in the dog. *J Am Vet Med Assoc* 1986;188:31–35.
65 Slocum B. L7–S1 fixation–fusion technique for cauda equina syndrome. In: Bojrab M (ed.) *Current Techniques in Small Animal Surgery*, 5th edn. Philadelphia, PA: Lea & Febiger, 1998: 861–864.
66 Smolders LA, Voorhout G, van de Ven R et al. Pedicle screw-rod fixation of the canine lumbosacral junction. *Vet Surg* 2012;41:720–732.
67 van de Ven R, Bergknut N, Voorhout G, Meij BP. Assessment of safe corridors for pedicle screw insertion in canine lumbosacral vertebras. Presented at European Veterinary Conference, Voorjaarsdagen, 2009. Available at http://www.voorjaarsdagen.eu/conference-info/european-veterinary-conference-voorjaarsdagen/proceedings/category/39-companion-animal-posters-2009
68 Fitzpatrick N. The FITS–Fitz intervertebral traction screw. In: *ACVS Symposium Proceedings 2011*. Germantown, MD: American College of Veterinary Surgeons, 2012: 241–243.
69 Fitzpatrick N, Jovanovik E. Evaluation of early effects of a novel lumbosacral distraction–fusion stabilization system for the treatment of degenerative lumbosacral stenosis over six months using computed tomography. Presented at the 42nd Annual Veterinary Orthopedic Society Conference, February 28 to March 7, 2015. *Vet Comp Orthop Traumatol* 2015;28:A2 (Abstract 7).
70 Cariou MP, Störk CK, Petite AF, Rayward RM. Cauda equina syndrome treated by lumbosacral stabilisation in a cat. *Vet Comp Orthop Traumatol* 2008;21:462–466.
71 Danielski A, Bertran J, Fitzpatrick N. Management of degenerative lumbosacral disease in cats by dorsal laminectomy and lumbosacral stabilization. *Vet Comp Orthop Traumatol* 2013;26:69–75.
72 Linn LL, Bartels KE, Rochat MC, Payton ME, Moore GE. Lumbosacral stenosis in 29 military working dogs: epidemiologic findings and outcome after surgical intervention (1990–1999). *Vet Surg* 2003;32:21–29.
73 Van Klaveren NJ, Suwankong N, De Boer S et al. Force plate analysis before and after dorsal decompression for treatment of degenerative lumbosacral stenosis in dogs. *Vet Surg* 2005;34:450–456.
74 Suwankong N, Meij BP, Voorhout G, de Boer AH, Hazewinkel HA. Review and retrospective analysis of degenerative lumbosacral stenosis in 156 dogs treated by dorsal laminectomy. *Vet Comp Orthop Traumatol* 2008;21:285–293.
75 De Risiò L, Sharp NJH, Olby NJ, Muñana KR, Thomas WB. Predictors of outcome after dorsal decompressive laminectomy for degenerative lumbosacral stenosis in dogs: 69 cases (1987–1997). *J Am Vet Med Assoc* 2001;219:624–628.
76 Suwankong N, Meij BP, Van Klaveren NJ, Van Wees AM, Meijer E, Van den Brom WE. Assessment of decompressive surgery in dogs with degenerative lumbosacral stenosis using force plate analysis and questionnaires. *Vet Surg* 2007;36:423–431.
77 Janssens L, Moens Y, Coppens P, Peremans K, Vinck H. Lumbosacral degenerative stenosis in the dog: the results of dorsal decompression with dorsal anulectomy and nuclectomy. *Vet Comp Orthop Traumatol* 2000;13:97–103.
78 Watt PR. Degenerative lumbosacral stenosis in 18 dogs. *J Small Anim Pract* 1991;32:125–134.
79 Denny HR, Gibbs C, Holt PE. The diagnosis and treatment of cauda equina lesions in the dog. *J Small Anim Pract* 1982;23:425–443.
80 Chambers J, Selcer B, Oliver J. Results of treatment of degenerative lumbosacral stenosis in dogs by exploration and excision. *Vet Comp Orthop Traumatol* 1988;3:130–133.

27 Surgical Management of Spinal Neoplasia

Mark S. Levy

Introduction

Spinal neoplasia is an infrequent diagnosis for the ataxic, paretic, or plegic patient. Some patients with spinal neoplasia present with pain as the only sign. Spinal neoplasia can imply tumors associated with the CNS neuropil, the spinal nerves, peripheral nerves, or the vertebrae. Dogs reportedly have a higher incidence than cats. Nonneoplastic conditions such as intervertebral disc disease are far more common in the dog. Nonneoplastic myelopathies are less common in cats.

Spinal tumors occur in all segments of the spinal cord and all of the vertebral regions. Tumors can be benign or malignant, but all present with a less than favorable prognosis based on the involvement of the nervous system. Benign tumors, even though they do not have the threat of metastasis, can form space-occupying lesions. Metastatic spinal tumors originate in tissues elsewhere and then spread to the spinal cord region. Even very small tumors can have devastating consequences within the confines of the spinal cord or vertebral canal. Space-occupying lesions can also disrupt blood supply to the cord and cause pain and inflammation.

Spinal tumors are divided into three groups based on their relative location: extradural, intradural/extramedullary, and intramedullary (Figures 27.1, 27.2 and 27.3). In cats, lymphomas and meningiomas are more common [1]. In dogs, menigiomas (Figure 27.2) are the most common spinal cord tumor and osteosarcoma is the most common vertebral tumor. Spinal neoplasia can present as an acute or chronic scenario. In general, if a patient has progressive clinical signs located to the spinal cord for more than a few weeks, spinal neoplasia should be higher on the differential list. An exception to this rule could be degenerative myelopathy in dogs.

The main factors in assessing the patient with suspicion of spinal neoplasia are history, signalment, complete physical examination, and neurological examination. For most patients complete blood work and urinalysis may also be appropriate. Additional basic diagnostics such as three-view thoracic radiographs, abdominal radiographs, and abdominal ultrasound may also be indicated.

In humans, primary nonlymphoproliferative tumors of the spine are uncommon, accounting for less than 5% of bone neoplasms and comprising less than 2.5–8.5 primary spine tumors per 100,000 people per year. Metastatic spinal tumors are much more common. As many as 40–80% of people are estimated to have skeletal metastasis, with the spinal column the most common location at the time of death [2].

History

One of the most important aspects of diagnosing spinal neoplasia, or for that matter many other abnormalities, is collecting the medical history. As a general rule, the clinical signs relating to spinal neoplasia have more of a chronic nature. If signs have been progressing for more than 2 weeks and steadily worsening, then spinal neoplasia is strongly considered as a main differential. The signs caused by the spinal tumor vary and are dependent on many factors: tumor location, rate of growth, and its effect on spinal stability to name a few. History often contains the answer or at least a short differential. Things to look for in the history with a patient with spinal neoplasia are (i) slow progression of weakness in the limbs (thoracic, pelvic or both depending on the location of the tumor); (ii) asymmetric weakness and/or muscle mass; (iii) presence of progressive pain experienced by the patient; (iv) increased thirst and/or urination prior to and during these episodes; (v) the lack of presence of pain either steadily or on manipulation/palpation; and (vi) and lack of any history of trauma. While none of these signs are exclusive to spinal neoplasia, the presence of more than one should lead to higher suspicion. In general, age would also be a factor but it does not make for a definitive differential. Intervertebral disc disease has been reported most commonly in dogs between 3 and 5 years of age. However, a

Current Techniques in Canine and Feline Neurosurgery, First Edition. Edited by Andy Shores and Brigitte A. Brisson.
© 2017 John Wiley & Sons, Inc. Published 2017 by John Wiley & Sons, Inc.
Companion website: www.wiley.com/go/shores/neurosurgery

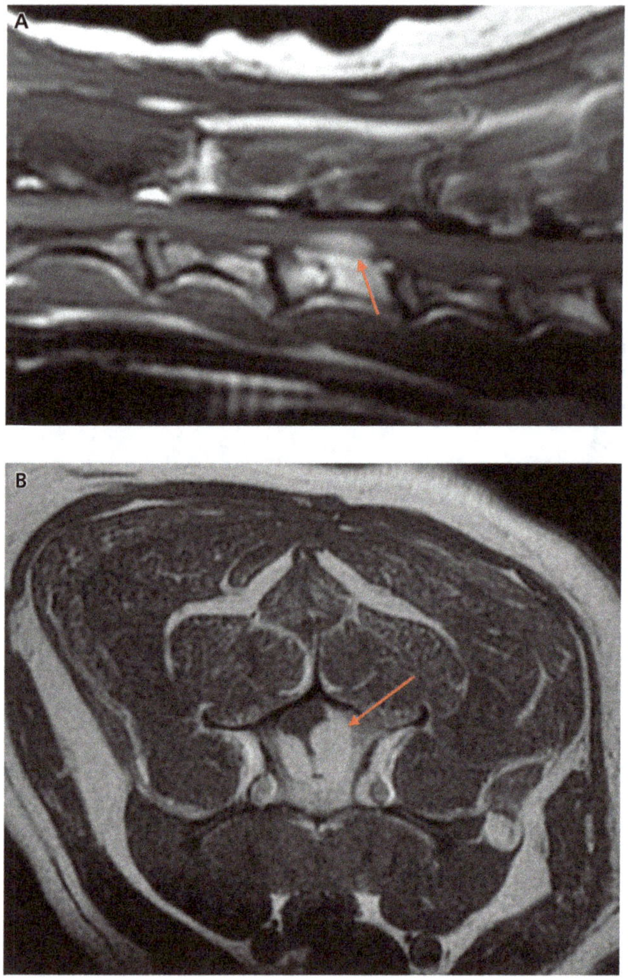

Figure 27.1 Extramedullary tumor at C4 (arrows in A, B): (A) sagittal T1-weighted MRI; (B) transverse T1-weighted MRI with contrast.

dog with intervertebral disc disease aged less than 2 years and certainly older than 6 is also common. Young and middle-aged cats can have disc disease as well, but far less commonly.

Physical and Neurological Examinations

A complete general physical examination is very important in addition to the neurological examination. Differentiating orthopedic from neurological abnormalities is important and often challenging. Discovering coexisting medical or surgical disorders may affect prognosis or change the client's resolve to pursue additional diagnostics. The neurological component also has to be separated from other conditions into those localized to the spinal cord. Ruling out intracranial disease as well as peripheral nerve disease will better help focus on what proper testing to perform. Perhaps the most challenging finding in older or even in more active patients is pre-existing orthopedic diseases, including elbow dysplasia, stifle disease, and hip diseases.

Terms often used in describing the spinal patient are paresis, paralysis (plegia), ataxia, and proprioception [3]. Paresis is defined as a deficit of voluntary movements. Paresis can be further differentiated into monoparesis, hemiparesis, and quadraparesis or tetraparesis. Plegia or paralysis means complete loss of voluntary motor function and, unlike in bipedals, does not imply both motor and sensory loss. A paraplegic quadruped must be further defined with regard to presence or absence of nociception. Ataxia is defined as the lack of coordination without spasticity, paresis or involuntary movements. However, each of these conditions can be seen in association with ataxia. Proprioception ("position sense"; Figure 27.4) is the ability of the body to recognize where the limbs are in relation to the body [3]. The complete neurological examination and associated differentials are well documented and can be found in several other resources.

Based on the level of suspicion for each case, various testing should be considered prior to the more definitive radiological studies. Diagnostic testing is oftentimes normal in cases of primary spinal tumors. Often, metastatic spinal neoplasia (Figure 27.5) or

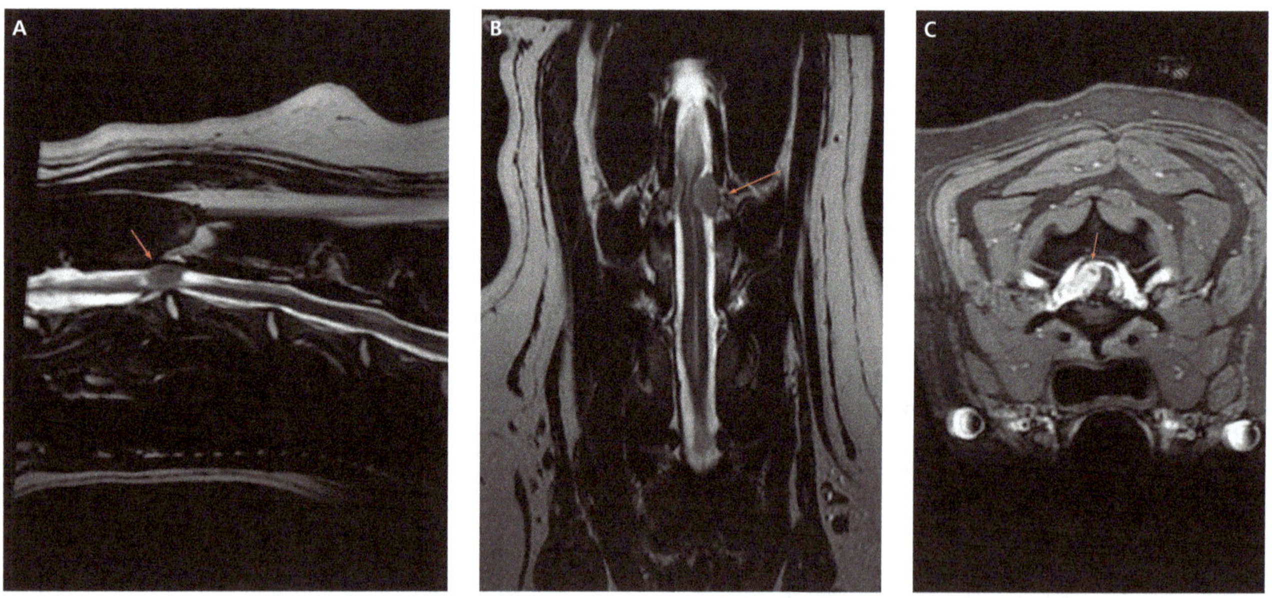

Figure 27.2 Intradural/extramedullary meningioma at C3 (arrows in A, B, C): (A) sagittal T2-weighted MRI; (B) dorsal T2-weighted MRI; (C) transverse T1-weighted MRI plus contrast. Note the typical "golf tee" appearance in (A) and (B).

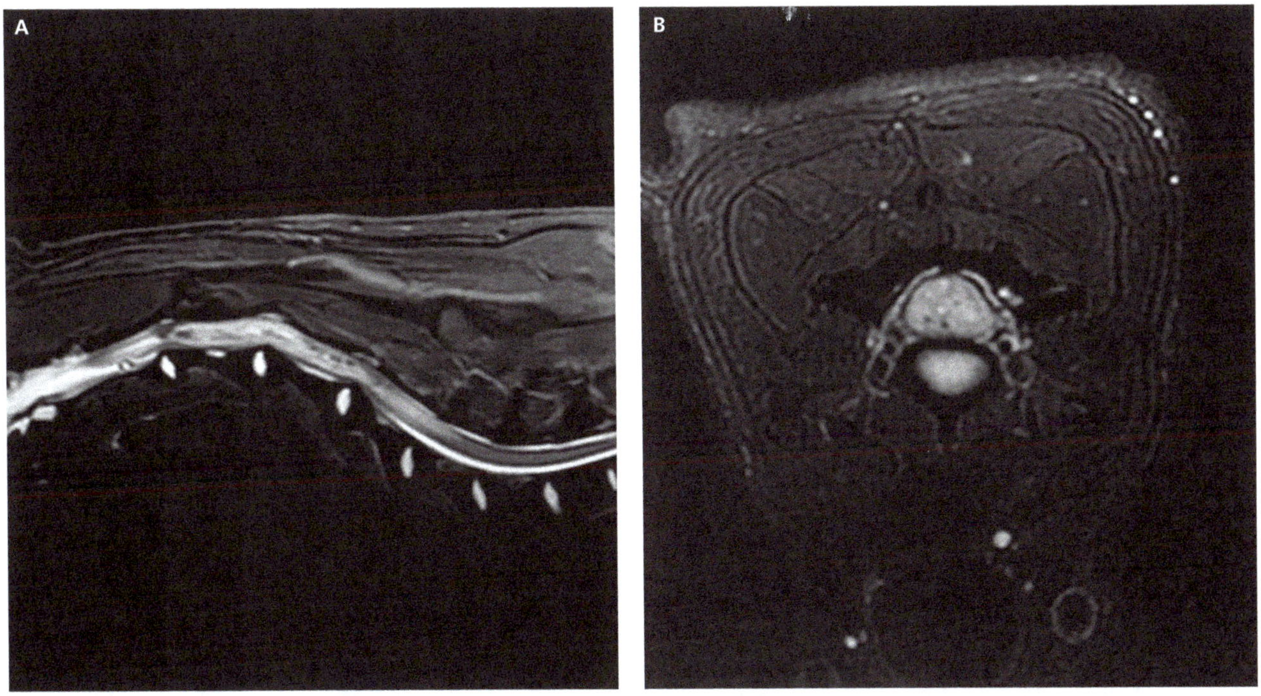

Figure 27.3 Intramedullary cervical spinal glioblastoma in a young dog: (A) sagittal T2-weighted short-tau inversion recovery (STIR) MRI; (B) transverse T1-weighted MRI with contrast.

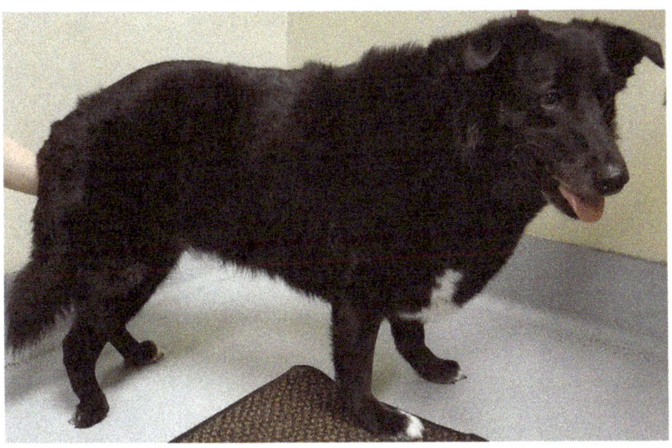

Figure 27.4 Dog demonstrating proprioceptive deficit involving the right pelvic limb.

patients that are otherwise systemically ill may have various abnormalities on diagnostic tests. A complete list of differentials for patients that present ataxic, progressively weak, with muscle atrophy can be found in the literature but some of the more common clinical examples include hypothyroidism, diabetes mellitus, hypercalcemia, hypertension, tick-borne diseases, Addison's disease, and lead toxicity. Neoplasms such as pheochromocytoma, lymphoma, plasma cell tumor, and metastatic carcinoma or sarcomas can all have systemic effects. Many of these disorders can be uncovered when the clinician performs a thorough initial work-up including complete blood cell count, serum chemistry and electrolytes, urinalysis, chest and abdominal radiographs, and ultrasound as indicated. In addition, blood pressure measurements and fundic examination may be indicated.

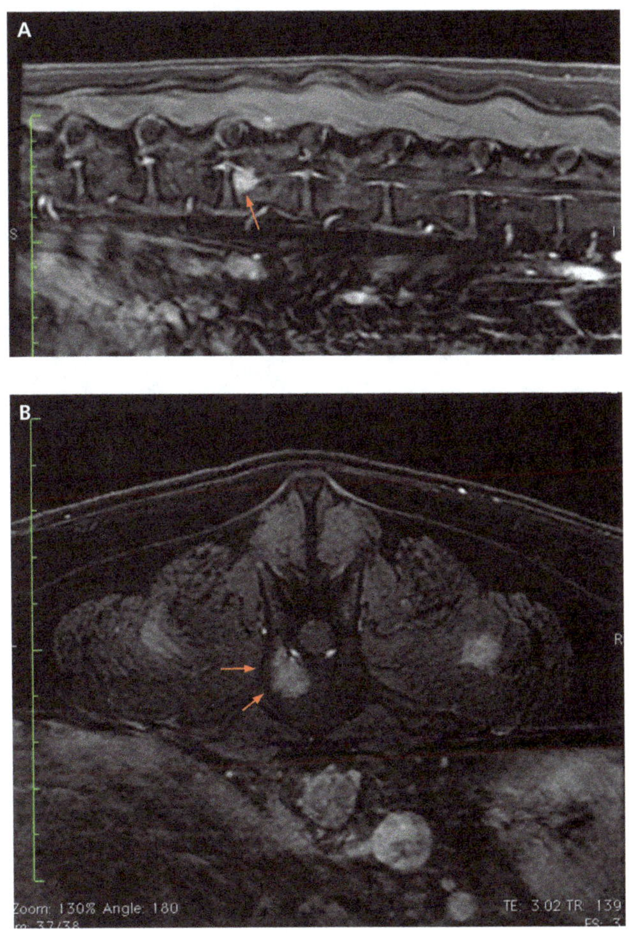

Figure 27.5 Metastatic sarcoma in the lumbar spine of a dog (arrows in A, B): (A) sagittal and (B) transverse T1-weighted fast-spin gradient MRI with contrast.

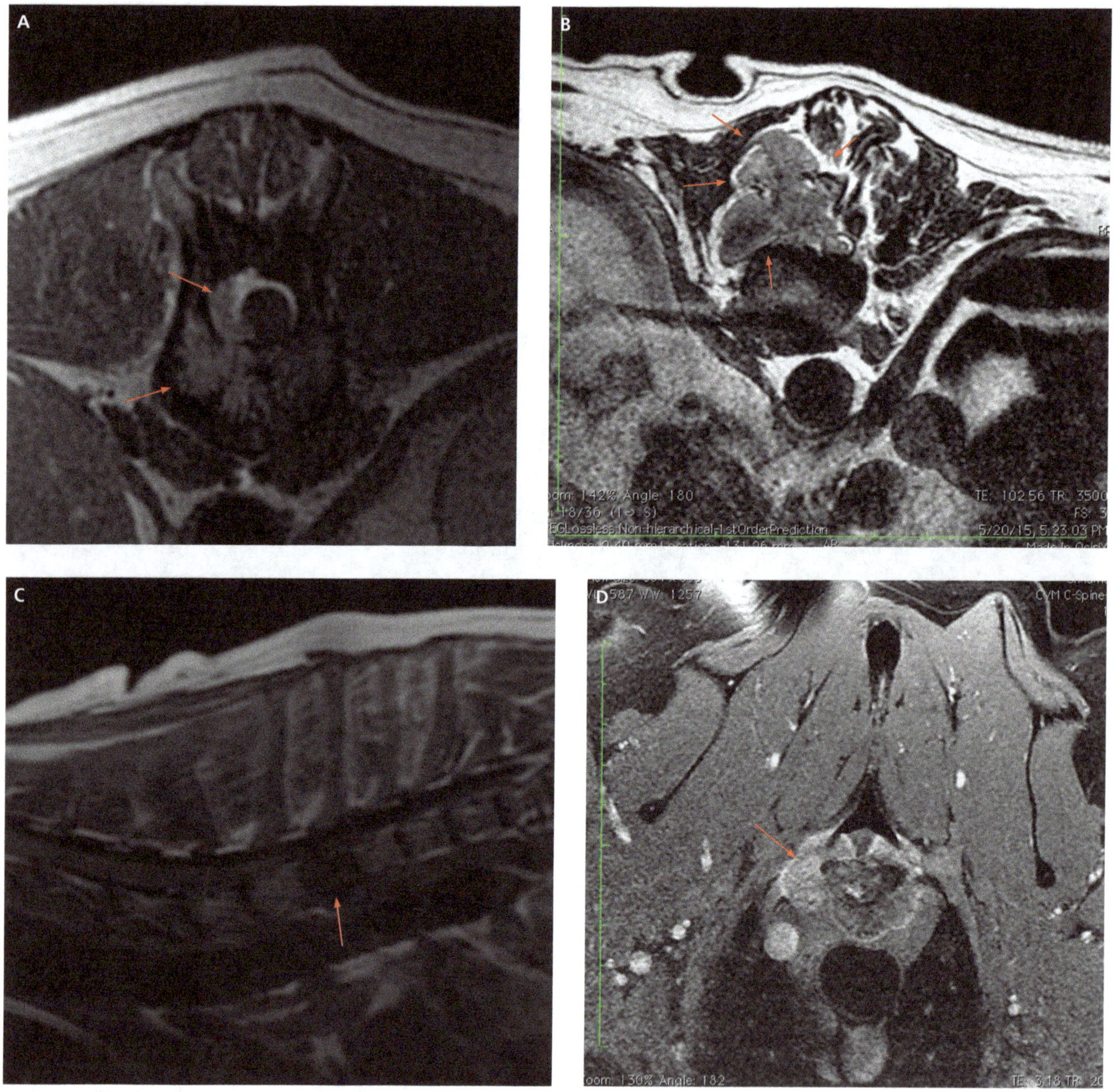

Figure 27.6 (A) Osteosarcoma of a lumbar vertebral body (arrows): transverse T1-weighted MRI with contrast. (B) Primary vertebral body tumor (sarcoma) in the thoracic spine (arrows): transverse T2-weighted MRI. (C, D) Vertebral body fibrosarcoma (arrows): (C) sagittal T1-weighted MRI and (D) T1-weighted MRI with contrast.

In humans, pain, numbness or change in sensory function, motor function or loss of muscle control are common initial complaints in patients with spinal tumors. Pain may be localized or extend to hips, legs or fingers. Oftentimes a burning or aching sensation is reported. Motor function could be weakness, spasticity, loss of bladder control or, if left untreated, muscle atrophy, loss of muscle strength, ataxia, and later paralysis [4].

Spinal Tumor Location

Understanding the location of spinal tumors in relation to the spinal cord can also help with the diagnosis and related clinical signs. Furthermore, it can help decide which radiological test is most likely to yield the most valuable and accurate results. As previously mentioned, spinal tumors can be divided into three main locations based on the relation to the spinal cord (extradural, intradural/extramedullary, and intramedullary).

Extradural tumors are usually within or associated with the vertebral spinal canal. Extradural tumors are the most common location of primary spinal cord tumors. Tumors in this location cause pain by compressing or irritating the cord and meninges. Approximately 50% of all spinal tumors are located in the extradural space. Sarcomas (osteosarcoma, hemangiosarcoma, fibrosarcoma, and chondrosarcoma) and plasma cell tumors are the most common types of primary extradural bone tumor (Figure 27.6) [5]. Osteosarcoma, hemangiosarcoma, fibrosarcoma, chemodectoma, anaplastic tumors, aortic body tumors, bronchogenic carcinoma, ganglioneuroma, malignant melanoma, mammary carcinomas,

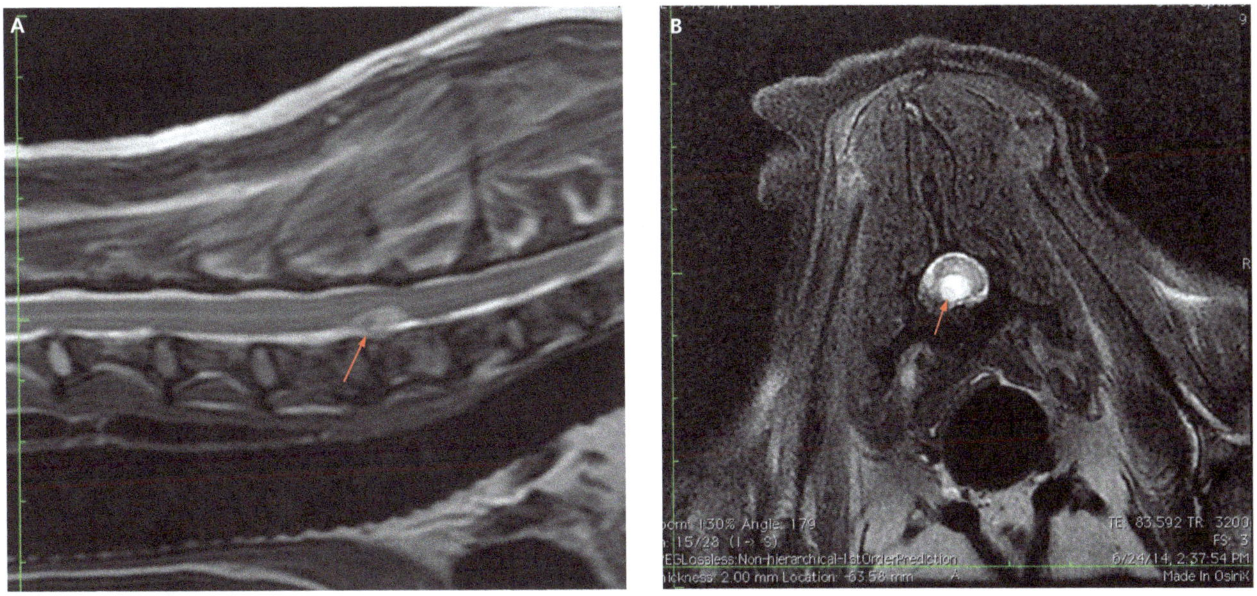

Figure 27.7 Intradural/extramedullary peripheral nerve sheath tumor (arrows in A, B) in a dog: (A) sagittal and (B) transverse T2-weighted MRI.

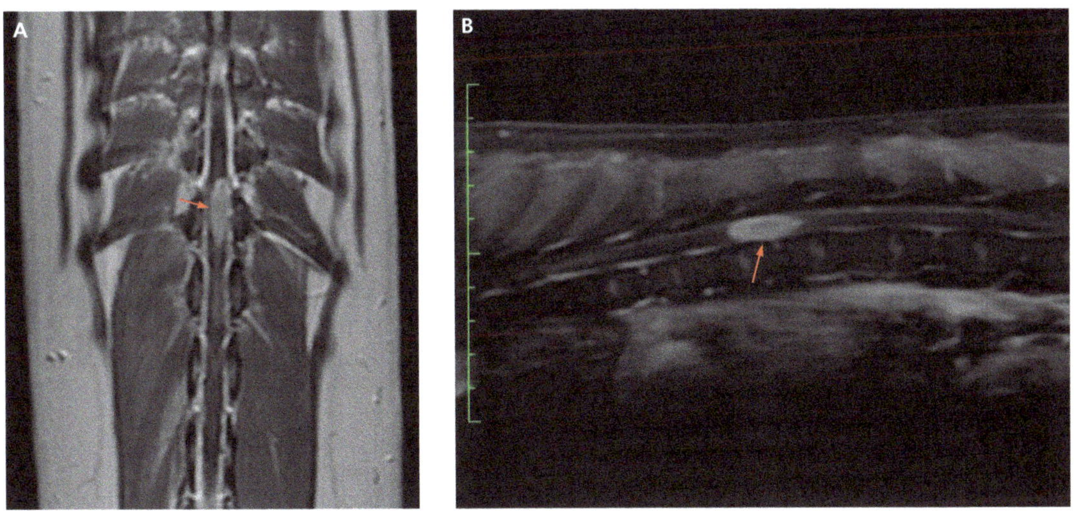

Figure 27.8 Nephroblastoma (arrows in A, B) in a dog: (A) dorsal T1-weighted MRI; (B) sagittal T1-weighted fluid-attenuated inversion recovery (FLAIR) MRI.

pancreatic adenocarcinoma, rhabdomyosarcoma, Sertoli cell carcinoma, squamous cell carcinoma, transitional cell carcinoma, prostatic carcinoma, and thyroid carcinoma have all been reported to metastasize to the spine [6]. Therefore additional testing (such as chest and abdominal radiographs, abdominal ultrasound and, if possible, thoracic CT when appropriate) should be considered if primary or metastatic disease has occurred in the specific patient. Of the primary soft tissue extradural spinal tumors, lymphoma is the most common seen in dogs. Meningioma and nerve sheath tumors are also common in the dog. Other soft tissue tumors reported in this location in dogs are myxosarcoma, myxoma, lipoma, and plasma cell tumor [7].

Intradural/extramedullary tumors are the second most common spinal tumor, accounting for about 35% of cases. They are found in the subarachnoid space, being confined by the dura mater. While some of the tumors in this location can be associated with pain from compression, not all of these dogs and cats exhibit pain. Hemangiomas, meningiomas (Figure 27.2), and nerve sheath tumors (Figure 27.7) are the most common type found in this location [6,7].

Intramedullary tumors (Figure 27.3) are the least common, accounting for about 15% of cases. Clinically, patients with tumors in this location typically do not present with pain. These tumors usually arise from cellular components of the normal spinal cord. Primary glial tumors such as astrocytoma, choroid plexus papilloma, ependymoma, oligodendroglioma, and undifferentiated sarcoma have all been reported [8].

Extrarenal nephroblastomas (Figure 27.8) are rare tumors that have been located either in the intradural/extramedullary space or intramedullary. They have also been termed as ependymoma, neuroepithelioma, and medulloepithelioma. They are most common in young dogs (5–36 months old), especially the German Shepherd. Typically, these tumors are found between T10 and L2. In general they are located dorsal or lateral to the spinal cord [6,9–11].

Diagnostic Evaluation

As with most disease syndromes, the clinician's main goal is to localize the underlying problem. As previously mentioned, the history and physical examination are paramount. The next step is deciding the most appropriate diagnostic tests and their order. A complete blood count, biochemical profile, and urinalysis are usually the initial part of a basic work-up. In many cases of spinal neurological disease all these results will be normal. In practice, veterinarians find themselves differentiating spinal neoplasia from the more common syndromes such as disc disease, degenerative myelopathy, fibrocartilagenous emboli, cervical vertebral instability or similar disorders. Certain basic testing results may reveal "red flags" that preclude the more common differentials. For example, elevated calcium (lymphoma), low hematocrit (anemia of chronic disease), and significantly elevated globulins (plasma cell tumor) signal underlying issues that are strongly indicative of a possible neoplastic process. Radiographs would be the next step in the process. While many spinal tumors are primary in origin, it is still imperative to exclude the possibility of a metastatic lesion. Radiological studies should include three-view thoracic radiographs. Abdominal radiographs and possibly abdominal ultrasound may also be indicated. Radiographs of the spinal column are the next logical step. Patients are sedated to allow proper positioning. In some cases radiographs of the pelvis and hips are also done at this time. Advanced imaging of the spine generally confirms the diagnosis: MRI, CT, and myelography are the mainstays. Each has advantages and disadvantages and not everyone has easy access to every modality. MRI, CT and myelography are all very good at evaluating extradural lesions. If bony involvement is suspected, then some of the older lower-quality MRI machines may give underwhelming results when compared with CT and myelography. Generally, MRI or CT myelography will provide the necessary imaging. CT can detect changes in physical bone density as small as 0.5%, whereas radiographs need about a 10% change in density before it becomes obvious [9]. One clear advantage of using CT to scan a bony vertebral tumor is the ability to reconstruct an image for use in surgical planning. Intramedullary tumors would be best evaluated with MRI and myelography. Tumors caudal to the L6 region are typically better evaluated with MRI and/or CT with epidurography. Myelograms and epidurograms are less sensitive in this area due to lack of the dural sac in this location. Intradural/extramedullary tumors and intramedullary tumors from C1 to L6 are usually well defined with a myelogram.

Intradural/extramedullary tumors often appear as expanded and outlined masses on one side of the spinal column. The other side of the column often deviates abaxially due to spinal cord swelling. This phenomenon is known as the "golf tee" sign (see Figure 27.2). In contrast, intramedullary tumors appear expansile and give the spinal cord the impression of being "fat" due to the bilateral deviation of the contrast column in the affected area. Bone scintigraphy can also be used to detect early signs of bony vertebral neoplasia [9]. However, this is rarely used in private referral practice and is not widely available in the university teaching hospital setting.

Cytology/Biopsy

When possible, cellular evaluation prior to any major surgical therapy is important. Cerebrospinal fluid (CSF) analysis, with the exception of spinal lymphoma, does not typically give a definitive diagnosis. Dogs have a higher chance of lymphoma cells being noted in the CSF compared with cats since dogs typically have lymphoma associated with the leptomeninges more commonly than cats. Elevated protein levels without concurrent increased cellularity is the most common result (albuminocytologic dissociation) [9].

Obtaining either a cytological or small Trucut biopsy when possible can often help with the overall plan and prognosis prior to definitive treatment options. Typically, aspiration and/or small Trucut biopsies are only practical and safe for extradural tumors involving the vertebrae or surrounding supporting structures. Cytology is usually safer and less traumatic with less risk but may not be as sensitive as a biopsy and certainly not as specific in providing the grade of tumor. Histological grade may be very important in treatment options and certainly with prognosis [17]. Depending on the size, location and involvement of the vertebral tumor, blind aspirates or Trucut biopsies can be obtained. Ultrasound guidance and CT-assisted biopsy are other more accurate means of obtaining preoperative samples.

If lymphoma specifically is suspected, then other diagnostics may obtain a definitive diagnosis when the CSF does not yield a conclusive answer. If enlarged lymph nodes are detected on physical examination, abdominal ultrasound or chest radiographs and aspiration of an abnormal/enlarged lymph node may be beneficial. Liver, splenic or bone marrow cytology may also give a definitive answer.

Treatment Options

Surgical intervention is of paramount importance in the treatment of spinal neoplasia. Spinal lymphoma, which responds very favorably to radiation therapy, might be the only or one of the few exceptions to this rule. Three important aspects of treatment are deciding on the best approach for removal or debulking the mass, seeking the input of an oncologist for adjunctive therapy, and considering the risk–benefit ratio of the surgery. How best to remove or debulk the tumor can influence the success and long-term comfort for the patient. Working with an oncologist will provide the most effective and current follow-up therapy. The potential effectiveness of radiation and chemotherapy can be a consideration in the aggressiveness of the surgery and in some instances the procedure to perform. In most cases complete removal is the ideal result but this must be weighed against possible permanent damage to the spinal cord and the risks of fracture, luxation or generalized instability as a result of surgical removal of supporting structures. The surgeon must act as a patient advocate and evaluate as fully as possible the risk–benefit ratio in performing a specific surgery. In many cases long-term results are significantly improved with follow-up radiation and/or chemotherapy and owners should be made aware of this prior to surgical intervention. Specific approaches to spinal tumors are described elsewhere in this book as well as many other sources. In general, surgeons should use the approach that allows the best visualization of the tumor as well as allowing the best chance for removal with least possible untoward complications.

Sometimes, performing a rhizotomy is necessary to either gain better access to the tumor or for alleviating regional pain. Rhizotomies in the lumbosacral and caudal cervical region can, of course, have possible neurological consequences. Removal of tumors within the dura require a durotomy. This is best achieved using a #11 or #12 scalpel blade. The tumor can often be "teased" from the spinal cord (Figure 27.9). Ultrasonic surgical aspirators have also been employed. The surgeon attempts as complete removal as possible while at the same time balancing the risk–benefit ratio of removal. Surgery alone for dogs with spinal tumors can result in prolonged survival in some instances. Nerve sheath tumors (see Figure 27.7) typically have a much worse long-term prognosis with surgery alone [7]. In general, cats with nonlymphoid spinal neoplasia tend to have a much better prognosis than cats with spinal lymphoma [1].

As with any tumor of the bone, the more complete the resection the better the chances of a longer-term prognosis. The location of the tumor in the vertebral body plays a large part in the overall success of removal. In general, tumors located dorsally or Zone 1 [12] are the easiest to remove and therefore probably have the best chance of complete excision. With regard to vertebral tumors, the biggest prognostic indicator is length of time to treatment. Dogs with the shortest duration of clinical signs and therefore the less time for invasion and metastasis had the best long-term survival.

Overall, primary spinal cord tumors occur infrequently in dogs. Meningiomas are the most common primary spinal tumor in dogs, and these seem to have a predilection for the cervical region. In a recent study of 34 intraspinal meningiomas, they were further classified into three different histological categories. These categories, as previously noted in humans, show a significant correlation with both tumor location and long-term survival. Moreover, cervical meningiomas tended to exhibit the less aggressive grade I form, whereas thoracolumbar and lumbar meningiomas tended to be grade II or III. In general, the higher the grade the worse the prognosis for patients with spinal meningioma. Grade III tumors are much less common than grade I or II. Higher cervical meningiomas (i.e., C3 or cranial) while having a lower grade can often make surgery more hazardous because of the critical location (brainstem) and more difficult resection [13]. Younger dogs were more likely to have grade II meningiomas and these grade II tumors tended to be in the thoracolumbar region. Older dogs tended to have grade I tumors and these tended to be in the cervical region. In comparison with humans, most spinal meningiomas are grade I and are usually well encapsulated. The most common location in humans is the thoracic spine, the hypothesis being that arachnoid cap cells are believed to be the progenitor cell for meningiomas and that these cells, which are found within arachnoid proliferations, are most commonly located in the thoracic spine in humans [13]. This makes surgical resection the treatment of choice and the need for follow-up therapy such as radiation unusual. In humans, recurrence of spinal meningiomas after surgical resection has been reported to be as low as 3–15% [14]. In humans, about 25% of all primary spinal cord tumors are meningiomas, and these usually occur in people in their fourth decade [4]. Young dogs, usually less than 3 years of age, have a propensity to form primitive neuroectodermal tumors (PNETs). These tumors are all considered biologically malignant and are able to differentiate into neuronal, glial, or ependymal cell lines [15]. Recently, some of these PNETs have been differentiated with the aid of positive immunohistochemical staining for Wilms tumor gene product (WT1) which is a human marker for human nephroblastoma (Wilms tumor) into extrarenal nephroblastomas. Typically, extrarenal nephroblastoma occurs in younger dogs aged between 5 months and 7 years, with 6–36 months the most common age. They are also found almost exclusively between T10 and L2 spinal vertebrae [6,10,11,15,16]. German Shepherds and Golden Retrievers are the most common breeds. The most common type of spinal tumor in cats is spinal lymphoma, and usually occurs in younger patients. Other types of spinal tumors in cats have been reported as well but they usually occur in older cats [1]. Osteosarcoma is the most common vertebral bone tumor in dogs and cats while in humans it is rare. Dogs and humans tend to have a much poorer prognosis than cats with osteosarcoma [2,11].

Nonsurgical Therapy

Other forms of therapy such as radiation therapy, chemotherapy and symptomatic care have been used. Radiation therapy is often recommended in addition to surgery or when surgery is not possible or viable. Radiation typically is used for local control. Depending

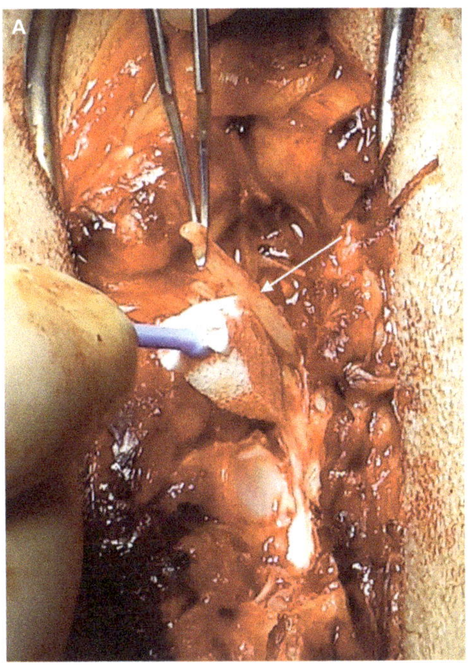

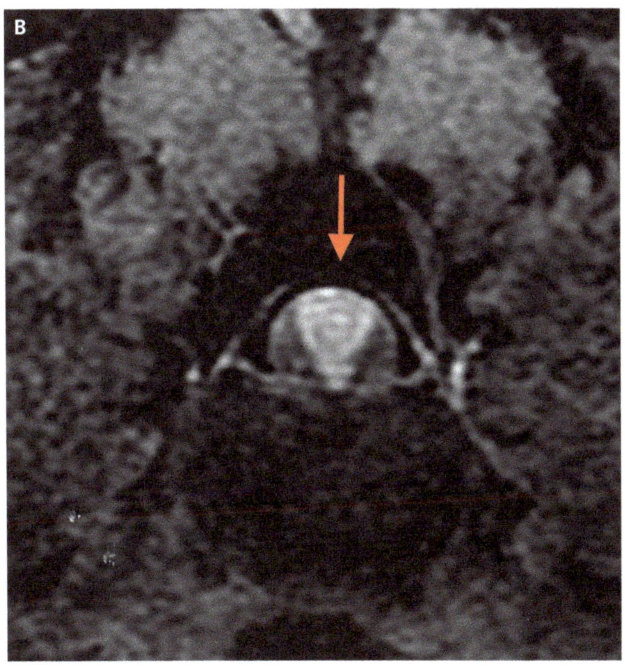

Figure 27.9 (A) Surgical removal of an intramedullary mass in the lumbar region of a dog following a dorsal laminectomy and durotomy. (B) Preoperative transverse T1-weighted MRI with contrast showing the mass (arrow).

on the specific case and situation, radiation will either definitively control the tumor or palliate its growth. High-dose radiation is usually good at killing tumor cells. Unfortunately, it can also damage the surrounding healthy spinal cord. Radiation oncologists and radiotherapy physicists are well-informed resources for planning therapies and intensity-modulated radiation therapy is often used in treatment of spinal neoplasms. In infrequent cases of spinal inflammation or necrosis, radiation therapy should be stopped as soon as neurological deficits are noted. Transient demyelination, known as Lhermitte's syndrome in humans, is usually reversible. In animals it could manifest itself with the animal either licking at the radiation therapy site or turning and looking at this site. This syndrome can resolve and is sometimes treated with steroids. It can be important to differentiate Lhermitte's syndrome with recurrence of disease [11]. Sometimes a follow-up advanced imaging technique such as MRI may be required to differentiate this from recurrent disease. Chemotherapy is generally not recommended for primary treatment of nonhematopoietic spinal tumors. Lymphoma, leukemia, disseminated histiocytic sarcoma, multiple myeloma, and to some extent osteosarcoma are responsive to chemotherapy. Palliative therapy is often indicated in dogs with spinal neoplasia. Corticosteroids may help alleviate peritumoral inflammation and edema. Steroids need to be considered based on the overall picture. They would likely not be indicated if the patient was Cushingoid or had an undiagnosed lymphoma. Some controversy exists over the risk–benefit ratio of using steroids. Unwanted side effects such as polyuria/polydipsia, gastrointestinal ulceration, weight gain, inhibition of tissue healing postoperatively, or higher risk of infection need to be weighed against the benefits of steroid use. Other medications such as tramadol, nonsteroidal antiinflammatory drugs (NSAIDs), amantadine, and gabapentin should be considered. Alternative therapies such as acupuncture might also help alleviate some of the pain associated with spinal tumors.

Spinal tumors offer a challenging dilemma. Because the physical examination findings are often similar to less life-threatening diseases like intervertebral disc disease and degenerative myelopathy, the clinician needs to be astutely aware of this on the differentials. Many times animals are sent home with palliative therapy on the assumption of the more benign syndromes. As with most cancers, the sooner they are diagnosed and treated the better potential for a more positive long-term outcome. Patients with a chronic or recurrent presentation or those not responding to traditional therapy should be regarded as highly suspicious for the presence of spinal neoplasia. Thorough work-ups are recommended. The best outcome can often come when doctors work as a team, which should consist of the primary veterinarian, a surgeon or neurologist with experience in neurosurgical oncology, the oncologist, radiation oncologist, and radiologist. Most importantly the owner/caregiver needs to be well informed throughout the entire process.

Video clips to accompany this book can be found on the companion website at:
www.wiley.com/go/shores/neurosurgery

References

1 Levy MS, Mauldin G, Kapatkin AS, Patnaik AK. Nonlymphoid vertebral canal tumors in cats: 11 cases (1987–1995). *J Am Vet Med Assoc* 1997;210:663–664.
2 Sama AA. Spinal tumors. Medscape. Available at http://Emedicine.Medscape.Com/Article/1267223-Overview (accessed May 15, 2012).
3 Oliver JE, Lorenz MD. *Handbook of Veterinary Neurological Diagnosis*. Philadelphia, PA: WB Saunders, 1983.
4 National Institute of Neurological Disorders and Stroke, NINDS. Brain and spinal tumors: hope through research. Available at https://www.ninds.nih.gov/Disorders/Patient-Caregiver-Education/Hope-Through-Research/Brain-and-Spinal-Tumors-Hope-Through (accessed May 15, 2012).
5 Bagley RS, Kornegay JM, Page RL et al. Central nervous system. In: Slatter D (ed.) *Textbook of Small Animal Surgery*, 2nd edn. Philadelphia, PA: WB Saunders, 1993: 2137–2166.
6 Smith AN. Overview of neoplasia of the nervous system. In: *The Merck Veterinary Manual*. Available at http://www.msdvetmanual.com/nervous-system/neoplasia-of-the-nervous-system/overview-of-neoplasia-of-the-nervous-system
7 Levy MS, Kapatkin AS, Patnaik AK, Mauldin GE. Spinal tumors in 37 dogs: clinical outcome and long-term survival (1987–1994). *J Am Anim Hosp Assoc* 1997;33:307–312.
8 Morrison WB. *Cancer in Dogs and Cats: Medical and Surgical Management*, 2nd edn. Jackson, WY: Teton NewMedia, 2002.
9 Seguin B, Bagley R, Silver G. Diagnosis and treatment of spinal neoplasia in dogs and cats. *Waltham Focus* 2000;10:4–9.
10 South Texas Veterinary Specialists. Spinal cord tumors. Available at http://www.stvetspecialists.com/index.php?option=com_content&task=view&id=23&Item (accessed March 26, 2012).
11 Kent M, Northrup N. Spinal neoplasia. In: Tobias KM, Johnston SA (eds) *Veterinary Surgery: Small Animal*. St Louis, MO: Elsevier Saunders, 2012: 537–551.
12 Gilson SD. Neuro-oncological surgery of the vertebral column and spinal cord. In: Slatter D (ed.) *Textbook of Small Animal Surgery*, 3rd edn. Philadelphia, PA: WB Saunders, 2003: 1277–1286.
13 Petersen SA, Sturges BK, Dickinson PJ, Higgind RJ. Canine intraspinal meningiomas: imaging features, histopathologic classification, and long-term outcome in 34 dogs. *J Vet Intern Med* 2008;22:946–953.
14 Gottfried ON, Gluf W, Quinones-Hinojosa A, Kan P, Schmidt MH. Spinal meningiomas: surgical management and outcome. *Neurosurg Focus* 2003;14(6):Article 2. Available at http://thejns.org/doi/pdf/10.3171/foc.2003.14.6.2
15 LeCouter RA. Tumors of the nervous system. In: Withrow SJ, MacEwen EG (eds) *Small Animal Clinical Oncology*. Philadelphia, PA: WB Saunders, 2001: 500–531.
16 National Canine Cancer Foundation. Spinal cord neoplasia. Available at http://wearethecure.org/learn-more-about-canince-cancer/canine-cancer-library/spinal-cord-neoplasia/(accessed March 26, 2012).
17 Wright JA., The Pathological Features Associated with Spinal Tumours in 29 Dogs. *J.Comp. Path* 1985; 95: 549–556.

SECTION IV

Postoperative Care and Rehabilitation

28 Guidelines for Postoperative Medical Care of the Neurosurgical Patient

Debbie Reynolds and Brigitte A. Brisson

Introduction

The level of postoperative care required for neurosurgical patients depends on the type of surgery performed and the neurological status of the patient. Important components of management include provision of adequate analgesia, meeting nutritional and fluid requirements, providing adequate bladder and defecation management, nursing care to prevent respiratory and skin complications, and physical therapy to limit muscle mass loss, maintain joint range of motion and health, and improve circulation.

Immediate Postoperative Care

In the immediate postoperative period it is important to provide appropriate analgesia maintain appropriate body temperature, oxgenation and hydration (Figure 28.1). Patients should be closely monitored to ensure that they are recovering without evidence of seizures (especially after myelography or intracranial surgery), hypotension, or inappropriate ventilation. Bladder and nutritional management should also be considered in this period.

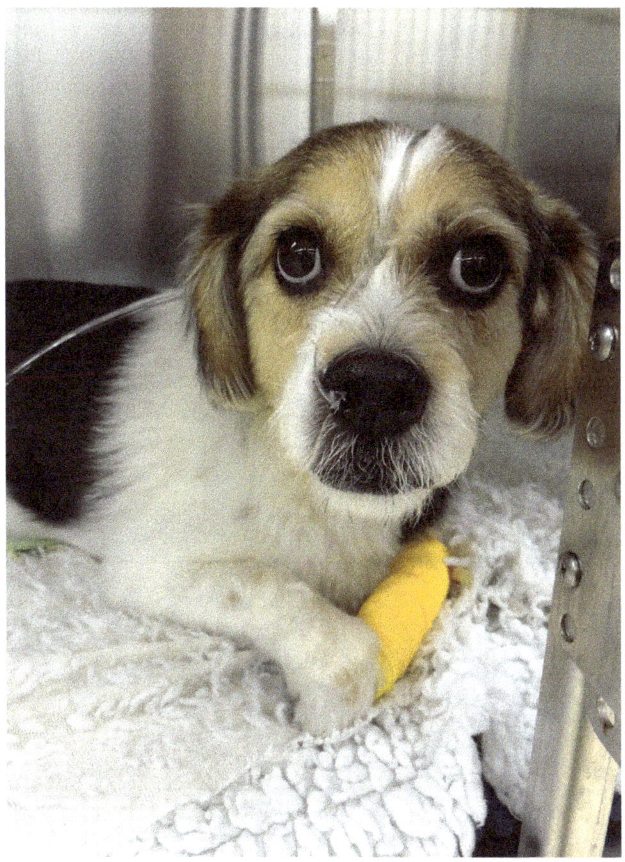

Figure 28.1 Postoperative patient with nasal cannula for oxygen supplementation and intravenous catheter for fluid administration.

Intravenous Fluids

Postoperative fluid therapy is important for maintaining hydration, replacing insensible losses, and allowing easy administration of medications until the patient is eating and drinking. A balanced electrolyte solution is selected, with the rate of administration based on the type and amount of fluids needed to correct dehydration over a 24-hour period, provide for maintenance and insensible losses, and to correct electrolyte and acid-base imbalances. Patients who receive corticosteroids or osmotic diuretics, such as mannitol, have higher fluid losses and this should be considered when

Current Techniques in Canine and Feline Neurosurgery, First Edition. Edited by Andy Shores and Brigitte A. Brisson.
© 2017 John Wiley & Sons, Inc. Published 2017 by John Wiley & Sons, Inc.
Companion website: www.wiley.com/go/shores/neurosurgery

calculating fluid rates. Daily maintenance fluid requirements are calculated as $(BW_{kg} \times 30) + 70$ (mL per day). For animals weighing less than 2 kg or more than 50 kg an alternative calculation should be used: $(BW_{kg}^{0.75}) \times 70$.

Spinal patients often fail to maintain adequate fluid intake prior to surgery due to stress, pain, or lack of mobility and may be mildly to moderately dehydrated on presentation. For acute spinal cord injuries, fluid therapy is indicated as hydration of the spinal cord and prevention of hypotension is thought to be an important component in the health and recovery of neurons [1]. Intraoperative blood losses can be significant, especially in small-breed dogs, and need to be considered when assessing a patient's fluid requirements. The venous sinuses run along the ventral aspect of the spinal column and can be disrupted during hemilaminectomy, mini-hemilaminectomy, corpectomy, or ventral slot procedures. During craniotomy, there can be blood loss from compromise to the dorsal sagittal and transverse sinuses. If greater than 10–15% of blood volume is lost intraoperatively or packed cell volume is below 22%, use of replacement blood products is indicated [2].

Specific blood products can also be indicated for thrombocytopenia (platelet-rich concentrate), prolonged clotting times as with von Willebrand disease (cryoprecipitate, fresh frozen plasma, and DDAVP or desmopressin acetate), and hypoalbuminemia (fresh frozen plasma). Alternatives to increase oncotic pressure include colloids such as Pentaspan® and Voluven®. Blood typing should be performed prior to transfusion and cross-matching should occur if the patient has previously received blood products to prevent acute transfusion reactions.

Analgesia

Postoperative pain associated with surgery is typically controlled with multimodal analgesia protocols. A large number of neurological patients will present having already received either nonsteroidal antiinflammatory drugs (NSAIDs) or corticosteroids, which may affect the options for postoperative analgesia (see discussion below). The mainstay of postoperative pain management following neurosurgery should be opioids. The selection of opioid will depend on the type of surgery performed, the availability of opioids, and level of postoperative care that is available in your practice. Postoperative analgesia is typically provided by a continuous-rate infusion of opioids (Table 28.1). For patients undergoing craniotomy, bolus dosing of opioids such as morphine and hydromorphone should be used with caution, as vomiting can be associated with its administration, which may increase intracranial pressure [3,4].

Table 28.1 Continuous-rate infusion doses for analgesics commonly used in dogs and cats.

Drug	Dose
Fentanyl	2–6 μg/kg per hour
Morphine	0.1–0.2 mg/kg per hour
Butorphanol	0.1–0.4 mg/kg per hour
Ketamine	0.1–2.0 mg/kg per hour
Lidocaine*	20–80 μg/kg per min
Dexmedetomidine	0.5–1 μg/kg per hour

* Care when using with cats as increased risk of toxicity.
Source: Doses modified from *Plumb's Veterinary Drug Handbook* [20].

Alternatively, intermittent use of longer-acting opioids can be used effectively (Table 28.2). Methadone is also an appropriate choice for analgesia, when available. Methadone is a μ-receptor agonist that has 10 times the potency of morphine but is also an *N*-methyl-D-aspartate (NMDA) receptor antagonist that reduces reuptake of norepinephrine and serotonin, which may make it ideal for neuropathic pain [5,6].

Adjunctive analgesics that can also be used based on response to opioids include continuous-rate infusions of ketamine (an NMDA receptor antagonist), lidocaine (local anesthetic), or dexmedetomidine (an α_2 agonist that provides both analgesic and sedative effects) (Table 28.1).

Several recent studies have evaluated the use of topical analgesia following hemilaminectomy with either morphine alone [7] or morphine and dexmedetomidine administered using gel foam as a carrier [8]. Both studies concluded that the topical use of analgesics reduced the need for systemic administration. However, temporary loss of nociception has been reported following topical intrathecal morphine administration using gel foam as a carrier [9]. Further studies comparing the use of directly applied analgesics versus those administered in a carrier and their long-term safety are required.

NSAIDs versus Corticosteroids

The use of corticosteroids in spinal surgery and in most cases of intracranial surgery has shown no benefit and may possibly be detrimental. A large proportion of neurosurgical patients presenting to referral centers for surgery have already received NSAIDs or corticosteroids. The decision is then whether to continue with the current protocol or stop it and use alternate drugs.

Corticosteroids

There is little evidence to support the use of corticosteroids in intervertebral disc (IVD) surgery. The previously recommended protocol of methylprednisolone sodium succinate 30 mg/kg within the first 6 hours followed by 15 mg/kg every 6 hours for 24–48 hours may provide some benefit in neurological recovery, although recent evidence suggests that there is no difference in outcome [10]. In addition, using this protocol greater than 8 hours after the initial spinal injury has been shown to have a detrimental effect in humans [11].

The use of corticosteroids may also predispose nonambulatory dogs undergoing neurosurgery to urinary tract infections (UTIs),

Table 28.2 Opioid doses that can be administered intermittently in dogs and cats.

Drug	Dose	Frequency	Route
Hydromorphone	0.025–0.05 mg/kg	4–6 hours	IV, IM, SC
Morphine	0.2–1.0 mg/kg	3–4 hours	IV, IM, SC
Methadone	0.1–0.5 mg/kg	4–6 hours	IV, IM, SC
Buprenorphine	0.01–0.03 mg/kg	6–8 hours	IV, IM, buccal

Source: Doses modified from *Plumb's Veterinary Drug Handbook* [20].

in some reports up to three times more than dogs that do not receive corticosteroids [12]. Another major concern with the use of corticosteroids in dogs with IVD disease is gastrointestinal hemorrhage. Dogs with IVD have been shown to be predisposed to gastrointestinal ulceration, and in a randomized study looking at high doses of methylprednisolone sodium succinate, all dogs that received the steroid had evidence of gastric hemorrhage on endoscopy, whereas those in the control group did not [13]. Rare but fatal colonic perforation has also been reported in dogs receiving dexamethasone for IVD herniation with or without surgery [14,15]. Whether they are effective or not, gastroprotectants should be used in patients that receive corticosteroids. Corticosteroids can also lead to increased metabolic requirement, nitrogen losses, and hyperglycemia [16].

Corticosteroids are often used for intracranial disease including neoplasia and inflammatory conditions. In neoplasia it often improves preoperative clinical status, which is thought to be due to a reduction in peritumoral edema. Vasogenic edema occurs secondary to the compressive effects of the tumor and responds well to antiinflammatory doses of corticosteroids [17]. Whether to continue with steroids postoperatively, what doses to use, and for how long are typically personal preferences with no strict guidelines or clinical controlled studies published. Doses of steroids used for vasogenic edema in intracranial disease are typically antiinflammatory: dexamethasone 0.25 mg/kg every 24 hours or prednisone 0.25–0.5 mg/kg every 12–24 hours.

NSAIDs

NSAIDs are widely used in both human and veterinary medicine to provide analgesia. As understanding of the biological effects of prostaglandins evolves, there has been development of drugs more selective for cyclooxygenase (COX)-2 in an attempt to limit the adverse effects such as gastrointestinal ulceration while providing adequate antiinflammatory and analgesic effects. There are several NSAIDs that are currently approved for short- and longer-term use in dogs including carprofen, deracoxib, etodolac, firocoxib, meloxicam, and tepoxalin. The most common adverse event reported in conjunction with the use of NSAIDs in dogs is gastrointestinal upset manifesting as vomiting and diarrhea. NSAIDs should also be used with caution in patients with bleeding disorders, renal insufficiency, hepatic disease, or inflammatory bowel disease. Other adverse events that have been reported with the use of NSAIDs include idiopathic hepatic failure (carprofen), especially in Labrador Retrievers. In feline patients, the long-term use of NSAIDs has not been approved by the Food and Drug Administration (FDA). Carprofen is approved as a single dose perioperatively (USA), meloxicam as a single injectable dose (USA and Canada) followed by 3 days of oral dosing (Canada), and more recently robenacoxib for up to 3 days (USA). Longer-term use of meloxicam has been reported in cats in Europe [18]. As the labeled dosing schedule for NSAIDs in cats varies for each region, the reader is referred to the drug monographs when considering dose rates and intervals.

The duration of postoperative pain management is typically limited to 5–7 days. If spinal hyperesthesia persists beyond this time, repeat imaging of the patient is recommended as residual disc material or further disc extrusion may have occurred [19]. Other complications such as surgical site infection and discospondylitis may also need to be considered.

Alternative or Adjunctive Analgesics

There is a variety of alternative or adjunctive analgesics that have been used in both veterinary and human patients. In some cases there is limited scientific literature on the efficacy of these medications in veterinary medicine and their use has been translated from the human literature. In most cases their use is associated with minimal adverse effects and may provide adjunctive or alternative therapy for surgical patients, particularly if the use of corticosteroids precludes the use of NSAIDs.

Codeine

Oral codeine is an alternative analgesic for patients that cannot receive NSAIDs or for patients that do not respond well to tramadol. Codeine is an opiate with 60% oral absorption in dogs. Codeine is less potent than morphine. The dose of codeine for analgesia in dogs and cats is 0.5–2 mg/kg orally every 6–12 hours [20].

Tramadol

Tramadol is a synthetic analgesic with weak μ-opioid receptor agonist effects that also inhibits the reuptake of serotonin and norepinephrine. Tramadol has good oral absorption (around 65%) with a potency between that of codeine and morphine. Side effects of tramadol are often related to the use of adjunctive drugs that increase serotonin levels. Dosages reported in dogs are 4–10 mg/kg orally every 6 hours and in cats 1–2 mg/kg every 12 hours [20].

Gabapentin

Gabapentin is a γ-aminobutyric acid (GABA) analog that has been shown to have some success in treating chronic pain, in particular neuropathic pain [21]. Gabapentin also has some anticonvulsant activity [22]. Oral antacids should not be administered with gabapentin as it may decrease its bioavailability. Analgesic doses used in dogs and cats vary, with recommended doses of 5–10 mg/kg every 8–12 hours. In cats, treatment should start at the lower dose and gradually increase if no adverse effects are noted within 2 hours [20]. Adverse effects that can be seen with administration of gabapentin include sedation and ataxia, which are usually self-limiting.

Amantadine

Amantadine is an antiviral drug that has NMDA receptor antagonistic properties. It has recently been purported to be useful as an adjunctive therapy for chronic pain [23]. The pharmacokinetics of amantadine have not been described in dogs or cats and it therefore should be used with caution in patients with renal or hepatic insufficiency. It is often used in addition to NSAIDs, which reportedly improves its efficacy [23]. Doses reported for use in both dogs and cats are 2–5 mg/kg orally once daily, although 3 mg/kg is most common in cats [20]. Long-term use and its side effects are unknown in dogs and cats. Adverse effects are generally related to the gastrointestinal tract, but some patients may exhibit agitation.

Methocarbamol

Methocarbamol is a centrally acting muscle relaxant approved for use in acute inflammatory and traumatic injuries to the skeletal muscle and to reduce muscle spasms. The mechanism of action is unknown and its use in managing spinal patients for muscle pain and to assist bladder expression is anecdotal with little evidence to suggest efficacy in either the human or veterinary literature [24,25]. Doses that have been reported for muscle relaxation in dogs are

15–20 mg/kg orally every 8 hours, and in cats 61–132 mg/kg orally divided every 8–12 hours [20].

Gastroprotectants

Gastric ulceration has been reported to occur at a higher incidence in patients with neurological disease [26,27]. This can be compounded by the use of high doses of corticosteroids that are sometimes administered prior to referral for surgery. The development of gastric ulceration following the use of corticosteroids may not be prevented by the use of gastroprotectants. A study evaluating the efficacy of omeprazole and misoprostol in dogs with naturally occurring IVD disease that were administered dexamethasone and prednisone revealed no difference in the degree of gastric ulceration in either group [26]. These findings were similar to the study evaluating misoprostol, cimetidine and sucralfate with methylprednisolone sodium succinate [28].

There is limited information in companion animals regarding the benefits of gastroprotectants in preventing gastric ulceration with concurrent NSAID use, with most recommendations extrapolated from human medicine. Misoprostol, a prostaglandin E1 agonist, has been shown to significantly decrease gastric ulceration associated with the use of NSAIDs [29]. Misoprostol has not been shown to have any advantage over other gastroprotectants in treating ulcerations not related to NSAIDs and is more expensive than other gastroprotectant drugs. Misoprostol doses that have been recommended are 2–5 μg/kg orally every 6–8 hours [20]. Gastroprotectants that have been shown to reduce gastric acidity in dogs and which may help prevent gastric ulceration include histamine antagonists (famotidine, 0.5 mg/kg every 12 hours) and proton pump inhibitors (omeprazole, 0.5–1.0 mg/kg orally once daily; pantoprazole, 0.5–1.0 mg/kg intravenously once daily). If ulceration is suspected due to the presence of melena, then sucralfate (0.5–1.0 g orally every 8 hours) should also be administered. In a study evaluating the effects of famotidine, ranitidine, omeprazole, and pantoprazole on gastric pH levels in normal dogs, it was found that famotidine, omeprazole, and pantoprazole significantly decreased gastric acidity compared with saline or ranitidine [30]. Oral omeprazole was also found to decrease gastric acidity faster than both famotidine and pantoprazole and for longer durations throughout the day. The higher efficacy of omeprazole in increasing gastric pH compared with famotidine was also found in the study by Tolbert et al. [31].

Antibiotics

The incidence of postoperative infection following spinal or intracranial surgery is low (1.3%) [32] compared with routine clean surgeries (2–5.8%) [33,34]. However, perioperative prophylactic antibiotics should be used to limit incisional infections. The most commonly used prophylactic antibiotic is cefazolin, a first-generation cephalosporin. It should be administered 30 min prior to surgery and then every 90 min throughout the duration of surgery at a dose of 22 mg/kg. Continuation of antibiotics following surgery is not indicated except in cases of intracranial surgery where the frontal sinus has been opened or when treating traumatic contaminated wounds that involve the CNS. In cases where bone cement is used intraoperatively, some surgeons administer a 7–10 day postoperative course of antibiotics as the development of infection in these cases could lead to surgical failure and would necessitate implant removal.

Managing the Recumbent Patient

Patients with paraparesis or tetraparesis or that are unconscious (craniotomy or trauma patients) are unable to change position and may be unable to ventilate appropriately. Until they become ambulatory, dry soft padded bedding should be provided to reduce the risk of developing decubital ulcers (Figure 28.2). The patient should be maintained in sternal recumbency or the side of recumbency should be changed every 4–6 hours depending on the size of the patient, always ensuring appropriate padding under bony prominences. If unconscious or heavily sedated, the patient's head should be elevated 30° above the body to limit the potential for aspiration pneumonia and to reduce intracranial pressure [35].

Physiotherapy for the Recumbent Patient

Passive range of motion (ROM) and muscle strengthening exercises are recommended in the short- and long-term postoperative neurological patient. Passive ROM exercises should be initiated as soon as the patient is comfortable enough to allow it and should be performed three to four times daily in recumbent patients to reduce limb edema and assist in peripheral perfusion (Figure 28.3). More details on rehabilitation are discussed in Chapter 29.

Thoracic percussion and neubulization as well as oral care should be performed three to four times daily, particularly in patients that

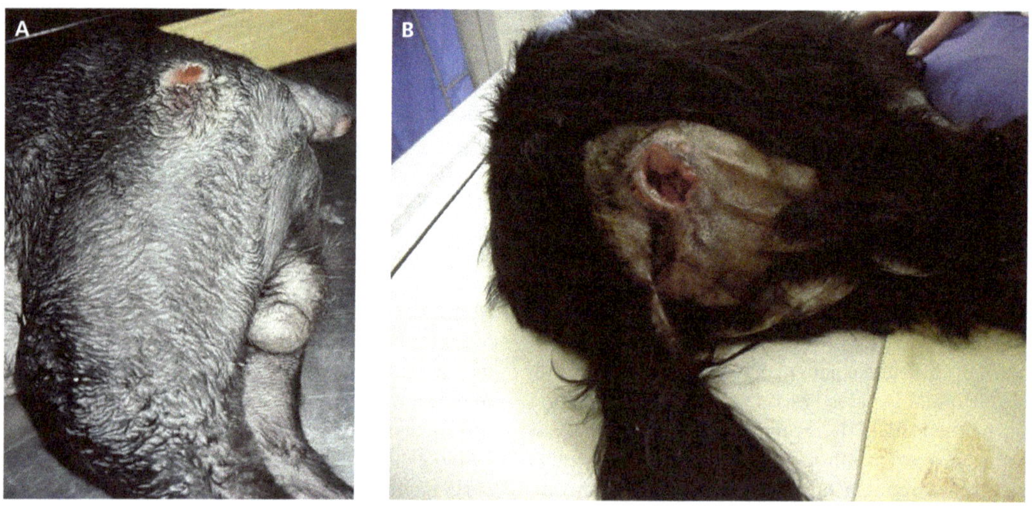

Figure 28.2 (A) Cutaneous erosion over the left hip of a paralyzed dog. (B) Decubital ulcer over the right ischium of a paralyzed dog.

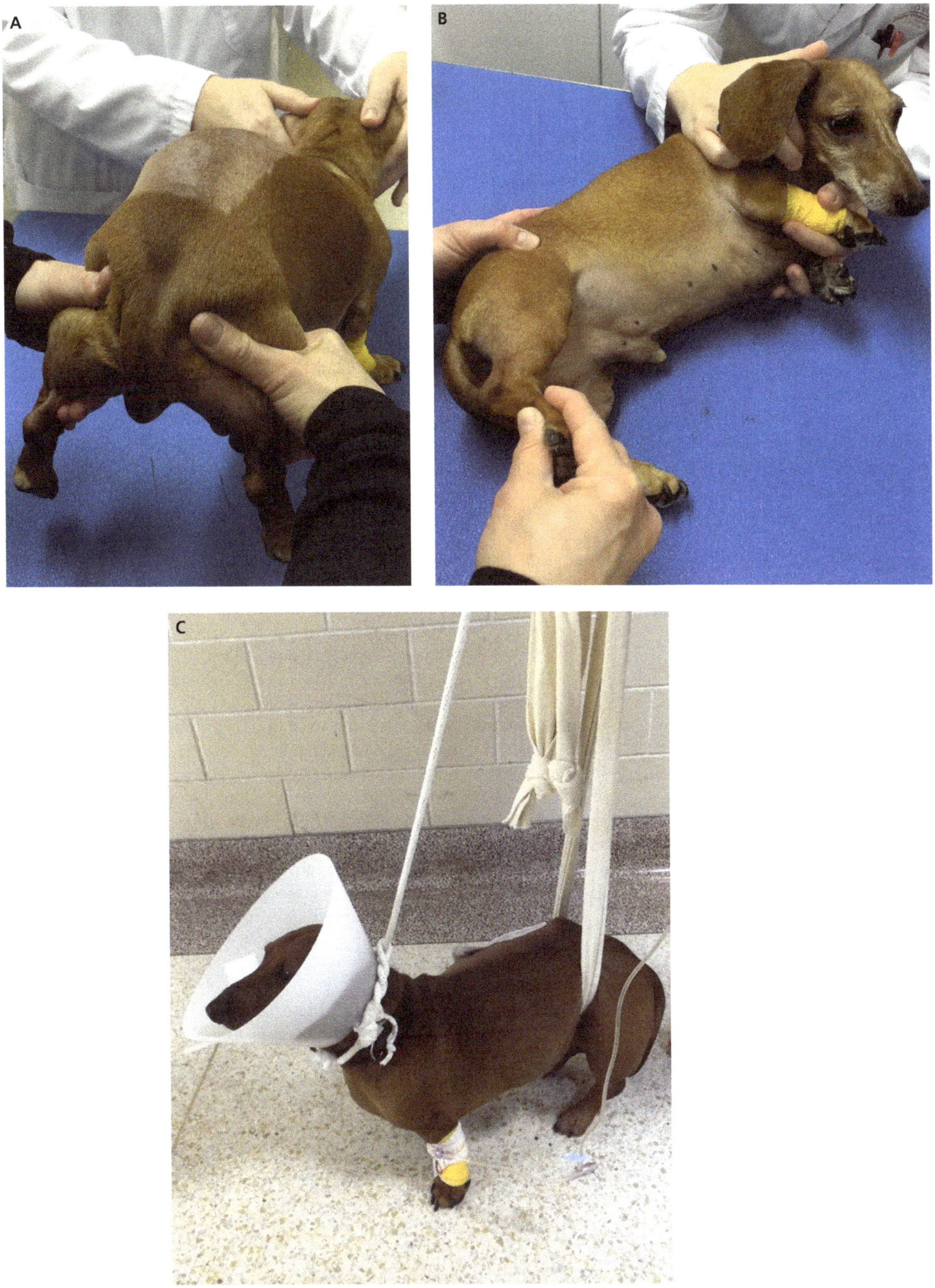

Figure 28.3 Postoperative physical exercises. (A) Passive range of motion exercises: abduction of the pelvic limbs. (B) Passive range of motion exercises: cycling of each individual pelvic limb. (C) Assisted walking with a towel or sling.

require assisted ventilation, and can be used in recumbent patients to try to limit thoracic congestion and development of aspiration pneumonia [36].

Mechanical Ventilation

Mechanical ventilation of neurological patients can be required prior to surgery, particularly in dogs with high cervical lesions (discs, tumors, and luxations/fractures) or in patients that have intracranial disease that is affecting respiratory function. Indications for mechanical ventilation include the lack of spontaneous respiration due to the location of the cervical lesion, to prevent hypercapnia in intracranial disease, to minimize cerebral edema, and in patients that have developed aspiration pneumonia and have reduced oxygenation. Triggers on blood gas analysis for mechanical ventilation are $Pa\text{o}_2$ below 60 mmHg or $Pa\text{co}_2$ above 60 mmHg [37]. In cases of intracranial disease, hyperventilation and reduction of CO_2 to around 35 mmHg is often indicated to minimize changes in intracranial pressure. If mechanical ventilation is required, positive end-expiratory pressure (PEEP) should be avoided as it may lead to increases in intracranial pressure due to impaired venous outflow secondary to increased intrathoracic pressure [38].

The prognosis for patients that require mechanical ventilation depends on the underlying pathology, the type of surgical procedure performed, and the development of ventilator-associated complications such as pneumonia and sepsis.

Bladder Management

One of the most important aspects of managing the neurological patient is management of the urinary bladder. Voluntary bladder control will depend on the neurological status of the patient at the time of presentation or postoperatively. If bladder function is not adequately managed, the patient is likely to develop a UTI, detrusor atony, and also severe and debilitating skin lesions secondary to urine scalding that can lead to sepsis. There are several alternatives to physically and medically manage the urinary bladder for both the short- and long-term neurology patient.

Urinary Catheters

Urinary catheters can be indwelling or placed intermittently. The decision to place a urinary catheter is based on the preoperative neurological status of the patient and can also be dependent on the gender and demeanor of the patient. The greatest risk associated with urinary catheterization is the development of UTIs, which can ultimately lead to pyelonephritis. However, this risk is also present if the patient is allowed to develop overflow incontinence. The risk of developing UTIs has been found to be unrelated to the use of indwelling or intermittent catheterization, but rather is related to the duration of catheter placement or urinary dysfunction [39]. Dogs that are nonambulatory have been shown to be twice as likely to develop a UTI [12]. The development of UTIs has also been reported in a population of dogs with indwelling urinary catheters in an intensive care setting [40]. In this study, female dogs had an overall higher incidence of UTIs than male dogs, with an increased risk of infection after 3 days of catheterization [40].

For patients without nociception preoperatively and postoperatively, and which may never fully regain voluntary urination, bladder expression is required and the owners need to be taught this technique. In some of the nociception-negative patients, reflex urination may develop between 4 and 6 weeks. Voluntary urination in the thoracolumbar spinal patient is typically possible if the patient retains or regains voluntary motor function; many patients remain nonambulatory for a variable period of time after regaining motor and voluntary urinary function.

Indwelling Catheterization

Indwelling urinary catheters are recommended for the intracranial patient or the tetraparetic or paraparetic patient with no loss of nociception or voluntary motor function in the immediate postoperative period until the change in neurological status and potential for recovery can be evaluated. In cases where the patient is experiencing pain and is finding it difficult to express urine in the immediate postoperative period, the use of an indwelling urinary catheter to prevent over-distension, overflow incontinence, and urine scalding is also recommended. The average time a urinary catheter can remain in place prior to development of a UTI has been shown to be approximately 3 days [39,40].

If possible, antibiotics should be avoided in patients while the catheter is in place and the urine should be cultured around 24 hours following removal of the catheter to determine if a UTI is present. If an infection is suspected during catheterization, appropriate antibiotics are selected based on bacterial culture and sensitivity. In the guidelines developed for managing UTIs in dogs and in cats, it is recommended to remove the urinary catheter whenever possible if infection has developed and to culture the urine via cystocentesis [41]. Prophylactic use of antibiotics is not recommended while the catheter is in place [41].

Indwelling urinary catheters should be placed using aseptic technique (catheter, gloves, lubricant, etc.). The vulva or prepuce should be prepared with an aqueous chlorhexidine solution or soap to limit retrograde introduction of bacteria during catheter placement. Some clinicians perform a complete surgical clip and preparation of the perivulvar or peripreputial region prior to placing a urinary catheter. Following placement, the sterile closed collection system should be kept as clean as possible (e.g., off the ground while allowing for drainage by gravity) (Figure 28.4). The urinary catheter, plus or minus vulva or prepuce, should be wiped every 8 hours with an aqueous chlorhexidine solution and the urine collection system should be replaced every 48 hours until the catheter is removed [37,42].

Intermittent Catheterization

Intermittent catheterization can be used to manage the urinary bladder and can be taught to an owner if manual expression is not tolerated in male patients. This is not typically a viable option in a female patient due to the increased difficulty of catheterization without sedation. The frequency of catheterization depends on whether the patient is on intravenous fluids and whether corticosteroids or mannitol are being administered. With the owners following aseptic technique, it is recommended catheterization be performed three to four times per day using a sterile catheter each time.

Manual Bladder Expression

Intermittent bladder expression can be performed for short- or long-term management of the neurological patient that does not have voluntary urination. If the patient is receiving intravenous fluids, this may need to be as frequently as every 3–4 hours to ensure that there is no over-distension of the bladder or overflow of urine that could cause urine scalding. If the patient is not

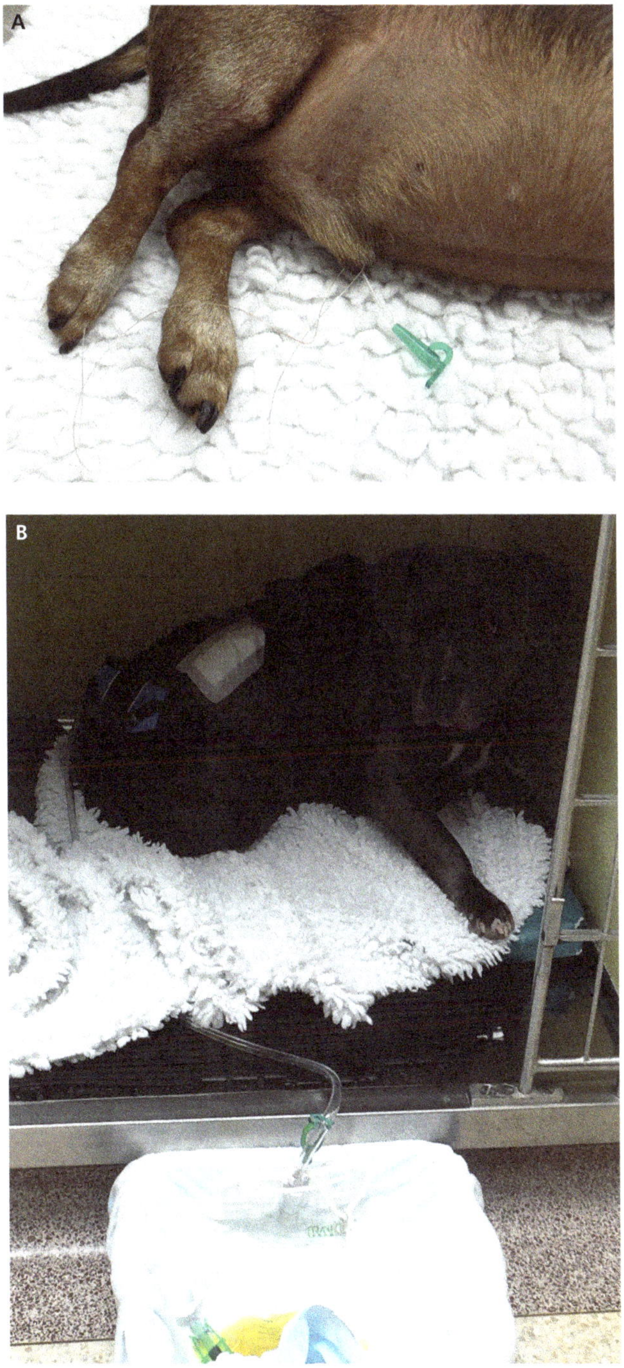

Figure 28.4 (A) Indwelling male urinary catheter immediately after aseptic insertion but prior to suturing and installation of the drainage system. (B) Closed sterile urinary collection system attached to an indwelling urinary catheter. Notice that the collection system is placed in a clean container, not on the floor.

polydipsic or polyuric, and no longer on intravenous fluids, bladder expression can typically be performed at 6–8 hour intervals. It is important to monitor the patient for complete voiding of the bladder as partial expression or overflow incontinence is often mistaken for voluntary urination. If urine is found in the cage, bed or following voluntary urination, the bladder size should be verified by manual palpation or ideally using ultrasound to ensure complete voiding has occurred.

Table 28.3 Pharmacological agents used in bladder management.

Drug	Dogs	Cats
Phenoxybenzamine	0.25–0.5 mg/kg PO every 12–24 hours	2.5–7.5 mg/cat PO every 12–24 hours
Prazosin	1 mg/15 kg PO every 8 hours	0.25–0.5 mg/cat PO every 12–24 hours
Diazepam	0.25–1.0 mg/kg PO every 8 hours; 0.5 mg/kg IV	0.5 mg/kg IV
Bethanechol	5–15 mg PO every 8 hours	1.25–7.5 mg PO every 8 hours

Source: Doses modified from *Plumb's Veterinary Drug Handbook* [20].

Long-term Management of the Bladder

In cases of IVD herniation where there is loss of deep pain, return of voluntary urination can be variable, with some patients never regaining normal function. In these cases, the owners need to learn to express the urinary bladder to limit complications from overflow including urine scalding, atonic bladder, and recurrent UTIs. Owners can develop the necessary skills to express the urinary bladder and also to assist in defecation if desired. Early instruction in bladder expression is recommended when long-term urinary dysfunction is expected.

Pharmacological agents that can be used to assist in bladder expression and treatment of urethral spasm and atonic bladder include phenoxybenzamine, prazosin, diazepam, and bethanechol (Table 28.3).

Phenoxybenzamine is an α-adrenergic blocker used for detrusor areflexia that acts by reducing internal urethral sphincter tone, but can also cause hypotension. Alternatively, prazosin, an α_1 blocker, has been used in both dogs and cats to decrease urethral resistance. Diazepam has been used as a muscle relaxant for functional urethral obstruction and urethral hypertonus. Use of oral diazepam in cats is controversial as there is a risk of hepatotoxicity if given orally over prolonged periods. Bethanechol is a synthetic cholinergic ester that is used to increase bladder contractility. It has also been used previously as a general gastrointestinal stimulant. Side effects that can be seen with its use are secondary to its muscarinic effects and include salivation, lacrimation, urination, and defecation. Bethanechol should be used in conjunction with medications that decrease urethral tone to reduce the risk of bladder rupture [20].

Despite the best efforts to completely evacuate the bladder, in some cases UTIs can recur. A UTI should be treated early with antibiotics based on urine bacterial culture and sensitivity of a sample obtained by cystocentesis [41]. If there are recurrent UTIs, longer-term management using nitrofurantoin or cranberry tablets can be considered. At low doses, nitrofurantoin is a bacteriostatic antimicrobial that is considered a urinary antiseptic (prophylactic dose 3–4 mg/kg orally every 24 hours) [37]. Approximately 40% of the drug is eliminated in the urine unchanged with no gastrointestinal side effects.

Nutritional Requirements

The need for postoperative nutritional supplementation is influenced by the preoperative neurological status, the type of surgery performed, and the expected time until appropriate nutritional intake returns. In most cases of IVD disease, the patient was neurologically normal prior to herniation of the disc and the period of perioperative anorexia is short. Nutritional supplementation in these patients is typically not necessary as normal appetite returns relatively soon after surgery. However, if anorexia is expected to persist beyond 3 days from the last meal, then supplementation should be considered.

In patients that have had prolonged periods of anorexia, such as those with intracranial disease or when it is unknown whether normal neurological status will be maintained postoperatively, nutritional supplementation should be considered as part of the perioperative management. Enteral nutrition is preferred over parenteral nutrition as it has been shown to be superior in maintaining enterocyte health and promoting gastrointestinal motility. Enteral nutrition should be used any time the intestinal tract is functional. Another consideration is when to start feeding patients following surgery, particularly when intracranial surgery has been performed. This depends on the period of anorexia prior to surgery, the postoperative neurological status, and method of nutritional supplementation.

Enteral Nutrition

There are several ways of providing enteral nutrition with varying degrees of invasiveness. The ability to prehend and swallow without risk of aspiration may be a concern in the immediate postoperative period in patients that have undergone intracranial surgery. The presence of megaesophagus or vomiting and regurgitation as well as having undergone intracranial surgery are risk factors for the development of aspiration pneumonia [43].

The simplest method of providing enteral nutrition is with a nasogastric tube. Tube placement is minimally invasive and can be performed under sedation. A tube is passed from the nares into the stomach with confirmation of tube placement via a lateral thoracic radiograph to ensure that the tube is in the stomach. An advantage of the nasogastric tube is the ability to aspirate stomach contents if there is delayed gastric emptying, which can otherwise lead to vomiting and regurgitation. A limitation of nasogastric tube feeding is the type of food that can be placed down the tube, with only liquid diets such as Clinicare® or Ensure® being appropriate. This method of feeding is considered temporary and if the patient is conscious the tube can cause some irritation leading to sneezing (increasing intracranial pressure) and pawing at the face, so caution should be exercised for craniotomy patients (Figure 28.5).

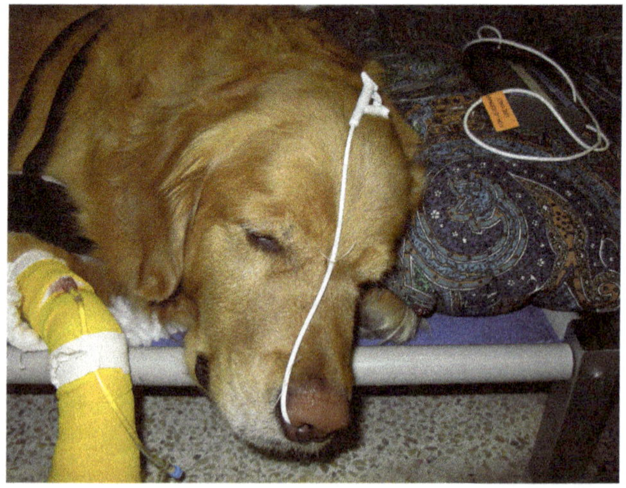

Figure 28.5 Postoperative patient with a nasogastric tube secured in place (right nostril). *Source*: Courtesy of Andrea Steele.

For provision of longer-term nutritional supplementation or when intracranial surgery has been performed, placement of an esophagostomy tube (E-tube) should be considered while the patient is under general anesthesia. This is especially important if prolonged anorexia or delayed neurological recovery is expected. Esophagostomy tubes are easy and quick to insert, are associated with few complications, and have the advantage of allowing foods with increased consistency, such as Hill's a/d®, to be fed through them along with any oral medication. The tube is typically placed on the left side of the neck and extends down to just past the base of the heart, which is confirmed by thoracic radiography. An E-tube can remain in place for short or long periods of time, with abscessation around the tube stoma being the most frequent complication. This tube can be converted into an esophagogastric tube if desired.

A gastrostomy tube could be considered to provide longer-term nutrition to patients. They can be placed either surgically via a celiotomy or percutaneously using endoscopic guidance (PEG tube). Percutaneously placed gastrostomy tubes should remain in place for a minimum of 10 days to allow adhesion of the stomach to the abdominal wall and a stoma to form. A potential complication of the gastrostomy tube is septic peritonitis if there is leakage around the tube or the tube is removed prior to a permanent adhesion forming to the abdominal wall. Complications that can be seen with either esophagostomy or gastrostomy tubes is infection around the stoma. Daily inspection and stoma care should be performed, with bandaging of the site recommended.

Whenever possible, bolus feeding (versus continuous-rate infusion feeding) should be considered for nutritional supplementation. If the patient is conscious and not vomiting, bolus feeding is recommended as it is more physiological and stimulates normal gastrointestinal motility. The maximum amount of food that is currently recommended to be fed to critically ill and postoperative patients is based on a patient's resting energy requirement (RER). It is not currently recommended to feed more than RER, with increasing evidence to suggest that overfeeding of patients can compound the metabolic alterations of the stress response leading to hyperglycemia [44]. Although it is unknown whether this translates to other species or to naturally occurring disease processes, restrictive feeding on an every other day schedule was shown to be neuroprotective in a rat cervical spinal cord model [45].

The following formula can be used to calculate RER:

$$\text{RER} = 70\,\text{kcal} \times \text{body weight in kg}^{0.75}$$

Depending on the period of anorexia, begin with feeding one-third to half the RER. The amount of food to be fed can be initially divided into six to eight bolus feedings over a 24-hour period or divided over the 24-hour period if continuous-rate feeding is used.

Prior to feeding bolus amounts, residual volumes should be checked by aspirating the feeding tube. Residual volumes that are considered normal in veterinary patients have not been established, although 4-hour residual volumes exceeding 50% of what was administered over the preceding 4 hours (or at last feeding) is considered excessive. For nasogastric tubes, if there are large residual volumes in the stomach, this could indicate poor gastric motility and may lead to increased nausea and risk of vomiting and regurgitation. If aspirating residual volumes for removal, approximately 1–2 mL/kg of the volume should be returned to prevent development of metabolic alkalosis. If there are large residual volumes or vomiting, addition of gastric motility agents should be considered (Table 28.4).

Table 28.4 Common gastric motility agents and their dose rates.

Drug	Continuous-rate infusion	Individual doses
Metoclopramide	1–2 mg/kg daily	0.3 mg/kg IV every 8 hours
Cisapride	–	0.1–0.5 mg/kg PO every 8 hours
Erythromycin	–	0.5–1.0 mg/kg PO, IV every 8 hours

Source: Doses modified from *Plumb's Veterinary Drug Handbook* [20].

Parenteral Nutrition

Parenteral nutrition is indicated whenever the gastrointestinal tract is not working well enough to digest or absorb sufficient nutrients, there is persistent vomiting or gastric stasis, or the risk of aspiration is high due to coma or mechanical ventilation. Parenteral nutrition consists of either total parenteral nutrition (TPN), which essentially provides most of the caloric and amino acid requirements, or partial parenteral nutrition (PPN), which provides only a portion of the caloric and amino acid requirements. PPN can be administered via peripheral veins. TPN requires a central venous line due to the high osmolarity of the solution and will cause severe phlebitis and thrombosis if administered through a peripheral vein [46]. Serial monitoring of blood glucose is recommended when TPN or PPN is initiated in patients with intracranial disease in which hyperglycemia should be avoided.

Parenteral nutrition solutions need to be mixed aseptically and can be stored refrigerated for up to 7 days and at room temperature for up to 2 days. The solution should be protected from light and no other medications should be mixed into the solution administration set/line. One of the complications associated with parenteral nutrition is sepsis due to growth of contaminants in the solution, which is reported in 5–8% of patients [47].

Monitoring Neurological Status

Following both intracranial surgery and spinal surgery, there is an expected course of recovery. If a patient does not follow the expected course of improvement or has significant deterioration in neurological status, repeat imaging may be indicated. In humans, postoperative imaging following spinal or intracranial surgery is standard to ensure adequate removal of the tumor or that decompression has occurred. In veterinary medicine, immediate postoperative imaging is rarely performed due to the associated financial cost.

Following intracranial surgery, progressive brain edema can occur for up to 48 hours and can persist for a week or more. During this time, the patient should be monitored for neurological deterioration. General physical parameters that should be assessed include heart rate and rhythm, respiratory rate and character, blood pressure, blood gases, oxygenation, and urine production. Neurological parameters that can be evaluated to assess changes in neurological status include pupil size and responsiveness to light, level of consciousness, and ability of the patient to move or walk. Individual cranial nerves can also be assessed to determine if there is underlying neurological deterioration.

Ascending Myelomalacia

Another cause of deteriorating neurological status in patients that are nociception-negative prior to or following decompressive thoracolumbar spinal surgery is ascending/descending myelomalacia. In the early postoperative period, dogs are typically comfortable following the removal of the compressive disc. In patients with ascending/descending myelomalacia, uncontrollable pain typically develops. Monitoring for myelomalacia involves twice-daily monitoring of the neurological status or more frequently if it is suspected. Evaluation of the cutaneous trunci muscle reflex (panniculus "cut-off") is important as ascending loss of this reflex is an early sign of myelomalacia [48]. Progression from upper motor neuron signs to lower motor neuron signs with loss of patella reflex is also an indication of possible myelomalacia. There is currently no known treatment or prevention for myelomalacia, and euthanasia is usually recommended prior to development of respiratory failure.

Repeat Imaging

Residual disc material was found to be present in 100% of dogs after hemilaminectomy for thoracolumbar disc herniation [49]. A more recent study found residual material in 44% of dogs following mini-hemilaminectomy [50]. Although the majority of these patients progress normally postoperatively, if a patient fails to improve as expected or shows deterioration in neurological status, early repeat imaging is recommended to document adequate decompression and removal of disc material or tumor or rule out the presence of a compressive hematoma.

Incisional Care

Following surgery, the incision should be monitored twice daily for signs of pain, redness, swelling, or discharge. A protective bandage can be applied to cover the incision for the first 24 hours until maturation of the fibrin clot (Figure 28.6). If skin sutures have been used, they are typically removed at 10–14 days.

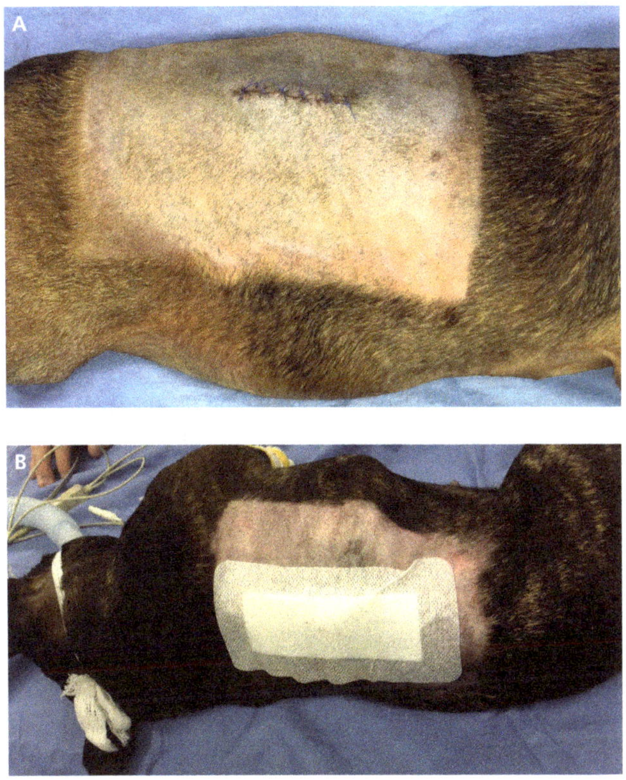

Figure 28.6 (A) Immediate postoperative incision following dorsolateral approach to the thoracolumbar spine for pediculectomy. (B) Semi-occlusive dressing used to cover incisions in the immediate postoperative period after spinal surgery.

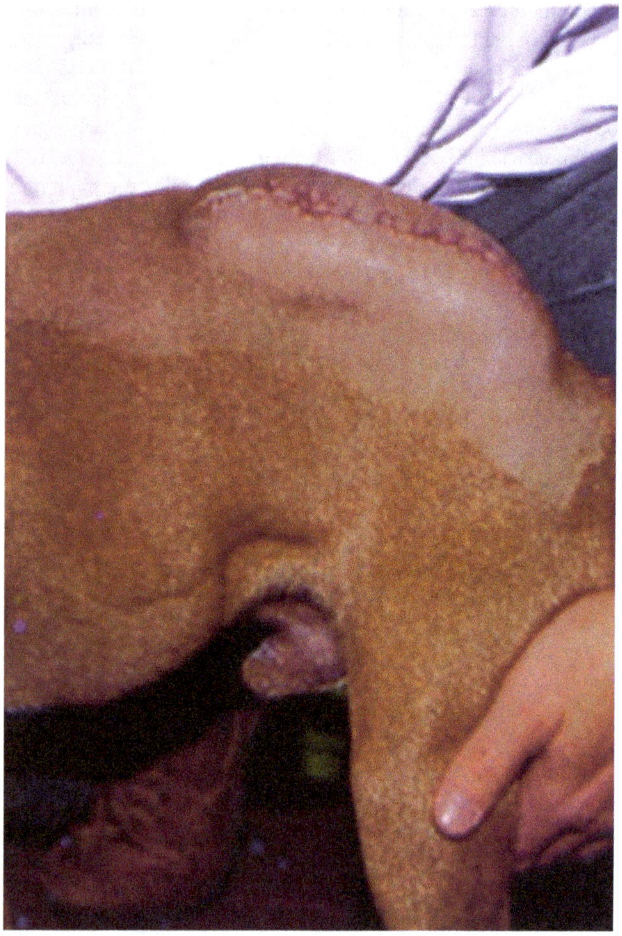

Figure 28.7 Postoperative incisional seroma/abscess noted 2 weeks following fixation of a lumbar fracture/luxation.

In the immediate postoperative period, the use of hypothermia in the form of cold packing can be employed to provide adjunctive analgesia and reduce postoperative swelling and inflammation. Hypothermia is recommended three to four times per day for 20 min for the first 3 days following surgery. After this period warm compresses can be used to help reduce swelling.

Complications that can be seen with incisions include dehiscence due to self-trauma, seroma formation due to inadequate obliteration of dead space or excessive motion, and incisional infections. Elizabethan collars can be used when appropriate to prevent self-trauma. In mild superficial incisional dehiscence with no evidence of infection, the incision can be treated conservatively with wound cleaning using a 0.05% aqueous chlorhexidine solution twice daily and the use of a wound dressing to prevent further contamination. If there is dehiscence of deeper tissue layers or evidence of infection, the wound can be initially managed as an open wound until infection has resolved and then general anesthesia, surgical debridement, and closure is recommended. This course of action is not acceptable when deep tissues are exposed, especially in patients with implants. In a large restrospective study the most common surgical wound complications were swelling and discharge in 7.5% and 5.3% of cases, respectively [51].

Seroma formation is common following dorsal approaches to the cervical spine and with excessive postoperative motion. Uncomplicated seromas are typically managed with exercise restriction, the use of warm packing and, if appropriate, a compressive bandage can be used to reduce potential dead space. Aspiration of the seroma is avoided unless infection is suspected, to limit the potential for bacterial seeding and abscess formation. If aspiration is performed, the area should be clipped and aseptically prepared prior to aspirating the fluid for cytology, and bacterial culture and sensitivity. Infected seromas typically require active drainage with appropriate antibiotic administration. Surgical site infections are uncommon in neurological surgery, but when they occur they need to be aggressively treated to prevent development of ascending infections into the CNS (Figure 28.7).

Laser Therapy

Laser therapy has been well described in both the human and veterinary literature as a technique for improving healing of tissues and wounds. For more information regarding the technique of laser therapy for incision and wound management, readers are referred to Chapter 29.

Antiepileptics

Seizures are often a presenting sign in patients with intracranial diseases. In many cases antiepileptic medications such as phenobarbitone, potassium bromide, levetiracetam, or pregabalin have been administered preoperatively to reduce the frequency or severity of seizures. Although not proven to be beneficial, antiepileptic medications have also been recommended for patients undergoing intracranial surgery to remove mass lesions. When antiepileptics have been administered prior to surgery, it is recommended to continue in the postoperative period and gradually taper the medications over a 4–6 week period to prevent seizure development.

The doses, frequency, and specifications of the individual antiepileptic medications are beyond the scope of this chapter and readers are referred to a veterinary drug handbook [20] for more information regarding available drugs.

Physiotherapy and Exercise Restriction

Physiotherapy is an important component of rehabilitation following neurosurgery and should be initiated as soon as the patient is comfortable. Although some concern for early reherniation has been expressed when physiotherapy is initiated in the early postoperative period [52], the benefits of early mobilization and controlled activity outweigh these concerns until there is further evidence of adverse effects. In a recent study [52], the early recurrence rate was reported at 2%, which is similar to that reported in older studies, and although not mentioned it is assumed that all the population of patients that underwent decompressive surgery during the study period also underwent a similar postoperative rehabilitation program without an increased incidence of recurrence.

Physiotherapy exercises that should be initiated in the early postoperative period include passive ROM exercises and muscle massage. Flexion and extension of all joints should be performed 10 times per joint, three to four times per day. For a complete discussion on physical rehabilitation of the neurosurgery patient, see Chapter 29.

Exercise Restriction Following Spinal Surgery

The duration of exercise restriction depends on the neurological status of the patient and the surgical procedure performed. Patients that have undergone decompressive surgery for IVD herniation are typically restricted for 4 weeks. Patients should be confined to a crate or small area to prevent running, jumping, or excessive rough play. Stairs are not recommended so when possible patients should be carried outside for voiding or provided with assisted walking to prevent falling.

For patients that have had spinal fracture/luxation stabilization using implants, exercise restriction should be implemented until there is evidence of osseous healing or fusion, typically 6–8 weeks postoperatively. Radiographs should be performed at 4 weeks to evaluate implant position and repeated every 4–6 weeks until satisfactory healing is evident. Healing may be difficult to assess if bone cement was used. If evidence of implant loosening or periosteal reaction is noted, more frequent radiographs may be required to determine if there is progression of implant failure or evidence of infection. Exercise restriction should be enforced until healing has occurred.

Video clips to accompany this book can be found on the companion website at:
www.wiley.com/go/shores/neurosurgery

References

1 Hurlbert RJ. Strategies of medical intervention in the management of acute spinal cord injury. *Spine* 2006;31:S16–S21.

2 Seeler DC. Fluid, electrolyte and blood component therapy. In: Tranquilli WJ, Thurmon JC, Grimm KA (eds) *Lumb and Jones' Veterinary Anesthesia*, 4th edn. Ames, IA: Blackwell Publishing, 2007:185–201.

3 Habib AS, Keifer JC, Borel CO, White WD, Gan TJ. A comparison of the combination of aprepitant and dexamethasone versus the combination of ondansetron and dexamethasone for the prevention of postoperative nausea and vomiting in patients undergoing craniotomy. *Anesth Analg* 2011;112:813–818.

4 Watcha M, White PF. Postoperative nausea and vomiting: its etiology, treatment and prevention. *Anesthesiology* 1992;77:162–184.

5 Ingvast-Larsson, Holgersson A, Bondesson U, Olsson K. Clinical pharmacology of methadone in dogs. *Vet Anaesth Analg* 2010;37:48–56.

6 Smith HS. Opioids and neuropathic pain. *Pain Physician* 2012;15:ES93–ES110.

7 Aprea F, Cherubini GB, Palus V, Vettorato E, Corletto F. Effect of extradurally administered morphine on postoperative analgesia in dogs undergoing surgery for thoracolumbar intervertebral disk extrusion. *J Am Vet Med Assoc* 2012;241: 754–759.

8 Barker JR, Clark-Price SC, Gordon-Evans WJ. Evaluation of topical epidural analgesia delivered in gelfoam for postoperative hemilaminectomy pain control. *Vet Surg* 2013;42:79–84.

9 Chamisha Y, Shamir MH, Merbl Y, Chai O. Reversible paralysis and loss of deep pain sensation after topical intrathecal morphine administration following durotomy. *Vet Surg* 2015;44:41–45.

10 Boag AK, Otto CM, Drobatz KJ. Complications of methylprednisolone sodium succinate therapy in Dachshunds with surgically treated intervertebral disc disease. *J Vet Emerg Crit Care* 2001;11:105–110.

11 Bracken MB, Shepard MJ, Collins WF et al. Methylprednisolone or naloxone treatment after acute spinal cord injury: 1-year follow-up data. Results of the second National Acute Spinal Cord Injury Study. *J Neurosurg* 1992;76:23–31.

12 Stiffler KS, McCrackin Stevenson MA, Sanchez S, Barsanti JA, Hofmeister E, Budsberg SC. Prevalence and characterization of urinary tract infections in dogs with surgically treated type 1 thoracolumbar intervertebral disc extrusion. *Vet Surg* 2006;35:330–336.

13 Roher CR, Hill RC, Fischer A, et al. Gastric hemorrhage in dogs given high doses of methylprednisolone sodium succinate. *Am J Vet Res* 1999;60:977–9981.

14 Bellah JR. Colonic perforation after corticosteroid and surgical treatment of intervertebral disk disease in a dog. *J Am Vet Med Assoc* 1983;183:1002–1003.

15 Toombs JP, Caywood DD, Lipowitz AJ, Stevens JB. Colonic perforation following neurosurgical procedures and corticosteroid therapy in 4 dogs. *J Am Vet Med Assoc* 1980;177:68–72.

16 Blackburn GL. Metabolic considerations in management of surgical patients. *Surg Clin North Am* 2011;9:467–480.

17 Wen PY, Schiff D, Kesari S, Drappatz J, Gigas DC, Doherty L. Medical management of patients with brain tumors. *J Neurooncol* 2006;80:313–332.

18 Bennet D, Ariffin Z, Johnston P. Osteoarthritis in the cat. 2. How should it be managed and treated. *J Feline Med Surg* 2012;14:76–84.

19 Forterre F, Gorgas D, Dickomeit M, Jaggy A, Lang J, Spreng D. Incidence of spinal compressive lesions in chondrodystrophic dogs with abnormal recovery after hemilaminectomy for treatment of thoracolumbar disc disease: a prospective magnetic resonance imaging study. *Vet Surg* 2010;39:165–172.

20 Plumb DC. *Plumb's Veterinary Drug Handbook*, 8th edn. Ames, IA: Wiley-Blackwell, 2015.

21 Aghighi SA, Tipold A, Piechotta M, Lewczuk P, Kästner SBR. Assessment of the effects of adjunctive gabapentin on postoperative pain after intervertebral disc surgery in dogs. *Vet Anaesth Analg* 2012;39:636–646.

22 Dewey CW, Cerda-Gonzalez S, Levine JM et al. Pregabalin as an adjunct to phenobarbital, potassium bromide, or a combination of phenobarbital and potassium bromide for treatment of dogs with suspected idiopathic epilepsy. *J Am Vet Med Assoc* 2009;235:1442–1449.

23 Lascelles BDX, Gaynor JS, Smith ES et al. Amantadine in a multimodal analgesic regimen for alleviation of refractory osteoarthritis pain in dogs. *J Vet Intern Med* 2008;22:53–59.

24 See S, Ginzburg R. Choosing a skeletal muscle relaxant. *Am Fam Physician* 2008;78:365–370.

25 Chou R, Peterson K, Helfand M. Comparative efficacy and safety of skeletal muscle relaxants for spasticity and musculoskeletal conditions: a systematic review. *J Pain Symptom Manage* 2004;28:140–175.

26 Neiger R, Gaschen F, Jaggy A. Gastric mucosal lesions in dogs with acute intervertebral disc disease: characterization and effects of omeprazole or misoprostol. *J Vet Intern Med* 2000;14:33–36.

27 Dowdle SM, Joubert KE, Lambrechts NE, Lobetti RG, Pardini AD. The prevalence of subclinical gastroduodenal ulceration in Dachshunds with intervertebral disc prolapse. *J S Afr Vet Assoc* 2003;74:77–81.

28 Hanson SM, Bostwick DR, Twedt DC, Smith MO. Clinical evaluation of cimetidine, sucralfate and misoprostol for prevention of gastrointestinal tract bleeding in dogs undergoing spinal surgery. *Am J Vet Res* 1997;58:1320–1323.

29 Johnston SA, Leib MS, Forrester SD, Marini M. The effect of misoprostol on aspirin-induced gastroduodenal lesions in dogs. *J Vet Intern Med* 1995;9:32–38.

30 Bersenas AME, Mathews KA, Allen DG, Conlon PD. Effects of ranitidine, famotidine, pantaprazole, and omeprazole on intragastric pH in dogs. *Am J Vet Res* 2005;66:425–431.

31 Tolbert K, Bissett S, King A et al. Efficacy of oral famotidine and 2 omeprazole formulations for the control of intragastric pH in dogs. *J Vet Intern Med* 2011;25:47–54.

32 Rossimeisl JH, White C, Pancotto TE, Bays A, Henao-Guerrero PN. Acute adverse events associated with ventral slot decompression in 546 dogs with cervical intervertebral disc disease. *Vet Surg* 2013;42:795–806.

33 Vasseur PB, Levy J, Dowd E, Eliot J. Surgical wound infection rates in dogs and cats: data from a teaching hospital. *Vet Surg* 1988;17:60–64.

34 Eugster S, Schawalder P, Gaschen F, Boerlin P. A prospective study of postoperative surgical site infections in dogs. *Vet Surg* 2004;33:542–550.

35 Meyer MJ, Megyesi J, Meythaler JM et al. Acute management of acquired brain injury. Part I: An evidence-based review of non-pharmacological interventions. *Brain Injury* 2010;24:694–705.

36 Pattanshetty RB, Gaude GS. Effect of multimodality chest physiotherapy in prevention of ventilator-associated pneumonia: a randomized clinical trial. *Indian J Crit Care Med* 2010;14:70–76.

37 Hopper K, Haskins SC, Kass PH, Rezende ML, Aldrich J. Indications, management and outcome of long-term positive-pressure ventilation in dogs and cats: 148 cases (1990–2001). *J Am Vet Med Assoc* 2007;230:64–75.

38 Bein T, Kuhr LP, Bele S, Ploner F, Keyl C, Taeger K. Lung recruitment maneuver in patients with cerebral injury: effects on intracranial pressure and cerebral metabolism. *Intensive Care Med* 2002;28:554–558.

39 Bubenik L, Hosgood G. Urinary tract infection in dogs with thoracolumbar intervertebral disc herniation and urinary bladder dysfunction managed by manual expression, indwelling catheterization or intermittent catheterization. *Vet Surg* 2008;37:791–800.

40 Ogeer J, Mathews K, Weese JS, Prescott JF, Boerlin P. Evaluation of catheter-associated urinary tract infections and multi-drug resistant *Escherichia coli* isolates from the urine of dogs with indwelling urinary catheters. *J Am Vet Med Assoc* 2006;229:1584–1590.

41 Weese JS, Blondeau JM, Boothe D et al. Antimicrobial use guidelines for treatment of urinary tract disease in dogs and cats: Antimicrobial Guidelines Working Group of the International Society for Companion Animal Infectious Diseases. *Veterinary Medicine International* 2011; Article ID 263768. doi: 10.4061/2011/263768

42 Smarick S. Urinary catheterization. In: Silverstein DC, Hopper K (eds) *Small Animal Critical Care Medicine*. St Louis, MO: Saunders, 2009:603–606.

43 Fransson BA, Bagley RS, Gay JM et al. Pneumonia after intracranial surgery in dogs. *Vet Surg* 2001;30:432–439.

44 Boitano M. Hypocaloric feeding of the critically ill. *Nutr Clin Pract* 2006;21:617–622.
45 Plunet WT, Streijger F, Lam CK, Lee JHT, Liu J, Tetzlaff W. Dietary restriction started after spinal cord injury improves functional recovery. *Exp Neurol* 2008;213:28–35.
46 Michel KE, Eirmann L. Parenteral nutrition. In: Silverstein DC, Hopper K (eds) *Small Animal Critical Care Medicine*. St Louis, MO: Saunders, 2009:58–62.
47 Queau Y, Larsen JA, Kass PH, Glucksman GS, Fascetti AJ. Factors associated with adverse outcomes during parenteral nutrition administration in dogs and cats. *J Vet Intern Med* 2011;25:446–452.
48 Muguet-Chanoit AC, Olby NJ, Lim JH et al. The cutaneous trunci muscle reflex: a predictor of recovery in dogs with acute thoracolumbar myelopathies caused by intervertebral disc extrusions. *Vet Surg* 2012;41:200–206.
49 Roach WJ, Thomas M, Weh M, Bleedorn JA, Wells K. Residual herniated disc material following hemilaminectomy in chondrodystrophic dogs with thoracolumbar intervertebral disc disease. *Vet Comp Orthop Traumatol* 2012;25:109–115.
50 Huska JL, Gaitero L, Brisson BA, Nykamp S, Thomason JJ, Sears WC. Presence of residual material following mini-hemilaminectomy in dogs with thoracolumbar intervertebral disc extrusion. *Can Vet J* 2014;55:975–980.
51 Hosgood G. Wound complications following thoracolumbar laminectomy in the dog: a retrospective study of 264 procedures. *J Am Anim Hosp Assoc* 1992;28: 47–52.
52 Hettlich BF, Kerwin SC, Levine JM. Early reherniation of disk material in eleven dogs with surgically treated thoracolumbar intervertebral disk extrusion. *Vet Surg* 2012;41:215–220.

29 Physical Rehabilitation of the Neurological Patient

María Pérez Hernández and Ruby Lynn Carter

Introduction

Many veterinarians in the neurology field have felt the need to improve postoperative care for the neurological patient. Although veterinary physical therapy started more than 30 years ago, its credibility has only been widely recognized during the last 10 years.

There is only a slight difference in the definitions of "physical therapy" (applied in humans) and "rehabilitation" (applied in veterinary medicine).

- *Physical therapy* includes the examination and evaluation of human patients with impairments, functional limitations, disability, and other health-related conditions to determine a diagnosis, prognosis, and intervention as defined by the American Physical Therapy Association.
- *Rehabilitation* is the set of noninvasive techniques, excluding veterinary chiropractic, for the rehabilitation of injuries in non-human animals as defined by the AVMA House Delegates.

According to these definitions, the rehabilitation should be performed by a licensed technician or physical therapist, certified or not in rehabilitation, under the supervision of a veterinarian, whereas in human medicine supervision by a doctor might not be needed if the therapy is performed by a physical therapist. These concepts may be modified in different countries, with disagreement about who should perform the rehabilitation and the regulation of rehabilitation centers with regard to preventing intrusiveness and the employment of unqualified personnel.

Rehabilitation includes all noninvasive physical therapies used in the functional recovery of orthopedic and neurological patients, as well as management and performance of geriatric, overweight, or sport dogs. In this chapter, we focus on rehabilitation that aids recovery from nervous system injury, also termed *neurorehabilitation* (NR).

Neurorehabilitation

Unlike rehabilitation, NR pursues recovery beyond musculoskeletal restoration. NR also pursues neurological recovery and includes additional exercises for the patient with neurological deficits. The patient's complete history should be considered in order to plan individual functional recovery according to each specific brain, spine or neuromuscular injury, and should also take into account the house environment and owner's willingness to handle the pet at home and guarantee quality of life.

Another concept must be introduced for a complete understanding of NR. *Neuroplasticity*, or brain plasticity, is characterized as the spontaneous ability of neurons to adapt to a new environment by transforming neural pathways ("rewiring") in response to changes that have occurred in the process of a neurological injury and during recovery. Spinal injuries may force the patient to move differently, change its environment, or develop different sanitary habits. Neuroplasticity will occur after the repetition of a new pattern and it can be either positive or negative. This is a very important concept to keep in mind when beginning NR in order to prevent bad habits and promote function and positive recovery. For example, a patient that suffered a severe back injury and remained paraplegic with intact nociception after surgical intervention will tend to move by dragging its rear, and recovery might take longer because the patient does not try to walk on all four limbs even after recovering some motor function. Days or weeks of repetition of this new pattern will encourage negative neuroplasticity and therefore institute a bad habit, also called *maladaptative change or compensation*, that might be difficult to reverse.

Understanding that the nervous system has neuroplastic mechanisms allows us to recognize how it tries to repair itself [1]. Listed

Current Techniques in Canine and Feline Neurosurgery, First Edition. Edited by Andy Shores and Brigitte A. Brisson.
© 2017 John Wiley & Sons, Inc. Published 2017 by John Wiley & Sons, Inc.
Companion website: www.wiley.com/go/shores/neurosurgery

below are some general principles to remember during the rehabilitation of the neurological patient.

- Body parts can compete for representation in the brain and use of a body part can enhance its representation, in the same way as lack of use will shrink its representation in the CNS [1–3].
- The premotor cortex can substitute for the motor cortex to control motion. It has been demonstrated that although the main output of the premotor cortex is ordinarily the primary motor cortex, it can also be the source of supraspinal control signals [1,2].
- The contralesional hemisphere can take over motor control if all else fails. Ipsilateral corticospinal neural pathways have been documented, especially for more proximal muscles. In severe unilateral hemisphere lesions, the undamaged hemisphere could take over and enhance the use of this pathway, although the exact mechanism is unkown [1,5,6].
- Neuroplastic mechanisms can be facilitated and this is a good basis for intervention. Early, intensive and focused NR is greatly advocated [1]. The neuroplasticity of the patient underlies all learning and will be enhanced by following five principles: practice, specificity, repetition, intensity, and motivation [7,8].

Physical Modalities

Physical modalities refer to a group of therapies applied in patients with neurological and motor rehabilitative dysfunction. These modalities are characterized by specialized exercises and application of noninvasive equipment with precise purposes in the restoration or maintenance of the debilitated patient. This chapter focuses on the rehabilitation of neurological diseases (intracranial, spinal, or neuromuscular disorders). Some of the most common therapies are described in the following sections.

Electrical Stimulation

Mechanism of Action

Electrical stimulation is applied by an electrical stimulator that transmits a current from one electrode to another in a specific area of the body. The stimulator parameters (frequency, amplitude, duty cycle, and intensity) are modified to achieve a specific function and purpose.

Goals

To increase muscle strength, control pain, and reduce muscle spasms and edema; and to provide neurological stimulation (sensory).

Applications

To prevent muscle atrophy, to build up muscle mass, and reduce neuropathic pain and pain associated with osteoarthritis, muscle spasms, edema, and decreased nociception.

Contraindications

Over areas of neoplasia or infections; patients with pacemakers [9,10].

Laser Therapy

Mechanism of Action

The term "laser" is an acronym for "light amplification by stimulated emission of radiation." A laser is an instrument that produces stimulated emission of photons. The proper application of laser therapy to the target allows each individual cell the opportunity to absorb as many photons as possible, and this photobiostimulation increases cellular health and energy.

Goals

Relieves pain, reduces inflammation, and accelerates tissue repair and cell growth.

Applications

Musculoskeletal pain, nonhealing wounds, and pressure sores.

Contraindications

Over areas of infections or neoplasia [11].

Thermotherapy

Mechanism of Action

Superficial heat and cold are used therapeutically to manage soft tissue and joint injuries, altering the inflammatory response. The most important physiological effects are as follows.

- *Superficial heat*: vasoconstriction, decreases blood flow, decreases swelling, reduces enzyme-mediated tissue damage, analgesia.
- *Superficial cold*: vasodilation, increases blood flow, relieves pain, increases soft tissue extensibility, relaxation of muscle spasm.

Goals

- *Superficial heat*: pain relief in chronic lesions, increase in elasticity of muscles, tendons and ligaments, and relief of muscle spasms.
- *Superficial cold*: pain relief in acute lesions.

Applications

- *Superficial heat*: chronic lesions, chronic pain, decrease in range of motion, and muscle spasms.
- *Superficial cold*: acute lesions and acute pain.

Contraindications

Over areas of infections, neoplasia, and open wounds [9,10].

Therapeutic Ultrasound

Mechanism of Action

A deep heating modality that can elevate tissue temperature at depths of 2 cm. The mechanism of action is the same as that for superficial heat but at a deeper level. Additionally, this modality has nonthermal effects caused by cavitation and acoustic streaming.

Goals

Vasodilation, pain relief in chronic lesions, increase in elasticity of muscles, tendons and ligaments, relief of muscle spasms, and stimulation of healing.

Applications

Chronic lesions at deeper locations or affecting large muscles (i.e., quadriceps muscle; Figure 29.1), fibrosis of soft tissue and ankylosis due to prolonged immobilization, and nonhealing ulcers or fractures.

Contraindications

Over areas of infections and neoplasia and areas with a metal implant [9,10].

Massage

Mechanism of Action

Massage is the manipulation of soft tissues of the body by the therapist's hands and by use of other instruments. There are multiple techniques directed towards a specific purpose but, basically, all of them apply pressure for tissue movement.

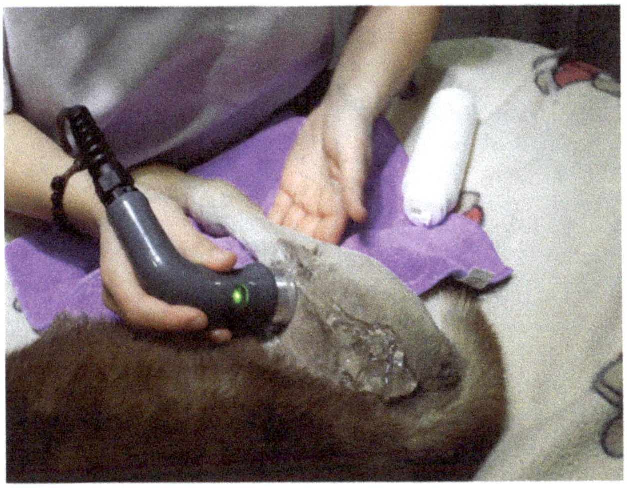

Figure 29.1 Therapeutic ultrasound applied to young shepherd dog with severe quadriceps contracture, severely decreased range of motion, and sciatic damage due to femur fracture.

Goals
Increases lymph flow, increases blood flow, relaxation, relieves muscle spasm, increases range of motion, breaks down fibrous tissue, relief of trigger points.

Applications
Muscle spasms and contractures, nervous patients, subcutaneous fluid accumulation in patients with diminished mobility, decreased range of motion and ankylosis.

Therapeutic Exercises

Therapeutic exercises include all types of passive, assisted-active, or active exercises that maintain or improve the patient's range of motion, muscle mass, and joint and bone health, as well as stimulate neurological function, without the use of physical therapies. Passive exercises involve an applied force, whereas assisted-active or active exercises result from voluntary contraction and relaxation of the muscles, with or without some support by the therapist. These exercises should not cause pain in the patient, although they might be challenging and cause discomfort for those with decreased range of motion or increased tone. Some animals will need some incentive (treats) and sedation might be needed for the most aggressive individuals. Specific rehabilitation equipment and accessories may be needed for some of the exercises as well as creativity and motivation to encourage the neurological patient to perform the exercises and accomplish specific goals. A specific rehabilitation plan is designed for each patient and will include exercises performed either on the ground (dry rehabilitation) or on the underwater treadmill (UWTM) or in the pool (water rehabilitation), depending on the patient and type and location of the injury.

Each of the exercises should be designed according to the neurological dysfunction and the patient's needs, paying attention to other possible concurrent conditions (e.g., an overweight patient would also need a low-calorie diet). Further, the rehabilitation tasks should follow the five principles of neuroplasticity. Repetition of a specific exercise with the adequate intensity and motivation, minimizing compensation, allows the patient to develop positive neuroplasticity to relearn the lost skill, so as not to end up a "functional pet" that can only move around at home but to aid optimal recovery in the shortest time possible. Many of these exercises are demonstrated in Video 29.1.

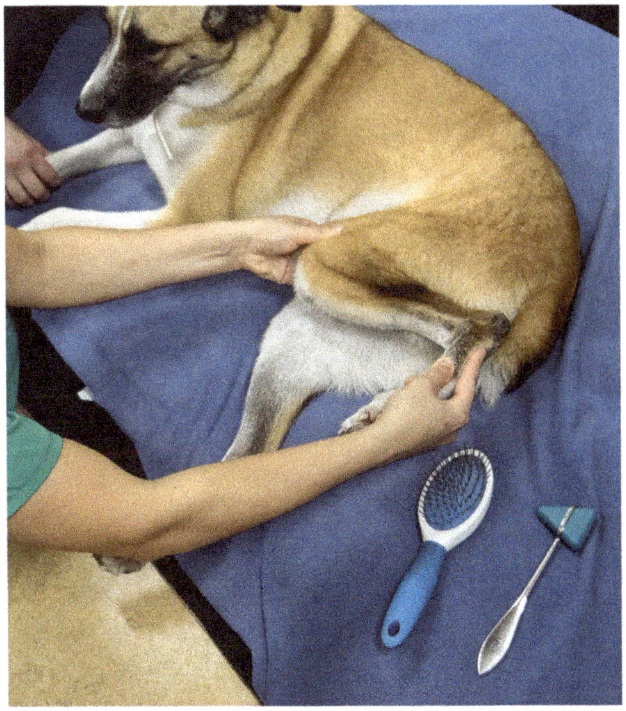

Figure 29.2 How to perform passive range of motion on a canine patient. A therapist performs flexion of the stifle and tarsal joints with both hands, one to hold and give support to the limb, the other to perform flexion of the joint.

Passive Exercises with Patient in Lateral Recumbency

Passive Range of Motion with Stretching

Move the front and/or hind limbs through a full range of motion by gently flexing and extending every joint of the limb independently (move nails, toes, carpus/hock, elbow/stifle, shoulder/hip). Hold flexion and extension of each joint for 3–5 seconds. Repeat three to five times per joint, two to three times daily.

Bicycle Movement

Move the front and/or hind limbs through a full range of motion by gently flexing and extending the whole limb with a forward bicycle movement. This movement should be performed as wide as possible. Perform 15–20 repetitions, two to three times daily.

Both passive range of motion (PROM) with stretching and bicycle movement should be performed using two hands; one hand holds the limb and gives support, the other performs the movement safely (Figures 29.2 and 29.3). These two exercises will maintain or improve range of motion in patients with decreased/absent motor function and/or increased tone.

Flexor Exercise

Gently pinch the webbing between the toes of the affected limb until the patient pulls the foot towards the body (Figure 29.4). Try to encourage the patient to withdraw and achieve full flexion of the limb before releasing the toe. This exercise stimulates sensory and motor pathways and at the same time activates the musculoskeletal system. Perform 10–15 repetitions, two to three times daily.

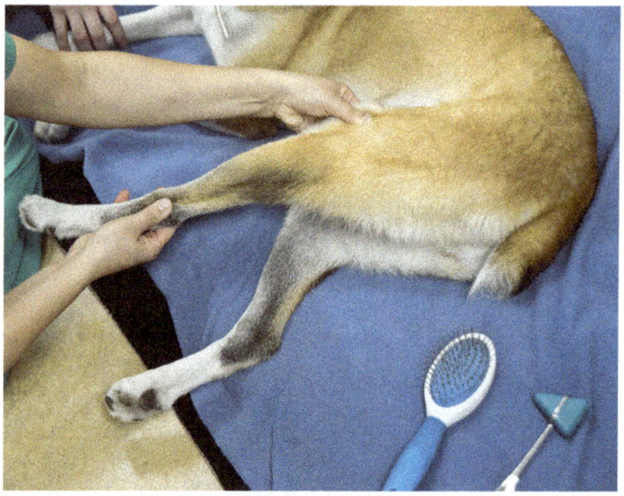

Figure 29.3 How to perform passive range of motion with two hands during extension of the stifle and tarsal joints. These two joints move together and full extension or flexion of one joint involves flexion or extension of the other.

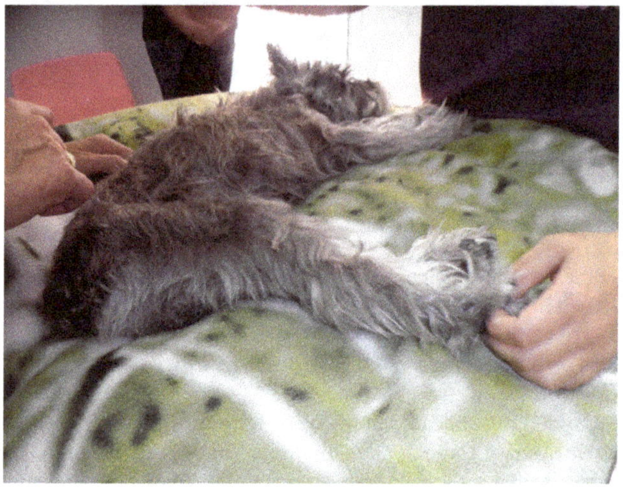

Figure 29.4 Flexor exercise or stimulation of the withdrawal reflex elicits sensory and motor function. Pinching the webbing between the toes is a noxious stimulus and therefore elicits flexion of the limb.

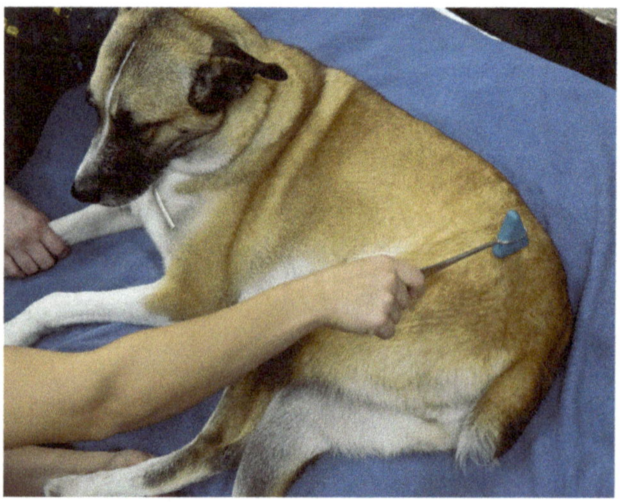

Figure 29.5 Tapping along the paraspinal dorsal muscles and limbs stimulates reflexes. As a result, muscle twitching will be seen. This exercise is especially important for patients with LMN lesions.

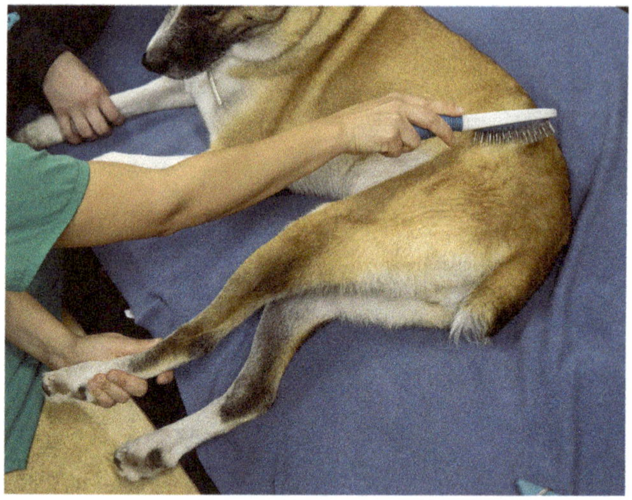

Figure 29.6 Brushing and scratching the patient along the back and limbs, including paws, stimulates sensory pathways. Some patients may react with muscle twitches or withdrawals.

Tapping to Stimulate Reflexes

Tap along the spine and along the affected limb while observing for muscle reactions and twitches in the belly and limbs (Figure 29.5). This exercise stimulates reflexes and the musculoskeletal system, which is especially beneficial in patients with lower motor neuron (LMN) signs. It should be performed for 2 min on each side, two to three times daily.

Brush/Scratch

Brush/scratch the area of the spine and/or limbs (inside and outside), trying to elicit muscle reactions and twitches in the abdominal and hind limb musculature with more sensory stimulation (Figure 29.6). This task should be performed for 2 min on each side, two to three times daily.

Passive/Assisted-Active Exercises with Patient in Standing Position

All standing exercises should be performed on a carpet, a rug, or other surface with good traction. The use of different surfaces (foam, carpet, grass, gravel, etc.) will also stimulate proprioception. Pinching or scratching of the tail with gentle fingertips might be helpful in patients with upper motor neuron (UMN) signs and/or intact nociception to simulate the mass reflex and/or sensation. It will require more than one person to perform these exercises in large dogs. Confirmation by the doctor involved in the case is highly recommended to ensure that all exercises are performed in a safe manner and that none are likely to increase the risk of deterioration. Neck leashes should be avoided at all times to prevent further damage.

Lateral Flexion of the Spine

Place the patient in lateral recumbency and encourage a lateral flexion of the spine by offering a treat or a toy at the tail, hip or stifle to work on range of motions (Figure 29.7). This exercise is especially important in nonambulatory tetraparetic patients to strengthen the core muscles and spine. Repeat the lateral flexion 3–10 times on both sides, one to three times daily.

Standing Exercise

Maintain the standing position by placing the limbs of the patient correctly. If still weak, the patient should be supported with a sling or the therapist's hands under the belly and/or chest. An inflatable round or peanut-shaped ball can be used for support. Ensure the ball is the correct size for the patient so that the animal can touch the ground with all four paws and split the weight uniformly. This task stimulates proprioception and encourages posture. Maintain the standing position for 10–60 seconds (depending on the patient's strength). Perform four sets of 1 min each, one to three times daily.

Sit-to-Stand Exercise

Help the patient to sit and hold this position for 10–40 seconds and then help the patient to stand and hold that standing position for another 10–60 seconds (Figure 29.8). Ensure the patient maintains the limbs in the correct position at all times to encourage proprioceptive input and postural rehabilitation in order to prevent the development of bad habits (Figure 29.9). This exercise should be performed 5–20 times, twice daily.

Weight Shifting

With the dog standing, perform gentle weight-shifting back and forth, as well as side to side. The patient may be supported by a harness/sling and the therapist's hands under the belly and/or chest. An inflatable round or peanut-shaped ball can be used for support. The ball can be sized to fit under the body so that the animal can still touch the ground with all four paws; alternately, the ball can be larger so that weight is shifted to the front or hind limbs when the hind or front limbs are lifted onto the ball (Figure 29.10). This exercise can also be performed on balance boards to provide an extra challenge (Figure 29.11). This helps the patient to maintain posture and balance. Perform four sets of 1 min each, one to three times daily.

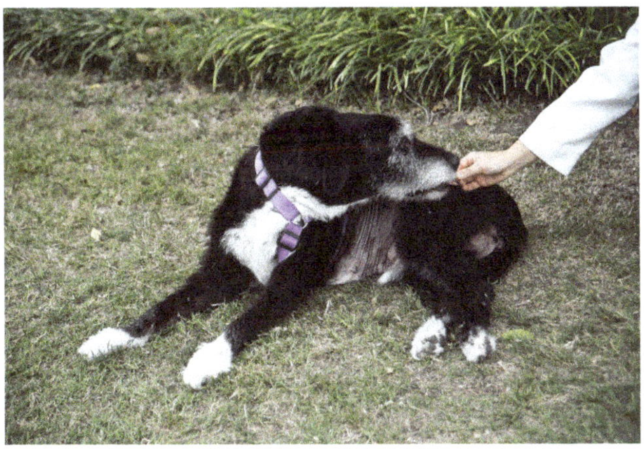

Figure 29.7 Lateral flexion of the spine can be encouraged with treats or toys.

Walks

Walk the patient with a harness or a sling for balance and support as needed. Use different surfaces for additional proprioceptive input. Further tail stimulation can be helpful for stimulating the mass reflex and activating the hind limbs. In some cases, especially patients with UMN signs, stimulation of the mass reflex can initiate involuntary movements that can be followed by voluntary motor movements. Walks on the treadmill can also be beneficial. This provides a consistent and uniform repetition of the gait, at an elected speed on a uniform surface. A walk on the treadmill also increases range of motion during hip extension. Walks can last from 2 to 10 min with 1–2 min breaks if the patient is tired; perform one to three times daily.

Paw Placement Stimulation

Gently drag the patient's paw backwards over a medium to rough surface that provides sensory/proprioceptive stimulation (Figure 29.12). If the patient does not place the paw correctly after the dragging, fingertip pinch the toes to elicit a withdrawal (Figure 29.13), and then help the animal drop it on the ground and place it correctly (Figure 29.14). The goal of this exercise is to stimulate sensory output, proprioception, and posture. Repeat 5–20 times each leg, one to three times daily.

Cavalettis

Set a few cavalettis in a row and have the patient walk through the obstacles, flexing one limb at a time; prevent the patient from bunny-hopping or skipping the obstacles (Figure 29.15). This exercise helps the patient to be aware of the position of the limbs in

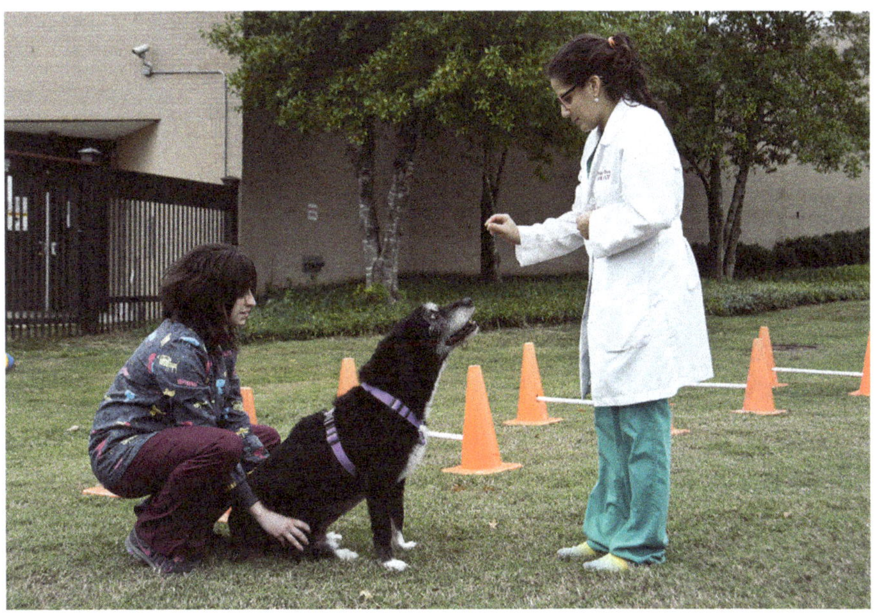

Figure 29.8 Sit-to-stand exercises should be performed with two people, one person in front of the patient to say "sit" and with treats if needed for motivation, the other behind the patient to position the hind limbs correctly during the exercise.

space, and to work on posture, balance and range of motion. Perform one to five sets of 1–5 min, one to three times daily.

Poles

Set a few poles in a row and have the patient walk through the obstacles in a zig-zag or figure-of-8 fashion in both directions while avoiding contact with the poles. This exercise encourages weight shifting to the limbs, and stimulates balance, proprioception and posture. It also increases range of motion and flexibility of the spine. Perform one to five sets of 1–5 min, one to three times daily.

Cart-work

The patient needs to be fitted for a cart that contributes to postural correction and allows the animal freedom to move around. Several wheelchairs for small animals with different indications are available on the market. Front-wheel, back-wheel, or four-wheel carts (Figure 29.16) are most common for neurological rehabilitation and they can be permanent or temporary (Figure 29.17) depending on the severity of the lesion. In stable lesions, it is recommended that cart-work exercises begin as soon as possible. Some dogs might need some time to adapt but most will get used to it very quickly. Cart-work exercise can start with 2–5 min walks and be increased up to 30–60 min.

Passive/Assisted-Active Exercises with Patient in the Water

Exercises in water provide additional benefits derived from the physical characteristics of water, flotation and viscosity being the two main properties of hydrotherapy [10]. Water stabilizes the patient and increases the resistance against movement, thus

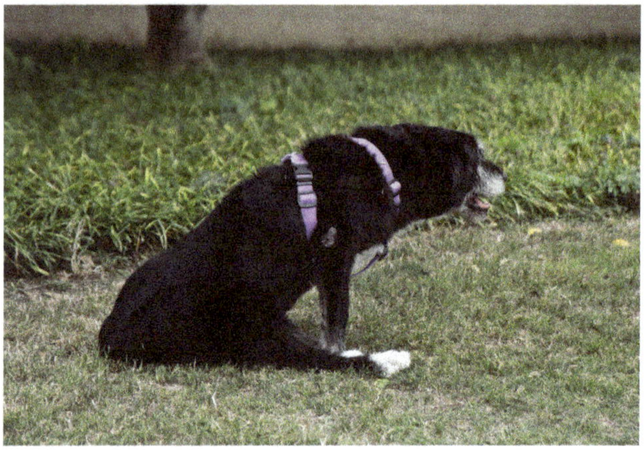

Figure 29.9 Example of a paraparetic patient in the sitting position with the hind limbs positioned abnormally. This is a common bad habit in patients with hind limb issues. If the orthopedic examination is unremarkable, this posture could be a result of maladaptive changes and should be corrected immediately.

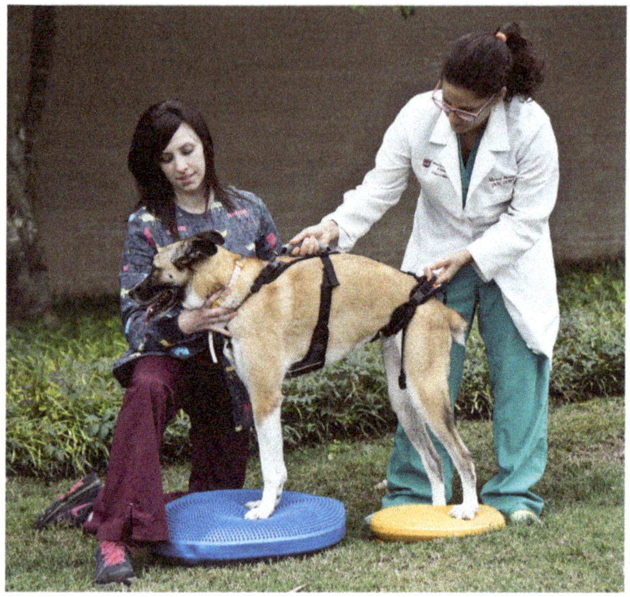

Figure 29.11 Weight-shifting exercise performed on balance boards for extra balance and proprioceptive training.

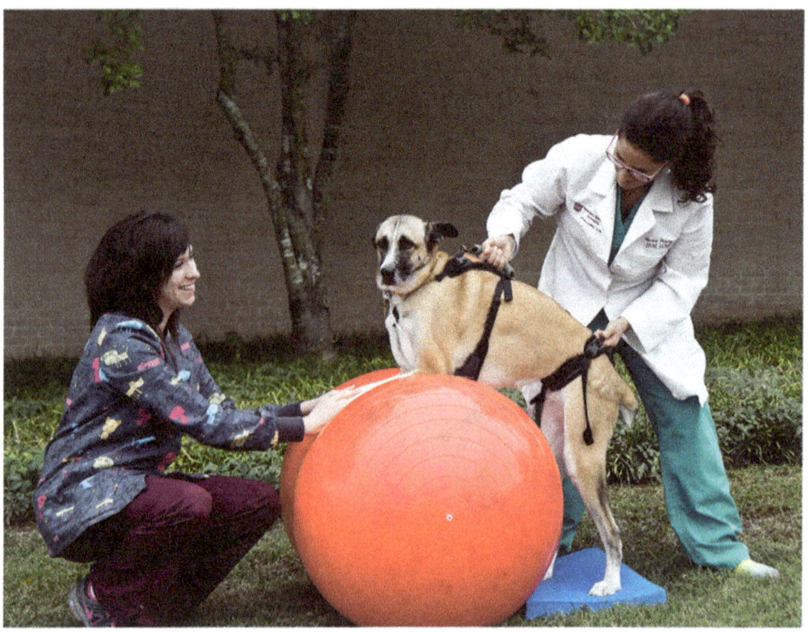

Figure 29.10 Weight-shifting exercises performed on a therapeutic peanut-shaped ball. Patient is shifting the weight to her hind limbs while the front limbs are on the ball. Her hind limbs are on a foam board for additional balance training. One of the therapists is in front of the patient for support and encouragement, the other is holding the patient from a therapeutic two-piece harness and doing some gentle rhythmic weight shifting side-to-side and forward/backward.

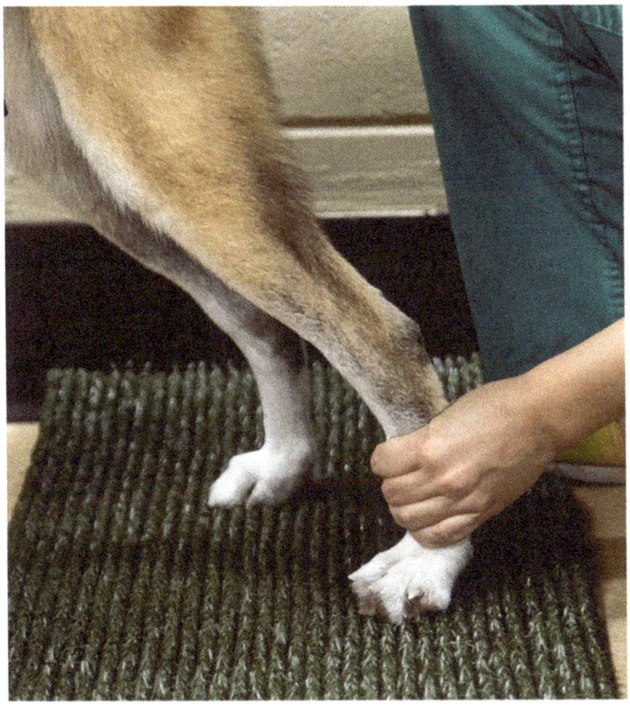

Figure 29.12 Paw placement stimulation exercise (1 of 3). The paw is dragged backwards for sensory and proprioceptive stimulation.

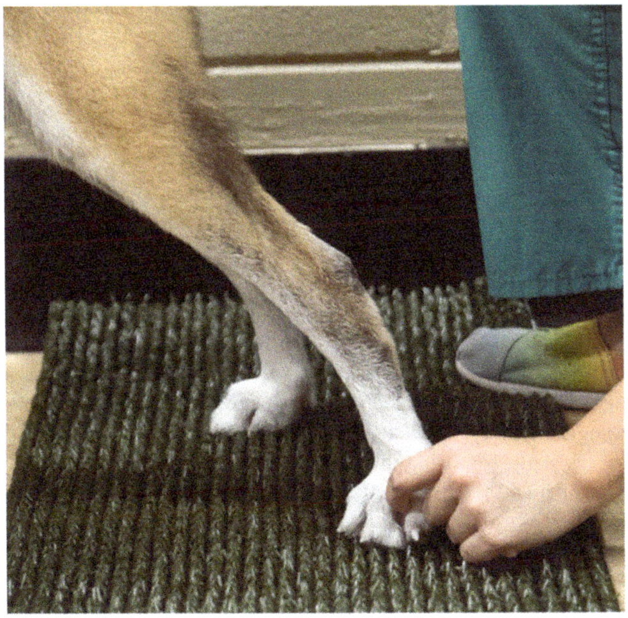

Figure 29.13 Paw placement stimulation exercise (2 of 3). Patients with decreased/absent proprioception will not place the paw correctly. Withdrawal reflex stimulation encourages the patient to pick up the limb and be aware of it.

strengthening in a low-impact manner. A life-jacket is recommended for safety purposes in most cases. Dogs with skin issues or healing incisions may not be able to enter the water until healed. There are some risks associated with hydrotherapy: aspiration pneumonia, skin reactions to the chemicals in the water, or falls around the pool area are three of the more common ones. Pay special

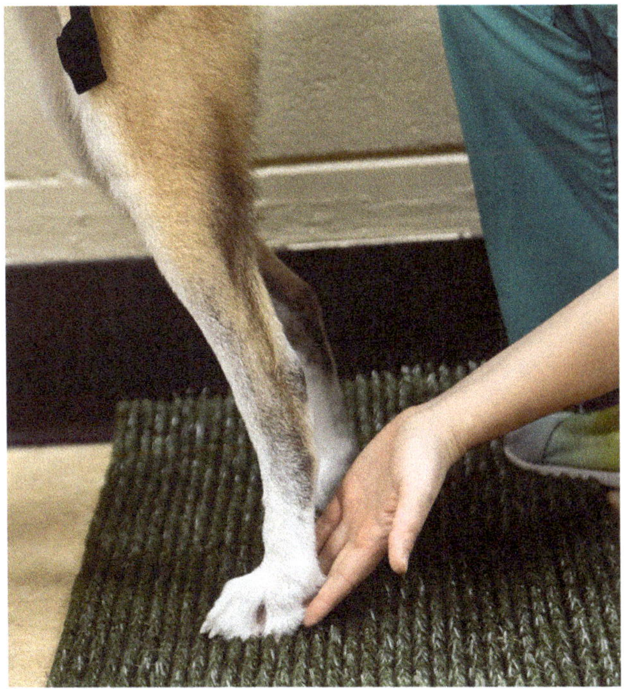

Figure 29.14 Paw placement stimulation exercise (3 of 3). The therapist helps the patient drop the limb and places it correctly for proprioceptive reinforcement as part of postural rehabilitation.

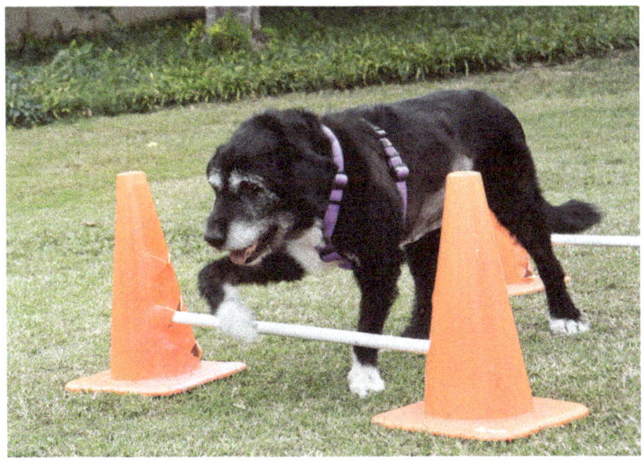

Figure 29.15 Cavalettis are recommended for encouraging the patient to flex and be aware of one limb at a time. This is especially recommended for correcting bunny-hopping.

attention to the airways in patients with severe motor dysfunction and difficulty in floating; in addition, check the skin regularly and prevent falls by providing an area of good traction around the pool, especially while the patient is still wet. Listed here are some of the more common exercises of hydrotherapy performed in the UWTM or swimming pool.

Swimming Pool

There are several types of pool but designing a pool at ground level eliminates the use of a hoist and decreases the risk of falls. Exercises in water provide an increased range of motion of the limbs with regard to the type of gait in the UWTM [10]. Some patients may do better in the pool than in the UWTM, so swimming will be chosen

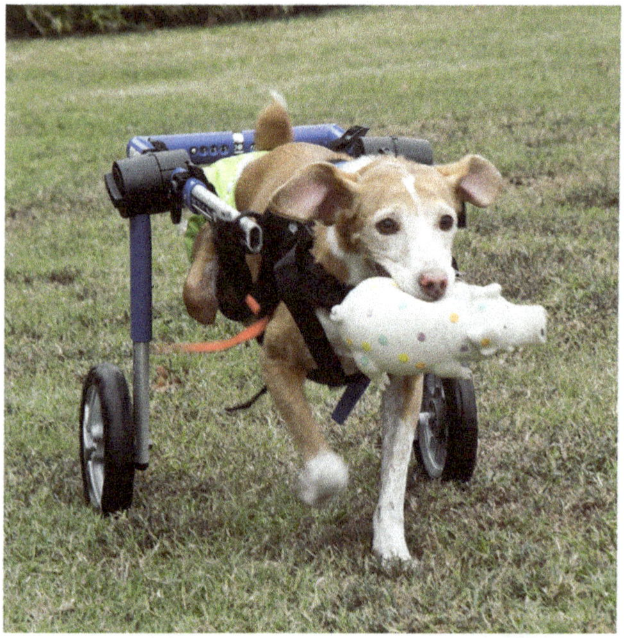

Figure 29.16 Temporary carts are used for patients during the recovery period. These can provide the patient with exercise, conditioning, and mental stimulation.

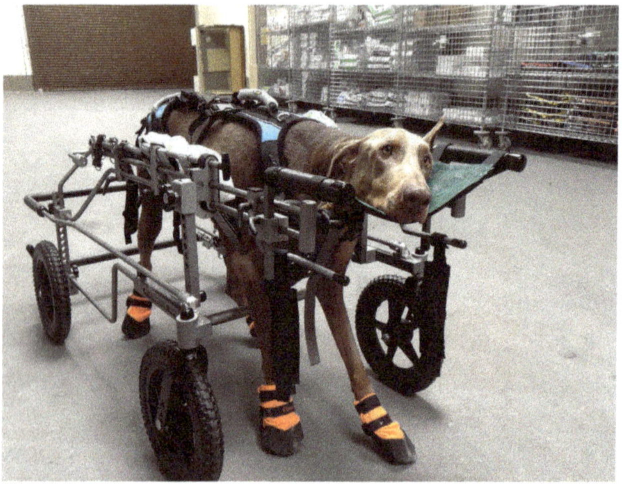

Figure 29.17 Four-wheel carts are designed for tetraparetic/tetraplegic patients. They may need to be pushed while the patient is recovering motor function, and additional accessories or maneuvers are recommended for maximum benefit of cart-work (e.g., boots for protection, elastic bands to help movement of the limbs, tail clip for mass reflex stimulation).

over walking on the treadmill. Patients with no motor function can obtain PROM of the affected limbs in the water, stimulation of withdrawal by touching or gently pinching the toes, or stimulation of the mass reflex by pinching the tail to initiate involuntary or voluntary motor function. Two people might be needed, so that one person can hold and give support while the other can be working on performing the exercises. Standing exercises can be performed on the entry and exit steps if they are safe and provide good traction. Turns and use of flotation devices attached to the limbs are some other examples of different exercises that can be performed in water. Use of treats or toys is recommended to make the therapy fun and stimulating for the patient.

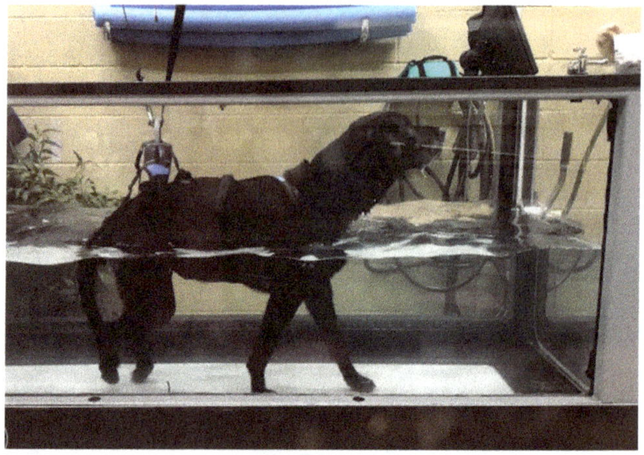

Figure 29.18 Underwater treadmill session.

Underwater Treadmill

The UWTM is an expensive piece of equipment that is frequently used for the rehabilitation of the neurological patient (Figure 29.18). The combination of controlled gait plus the benefits of water makes this technique very useful for recovery. Different water levels are used for different purposes [10]. For instance, low-level water will increase range of motion because the patient will instinctively pick up the legs when walking, whereas high-level water is recommended for patients needing more support. Some cases need two people, a person inside the tank manipulating the hind limbs or helping with balance, the other outside supervising and helping as needed. A hoist, slings, flotation devices, or elastic bands are some of the accessories that can be used in the session, with the goal of maximum benefit for the patient.

Prevention and Treatment of Bad Habits

Many patients present for their 3–6 week rechecks with fair neuromuscular function recovery but still with neurological deficits and abnormal gait and/or postures secondary to the development of bad habits. Bad habits in neurological patients can be defined as a negative patterned behavior or motor activity secondary to a neurological disease associated with loss of neuromuscular function that is acquired during the recovery through frequent repetition. Many patients recovering after back injury may present with severe kyphosis and/or scoliosis and bunny-hopping as a consequence of a new negative pattern that has been learnt during the post-injury period. These bad habits may not affect the patient's ability to move around and be functional but could influence quality of life a few months or years in the future. For example, a bunny-hopping gait is a result of increased tone and lack of dissociation in the hind limbs. These abnormalities may lead to muscles spasms in the hind limbs and back and other possible changes due to secondary compensation, so that avoidance of bad habits is paramount for full recovery.

Bad habits should be prevented because once the negative pattern becomes routine, it may take a long time to remove or may never be completely eliminated. The following sections list the most common bad habits that develop in the neurological patient, especially back-injured dogs, and some of the recommended exercises to prevent or remove them.

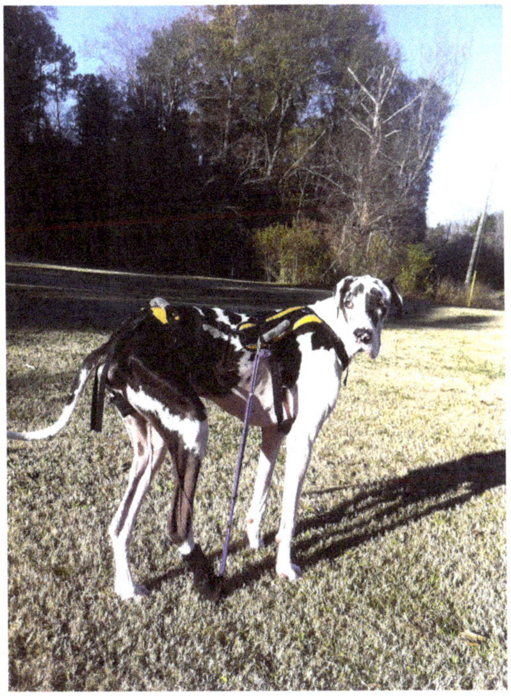

Figure 29.19 An elastic band that goes from the harness of the patient to the tip of boot is used to correct dragging of the limb due to proprioceptive deficits.

Dragging the Limbs

Dragging the limbs should be avoided in patients with potential for recovery of motor function. Cage confinement, cart walks, sling walks, splints (especially for brachial avulsion lesions), and postural rehabilitation (standing, sit-to stand, or ball-work) should be initiated from the beginning of recovery. Tail stimulation may help in some dogs with hind limb paralysis. Dogs with instability should be treated cautiously but keeping in mind the importance of maintaining range of motion and muscle/bone/joint mass. Patients with distal brachial plexus avulsion require strict PROM and splinting to maintain range of motion of the front limb, especially the carpal joint, which becomes irreversibly degenerated and ankylosed very promptly, possibly culminating in amputation of the limb, even in those cases that achieve relief from deep pain.

Abnormal Sitting Posture

Abnormal sitting posture should be discouraged in those patients with proprioceptive deficits in the hind limbs. Correction of the posture through repetitive sit-to-stand exercises should improve this and prevent abnormal position.

Knuckling Over

Knuckling over of any of the limbs should always be corrected and prevented. Use of rehabilitation accessories during walking or standing may help. Elastic bands that pull the tip of the paw through a wrap around the toes or a therapeutic boot (Figure 29.19), as well as splints, may be recommended in some cases. Usually, these accessories will be removed when the patient is back in the cage and special attention should be paid to pressure sores in theses cases. Tail stimulation might also help in patients with affected hind limbs, especially those with UMN signs in the hind limbs.

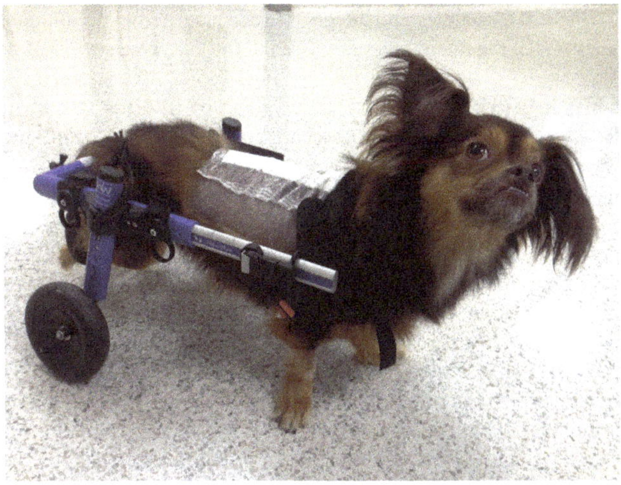

Figure 29.20 Patient is placed in cart during early recovery to prevent kyphosis. Encouraging the patient to lift the head up (cervical extension) while in the cart helps to stretch the back after back surgery.

Kyphosis

Kyphosis is commonly seen in patients with back injuries. Both back pain and gait difficulties play a role in the development of this bad habit. After a few weeks of kyphosis, the sublumbar and subthoracic muscles of the spine and core muscles shorten. This, in combination with weakness of the dorsal muscles, worsens the kyphosis. Adequate pain control and early prevention of kyphosis is recommended in all cases with back injuries. Cart walks (Figure 29.20), swimming or dry/water walking, and postural rehabilitation (standing, ball-work) all help in early prevention. Once kyphosis is present and the patient is healed, a few more exercises can be recommended.

- Lift the head of the patient during walks, sitting or standing (use treats for encouragement).
- Lateral flexion of the spine from side to side (use treats for encouragement).
- Gentle stretch of the back by putting some pressure over the dorsal aspect of the spine at the thoracolumbar region while the patient is standing. Previous warm packs will help with this stretch.
- Encourage the patient to lie on the back (a belly scratch might help) on a padded bed. While the animal is lying down, extension of front and hind limbs will help to achieve a better stretch of the back.

Bunny-hopping

Bunny-hopping is commonly seen in dogs secondary to a lack of dissociative movement of the hind limbs (ability of the patient to move one limb independently from the other limb or body) in patients recovering after back issues. Leash-walks and low cavalettis help the patient to use one a leg at a time. The animal may need some extra stimulation with doggie treats.

Management of the Recumbent Patient

Management of the recumbent patient can be challenging, especially when the patient is large and recumbency is prolonged. Specific preventive measures should be applied from the start of hospitalization of the neurological patient with motor dysfunction. Skin integrity, management of bladder function, assessment of permanent disabilities, and design of an adequate home environment are some of the main topics discussed in the following sections.

Skin Integrity

Skin infections and wounds are commonly found in the neurological patient but these could be reasonably prevented. A pressure ulcer characterized by full-thickness tissue loss is a concern during the long healing process and may indicate a worse prognosis or even become life-threatening if infected. This can change the direction of recovery of the patient, increase the cost, and limit the type of rehabilitation (restricting it to only dry rehabilitation); some owners may even decide to stop therapy and give up trying to get their pet better. Prevention is highly recommended in dogs at risk of pressure sores, principally those patients with thin skin and bony prominences, the two most frequent locations being the greater trochanter (Figure 29.21) and acromion. Urine scald is a potential issue in any patient with some degree of urine/fecal incontinence or movement disability. A patient leaking urine will lie on a wet bed and management of urinary incontinence and frequent bed changing will be necessary. Abrasion sores are frequent in patients with neurological deficits. For instance, decreased or lack of proprioception predisposes the patient to abrasion sores in the dorsal aspect of the toes and worn-down nails that bleed easily. Some of the prophylactic measures to apply in the recumbent patient are listed below.

- Keep bed clean, dry, and well padded at all times (Figure 29.22).
- Turn the patient every 4 hours when the animal cannot do it by itself. Right side, left side, and sternal (if possible) recumbency must be altered. The use of pillows might be needed to keep the patient in a comfortable position. Positioning the patient sitting up is recommended to prevent aspiration pneumonia, especially when eating or drinking. The patient should be looking out of the cage instead of facing the back of the cage or a wall so that it is stimulated by environmental interaction.
- Skin should be checked twice daily for early signs of pressure sores, especially in predisposed regions of the body. Pressure sores can be classified in four stages. Early lesions will appear as a small region of hyperemia over a bony skin region with intact skin (stage I). If this progresses, the small hyperemic region becomes a little larger and the hair will appear wet due to the exudate from the inflammatory skin process (stage II). Usually, this is the phase observed when the skin is checked regularly. The earlier hyperemic stage might not be seen because the hair will cover the skin. At this point, shaving the area and close monitoring is recommended. If the wound progresses, it becomes larger with a pale region at the center due to ischemia. This central region progresses to dark skin and necrosis involving the subcutaneous fat (stage III) or even muscle and bone tissues (stage IV). Do not forget bony regions in the medial aspects of the limbs. An additional pillow between the limbs is also recommended in patients with severe mobility problems. Pressure sores can also appear in non-bony regions due to position. For example, the skin in the cranial aspect of the elbows in patients kept too long in a sitting-up position with only turns of the hips are predisposed to ulcer.
- Check toes and nails regularly for early signs of abrasion sores. Patients with dysfunction of postural reactions drag the affected limb(s) and develop sores on the dorsal aspect of the toes and worn-down nails (Figure 29.23). Boots, socks, plastic fake nails, and elastic bands must be used in patients with these types of deficit.
- Prevent skin irritation by urine and feces. Management of bladder incontinence is essential to keep the neurological patient clean and dry. Patients predisposed to urine/fecal leakage, overflow or diarrhea should be monitored closely and medically treated as needed. If the skin appears hyperemic, wash with a soft wet sponge using water and soap, rinse well with water, dry

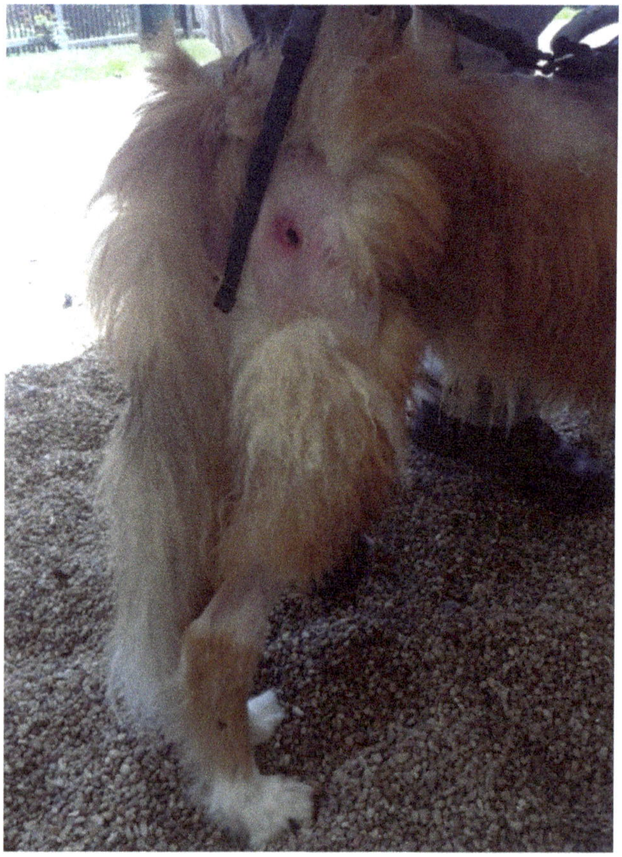

Figure 29.21 Pressure sore over the greater trochanter in recumbent patient with prominent bones. Note the dark round region over the hip due to necrosis of the skin covering the prominent lateral aspect of the femur.

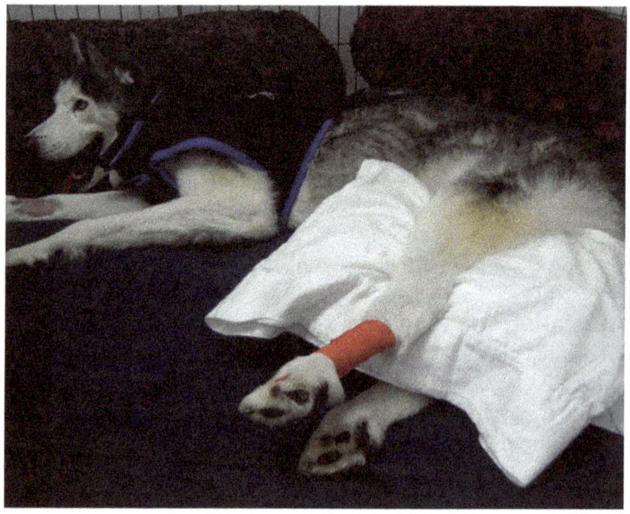

Figure 29.22 Recumbent patient with clean, dry and padded bed. Note the extra pillow between his hind limbs for protection of ulcers in the medial aspect of the hind limbs.

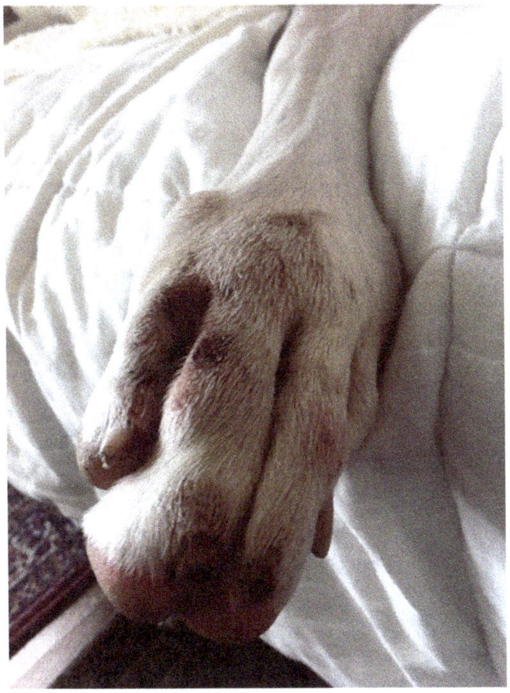

Figure 29.23 Severely worn down nails and skin abrasion wounds on the top of the toes in patient with absent nociception with severe sciatic lesion. Patient presented no proprioception and dragged the paw repetitively.

and shave the region until healthy skin is apparent, then apply ointment if needed (topical antibiotic, diaper rash ointment for fecal irritation). Consider male or female doggie diapers for some cases.

Bladder Management

Patients with neurological problems often have urinary and/or fecal incontinence and/or retention. Incontinence is the involuntary leakage of urine or feces, whereas retention is the involuntary holding of urine or feces within the bladder or rectum, respectively. Patients with UMN lesions present with increased tone of sphincters and bladder wall, while patients with LMN lesions or spinal shock exhibit decreased tone of both. In patients with UMN lesions, bladders that are not released adequately may show overflow incontinence, i.e., leakage of urine after the bladder becomes full and over-extended. This is commonly confused with voluntary urination in those cases where the dog is found in the cage with a wet bed. Palpation/ultrasound of the bladder is essential for assessment of bladder function in these cases. Patients unable to empty the bladder efficiently are predisposed to urinary tract infections, and urinary analysis and/or cultures may be indicated in those with difficult bladder management.

Urinary catheterization and/or medical management is frequently recommended in the early recovery stage of the patient with back problems to prevent complications (Figure 29.24). Parasympathomimetics (e.g., bethanechol) are used to increase detrusor muscle contractility in combination with muscle relaxants (e.g., diazepam) and α-adrenergic blockers (e.g., prazosin, phenoxybenzamine) in order to decrease the external or internal urethral resistance in those with severe UMN lesions. In cases with LMN lesions with decreased tone of the bladder wall, the use of parasympathomimetics can increase the tone of the detrusor

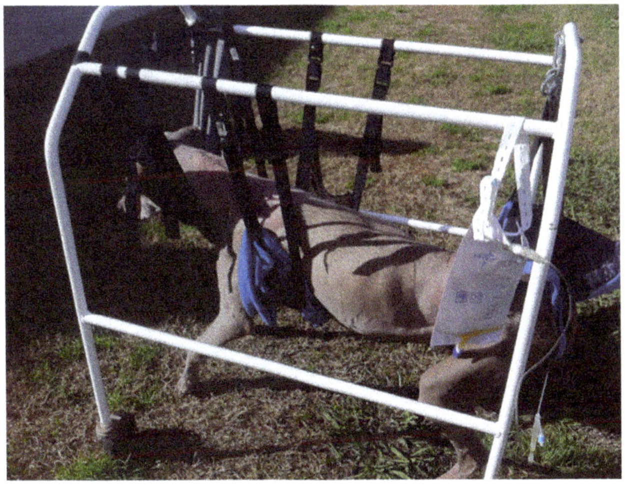

Figure 29.24 Critical tetraparetic patient placed on four-wheel cart for short outside walk for environmental enrichment, mental motivation, and posture rehabilitation. Note how the patient carries his urinary bag attached to his cart.

muscle and combination with other drugs to relax the sphincters might be indicated, especially in male dogs with a strong urethral muscle.

Permanent Disabilities

Currently, there are clients willing to take care of a pet with permanent neurological disabilities and it is our job to inform these owners about their pet's possible special care, cost, or complications to expect at home in a long-term setting. Monoplegia/paraplegia and incontinence are some of the most common conditions in the neurological patient. For owners that still want to keep their pet, these conditions can be overwhelming and our support and empathy is essential in order to ease adaptation to the new circumstances. Quality of life is a subjective concept and full understanding of a particular situation might not be possible. Some owners have a special bond with their pet and might not be ready to let them go, so it is our responsibility to ensure they receive sound advice to guarantee the best quality of life for the patient in a home environment. Hospice care may be necessary for the most severely affected patients, but many may be able to enjoy a fair quality of life with minimal extra care by the owner.

Multiple cart designs, harnesses, and other accessories are available to support the patient with permanent paralysis of the hind limbs, front limbs, or even all four limbs (Figure 29.25). Carts can be designed with two or four wheels according to the type and location of the lesion, size/weight, body condition, and any other health issues. Sturdy and durable carts are recommended for permanent disabilities. Some patients, especially toy or large breeds, might need custom carts that fit them correctly and provide comfort while moving around. Skin, toes, and nails should be checked frequently for any abrasions or sores from dragging, cart rubbing or pressure sores.

Adaptation of Environment

Recovery of a neurological patient may take weeks to months and never be complete. Owners need to be adequately educated so they can make changes at home promptly to prevent further damage and improve the quality of life of the patient. The individual management of each case is determined by the home environment and the

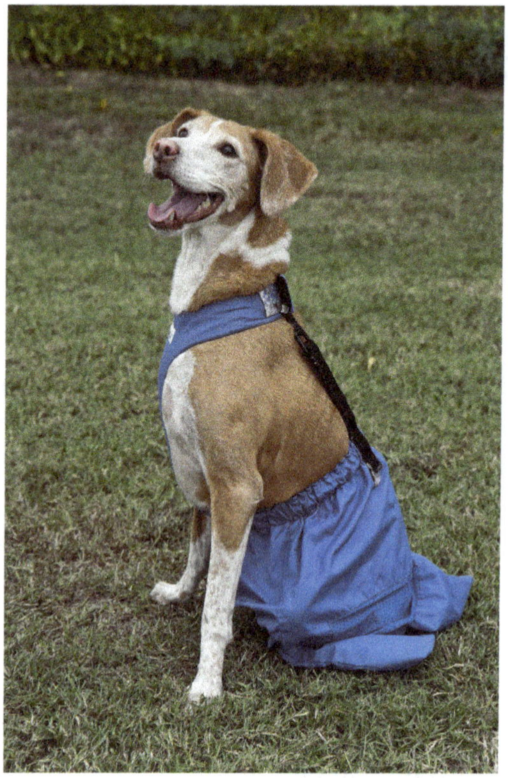

Figure 29.25 Patient with permanent paralysis of the hind limbs wearing a protective bag to prevent skin abrasion and diaper tearing. This accessory is ideal for incontinent patients that will stay at home for long hours. The patient in the picture usually wears a diaper but, when the owner stays at work for long periods, the dog wears this protective bag to prevent leakage at home.

capabilities of the owner: large dogs in homes where the owners have minimal ability to help their pet might be a challenging situation.

Some examples of patients in need of home environment changes are listed below:

- Patients with balance disorders (i.e., cerebellar, vestibular ataxia) require a padded cage/room to prevent further damage when falling over. The patient needs to be kept away from stairs or large windows and may need to be carried.
- Patients with balance disorders and postural reactions struggle walking on hard floors and this will necessitate rugs/carpets to be moved around. Most of these patients should be able to move better over grass or gravel.
- Owners of patients predisposed to back injuries (i.e., chondrodystrophic dogs) are advised to make permanent changes at home.
  - Ramps instead of steps.
  - Discourage the dog from jumping off furniture or from a car. This does not seem to be a problem for those owners with pets used to being on a couch or bed.
  - Confinement when pets are not supervised. This can be a large cage where the patient can turn around or a small room with good footing and without furniture.

Video clips to accompany this book can be found on the companion website at:
www.wiley.com/go/shores/neurosurgery

References

1 Hallet M. Neuroplasticity and rehabilitation. *J Rehabil Res Dev* 2005; 42(4): xvii–xxi.
2 Liepert J, Tegenthoff M, Malin JP. Changes of cortical motor area size during immobilization. *Electroencephalogr Clin Neurophysiol* 1995;97:382–386.
3 Nudo RJ. Functional and structural plasticity in motor cortex: implications for stroke recovery. *Phys Med Rehabil Clin North Am* 2003;14(1 Suppl):S57–S76.
4 Frost SB, Barbay S, Friel KM, Plautz EJ, Nudo RJ. Reorganization of remote cortical regions after ischemic brain injury: a potential substrate for stroke recovery. *J Neurophysiol* 2003;89:3205–3214.
5 Ziemann U, Ishii K, Borgheresi A et al. Dissociation of the pathways mediating ipsilateral and contralateral motor-evoked potentials in human hand and arm muscles. *J Physiol* 1999;518:895–906.
6 Johansen-Berg H, Rushworth MF, Bogdanovic MD, Kischka U, Wimalaratna S, Matthews PM. The role of ipsilateral premotor cortex in hand movement after stroke. *Proc Natl Acad Sci USA* 2002;99:14518–14523.
7 Byl NN, Merzenich MM. Principles of neuroplasticity: implications for neurorehabilitation and learning. In: Gonzalez ES, Myers S, Edelstein J, Lieberman JS, Downey JA (eds) *Downey and Darling's Physiological Basis of Rehabilitation Medicine*. Boston, MA: Butterworth-Heinemann, 2001.
8 Fisher BE. Principles of neuroplasticity: strategies for improving functions in patients with a neurologic injury. Presented at the 34th Anual Neurohabilitation Conference of Traumatic Brain Injury, Stroke and Neurologic disorders, Boston, MA, 2013.
9 Millis D, Levine D, Taylor R. *Canine Rehabilitation and Physical Therapy*. Philadelphia, PA: WB Saunders, 2004.
10 Millis DL, Levine D. *Canine Rehabilitation and Physical Therapy*, 2nd edn. Philadelphia, PA: Elsevier Saunders, 2014.
11 Riegel RJ. *Laser Therapy in the Companion Animal Practice: Mechanisms and Protocols for Class IV Laser Therapy*. Newark, DE: LiteCure LLC, 2008.

Index

Note: page numbers in *italics* indicate figures, and those in **bold** tables.

abdominal ultrasound
  intracranial surgery **24**, *24*, 24–25
  spinal surgery 59, 65–68, *67*, *68*
abdominal wall weakness, postoperative 188, *196*, 203, *203*
abrasion sores 266, *267*
acanthocytes 60
activated partial thromboplastin time (aPTT) 64
Adson-baby retractors 3–4, *5*
alanine aminotransferase 62
albumin, serum 62
alkaline phosphatase 62
amantadine 247
analgesia, postoperative *see* postoperative analgesia
anemia 61
angle-stable constructs 13, 16
antibiotics, perioperative 248
antiepileptics (anticonvulsants) 25–26, 254
apical ligament of the dens 141
arachnoid diverticula 135
Army–Navy retractor 4, *5*
arthrodesis
  atlantoaxial 146
  cervical spine 171–172, 176, *177*
  lumbosacral 229
aspergillosis 102
aspiration pneumonia 22, 23, 25, *25*
aspirin 64
atlantoaxial subluxation (AAS) 141–148
  anatomy 141
  clinical signs 142
  diagnosis 142, *142–143*
  medical management 143, *144*
  pathophysiology 141–142
  postoperative care *144*, 148
  surgical complications 146
  surgical procedures 143–146, *145–146*
  surgical prognosis 148
atlantooccipital overlap (AOO) 142
atlas (C1) 141
  dorsal atlantoaxial stabilization 144
  dorsal laminectomy/hemilaminectomy 155–156
  ventral atlantoaxial stabilization 144–145, *145*
  wings 55, *56*
Australian Shepherd, Pelger–Huët anomaly 61, *62*
axis (C2) 115, 141
  dorsal atlantoaxial stabilization 144
  dorsal laminectomy/hemilaminectomy 155–156
  laminotomy 155–156, *155–156*
  spinous process 55, 56, *56*
  ventral atlantoaxial stabilization 144–145, *145*
azotemia 23, 62, 63

bad habits 257
  preventing and treating 264–265, *265*
  sit-to-stand exercise 261, *262*
Balfour retractor, pediatric 3, *5*
bethanechol 251, **251**, 267
biceps femoris muscle biopsy 93, *94*, *95*, 95–96
bicortical pins
  cervical fracture/luxation repair 211
  thoracolumbar fracture/luxation repair 214–215, *215–216*
bicortical screws 14
  cervical distraction and stabilization *175*, 175–176
  cervical fracture/luxation repair 211–212

Current Techniques in Canine and Feline Neurosurgery, First Edition. Edited by Andy Shores and Brigitte A. Brisson.

© 2017 John Wiley & Sons, Inc. Published 2017 by John Wiley & Sons, Inc.

Companion website: www.wiley.com/go/shores/neurosurgery

bicortical spinal implants 18
  cervical stabilization 169–170
  thoracolumbar stabilization 213, **213**
bicycle movement exercises *249*, 259, *259–260*
bile acid concentrations 25
bilirubinuria 63
biochemistry, serum 23, **24**, 62–63
biopsy
  brain 48–50, *49*
  extracranial lesions 24–25, *25*, 30, *31*
  muscle and nerve 93–96
  skull tumors 121
  spinal neoplasia 240
  tract removal 123, *124*
bipolar electrosurgery 3, *4*
biventer cervicis muscle 166, *166*
bladder expression, manual 250–251
bladder management 250–251, **251**, *251*, 267
blade fenestration *191*, 191–192, 194–195, *195*
bleeding *see* hemorrhage/bleeding
bleeding disorders 64, 89
bleeding time, buccal mucosal 25, *25*, 63
blood component therapy 246
blood pressure 22, 23, 24, **24**
blood typing 23, **24**, 25
blood urea nitrogen (BUN) 62
bone cement *see* polymethylmethacrylate (PMMA) cement
bone grafts
  atlantoaxial stabilization 146, *146*
  cancellous, harvesting *173*
  cervical distraction and stabilization 170, *172*, 172–173, *174*
bone metastases, spinal 235, *237*
bone plates *see* plates, bone
bone screws *see* screws, bone
bone tap guide 14, *14*
bone tumors, primary
  skull *30*, 121–128
  spine 235, 238, *238*
bone wax 7, *7*
Boxers, cardiac disease 22
brachiocephalicus muscle 165, *165*
brachycephalic dogs
  congenital hydrocephalus 129
  frontal sinus 99, *100*
  transfrontal craniotomy *104*
brain biopsy 48–50, *49*
brain-heart syndrome 22
brain herniation
  clinical features 22, *22*
  CSF taps and 57, 88–89
  diagnostic imaging 38–39
brain masses
  extraaxial 37, 38, *38*, *39*
  image interpretation 37–39
  intraaxial 37, 38, *38*
  intraoperative ultrasonography 46–48, *47*, 110–112
  perilesional edema 37, *37*
  removal techniques 112, *113*
  suboccipital craniectomy *115*, *116*
  see also intracranial tumors
brain plasticity 257–258
Brainsight™ stereotactic system 48–50, *49*
brain spoons 7
brain tumors *see* intracranial tumors
brushing/scratching, therapeutic 260, *260*
Brussels Griffons, foramen magnum decompression 26
buccal mucosal bleeding time 25, *25*, 63
bunny-hopping gait 264, 265
buprenorphine **246**
burrs, drill *6*, *7*
butorphanol **246**

C1 *see* atlas
C2 *see* axis
calcium, plasma 62
cancellous bone
  pin–bone interface 12–13
  threaded pins 11, 13
cancellous screws 15
cardiac arrhythmias 68, *68*, 160–161
cardiac disease
  breeds at risk 22, 26
  preoperative evaluation 22–23, 25, *26*, 68
cardiovascular evaluation, preoperative 22–23
carprofen 247
carts, for permanent disabilities 267
cart-work exercises 262, *264*, *265*
Caspar retractors 171, *171*
casts, urinary 63
cauda equina 226
cauda equina syndrome *see* degenerative lumbosacral stenosis
cavalettis 261–262, *263*
Cavalier King Charles Spaniels (CKCS)
  cardiac disease 22, 26
  cerebral infarction 41
cefazolin 116, 131, 248
cellulose surgical spears *7*, 7–10
central canal dilation, with myelography 89
cerebral edema
  perilesional 37, *37*
  periventricular 130
  steroid therapy 247
cerebral infarction 39–43
  lacunar 41, *42*
  territorial 41, *42*
cerebro-cardiac syndrome 22
cerebromedullary puncture *see* cisternal cerebrospinal fluid tap
cerebrospinal fluid (CSF)
  cisternal tap 55–57
  failure to obtain (dry tap) 89–90
  lumbar tap 85–91
  over-drainage, VP shunts 134
  sample collection 56, *57*, 88
cerebrospinal fluid (CSF) analysis 57, 85
  hydrocephalus 130
  indications 90–91
  normal values in dogs **90**
  spinal neoplasia 240
cerebrovascular disease
  advanced imaging 39–43
  lateral rostrotentorial approach 109

transfrontal craniotomy 102
see also intracranial hemorrhage
cervical disc fenestration 192, 193
cervical disc herniation
dorsal approach 149, *150*
lateral approach 163–164, *164*
modified dorsal–lateral approach 166
prophylactic disc fenestration 192
ventral slot 157, 158–160
ventral vs dorsal approaches 149
cervical distraction and stabilization 169–178
additional decompression 172–173, *173*
complications 176–178
discectomy *171*, 171–172
intervertebral spacers 172, *172*
multiple spaces 176, *176*
positioning and approach 170, *170*
postoperative assessment 176
preoperative planning 169–170, *170*
stabilization techniques 173–176, *174–175*
surgical procedure 171–176
vertebral distraction 171, *171*
cervical fractures/luxations 211–213
decompression techniques 209
positioning and approach 211
reduction 211
stabilization techniques 211–213
cervical hemilaminectomy
cervical distraction and stabilization 173, *173*
dorsal approach to C1–C2 155
dorsal approach to C3–T1 *154*, 155
lateral approach 164
modified dorsal–lateral approach 166, *167*
vs dorsal laminectomy 149–150, *150–151*
cervical myelopathy
atlantoaxial subluxation 142, *143*
imaging *67*, 80–81
see also cervical spondylomyelopathy
cervical spine
postoperative instability 161, 167
prophylactic disc fenestration 192
surgical anatomy *153*, 164–165, *165*, 169, *170*
cervical spondylomyelopathy (wobbler syndrome)
cervical distraction and stabilization 169–178
dorsal laminectomy 153
dorsal vs ventral approaches 149
modified dorsal–lateral approach 164, *164*
ventral slot 157, 161
cervicoauricular–occipital complex 115
chemotherapy 240, 242
Chiari-like malformation 115, *117*
surgical procedure 117, 118–120, *119*
chisel pin tip 11, *11*, *12*
choline/creatine (Cho/Cr) ratio 35
choline:*N*-acetylaspartate (Cho:NAA) index (CNI) 36
choline/phosphocreatine–creatine (Cho/PCr-Cr) ratio 36
choroid plexus tumors 43, *115*
cisapride **253**
cisternal cerebrospinal fluid tap 55–57, 71
complications 57
contraindications 91
equipment 55, *56*
interpretation 57
preparation and positioning 55, *56*
sample acquisition 55–56, *56*, *57*
coagulation factors, inherited deficiencies 64
coagulation tests 25, 64
codeine 247
cold therapy, postoperative 254, 258
common peroneal nerve biopsy 93, *94*, *95*, 95–96
compensation *see* bad habits
complete blood count (CBC) 23, **24**, 60–62
complexus muscle 165, 166, *166*
computed tomography (CT)
atlantoaxial subluxation 142, *143*
cervical distraction and stabilization 176
cervical stenotic myelopathy 80–81
degenerative lumbosacral stenosis 225, *225*
extradural spinal lesions 81, *81*
-guided brain biopsy 48
head 32–33, *34*, 36–44
head trauma 27
intervertebral disc disease 78–80, *79*, *80*
lateralized cervical lesions 163
lumbosacral disease 80
myelography 74, *75*, 78–79, 80, *80*
skull tumors 121, *122*
spinal neoplasia 240
spine 74, **74**, *75*, 76–78
thoracic 65, *66*
congenital malformations, transfrontal craniotomy 102
contrast agents 71, 74
adverse reactions 23, 73, 74
cortical bone
pin–bone interface 12, 13
threaded pins 11, 13
cortical ring allografts, as intervertebral spacers 172, *172*
cortical screws 15
cervical fracture/luxation repair 211, *211*
see also bicortical screws; monocortical screws
corticosteroids 242, 246–247, 248
cough 22
cranial tibial muscle biopsy 93, *94*
craniectomy
instruments *6*, *7*
lateral (rostrotentorial) 109–114
skull tumors 121–128
suboccipital 115–120
craniotome *6*, 7
craniotomy
lateral (rostrotentorial) 109–114
transfrontal 99–107
creatinine, serum 62
crystalluria 63
CSF *see* cerebrospinal fluid
CT *see* computed tomography
curettes, surgical *8*, 195, *196*
CUSA ultrasonic tissue ablation system *see* ultrasonic surgical aspirator
Cushing's reflex 22
cycling exercises, passive *249*, 259, *259–260*
cytology *see* fine-needle aspiration cytology

D-dimer assays 65
decubital ulcers 248, *248*, 266, *266*
degenerative lumbosacral stenosis (DLSS) 223–230
  conservative and medical therapy 225
  diagnosis 224–225
  imaging 80, 224–225, *224–226*
  pathophysiology 223–224
  postoperative outcomes 229–230, **231**
  surgical treatment *see* lumbosacral decompression and foraminotomy
dens (odontoid process) 141
  developmental abnormalities 141, 142
  resection 146
dental tartar scraper 7, *8*
dentate ligament 181
depth gauges 14
desmopressin (DDAVP) 64
dexmedetomidine **246**
diazepam 251, **251**, 267
diffusion-weighted imaging (DWI) 41
diploic hemorrhage 154, *154*
Dirofilaria immitis larva *151*
disabilities, permanent 267, *268*
discospondylitis 90, 223–224
diverticuloperitoneal shunting 135, 136
Doberman Pinschers
  cardiac disease 22
  von Willebrand disease 25, 64, 160
dolichocephalic dogs
  frontal sinus 99, *100*
  transfrontal craniotomy *104*, *105*
Doppler ultrasonography
  intraoperative 46
  transcranial 32, *32*
dorsal approaches
  cervical spine 144, 149, 150–153
  occipital–atlantoaxial vertebral canal (medulla to C2) 155–156
  pediculectomy/mini-hemilaminectomy 185
  thoracolumbar disc fenestration 194
dorsal atlantoaxial ligament 117–118, 141
  dorsal laminotomy of C2 *155*, 155–156
  prosthetic replacement 144
dorsal decompression of cervical spine 149–156
  complete dorsal laminectomy 153–155
  dorsal surgical approach 150–153, *152*
  hemilaminectomy (C3–T1) 155
  indications 149
  laminectomy vs hemilaminectomy 149–150, *150–151*
  occipital–atlantoaxial region (medulla to C2) 155–156
dorsal laminectomy
  C1–C2 155
  C3–thoracic vertebrae *153*, 153–155, *154*, 173
  classification 205, *206*
  deep *206*, 207
  Funkquist A 206, *206*
  Funkquist B 205, 206, *206*
  indications 205
  lumbosacral region 226–228, *227–228*
  modified 205, *206*, 206–207
  spinal trauma 209
  surgical approach 205–206, *206*
  thoracolumbar region 183, 205–207
  vs cervical hemilaminectomy 149–150, *150–151*
dorsal–lateral approach to lateral cervical spine, modified
  indications 164, *164*
  surgical technique 166, *166–167*
dorsal longitudinal ligament *200*, 201, *201*
dorsal sagittal sinus 105, 123, *123*
dorsolateral thoracolumbar approaches
  disc fenestration 194
  lateral corpectomy 199
  pediculectomy/mini-hemilaminectomy *184*, 184–185, *185*, *186*
double myelographic line sign 78
dragging the limbs
  abrasion sores 266, *267*
  preventing and treating 265, *265*
draping 3, *4*
drill bits, size 14
drills, power *6*, 7
dry tap 89–90
dura mater
  closure of defects 114, *114*, 118, *118*
  lateral rostrotentorial craniectomy 110, *113*
  transfrontal craniotomy 105, 106
durotomy
  lateral cervical approach 166
  spinal neoplasia 240–241, *241*
  thoracolumbar hemilaminectomy 181–182

eccentrocytes 60, *60*
echinocytes 60
electrical stimulation 258
electrocardiogram (ECG) 22, **24**, 68, *68*
electrolytes, serum 23, **24**, 62
electromyography (EMG) 163
electrosurgical instruments 3, *4*
elevators, soft tissue 4, *6*
empyema, intracranial *44*, 102, *102*
endocrine evaluation, preoperative 23
endoscope-assisted minimally invasive surgery 160, 202
endoscopy 3, *4*
enteral nutrition 252, *252*
environment, adaptation of home 267–268
eosinophilia **61**
epidural abscess 90
epidural space
  inadvertent injection of contrast 72, *73*
  lumbosacral region 86
erythrocytes *60*, 60–61
erythrocytosis 61
erythromycin **253**
esophagostomy tube (E-tube) 252
exercise restriction, after spinal surgery 254–255
exercises, therapeutic 254, 259–264
  lateral recumbency 259–260, *259–260*
  standing position 260–262, *261–264*
  water-based 262–264, *264*
exoscopy 3, *4*
external skeletal fixation (ESF) 215
extradural spinal lesions
  diagnostic imaging 76–77, *77*, 81
  intervertebral disc disease 78, *79*
  neoplasia 235, *236*, 238–239

facetectomy
  cervical distraction and stabilization 173, *173*
  lateral cervical approach 165
  lumbosacral 225–226, 228–229
  modified dorsal–lateral cervical approach 164, *164*, 166
famotidine 116, 248
fasting, perioperative 23
fat grafts
  suboccipital craniectomy 116, 118, *118*
  thoracolumbar hemilaminectomy 179, *179*, 182
fecal incontinence 266, 267
feline infectious peritonitis (FIP) 43, *45*
fenestration *see* intervertebral disc fenestration
fentanyl **246**
fibrin–fibrinogen degradation products (FDPs) 65
fibrosarcoma, vertebral *238*
fine-needle aspiration cytology
  extracranial lesions 24–25, *25*
  skull tumors 121
  spinal tumors 240
flexor exercise 259, *260*
flexor withdrawal testing 163
fluid therapy, postoperative 245–246
foramen magnum decompression (FMD) 115–120
  indications 115, *115–117*
  minimum database **24**, 26
  patient positioning 115–116, *117*
  surgical anatomy 115, *117*
  surgical technique 116–120, *117–119*
foraminotomy
  extended thoracolumbar 183, *184*
  lumbosacral 225–226, 228–229
forceps, bone holding *9*, 10
fovea dentis 141
Frazier–Ferguson suction tip 7, *8*
Freer periosteal elevator 4, *6*
frontal bone
  anatomy 99, *99*, *100*
  bone flap closure 105, *105*, 107
  craniectomy defect 105, 107
  osteotomy *103*, 103–104, *104*
frontal lobes 99–100
  anatomy 99, *99*, *100*
  indications for surgery 100–102
  transfrontal approach *see* transfrontal craniotomy
frontal sinus
  anatomy 99, *99*, *100*
  transfrontal craniotomy 104–105
fucosidosis *35*

gabapentin 167, 247
gastric motility agents **253**
gastrocnemius muscle biopsy 93, *94*, *95*, 95–96
gastrointestinal evaluation, preoperative 23
gastroprotectants 247, 248
gastrostomy tube feeding 252
gelatin sponge *7*, 7–10, 187
Gelpi retractors 4, *5*, 171
glioblastoma, spinal *237*
gliomas
  intraoperative ultrasonography 46, *47*, 47–48
  magnetic resonance spectroscopy 35–36, *36*
glucose, plasma 62
glucosuria 63
golf ball sign 78, *78*
golf tee sign 78, *236*, 240
Gossett retractor 3, *5*
granulomatous meningoencephalomyelitis *90*
great auricular artery 115, 117

hand-held chucks 10, *10*
headache, post-lumbar puncture 86, 90
head trauma
  advanced imaging 43, *43*, *44*
  indications for surgery 27
  lateral rostrotentorial approach 109, *110*
  minimum database **24**, 26–27, *27*
  survey radiographs 27, 29
  transfrontal craniotomy 102, *102*
heartworm 21
heat therapy 258
Heinz bodies 60
hemangiosarcoma, metastatic *38*
hematological investigations 23, 60–62, 63–65
hematuria 63
hemilaminectomy *see* cervical hemilaminectomy; pediculectomy/mini-hemilaminectomy; thoracolumbar hemilaminectomy
hemophilia 64
hemorrhage/bleeding
  CSF taps 57, 89
  intracranial *see* intracranial hemorrhage
  laminectomy 154, *154*
  lateral rostrotentorial craniectomy 110
  modified dorsal–lateral cervical approach 166
  pediculectomy/mini-hemilaminectomy 188
  suboccipital craniectomy 118
  thoracolumbar lateral corpectomy 202–203
  thrombocytopenia 62, *62*
  ventral cervical decompression 160
hemorrhagic disorders 64, 89
hemostasis
  disorders of 64
  testing 25, *25*, 63–65
hemostatics, topical *7*, 7–10
hepatic failure 64
Hohmann retractors 4, *5*
Holter monitoring, preoperative 22
home environment, adaptations 267–268
Horner's syndrome 161
Howell–Jolly bodies 60
hydrocephalus 129–134
  acquired 43, *45*, 129
  advanced imaging 43–44, *45*, *46*
  clinical features 129
  compensatory (ex vacuo) 43–44, *46*, 129
  congenital 43, *45*
  diagnostic evaluation 129–130, *130*
  fenestration and marsupialization of lateral ventricles 136, *137*
  indications for surgery 130
  minimum database 26
  pediatric 129
  secondary to brain masses 38, *40*
  shunt surgery *see* ventriculoperitoneal (VP) shunt placement
  transcranial ultrasound 30, *31*

hydromorphone 246, **246**
hydrotherapy 262–264, *264*
hyperadrenocorticism 23
hypercalcemia 62
hyperglycemia 62
hyperkalemia 62
hypernatremia 62
hypocalcemia 62
hypoglycemia 62
hypokalemia 62
hyposthenuria 63
hypotension, intraoperative 160–161
hypothyroidism 23

iliocostalis lumborum muscle 185, 193, *193*
iliocostalis thoracis muscle 193
imaging
  intracranial *see* intracranial imaging
  intraoperative *see* intraoperative imaging
  postoperative 253
  skull tumors *30*, *121*, *122*
  spinal surgery 71–82
  see also computed tomography; magnetic resonance imaging; radiography; ultrasonography
Imex Miniature Interface® pins *13*
implant failure
  cervical distraction and stabilization 176, 177, 178
  thermal injury as cause 12
  vertebral fracture/luxation repair 212, 219, 220
implants, orthopedic 11–18
  bone plates 16–18
  bone screws 13–16
  instruments for placing 10, *10*
  pins and wires 11–13
incisional care, postoperative 253–254, *253–254*
incisional dehiscence 254
incontinence 266, 267
infections, postoperative 254
  cervical distraction and stabilization 177
  spinal surgery 59–60
  thoracolumbar lateral corpectomy 203
  VP shunts 134
inflammatory CNS disease 44, 90, *90*
instrumentation, neurosurgical 3–10
integument *see* skin
interarcuate ligaments *see* ligamentum flavum
interspinales muscle 85–86
interspinous ligaments 86
intervertebral disc fenestration 191–197
  blade *191*, 191–192, 194–195, *195*
  cervical 192, 193
  complications *196*, 196–197, *197*
  extent of nucleus pulposus removal 191–192, *192*
  indications 192
  postoperative care 197
  power-assisted 191–192, 195
  procedure 194–195, *195–196*
  surgical approaches 192–194
  thoracolumbar 193–197
  at time of hemilaminectomy 182
intervertebral disc herniation
  advanced imaging 78–80, 82
  bladder management 251
  cervical *see* cervical disc herniation
  CT 78–80, *79*, *80*
  extrusion vs protrusion 76, *78*
  lumbosacral 223, 228, *228*
  MRI *66*, 76, *76*, *78*, 80
  myelography 71, 78, *79*
  postoperative analgesia 246–247
  sinus tachycardia *68*
  thoracolumbar *see* thoracolumbar disc herniation
intervertebral space, distraction 171, *171*
intervertebral spacers
  cervical distraction 172, *172*
  complications 177
  lumbosacral distraction 229
intracranial abscess
  minimum database 26–27, *27*
  transfrontal craniotomy 102, *102*
intracranial hemorrhage
  contraindicating lumbar tap 89
  imaging 33–35, *34*, 39, **40**, *41*
  intraparenchymal *34*, 39
  presurgical investigations 23, 24
  transfrontal craniotomy 102
intracranial imaging, advanced 24, 29–50
  image interpretation 36–44
  intraoperative 44–50
  renal complications of contrast agents 23
  techniques 29–36
intracranial pressure (ICP), raised
  clinical features 21–22, *22*
  contraindicating lumbar tap 88–89
  imaging 38–39
  minimum database 21–22, 24
intracranial surgery
  advanced imaging 29–50
  indications 21
  minimum database 21–27
intracranial tumors
  diagnostic imaging *38*, 38–39, *39*
  hemorrhagic 39, *41*
  intraoperative ultrasonography 46–48, *47*
  lateral rostrotentorial approach 109, *109*
  magnetic resonance spectroscopy 35–36, *36*
  metastatic 38, *38*
  minimum database **24**, 24–26
  suboccipital craniectomy 115, *115*, *116*, 117–118
  transfrontal craniotomy 100, *101*, 105
intradural-extramedullary spinal lesions
  imaging 76, *77*, 77–78
  neoplasia 235, *236*, 239, *239*, 240
intramedullary spinal cord lesions
  imaging 76, 77, *77*, *81*, 81–82
  intervertebral disc disease 80
  tumors 235, *237*, 239, 240
intraoperative imaging 44–50
  image-guided brain biopsy 48–50, *49*
  lateral rostrotentorial craniectomy 110–112, *113*
  rationale 44–46
  ultrasonography 46–48, *47*

intravenous fluids, postoperative 245–246
intraventricular hemorrhage *34*, 39
iodinated contrast agents 71
iris scissors *9*, 10
iris spatula 7, *7*, *8*

Kern bone-holding forceps *9*, 10
Kerrison rongeurs 7, *8*
ketamine 246, **246**
ketonuria 63
Kirschner wires (K-wires) 11
  stapling of spinal injuries 216
  thoracolumbar fracture reduction 213
Kishigami device 144
knuckling over 265, *265*
kyphosis 265, *265*

lacunar infarcts 41, *42*
laminectomy
  dorsal *see* dorsal laminectomy
  lateral cervical approach 165
  modified dorsal-lateral cervical approach 166
  prophylactic disc fenestration 192
laminectomy spreaders *9*, 10
laminotomy, C2 155–156, *155–156*
Langenbeck retractors 4, *5*
laser therapy 254, 258
lateral cervical approach (C3–T1) 155, 163–167
  clinical evaluation 163
  diagnosis 163
  indications 163–164, *164*
  lateral approach 165
  modified lateral approach *165*, 165–166
  postoperative care 166–167
  surgical anatomy 164–165, *165*
  see also dorsal-lateral approach to lateral cervical spine, modified
lateral (rostrotentorial) craniotomy/craniectomy 109–114
  indications 109, *109*, *110*
  preparation and positioning 109, *111*
  quadrigeminal diverticula 136
  surgical technique 109–114, *112–114*
lateral flexion of spine exercise 260, *261*
lateral lumbosacral approach 229
lateral thoracolumbar approaches
  corpectomy *see* thoracolumbar lateral corpectomy
  disc fenestration 193–194, *193–194*
  pediculectomy/mini-hemilaminectomy 184, 185
lateral ventricles, fenestration and marsupialization 136, *137*
leukocytes 61
  circulating 61, *61*
  CSF **90**, *90*
leukocytosis 61, **61**
leukopenia 61, **61**
levator costae muscles 193
levetiracetam 25–26
Lhermitte's syndrome 242
lidocaine **246**
ligamentum flavum (interarcuate ligament) 86
  cervical dorsal laminectomy 153–154, *154*
  lumbosacral dorsal laminectomy 227

Limited Contact Dynamic Compression Plate (LC-DCP®) 16, *17*
liver function tests 23, 62
locking compression plate (LCP)
  cervical distraction and stabilization 175, *175*
  cervical fracture/luxation repair 212, *213*
locking plates 16–18, *17–18*
  fixed angle 16, 17, *17*
  variable angle 16, 17, *17*, 18
  see also plate fixation
locking screws 16, *16*, 18
longissimus capitis muscle *165*, 165–166, *166*
longissimus cervicis muscle 165, *165*
longissimus (thoracis and lumborum) muscle 185, *186*, 194
longus colli muscles 158
loupes, surgical 3, *3*
lumbar puncture (tap) 85–91
  anatomy 85–86
  complications 89–90
  contraindications 88–89
  dry 89–90
  indications 85, 90–91
  myelography 71–72, *72*, 85, 88
  patient positioning 86–87, *87*
  preparation and equipment 86, *86*
  technique *87*, 88, *88*, *89*
lumbosacral decompression and foraminotomy 223–230
  distraction and stabilization/fusion 229, *230*
  dorsal laminectomy 226–228, *227–228*
  foraminotomy and facetectomy 228–229
  indications 225
  postoperative care 229
  postoperative outcomes 229–230, **231**
  surgical anatomy 226, *227*
lumbosacral injuries 217–219
  decompression techniques 209–211
  fixation methods 219, *219*, *220*
  reduction 219
lumbosacral joint 223, *223*
  distraction and stabilization/fusion 229
  surgical anatomy 226, *227*
  transarticular fixation of fractures 219
lymphocytes, CSF **90**, *90*
lymphocytosis **61**
lymphoma
  nasopharyngeal *30*
  spinal 239, 240, 241
lymphopenia **61**

macrocytosis 61
magnetic resonance imaging (MRI)
  atlantoaxial subluxation 142, *143*
  brain 29, 33–35, 36–44
  cervical stenotic myelopathy 80–81
  contrast enhancement 33, 37
  degenerative lumbosacral stenosis 225, *226*
  extradural spinal lesions 81
  -guided brain biopsy 48–50, *49*
  hydrocephalus 43, *45*, 129–130, *130*
  intervertebral disc disease *66*, 76, *76*, *78*, 80
  intramedullary spinal cord lesions *81*, 81–82

magnetic resonance imaging (MRI) (*cont'd*)
  lateralized cervical lesions 163
  lumbosacral disease 80
  quadrigeminal diverticula 135, *135*
  spinal tumors *236–239*, 240
  spine 74–78, **76**
magnetic resonance spectroscopy (MRS) 35–36, *35–36*
magnetic susceptibility artifact 34
maladaptive change *see* bad habits
manual traction, cervical vertebral distraction 171
massage 258–259
mass effect, intracranial 37, *37*
mechanical ventilation 250
medulla oblongata, dorsal approach 155–156
megaesophagus 23, *65*
meloxicam 247
meningiomas
  diagnostic imaging 38, *38*
  intraoperative ultrasonography *47*, 47–48
  lateral rostrotentorial craniectomy *109*
  spinal *68*, 235, *236*, 239, 241
  suboccipital craniectomy *116*
  transfrontal craniotomy 100, *101*, 105
meningitis 90, *90*
meningocele 102
meningoencephalocele 102
mesocephalic dogs
  frontal sinus 99, *100*
  transfrontal craniotomy *104*
methadone 246, **246**
methocarbamol 247–248
methylprednisolone 225, 246, 247
metoclopramide **253**
microcytosis 61
micro-Doppler ultrasonography, intraoperative 46
middle cerebral artery 99, *99*
Miller–Senn retractors 4, *5*
mini-hemilaminectomy *see* pediculectomy/mini-hemilaminectomy
minimally invasive surgery, endoscope-assisted 160, 202
misoprostol 248
mitral valve disease 26
monocortical screws 14, 18
  cervical distraction and stabilization 170, 173–174, *174*, 176, *176*
  cervical fracture/luxation repair *211*, 211–212
monocytes, CSF **90**, *90*
monocytosis **61**
monopolar electrosurgery 3, *4*
morphine 246, **246**
MRI *see* magnetic resonance imaging
mucosal bleeding time 25, *25*, 63
multifidus cervicis muscle 165, *165*, 166, *166*
multifidus (thoracis and lumborum) muscles 85–86, 179–180, 185, 194
muscle biopsy 93–96
  pelvic limb 93–96, *94*, *95*
  thoracic limb *95*, 96, *96*
myelography 71–74
  artifacts 72, *73*
  atlantoaxial subluxation 142
  cervical stenotic myelopathy 80
  cervical technique 71
  CSF analysis prior to 90–91
  CT 74, *75*, 78–79, 80, *80*
  degenerative lumbosacral stenosis 225
  interpretation 76–78
  intervertebral disc disease 71, 78, *79*
  intramedullary spinal cord lesions 82
  lumbar technique 71–72, *72*, 85, 88
  lumbosacral disease 80
  MRI *75*
  normal variations 72–73
  side effects 72–73
  spinal tumors 240
  tips 73, *73*
myelomalacia
  imaging 80, 82
  postoperative monitoring 253
myocardial necrosis, acute 68, *68*

N-acetylaspartate/choline (NAA/Cho) ratio 35–36, *36*
nasogastric tube feeding 252, *252*
nasopharyngeal mass *30*
needles, bent 7, *7*
negative-profile threaded pins 11, *12*
nephroblastoma, extrarenal 239, *239*, 241
nerve biopsy 93–96
  pelvic limb 93–96, *94*, *95*
  thoracic limb *95*, 96, *96*
nerve hooks *9*, 10
nerve roots, surgical injury 188, 203
nerve sheath tumors 239, *239*, 240–241
neurogenic cardiomyopathy 68, *68*
neurological assessment 21–22, 253
neurological complications
  pediculectomy/mini-hemilaminectomy 188
  thoracolumbar lateral corpectomy 203
  ventral slot surgery 161
neuroplasticity 257–258
neurorehabilitation 257–258
neutrophils **61**, *90*
nitrofurantoin 251
non-steroidal anti-inflammatory drugs (NSAIDs) 246, 247, 248
nuchal ligaments 115, 117, 151
nutrition, postoperative 251–253

occipital–atlantoaxial vertebral canal, dorsal approach 155–156
occipital bone, craniectomy 118
occipital dysplasia 117, 118, *118*
odontoid process *see* dens
olfactory lobe
  indications for surgery 100, *101*
  surgical approach 102–105, 109
Oliver, J.E. 109, 115
omeprazole 248
omotransversarius muscle 165, *165*
opioid analgesics 246, **246**
osteosarcoma
  cranial *122*
  vertebral *66*, 235, *238*, 241
otitis media 29, *30*

packed cell volume (PCV) 22, 23, **24**, 60
pain management, postoperative *see* postoperative analgesia
pantoprazole 248
paradoxical contrast obstruction sign 78, *79*
paralysis, permanent 267, *268*
parenteral nutrition 253
passive/assisted-active exercises
  standing position 260–262
  water-based 262–264
passive exercises, lateral recumbency 259–260
passive range of motion (PROM) exercises
  recumbent patients 248, *249*
  techniques 259, *259–260*
paw placement stimulation exercise 261, *263*
pediculectomy/mini-hemilaminectomy 183–188
  complications 188
  dorsolateral approach *184*, 184–185, *185*, *186*
  indications 183
  lateral approach 184, 185
  partial 183, *184*, *188*
  patient positioning *184*
  postoperative care 188
  principles 183–184, *184*
  surgical closure 188
  surgical procedure 185–188, *186–187*
  with thoracolumbar lateral corpectomy 202
  traumatic injuries 209
Pelger–Huët anomaly 61, *62*
Pelorus Mark III Stereotactic System 48
percutaneous laser disc ablation (PLDA) 192
periosteal elevators 4, *6*
peripheral nerve sheath tumors 239, *239*, 240–241
phenobarbital 25–26
phenoxybenzamine 251, **251**, 267
physical examination
  presurgical 22–23, 59
  spinal neoplasia 236–238
physical therapy (physiotherapy)
  bad habits 264–265, *265*
  defined 257
  physical modalities 258–259
  recumbent patients 248–250, *249*
  therapeutic exercises 254, 259–264
  see also rehabilitation
pin fixation
  atlantoaxial subluxation 145, *145*
  cervical fractures/luxations 211
  lumbosacral injuries 219
  thoracolumbar fractures/luxations 213–215, *215–216*
pins, surgical 11–13
  bone cement interface 13, *13*
  bone interface *12*, 12–13
  insertion technique 12–13
  length of bone engagement 12–13
  negative-profile 11, *12*
  positive-profile 11, *12*
  thread design 13
  threaded 11, *12*, *13*
  tip types 11, *11*, 12
  unthreaded 11, *12*
plate fixation
  atlantoaxial subluxation 145
  cervical distraction and stabilization 170, 174–175, *175*
  cervical fractures/luxations 212–213, *212–213*
  lumbosacral injuries 219, *220*
  thoracolumbar fractures/luxations 215, *217*
platelet count 61–62, 63
plates, bone 16–18
  locking 16–18, *17–18*
  nonlocking 16, *17*
PMMA *see* polymethylmethacrylate
pneumocephalus
  after transfrontal craniotomy 105–107, *106*
  imaging 43, *44*
pneumothorax 196
poikilocytes 60
poles, walking through 262
polycythemia 61
polymethylmethacrylate (PMMA) cement 10, *10*
  atlantoaxial stabilization 145, *147*
  cervical distraction and stabilization 170, 173–174, *174*, 176, *176*
  cervical fracture/luxation repair *211*, 211–212
  lumbosacral injury repair 219
  screw fixation 15
  skull reconstruction 105, 107, 125–127, *126*
  stability of pin interface 13, *13*
  thoracolumbar fracture/luxation repair 214–215, *215–216*
polypropylene mesh, craniectomy defects 114, *114*
positioning, patient
  cervical distraction and stabilization 170, *170*
  cisternal tap 55, *56*
  dorsal cervical decompression 150, *152*
  dorsal laminectomy 205
  foramen magnum decompression 115–116, *117*
  lateral cervical approach 165, 166
  lateral (rostrotentorial) craniotomy/craniectomy 109, *111*
  lumbar puncture 86–87, *87*
  pediculectomy/mini-hemilaminectomy *184*
  recumbent patients 266, *266*
  shunt surgery 131, *132*
  skull tumors 123, *123*
  thoracolumbar disc fenestration 193
  ventral cervical decompression 157, *157*
  vertebral fracture/luxation repair 211, 213, 219
positive-profile threaded pins 11, *12*
postoperative analgesia **246**, 246–248
  alternative or adjunctive analgesics 247–248
  lateral cervical approach 166–167
  ventral slot surgery 161
postoperative care 245–255
  antibiotics 248
  antiepileptics 254
  bladder management 250–251
  exercise restriction 254–255
  gastroprotectants 248
  incisional care 253–254
  intravenous fluids 245–246
  mechanical ventilation 250
  monitoring neurological status 253
  nutritional support 251–253

postoperative care (*cont'd*)
  pain management *see* postoperative analgesia
  physiotherapy *see* physical therapy
  recumbent patients 248–250
potassium, serum 62
Potts scissors *9*, 10
power-assisted fenestration 191–192, 195
prazosin 251, **251**, 267
preanesthetic assessment, intracranial surgery 21–23
predrilling 12, 14
pregabalin 167
pressure ulcers 248, *248*, 266, *266*
primitive neuroectodermal tumors (PNETs) 241
proteinuria 63
prothrombin time (PT) 64
pseudohyperkalemia 62
pulmonary masses, multifocal *66*, *67*
pyuria 63

quadrigeminal diverticula (cysts) 135–136
  diverticuloperitoneal shunting 135, 136
  fenestration and marsupialization 135–136
  preoperative evaluation *32*, 135, *135*
  suboccipital craniectomy 115, *116*, 118, 135–136

radiation therapy, spinal tumors 240, 241–242
radiculopathies, CSF analysis 91
radiography
  atlantoaxial subluxation 142, *142*
  degenerative lumbosacral stenosis *224*, 224–225
  skull 27, 29, *30*
  spinal neoplasia 240
  thoracic *see* thoracic radiographs
recumbent patients 265–268
  bladder management 267
  environmental adaptation 267–268
  permanent disabilities 267, *268*
  physiotherapy 248–250, *249*
  skin integrity 248, *248*, 266–267, *266–267*
recurrent laryngeal nerve 148, 158
rehabilitation 254, 257–268
  bad habits 264–265
  defined 257
  physical modalities 258–259
  recumbent patients 265–268
  therapeutic exercises 259–264
renal disease, chronic 23
renal system, evaluation 23
rescue screw 14–15
respiratory assessment, preoperative 22
respiratory complications, cervical spinal surgery 160
resting energy requirements (RER) 252
resuscitation, preoperative 26–27
retractors 3–4, *5*
rhizotomy
  spinal tumor surgery 240
  thoracolumbar lateral corpectomy 200, 203
robenacoxib 247
rongeurs 7, *8*
root signature 163
rostral cerebral artery 99, *99*
Rottweilers, von Willebrand disease 160

sagittal sinus, dorsal 105, 123, *123*
saline irrigation
  dorsal cervical laminectomy 153
  pin insertion 12
  skull tumor resection *124*, 124–125
  thoracolumbar hemilaminectomy 180
sarcoma
  spinal *237–238*, 238
  sternal *68*
schistocytes 60
scissors *9*, 10
scoliosis, postoperative 188
scratching/brushing, therapeutic 260, *260*
screw fixation
  atlantoaxial subluxation 145, *146–147*
  cervical distraction and stabilization 169–170, 173–174, *174*
  cervical fractures/luxations *211*, 211–212
  lumbosacral decompression 229, *230*
  lumbosacral injuries 219, *220*
screws, bone 13–16
  cancellous 15
  core (minor) diameter 13, *14*
  cortical *see* cortical screws
  insertion 14–15
  locking 16, *16*
  main characteristics 13, *14*
  measuring hole length 14
  pitch 13, *14*
  predrilling 14
  rescue 14–15
  self-drilling 15, *15*, *16*
  self-tapping 15, *15*
  tapping 14, *14*
  thread (major) diameter 13, *14*
  types 15–16
seizures
  frontal lobe lesions 100, *101*, *106*
  post-myelographic 73
  prophylaxis 25–26, 254
self-drilling screws 15, *15*, *16*
self-tapping screws 15, *15*
seromas, postoperative 254, *254*
  cervical distraction and stabilization 177–178
  vertebral fracture/luxation repair 220
serratus ventralis muscle 165, *165*
serum biochemistry 23, **24**, 62–63
shunt passer 132, *133*
sinus tachycardia *68*
sitting posture, abnormal *262*, 265
sit-to-stand exercises 261, *261*, *262*
skin
  infections 23, 89
  integrity, recumbent patients 248, *248*, 266–267, *266–267*
skull
  caudal anatomy 115, *117*
  fractures 29, 43, *43*, *110*
  lateral anatomy *112*
  reconstruction 125–128, *126–128*

surgical anatomy 121–123, *123*
survey radiographs 27, 29, *30*
skull tumors 121–128
patient positioning 123, *123*
postoperative care 128
preoperative imaging *30*, 121, *122*
surgical anatomy 121–123, *123*
surgical technique 123–128, *124–128*
three-dimensional printing 121, *122*
Small Animal Coma Scale (SACS) 21
soft tissues
elevators 4, *6*
imaging 30, *31*, 37
infections 89
specific gravity, urine 63
spherocytes 60
spinal cord lesions
complicating lumbar tap 89
imaging *77*, *81*, 81–82
intramedullary *see* intramedullary spinal cord lesions
spinal imaging, advanced 71–82
interpretation 76–78
modalities 71–76
specific diseases 78–82
spinal instability, postoperative
cervical spinal surgery 161, 167
disc fenestration 197
thoracolumbar lateral corpectomy 202, 203
spinal needles
cisternal CSF tap 55–56, *56*
lumbar puncture 86, 88
myelography 71
spinal neoplasia 235–242
diagnostic evaluation 81, 240
extradural 235, *236*, 238–239
intradural/extramedullary 235, *236*, 239, *239*, 240
intramedullary 235, *237*, 239, 240
lateral cervical approach 164, *164*
localization 238–239
medical history 235–236
metastatic 66, 235, *237*
modified dorsal-lateral cervical approach 166
nonsurgical therapy 241–242
physical and neurological examination 236–238, *237*
surgical treatment 240–241
spinal nerves
disc fenestration 194
lumbosacral dorsal laminectomy *227*, 227–228
thoracolumbar lateral corpectomy 200, *201*
spinal stabilization procedures
atlantoaxial subluxation 143–146
degenerative lumbosacral stenosis 229, *230*
implants used 11–18
instrumentation *9*, 10
vertebral fractures/luxations 209, 211–213
see also cervical distraction and stabilization
spinal stapling, fractures/luxations 216–217, *217–218*
spinal surgery
advanced imaging 71–82
exercise restriction after 254–255
indications 59
minimum database 59–68
spinal trauma *see* vertebral fractures/luxations
splenius muscle 165, *165*
splinting, atlantoaxial subluxation 143, *144*
spondylosis deformans 223–224
standing exercise 260–261
stapling, spinal fractures/luxations 216–217, *217–218*
Steinmann pins 11, *11*
cervical stabilization *175*, *176*
stapling of spinal injuries 216–217, *217–218*
stereotactic brain biopsy 48–50
sternocephalicus muscle 158, *158*
sternohyoideus muscle 158, *158*
String of Pearls™ (SOP) plate system 18, *18*
cervical fracture/luxation repair 212, *212*
lumbosacral injuries *220*
thoracolumbar fractures/luxations 215, *217*
stroke 39–43
subarachnoid cyst 78, *78*
subarachnoid diverticulum *116*
subarachnoid hematoma 39, *43*
subarachnoid space
air bubbles 72
attenuation *75*, 76, 78, *79*
deviation 76, 77, *77*
focal dilation 78, *78*
imaging 72, 76, *77*
injection of contrast medium 71, 72, 73, *73*
lumbar tap 86, 88
subcutaneous tunneling, shunt surgery 132, *132*, *133*
subdural hematoma *34*, 39
suboccipital craniectomy 115–120
indications 115, *115–117*
patient positioning 115–116, *117*
quadrigeminal diverticula 115, *116*, 118, 135–136
surgical anatomy 115, *117*
surgical technique 116–120, *117–119*
sucralfate 248
suction, intraoperative 7, *8*
superficial digital flexor muscle biopsy 96, *96*
supraspinous ligament 86
swimming pool exercises 263–264

tapping
bone hole 14, *14*
to stimulate reflexes 260, *260*
temperature, intraoperative control 12, 14
temporalis muscle/fascia
lateral rostrotentorial approach 110, *112*, 114
skull tumor resection 123, *123*, *124*, 125
tenotomy scissors *9*, 10
thermal injury 12, 14
thermotherapy 258
thoracic computed tomography (CT) 65, *66*
thoracic radiographs
intracranial surgery 22, **24**, *24*, 25, *25–26*
spinal surgery 59, 65, *65*, *66*, *67*
three-view 65, *67*

thoracolumbar disc fenestration 193–197
  complications *196*, 196–197, *197*
  dorsal approach 194
  dorsolateral approach 194
  lateral approach 193–194, *193–194*
  with pediculectomy/mini-hemilaminectomy 188
  postoperative care 197
  preparation/positioning 193
  surgical procedure 194–196, *195–196*
thoracolumbar disc herniation
  dorsal laminectomy 183
  hemilaminectomy 180, 181, *181*, 199
  lateral corpectomy 199–203
  pediculectomy/mini-hemilaminectomy 183–188
thoracolumbar fascia 179, *180*
thoracolumbar fractures/luxations 213–217
  bicortical pin and PMMA fixation 214–215, *215–216*
  decompression techniques 209
  external skeletal fixation 215
  implant selection 213–214
  plate fixation 215, *217*
  positioning and approach 213
  reduction 214
  spinal stapling 216–217, *217–218*
thoracolumbar hemilaminectomy 179–182
  bilateral 181
  indications 179
  surgical approach 179–180, *179–180*
  surgical procedure *180–181*, 180–182
  traumatic injuries 209
  vs lateral corpectomy 199
thoracolumbar lateral corpectomy (TLLC) 199–203
  combined with other techniques 202
  complications 202–203
  instrumentation 200
  minimally invasive 202
  multiple consecutive 202
  results 202–203
  surgical approaches 199–200
  surgical technique 200–202, *200–202*
thoracolumbar myelopathies, CSF analysis 90
thoracolumbar pediculectomy/mini-hemilaminectomy *see* pediculectomy/mini-hemilaminectomy
thoracotomy, intercostal 199–200
3M craniotome 6, *7*
three-compartment concept, vertebral column 209, *210*
three-dimensional printed models
  aiding skull reconstruction 127, *127*
  planning skull tumor resection 121, *122*
thrombocytopenia 62, *62*
thrombocytosis 61–62
thromboelastography (TEG) *64*, 65, *65*
thyroid disease 23
tibial nerve biopsy 93–95, *94*, *95*
titanium implants 170, 176
titanium mesh, skull reconstruction *126–128*, 127–128
topical analgesia 246
towel clamps *9*, 10
toy-breed dogs
  atlantoaxial subluxation 141, 142, 143, 148
  congenital hydrocephalus 43, 129
tramadol 247
transfrontal craniotomy 99–107
  anatomy 99, *99*, *100*
  complications 105–107, *106*
  indications 100–102
  surgical technique 102–105, *103–105*
transiliac approach 200, 229
transverse atlantal ligament 141
transverse sinus 123, *123*
trapezius muscle 165, *165*
traumatic injuries *see* head trauma; vertebral fractures/luxations
treadmill walking 261
triceps brachii muscle biopsy 96
trocar pin tip 11, *11*, *12*

ulnar nerve biopsy *95*, 96, *96*
ultrasonic surgical aspirator (CUSA) *6*, 7
  brain tumor removal 112, *113*
  skull tumor resection 124, *124*
ultrasonography
  abdominal *see* abdominal ultrasound
  cranial 30–32, *31*, *32*
  intraoperative 46–48, *47*
ultrasound, therapeutic 258, *259*
underwater treadmill (UWTM) 264, *264*
urinalysis 23, **24**, 63
urinary catheterization 250, *251*, 267, *267*
urinary incontinence 266, 267
urinary tract infections (UTI) 23, 63, 250, 251
urine
  evaluation/inspection 63
  scald, preventing 266–267

ventilation, mechanical 250
ventral approaches
  atlantoaxial subluxation 144–145, *145*
  cervical disc fenestration 193
  cervical spine decompression *see* ventral cervical decompression
  thoracolumbar disc fenestration 196
ventral cervical decompression (ventral slot) 149, 157–161
  complications 160–161
  disc fenestration 192, 193
  inverted cone technique 159, *160*
  median approach 158, *158*
  paramedian approach 158, *158*
  postoperative care 161
  preparation 157, *157*
  slanted slot technique 159–160
  surgical procedure 158–159, *159*
  traumatic injuries 209
  video-assisted technique 160
ventral slot *see* ventral cervical decompression
ventricular premature complexes (VPCs) *68*
ventriculoperitoneal (VP) shunt placement 129–134
  complications 134
  equipment 130–131, *131*

indications 130
minimum database **24**, 26
postoperative care 134, *134*
preoperative preparation 131, *132*
prognosis 134
revision 134
surgical technique 131–133, *132–133*
see also hydrocephalus
ventrolateral thoracolumbar approaches
disc fenestration 196
lateral corpectomy 199, 200–202, *200–202*
vertebral arteries 153, *153*, 166
vertebral body plates
cervical distraction and stabilization 174–175, *175*
cervical fracture/luxation repair *212*, 212–213, *213*
thoracolumbar fractures/luxations 215, *217*
vertebral distractors 171, *171*
vertebral fractures/luxations 209–221
cervical 211–213
decompression techniques 209–211
diagnostic imaging 81, *81*
lumbosacral 217–219
mechanics 209, *210*
postoperative complications 220–221
postoperative imaging 219–220
preoperative planning 209, *210*
surgical instruments *9*, 10
thoracolumbar 213–217
three-compartment concept 209, *210*
vertebral instability, postoperative *see* spinal instability, postoperative
vertebral venous plexus, internal
lateral cervical approach 165, 166
thoracolumbar lateral corpectomy *200*, 201, 202–203
ventral cervical decompression 159, *159*, 160
vestibular disease 29, 142
Vetrix® BioSIS ECM 125
von Willebrand disease 25, 64, 160
von Willebrand factor (vWF) 64
VP *see* ventriculoperitoneal

walking, assisted *249*, 261
warfarin 64
water rehabilitation 262–264, *264*
weight-shifting exercises 261, *262*
Weitlaner retractors 3–4, *5*
wires, surgical *11*, 11–13
wobbler syndrome *see* cervical spondylomyelopathy

Yorkshire Terrier, atlantoaxial subluxation 142

www.ingramcontent.com/pod-product-compliance
Lightning Source LLC
LaVergne TN
LVHW082118200926
848484LV00008B/1977